Estimated Sodium, Chloride, and Potassium Minimum Requirements of Healthy Persons

Age	Weight (kg)	Sodium (mg)[a,b]	Chloride (mg)[a,b]	Potassium (mg)[c]
Months				
0-5	4.5	120	180	500
6-11	8.9	200	300	700
Years				
1	11.0	225	350	1,000
2-5	16.0	300	500	1,400
6-9	25.0	400	600	1,600
10-18	50.0	500	750	2,000
>18[d]	70.0	500	750	2,000

[a]No allowance has been included for large, prolonged losses from the skin through sweat.

[b]There is no evidence that higher intakes confer any health benefit.

[c]Desirable intakes of potassium may considerably exceed these values (~13,500 mg for adults).

[d]No allowance included for growth. Values for those below 18 years assume a growth rate at 50th percentile reported by the National Center for Health Statistics and averaged for males and females.

Estimated Safe and Adequate Daily Dietary Intakes of Selected Vitamins and Minerals[a]

Category	Age (years)	Vitamins		Trace Elements[b]				
		Biotin (µg)	Pantothenic Acid (mg)	Copper (mg)	Man-ganese (mg)	Fluoride (µg)	Chromium (µg)	Molybdenum (mg)
Infants	0-0.5	10	2	0.4-0.6	0.3-0.6	0.1-0.5	10-40	15-30
	0.5-1	15	3	0.6-0.7	0.6-1.0	0.2-1.0	20-60	20-40
Children and adolescents	1-3	20	3	0.7-1.0	1.0-1.5	0.5-1.5	20-80	25-50
	4-6	25	3-4	1.0-1.5	1.5-2.0	1.0-2.5	30-120	30-75
	7-10	30	4-5	1.0-2.0	2.0-3.0	1.5-2.5	50-200	50-150
	11+	30-100	4-7	1.5-2.5	2.0-5.0	1.5-2.5	50-200	75-250
Adults		30-100	4-7	1.5-3.0	2.0-5.0	1.5-4.0	50-200	75-250

[a]Because there is less information on which to base allowances, these figures are not given in the main table of RDA and are provided here in the form of ranges of recommended intakes.

[b]Since the toxic levels for many trace elements may be only several times usual intakes, the upper levels for the trace elements given in this table should not be habitually exceeded.

Daily Values established by the Food and Drug Administration as standards for nutrient labeling purposes

REFERENCE DAILY INTAKES (RDIs)[*‡§]

NUTRIENT	REFERENCE AMOUNT
Vitamin A[‖]	5000 International Units (IU)
Vitamin C[‖]	60 mg
Thiamin	1.5 mg
Riboflavin	1.7 mg
Niacin	20 mg
Calcium[‖]	1 g
Iron[‖]	18 mg
Vitamin D	400 IU
Vitamin E	30 IU
Vitamin B_6	2 mg
Folic acid	0.4 mg
Vitamin B_{12}	6 µg
Phosphorus	1 g
Iodine	150 µg
Magnesium	400 mg
Zinc	15 mg
Copper	2 mg
Biotin	0.3 mg
Pantothenic acid	10 mg

DAILY REFERENCE VALUES (DRVs)[‡§]

NUTRIENT	BASIS FOR CALCULATING DAILY REFERENCE VALUE
Total fat	30% of calories
Saturated fat	10% of calories
Carbohydrate	60% of calories
Dietary fiber	11.5 g of fiber per each 1000 calories
Protein[†]	10% of calories for adults and children over 4 years

NUTRIENT	2000 CALORIES	2500 CALORIES
Total fat[‖]	65 g	80 g
Saturated fat[‖]	20 g	25 g
Cholesterol[‖]	300 mg	300 mg
Sodium[‖]	2.4 mg	2.4 mg
Total carbohydrate[‖]	300 g	375 g
Dietary fiber[‖]	25 g	30 g
Protein[‖]	50 g	65 g
Potassium	3.5 mg	3.5 mg

[*] Based on the National Academy of Sciences' 1968 recommended dietary allowances (same as U.S. RDA used until 1994). Values are highest RDAs except for pregnancy and lactation.

[†] The DRV for protein does not apply to certain populations. An RDI for protein has been established for these groups: infants under 1 yr, 14 g; children 1-4 yrs, 16 g, pregnant women, 50 g; and nursing mothers, 66 g.

[‡] Some Daily Values (DVs) have been rounded to make label reading easier for consumers.

[§] DV as used on label includes both Reference Daily Intakes (RDIs) for vitamins and minerals and DRVs for macronutrients and electrolytes.

[‖] % DVs must be declared on label. % DV for other nutrients may be provided voluntarily.

Median Heights and Weights and Recommended Energy Intake

Category	Age (years) or Condition	Weight (kg)	Weight (lb)	Height (cm)	Height (in)	REE[a] (kcal/day)	Multiples of REE	Average Energy Allowance (kcal) Per kg body weight	Per day[b]
Infants	0.0-0.5	6	13	60	24	320		108	650
	0.5-1.0	9	20	71	28	500		98	850
Children	1-3	13	29	90	35	740		102	1,300
	4-6	20	44	112	44	950		90	1,800
	7-10	28	62	132	52	1,130		70	2,000
Males	11-14	45	99	157	62	1,440	1.70	55	2,500
	15-18	66	145	176	69	1,760	1.67	45	3,000
	19-24	72	160	177	70	1,780	1.67	40	2,900
	25-50	79	174	176	70	1,800	1.60	37	2,900
	51+	77	170	173	68	1,530	1.50	30	2,300
Females	11-14	46	101	157	62	1,310	1.67	47	2,200
	15-18	55	120	163	64	1,370	1.60	40	2,200
	19-24	58	128	164	65	1,350	1.60	38	2,200
	25-50	63	138	163	64	1,380	1.55	36	2,200
	51+	65	143	160	63	1,280	1.50	30	1,900
Pregnant	1st Trimester								+0
	2nd Trimester								+300
	3rd Trimester								+300
Lactating	1st 6 months								+500
	2nd 6 months								+500

[a]Resting energy expenditure (REE); calculation based on FAO equations, then rounded. This is the same as resting metabolic rate (RMR).
[b]Figure is rounded.

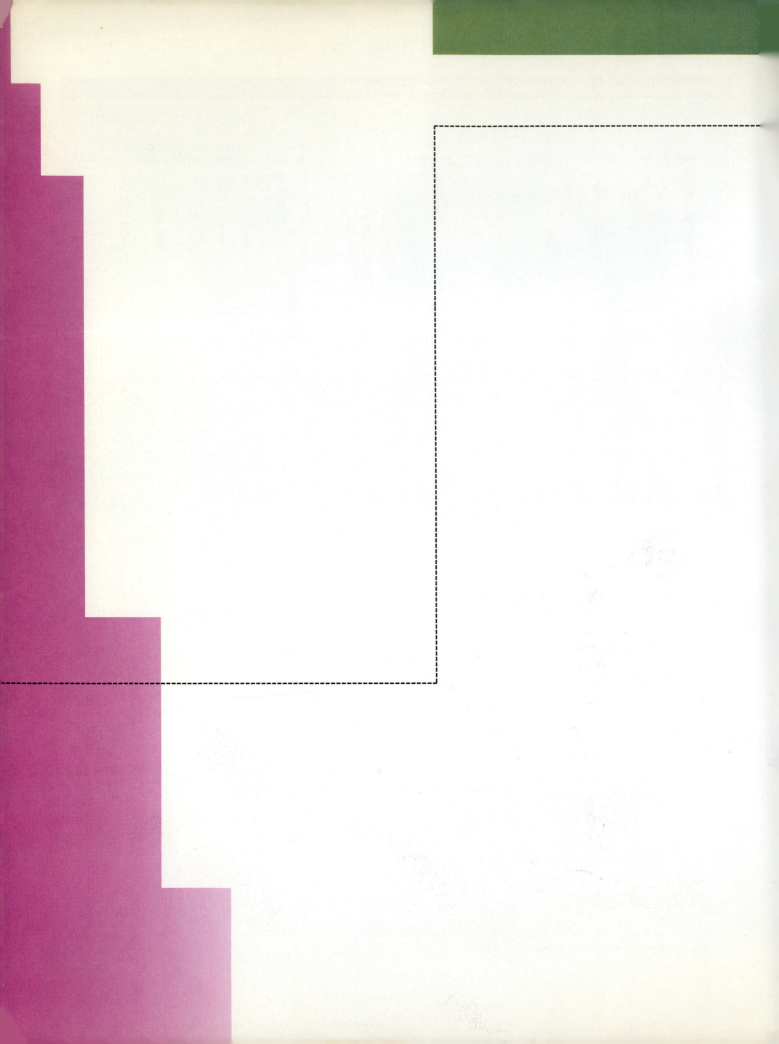

FOCUS ON NUTRITION

Nancy Anne DuPuy, MS
Solano Community College

Virginia Lee Mermel, PhD, CNS

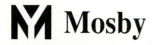 Mosby

St. Louis Baltimore Berlin Boston Carlsbad Chicago London Madrid
Naples New York Philadelphia Sydney Tokyo Toronto

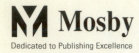
Mosby
Dedicated to Publishing Excellence

Publisher: *James M. Smith*
Acquisitions Editor: *Vicki Malinee*
Managing Editor: *Terry Eynon*
Project Manager: *Patricia Tannian*
Senior Production Editors: *John Casey, Suzanne Fannin*
Manuscript Editor: *Elisabeth Boone*
Manufacturing Supervisor: *Kathy Grone*
Design: *Jeanne Wolfgeher*
Art Researcher: *Elisabeth Boone*
Cover Illustration: *Andrew J. Zito*/The Image Bank

Printed in the United States of America
Composition by Graphic World, Inc.
Printing/binding by Von Hoffmann, Inc.

Mosby–Year Book, Inc.
11830 Westline Industrial Drive
St. Louis, Missouri 63146

Library of Congress Cataloging in Publication Data

DuPuy, Nancy A.
    Focus on nutrition   /   Nancy Anne DuPuy, Virginia Lee Mermel.
       p.   cm.
    Includes bibliographical references and index.
    ISBN 0-8016-7261-9
    1. Nutrition.   I. Mermel, Virginia Lee.   II. Title.
QP141.D798   1994
613.2—dc20
                                   94-36731
                                      CIP

94 95 96 97 98   /   9 8 7 6 5 4 3 2 1

CONTENTS IN BRIEF

Detailed Contents

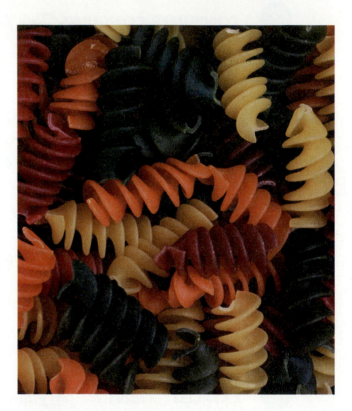

4 CARBOHYDRATES
The Staff of Life, 43

5 LIPIDS
Luxury and Necessity, 69

6 PROTEINS
The Body's Building Blocks, 95

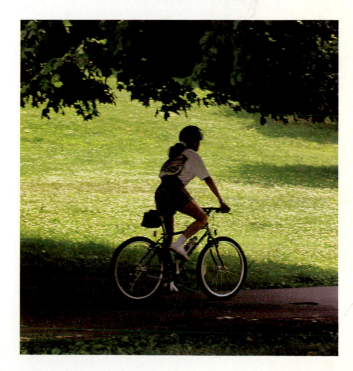

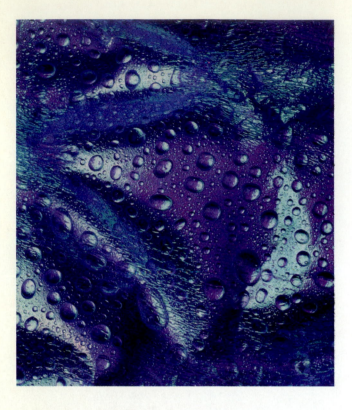

VITAMINS
Separating Fact From Fiction, 115

MINERALS
Gift From the Earth, 141

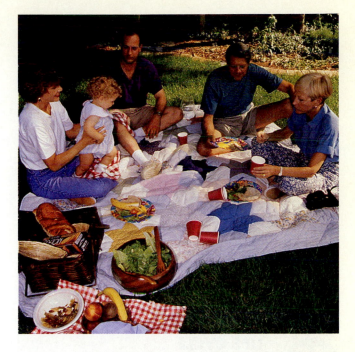

9 ENERGY
Putting Nutrients to Work. 165

10 EXERCISE
Fueling Up for Fitness. 185

11 WEIGHT CONTROL
Finding a Healthy Balance. 205

LIFE CYCLE
Nutrition From Infancy Through Adulthood, 219

LOOKING TO THE FUTURE
Issues and Trends, 239

APPENDICES

INSTRUCTOR'S PREFACE

Because food both feeds the body and nourishes the soul, the field of human nutrition considers the physiological, environmental, cultural, economic, and psychological factors that govern our individual food choices. The major challenge of writing a book for nonscience majors is making these key aspects of nutrition palatable and relevant to students with no scientific background. Writing a "chemistry free," "ecology free" book, as has been tried before, is like trying to teach history without talking about time and geography. Ecology, physiology, and scientific controversy are challenging but not impossible concepts to teach to novices. To help students master these aspects of nutrition *Focus on Nutrition* uses analogies to everyday experiences and takes advantage of a proven learning technique to reinforce comprehension of new information.

Since the typical student enrolls in a nonmajor's nutrition course to increase his or her personal nutrition IQ, *Focus* concentrates on giving students concrete examples of how to personalize and implement their newly learned nutrition and exercise knowledge, evaluate the impact of their dietary choices, and keep abreast of changes in the field of nutrition after they complete the course. *Focus* is more than just a nutrition text; it is a sound personal wellness plan, usable today and in the future.

WHAT'S DIFFERENT ABOUT FOCUS?

Focus on Nutrition uses a number of design and content features that are intended to present material in a clear, readable, and colorful way. Our goal was to help students enjoy learning, remember what they learn, and apply their new knowledge in everyday life.

SQ4R Learning System

Focus on Nutrition is designed according to the tenets of the SQ4R learning system (*S*urvey, *Q*uestion, *R*ead, *R*ecord, *R*ewrite, and *R*eview). Since using this system in our own courses, we've seen an immediate improvement in student satisfaction, self-esteem, retention, and grades. All of these benefits translate into enhanced instructor satisfaction, with favorable student course evaluations and high rates of student retention.

Why a learning system? Many students have not learned to read and critically evaluate text material. Many also lack good study and test-taking skills. Using the proven techniques of a single learning system rather than selected parts of different learning theories gave us the opportunity to coordinate text, pedagogy, and test elements. Here is how *Focus* puts SQ4R into action:

*S*URVEY: The Instructor's Resource Manual contains assignments designed to encourage students to survey the material in each chapter before it is discussed in class.

*Q*UESTION: Focus Questions introduce major concepts in each chapter to help guide students' critical thinking.

*R*EAD: Reading the text is obviously the student's responsibility. Definition boxes and a glossary enhance understanding of the material. Pronunciation is provided for unfamiliar or difficult terms.

*R*ECORD: Recording key points briefly at the end of each paragraph (either in the text itself or in a notebook) helps students reinforce and retain what they learn. To identify these key points, students can use headings, subheadings, and Focus Questions.

*R*EWRITE: The questions in Connections: Tying It All Together at the end of each chapter encourage students to integrate, review, and rewrite the material from a different perspective.

*R*EVIEW: Preview/Review tables appear throughout the text to help students make connections between the material they have just completed and the information they are about to cover. In addition, NutriQuiz questions placed throughout the text and the Test Yourself section at the end of each chapter help students review and test their understanding of concepts they have just studied.

The Student Preface explains the SQ4R features of the text to students, shows examples of the pedagogical elements, and gives practical study and test-taking tips.

Flexible Core Science and Applications Sections

Each chapter is divided into two sections. The first section explains science concepts relevant to that chapter. The second section, including In Today's World and In My Diet, examines ecological issues and gives students information they can use to put the science concepts they have learned to work in their personal environment. For example, the first section of Chapter 9, Energy, explains the physiological basis of energy utilization. The second section explores ecological concerns related to the energy used in food processing and gives examples of new uses of energy that students will encounter at the grocery store (irradiation) and in the kitchen (microwaving).

Organizing the chapters in this way offers several benefits. First, it helps students distinguish scientific/theoretical considerations from applications. It also allows you as the instructor the flexibility to teach the material in accordance with your individual preferences and circumstances. If lecture time is short, you can assign the second section of each chapter for out-of-class reading or simply make your students aware that the material is there if they would like to explore it. Alternatively, if you decide to take a very application-oriented approach to nutrition, you can use the second section of each chapter as the basis for your lectures and introduce just a few key scientific points from the first section.

A Separate Chapter Devoted Entirely To Water

Most texts combine water with minerals. As a result, many students leave introductory nutrition courses without realizing the essential role water plays in many body functions. In *Focus* we devote an entire chapter to this vital but often forgotten nutrient.

Foods vs. Nutrients

A major stumbling block for students in introductory nutrition courses is understanding the difference between foods and nutrients and appreciating the role digestion plays in nutrition. "People eat foods; cells eat nutrients" is a recurring theme throughout this text. The link among foods, digestion, and nutrients is explained this way: "Foods contain the nutrients our cells require. Digestion is the process that changes the foods we eat into the nutrients our cells require."

To reinforce the transformation of foods into nutrients, the first section of each nutrient chapter is divided into three areas: (1) In the Diet, (2) In Between—Digestion, and (3) In the Body. Each chapter contains pedagogical aids that categorize intake standards, including the Food Guide Pyramid and the RDA into either Food Intake Standards or Nutrient Intake Standards.

Functional Organization of Vitamin and Mineral Chapters

Nutrition texts traditionally present vitamins and minerals according to their solubility in water or prevalence in the diet. In *Focus* we take a different approach: we discuss these nutrients in terms of the functions they perform in the body, such as blood building, tissue synthesis, and energy utilization. This functions-oriented approach makes it easier for you to organize your lectures and helps students understand the physiological importance of these nutrients.

The vitamin chapter also contains up-to-date antioxidant information, including a plan for safely increasing antioxidant intake through dietary improvements rather than supplementation.

Up-to-date Meal Planning Information

Focus emphasizes using the Food Guide Pyramid, the new food label, simple calculations for determining individual kcalorie needs, and fat and sugar intake goals to help students develop a personalized menu.

Multicultural Examples

Multicultural examples of food intake patterns throughout the text help you introduce cultural diversity into your lectures. The Instructor's Resource Manual provides additional examples, including a brief culinary history of each of the 50 United States, and lists resources for delving further into the topic.

COPING WITH CHANGE AND CONTROVERSY

Like most scientific disciplines, nutrition is a rapidly evolving field. Understandably, the ongoing influx of new information gives rise to a number of changes as well as fueling some heated controversies.

The Food Guide Pyramid, 5-A-Day campaign, and new food labels required us as instructors to change the way we think about and present nutrition information. More difficult to resolve is how to teach controversial topics like the cholesterol–cardiovascular disease link, the sodium-hypertension connection, and the issues that surround antioxidant vitamin intake.

To provide balanced and accurate coverage of these controversies, we have relied on authoritative reports such as the Surgeon General's Report on Nutrition and Health; The National Academy of Sciences Reports: Diet and Health, Nutrition During Pregnancy, and the tenth edition of the RDAs; reports from FASEB's Life

Science Research Office; and position papers from the American Dietetic Association. We have supplemented the information in these documents with up-to-date scientific reviews and selected articles from basic science journals, most published since 1990. In addition, more than 60% of the references are from sources published since 1993. Thus *Focus* presents your students with the most balanced and accurate picture of nutrition today.

SUPPLEMENTARY MATERIALS

Instructor's Resource Manual and Test Bank

Prepared by the authors with the assistance of learning specialist Rob Simas, this teaching aid provides you with sample lesson plans for every chapter. Each plan includes key concepts and terms, suggestions for in-class activities and demonstrations (like teaching lipid chemistry with pipe cleaners), multicultural material, intriguing tidbits of information to spice up lectures, and suggestions for teaching difficult material. An example is the mnemonic "The fat on which you sat was a saturated fat," which helps students remember that animal fats tend to be saturated and solid. Because "a picture is worth a thousand words," the resource manual introduces a nonchemical technique to illustrate the configuration of dietary fats and how it affects their behavior in the body. With "bendable rod" illustrations, it is easy for students to understand that saturated fats stay straight, stackable, and solid, whereas unsaturated fats bend at their double bonds, which causes them to stay fluid. An instructor's "survival guide" chapter is also provided for new instructors.

The Test Bank features more than 750 test items: agree/disagree, multiple choice, short answer, and matching. The resource manual also includes 50 Transparency Masters of key illustrations from the text and other sources.

Computerized Test Bank

Qualified adopters of the text receive a computerized test bank package compatible with IBM or Macintosh computers. This advanced-feature test generator allows you to add, delete, or edit questions; save and reload tests; and print different versions of each test.

Computerized Instructor's Resource Manual

The resource manual is available on disk in both IBM and Macintosh formats.

Nutrient Analysis Software

Mosby offers easy-to-use interactive software that allows students to input food intake and physical activities to determine total kcalories consumed and expended in multiple 24-hour periods. A toll-free number is available for technical support for students and instructors.

Transparency Acetates

Full-color transparency acetates feature key illustrations from the text with large, easy-to-read labels.

Audiovisual Resources

Qualified adopters may choose from an excellent selection of videotapes and videodiscs. The Mosby Multimedia Library: Nutrition II Teaching Videodisc offers almost 50 spectacular 3-D animations of physiological processes, 280 colorful still images, and several short video clips that will help students apply nutrition concepts.

Nutri-News

Mosby offers a 16-page semiannual nutrition update with expert opinions on late-breaking or controversial nutrition topics. You'll find this interesting material to supplement lectures or to hand out to students.

ACKNOWLEDGMENTS

We would like to recognize and thank the reviewers and focus group participants whose direction and insight guided us in writing this text:

Mallory Boylan, PhD, RD, LD
Texas Tech University

Jeffrey E. Harris, DrPH, MPH, RD, CHES
West Chester University

Margaret C. Horvath, MA
Youngstown University

Rita M. Johnson, MS, RD
Indiana University of Pennsylvania

Noelle L. Kehrberg, PhD, RD
Western Carolina University

Karen R. Lowry, PhD, RD
Kent State University

Joan L. Magee, MS
Henry Ford Community College

Rose L. Martin, MS
Arizona State University

Suzanne Martin, PhD
College of the Ozarks

Nancy S. Maylath, HSD
University of Toledo

Constance G. Mueller, MS, RD
Illinois State University

Nell B. Robinson, PhD, RD, LD
Texas Christian University

Jimmy Tanaka, PhD
Solano Community College

We also want to thank our Mosby team for their invaluable assistance: Terry Eynon, managing editor, who helped us fine-tune our vision to the needs of our audience; Elisabeth Boone, manuscript editor, for her creativity and attention to detail; John Casey and Suzanne Fannin, senior production editors, for smoothly and patiently guiding our manuscript through the production process; and Vicki Malinee, acquisitions editor, and Jim Smith, publisher, for foreseeing the potential of our book in the first place.

We also extend thanks to FDA Press Officer Judith Foulks and FDA Label Technology Specialist Virginia L. Wilkening, RD, for helping us stay up to date with the latest developments regarding implementation of the 1990 Nutrition Labeling and Education Act. In addition we are grateful to Dr. Gordon Wardlaw for his generosity in sharing information and tips on the textbook authoring process.

Special thanks to Susan Messina for acquainting us with the principles of the new SQ4R learning system and to learning specialist Rob Simas for editing preliminary versions of the text, consulting with us regarding the application of SQ4R to our text, and developing many of the pedagogical elements in the text. And heartfelt thanks to our families, whose support and encouragement helped make this book possible.

Nancy Anne DuPuy
Virginia Lee Mermel

DEDICATION

Professionally to Rob Simas and Carol Bishop, colleagues and friends, who saw me through the conception and birthing of this book. Personally to granddaughter Meghan Marie Kelly, who often patiently waited while I worked.

NAD

To Gary and Matthew Mermel and Nancy Bjonerud.

VLM

STUDENT PREFACE

SQ4R: YOUR PASSWORD TO LEARNING

What in the world is SQ4R?   Although SQ4R looks like a secret code, it's really a not-so-secret learning system that anyone can use. SQ4R stands for **S**urvey, **Q**uestion, **R**ead, **R**ecord, **R**ewrite, and **R**eview. We've designed this text for you to use with the SQ4R system because in our experience as instructors it's proved to be the most effective method of learning for our students.

How does SQ4R work?   When introduced to new material, particularly in an unfamiliar subject area, many students simply try to memorize all of the information (facts) presented. There's no question that facts are essential: they are the very building blocks of our knowledge. But if you focus only on memorizing individual facts, your brain will soon be overwhelmed. How can you keep all the facts straight? How can you make sense of them?

Using the SQ4R system helps you see the BIG picture: how all the facts you're learning fit together. Like other students who use SQ4R or some variation, you can learn new information more quickly and completely and be more successful on exams than students who just try to memorize the facts. Here are some specific steps to put the SQ4R plan into action when you're using this and other textbooks.

S: Survey

At the beginning of each study session, determine how much material you can cover in the time available. It's better to read half a chapter thoroughly than to read an entire chapter quickly without gaining an understanding of the material.

Next look over the material you'll be covering—scan it from start to finish, searching for key topics. Your "alert" signals for these topics are the chapter title, the major headings and subheadings, and the outlines and summaries. Read the detailed table of contents and the final summary paragraph, if the chapter has one. At this

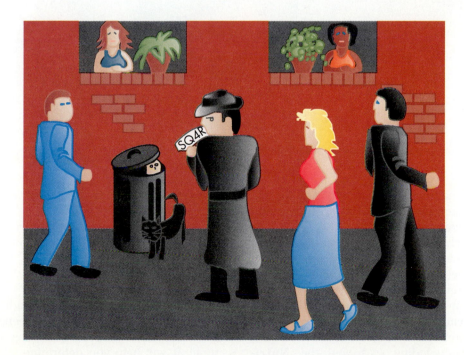

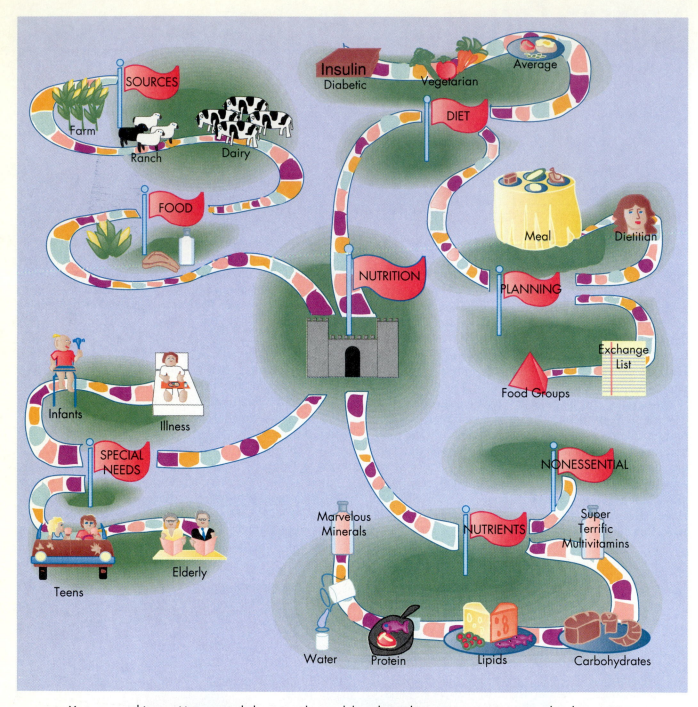

You can use this cognitive map to help you understand the relationships among major topics related to nutrition.

point you're not trying to read or understand all the material—you're just getting a general idea of the chapter's purpose and major topics.

As you skim a chapter in this text, watch for **Focus Questions** (in a different typeface from the text, highlighted in blue). Also look for **visual learning cues** (like Review/Preview tables and Intake Standards boxes) and for the boxes that contain **definitions of key terms.** All of these features pinpoint essential information. You'll also want to check out the **illustrations**—including cartoons—the **Nutri-** **nuggets, Nutralerts,** and other supplemental information.

Taking a few minutes to go through this procedure will help you recognize and organize the key ideas presented in each chapter.

Q: Question

List the major topics and subheadings in your notebook, leaving several lines between each. This list is the "blueprint" for your questions and notes on the topic. It will help you determine what information is relevant to the chapter's main ideas and guide you in organizing the information.

Every chapter in this text contains Focus Questions to direct your attention to key points. Add to these any questions that came to mind as you surveyed the material. These questions will become your guides during the next step.

R: Read

Read each section and answer the Focus Question that precedes it. Read the material carefully. Note the highlighted words (in italic or bold print). Also pay close attention to key qualifying words like *sometimes*, *always*, and *never*. Look up unfamiliar terms.

R: Record

This step forces you to slow down and process the text material in small bites. It also helps you create your own signposts back into the text material to assist you in finding and reviewing information.

After reading each paragraph, stop. In the margin at the top of the page, jot down a word or phrase that captures the main topic of the paragraph. Continue this process paragraph by paragraph until you complete an entire section of the chapter.

After completing the last paragraph of a section, stop again. Do you understand the information in the section and how it relates to other material you have covered? Did you find the answers to the questions you developed? If so, record them in your notes. What don't you understand? Write it down also. You may find clarification as you continue. If not, you can raise the issue in class.

A practical tip:

Always go back to highlight key words and main points *after* you have read and understood a section of material. If you highlight as you're reading, you'll tend to highlight everything; then nothing really stands out.

R: Rewrite

After you finish reading and taking notes on a chapter, the next step is to rewrite the material from memory in your own words, preferably by answering the questions you've developed and the questions in the text. Why rewrite? For several very good reasons.

1. Reading and writing use different parts of your body and therefore your brain. The more parts of yourself you involve in the learning process, the more "handles" you have to remember the information.
2. Rewriting the material gives you a chance to review the information again. The more frequently you go over material, the more likely you are to remember it.
3. Writing is a good way to practice generating information as you must do on subjective test items, such as essay or fill-in-the-blank questions.

Generating sentences is a higher level activity than passively recognizing written material as you do when you answer objective test items such as true or false, matching, and multiple choice questions.

R: Review

After completing the Rewrite step, review the entire chapter's content. Review it again before starting to study the next chapter, if you're not covering both in the same study session. Look at your topic outline and questions. Does everything look complete? Go back through all the material, scanning quickly to confirm your notes and answers and maybe to gain new understanding of various details of the topic. Cover your notes. Check your memory by reciting the major points of each section. Expose each major point and try to recall the subpoints under it.

Answer the questions at the end of the chapter. Find study partners so you can compare your answers with theirs.

Draw diagrams (cognitive maps) to show how main points relate to one another. Talk aloud as you work your way through a diagram. The diagram on p. xvi is a cognitive map outline of some major topics related to nutrition: food, diet, nutrients, and special needs.

Try Teamwork

A good way to reinforce what you're learning is to teach it to someone else. Consider joining a study group with two to five of your classmates. By participating in a study group you can practice explaining to someone the information you're studying (just as you have to do for your instructor on a test or in a paper). By listening to other students and comparing answers to the questions in the text, you can add different perspectives to the information you already know. What's more, you and your study partners can test each other to see how much you really remember and understand.

TAKING TESTS: PREPARING FOR THE INEVITABLE

How can I improve my test results? Follow the SQ4R system during your pretest study sessions. Note key differences between various concepts. Which areas did the instructor emphasize? Develop some of your own practice questions about these concepts.

Ask your instructor for copies of old tests and/or practice exams. Try to answer the questions on these exams.

All tests are not alike. Objective tests (multiple choice, true or false, matching, and fill in the blank questions) require that you be able to recognize a correct answer. In contrast, subjective tests (short answer

Test-Taking Tactics

1. **Try to find out ahead of time the general composition of the test.** Different types of questions demand different study techniques and answering strategies. Objective items usually require only visual recognition of information. Subjective questions require more detailed information. Prepare for these by outlining written or oral answers to likely questions.

2. **Budget your testing time.** Divide the time available by the total points on the test. For example, if you have 60 minutes to complete a 60-point test you can spend 1 minute per point. If the test contains 30 multiple-choice items worth 1 point each and two short essay items worth 15 points each, spend a maximum of 30 minutes on the multiple-choice section and 15 minutes on each of the two essay items. Try to allow a few minutes to review your answers. If you are stumped by a question, move on. Answering subsequent questions may provide clues to help you answer the question(s) that stumped you.

3. **Read the instructions carefully.** It is essential that you fully understand both the general test instructions as well as the specific instructions for completing each section. Where should the answers go? Is there a penalty for guessing? Can you use scratch paper to work out problems, or should all work be done on the test or answer sheet? Can you use any reference materials? When in doubt, ask your instructor or test proctor.

4. **Attack the test systematically.** Begin with the objective questions, as they are usually the easiest to answer. Next tackle the subjective section, if there is one.

5. **Read questions carefully.** For multiple-choice and matching questions, be sure you understand the question. Then read *all* of the alternative answers before making your selection. For essay questions, note all the key points to which you are being asked to respond. Briefly outline your response. Using the outline, write a brief essay, including specific facts and examples when possible. Check your answer, making sure you have responded to the entire question.

6. **Pay attention to qualifying words.** In objective questions, look for key words like *sometimes, always,* and *never.* An unqualified *always* or *never* suggests an answer is false; conditional qualifiers like *sometimes, usually,* or *almost* suggest an answer is true.

questions and essays) demand that you recall facts, integrate concepts, and formulate a correct response. Prepare for a subjective exam by briefly outlining major concepts and giving specific examples.

Avoid cramming. It's no substitute for real studying. Facts "learned" while cramming are easily confused and quickly forgotten. Cramming also adds to test anxiety. For test-taking triumphs, avoid last-minute cram sessions—and even last-minute crammers! Then follow the test-taking tips outlined in the box on the following page.

ORGANIZATION

This text is organized according to the principles of the SQ4R learning system outlined earlier. Getting acquainted with its special features will help you make the best use of your study time.

Sequencing of Chapters

Skim through the detailed table of contents to get an overview of the field of nutrition and to learn how the text is organized to cover each major topic.

The first two chapters, Nutrition Awareness and Consumer Concerns:

- Present an overview of the factors that influence our food choices
- Introduce the six nutrient classes and the standards used to make dietary recommendations
- Explain how our bodies extract the nutrients from foods

- Introduce the vital role of energy (kilocalories)

Each of the next six chapters covers one of the major nutrients:

1. **Water** is the first nutrient covered because it is a vital nutrient, in terms of both the quantity we require (approximately 64 ounces a day) and how quickly a deficiency will prove fatal.

2. **Carbohydrates** is presented second because it is our bodies' preferred energy source.

3. **Lipids** (fats and oils) follows carbohydrates because it is our bodies' other major energy source.

4. **Proteins** perform another vital role: they provide the materials needed to build body parts and many specialized chemicals.

5. **Vitamins** is presented fifth because although only tiny amounts are needed in our diets, these nutrients are "vital" to the regulation of carbohydrate, fat, and protein utilization.

6. **Minerals** is the last class of nutrients presented but is by no means the least important. Ongoing research is increasing our understanding of the exciting roles minerals play in metabolism and fluid balance.

The next four chapters—Energy, Exercise, Weight Control, and Life Cycle—focus on applied nutrition. Each chapter explores the ways in which the nutrients you learned about earlier are used in special situations. The text ends with Looking to the Future, in which we examine emerging trends in the field of nutrition.

TABLE 0-1   Outline Used in Nutrient Chapters of Text

I. FOOD SOURCES

What exactly is this nutrient?
A. INTRODUCTION—Science of Nutrition
Which foods contain this nutrient?
B. IN THE DIET—Food Sources

II. NUTRIENT USE

How is this nutrient removed from the food and moved into the cell where it is used?
A. IN BETWEEN—Digestion
Why does my body need it?
B. IN THE BODY—Metabolism

III. CONTEMPORARY CONCERNS

What contemporary concerns—personal, social, environmental—are linked to this nutrient?
A. IN TODAY'S WORLD—Processed Foods
How can I plan a diet that provides adequate amounts of each nutrient?
B. IN MY DIET—Menu Planning

VISUAL CUES

How can I find my way around all the information in this textbook?   We've developed several visual cues that will act as learning aids to help you organize new information.

Outline Style

Is there a logical pattern or order to this information?   In each chapter we use an outline format to help you **survey** the material, locate information, and identify major concepts. In general, the six nutrient chapters are organized according to the grid shown in the table below so that you can recognize the concerns that are common to all nutrients.

Each of the nutrient chapters is subdivided into sections. In the first and second sections we present the basic scientific facts about that class of nutrients. In the third section we explain how processing affects the nutrient class, examine environmental impacts on the nutrient class, and apply the scientific facts about the nutrient class to everyday diet choices. At the end of each In My Diet section we refer to the Menu Matrix. You can use this information to develop a personal Menu Matrix for weekly diet planning, one nutrient class at a time.

Chapters on other topics are divided into at least two main sections: The first presents the core concepts related to the chapter topic. In the second section, including In Today's World and In My Diet, we explore contemporary personal, social, and environmental issues related to the chapter topic. For example, the In Today's World section of Chapter 11, Weight Control, explores ways in which people who tend to overeat can learn to cope with holidays and other celebrations that are full of tempting foods.

Questions

What is the purpose of the questions built into the chapter outline shown above?   Each chapter contains four kinds of questions:

1. **Focus Questions,** in a larger typeface and highlighted in blue (like the question above), are placed throughout each chapter to direct your attention to the core concepts and help you *survey* the material. You should be able to answer some of these questions from earlier material, others from reading the section.
2. **NUTRIQUIZ questions,** found in yellow boxes throughout each chapter, help you review and also understand how to turn nutritional theory into practical dietary changes.
3. **Test Yourself** questions right after the text in each chapter serve as a built-in study guide to help you check your grasp of the factual information in the chapter (see p. xxi).
4. **Connections—Tying It All Together questions** at the end of each chapter help you determine how well you have understood the material by asking you to apply what you have learned (see p. xxi).

Tables, Illustrations, and Boxed Features

Each chapter also contains a variety of features to supplement and reinforce what you're learning. We describe each of these learning aids in the sections that follow.

Tables and Boxes

The tables, boxes, and illustrations condense and highlight core concepts. They also provide a framework you can use to arrange the new information being presented, to relate it to material you've already mastered, and to review the material.

Review/Preview tables summarize the core concepts related to nutrients. Table 0-2 below is an example of this kind of summary table you'll find near the beginning of the six nutrients chapters.

Vocabulary

Which words are important?   A major challenge of learning a new subject is to grasp the special terminology used. To help you master the vocabulary of nutri-

---

oligosaccharide   a sugar that contains a known small number of monosaccharide units (from Greek *oligos,* "few, little," and *sakkharon,* "sugar")

TABLE 0-2 Review/Preview

Core Concepts	Nutrient		
	Carbohydrates	Lipids	Proteins
Building block	Monosaccharides	Mostly fatty acids and glycerol	Amino acid
Kcalorie content	4 kcal/gram	9 kcal/gram	4 kcal/gram
Source	Breads, cereals, grains	Oils, fats	MFP, legumes, dairy products
Nutrient intake standard	Exchange Lists	Dietary Goals	RDA
Food intake standard	Dietary Guidelines, Food Guide Pyramid	Dietary Guidelines, Food Guide Pyramid	Food Guide Pyramid
In the body	Fuel (blood glucose), mucus	Cell membranes, fuel storage, hormones	Structural proteins, functional proteins
Deficiency	Ketosis, gluconeogenesis	(Unlikely) Flaky dermatitis	Decreased growth, anemia, edema, impaired immune function
Excess	Stored as glycogen and fat	Obesity, CVD, some cancers	Excess urea, excess kcal stored as fat

tion, selected words throughout the text are **boldfaced** for added emphasis. Terms that appear in ***bold italicized*** print are defined in special vocabulary boxes in the text, often accompanied by pronunciation and derivation of the word. Learning the roots of words can often help you remember their meaning. Both **boldfaced** and ***boldface italic*** terms appear in the glossary.

Intake Standards Boxes

How much of which foods should I eat? A variety of intake standards have been developed to help nutrition professionals and consumers alike determine how much of which foods and nutrients a healthy

TABLE 0-3 Intake Standards

Foods	Nutrients
Dietary Guidelines	RDA
Food Guide Pyramid	% Daily Value (labels)
5-A-Day Program	
American Heart Association	Dietary Goals
American Cancer Society	
People eat foods.	***Cells eat nutrients.***

person needs. Beginning nutrition students are frequently confused by which standard applies to which class of nutrients and how nutrient standards relate to food intake standards. To clarify this information, the six nutrient chapters each contain an Intake Standards table like the one shown in Table 0-3. We use **boldface** type to highlight the nutrition and food intake standards most closely linked to the nutrient class being studied.

Nutralerts

These features provide pertinent nutrition-related health warnings. They appear in yellow boxes with orange type and a bright yellow and orange heading.

Cycles and Recycling

Is there more to nutrition than what I eat? Life on Earth depends on recycling, a concept that is basic to an understanding of the field of nutrition. In fact, nutrition can be approached in terms of interrelated recycling processes. Energy, water, and specific nutrients are all recycled.

FYI

Are there any other features I'll find helpful? Nutrinuggets and A Closer Look boxes are items of interest that are not required for mastery of basic nutrition concepts. Your instructor may assign some of these features for study and class discussion.

Nutrinuggets

Nutrinuggets are designed to tie course content to everyday life. They appear throughout the text in blue type and are identified by a gold nugget icon.

NUTRI NUGGET **The size and shape of a molecule affect the way our taste buds perceive it.**

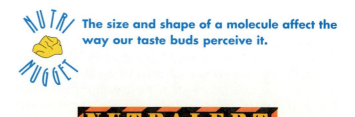

NUTRALERT

Although some fitness experts advise people to use hand or ankle weights to increase the intensity of their workout, many others caution against this practice because these kinds of weights increase stress on ankle, back, knee, and hip joints, increasing the potential for injury. A safer approach: wear a weight belt!

A Closer Look

A Closer Look boxes present selected topics in more depth than you need for a basic understanding of the field of nutrition.

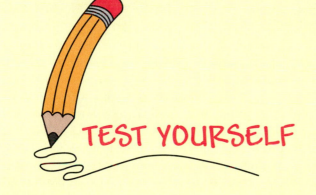

Each chapter contains one or more of these boxed features. They provide more in-depth information on a given topic than you need for a basic understanding of nutrition. They help you put what you're learning about nutrition into a larger, real-world context and illuminate historical or behind-the-scene aspects of specific topics and issues. Instructors may assign this material at their discretion.

TEST YOURSELF

True or False. Put a **T** for true or an **F** for false in the space beside each question.

___ 1. It doesn't matter *how* you study; it only matters *if* you study.

___ 2. Cognitive maps help you connect different aspects of related information.

___ 3. Working with study partners can give you a chance to test your knowledge.

___ 4. You should review old material before beginning to study new information.

___ 5. Study only if you have time to read the entire chapter.

___ 6. Highlight important words as you come across them.

___ 7. Pause after each paragraph and explain to yourself what you have just read.

___ 8. When studying, pay close attention to qualifying words like *always*, *sometimes*, and *never*.

Short Answer

___ 9. What does **SQ4R** stand for?

___ 10. List two learning aids built into this book.

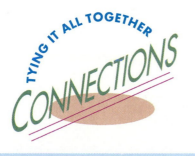

TYING IT ALL TOGETHER
CONNECTIONS

1. Read each of the Focus Questions in this chapter and answer each in your own words.

2. List the steps you normally have followed when studying textbooks.

3. What changes would you have to make to follow the SQ4R approach?

4. List the general procedures you would use in the SQ4R approach to studying.

The purpose of this section is to test your understanding and application of the chapter material. The questions that follow will help you try out the SQ4R learning process.

Food is an important
part of a balanced diet.

— *Fran Lebowitz*

CHAPTER

1

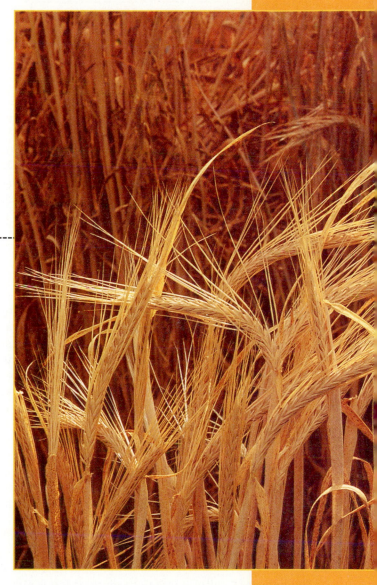

NUTRITION
AWARENESS

Food, Fuel, and Fitness

What is nutrition?   The first thought that comes to most people's minds is "health food." But knowing how much of what foods to eat to ensure good health is only part of the story. Technically, **nutrition** is defined as "the sum of the processes involved in eating, digesting, absorbing, and using nutrients." The science of nutrition studies the processes by which the body uses food for energy, maintenance, and growth. It is particularly concerned with identifying those nutrients and substances in foods that foster the development of a strong body and promote good health.[2]

INFLUENCES ON HUMAN NUTRITION

"The first thing I remember liking that liked me back was food."

— *Valerie Harper*
Rhoda, *1970s*

Because food both feeds the body and nourishes the soul, the field of human nutrition also considers the *environmental, cultural, economic,* and *emotional* factors that govern our individual food choices.[13] In the sections that follow, we'll discover how these factors affect what we eat.

Environment

Before the days of a worldwide transportation network and sophisticated agricultural practices, people's physical environment (tropical island, snow-covered mountain, or arid plains) determined what foods were available to them. In developing nations this is still largely true. However, people in industrialized countries have an almost limitless variety of food choices. Theoretically, choice should improve a person's nutritional status. In reality, people often end up eating unbalanced diets or relying heavily on processed foods despite access to a wide variety of fresh items. Added to the personal impact of such food choices is the environmental effect. Modern agricultural, food preservation, packaging, and shipping practices all have taken a toll on the Earth's environment. Environmental problems specific to each of the nutrient classes are discussed in detail in the appropriate chapters.

Culture

The impact of cultural practices on nutrition is almost inseparable from the impact of nutrition on culture. In addition to food's role in religious rituals, community celebrations, folk medicine, and superstitions, the need to establish and maintain a reliable food supply spurred some of humankind's most significant achievements. Modern humans have been on Earth for at least 50,000 years. For most of this time people lived the nomadic

life of hunter-gatherers, covering vast territories in pursuit of migrating animal herds and in search of maturing plants.[3,10]

Cities

Purposeful agriculture first appeared about 10,000 years ago in an area of the Middle East known as the Fertile Crescent. It was here that people began to cultivate barley and wheat. Shortly thereafter they domesticated certain animal species to provide a ready and reliable source of meat. The significance of these events in human history is that they freed people from the need to wander in search of food and allowed them to begin developing permanent encampments. These encampments in turn gave rise to cities; and with a stable food supply available, people could devote time to a wide range of other activities: religion, storytelling, arts and crafts, scientific inquiry, and engineering.

NUTRI NUGGET Flowers, not food crops, were the first plants that people purposely cultivated, according to cultural nutritionist Dr. Louis Gravetti.

Writing

As life in the cities grew more complex, it became necessary to develop a system of record keeping. Once again, food seems to have provided the impetus for a major development in human culture. To date, the earliest known piece of writing is a clay tablet dating back over 5000 years from the ancient city of Urok in what is now Iraq. It details the distribution of food items from a community supply over a 5-day period. The ability to create a permanent record of ideas, experiences, agreements, transactions, and plans[10] helped fuel the next major development in human culture: the shift from a predominantly agricultural to a predominantly industrialized society.

Agricultural Society

"Farming looks mighty easy when your plow is a pencil and you're a thousand miles from the cornfield."

— *Dwight D. Eisenhower*

Until the beginning of the industrial era in the mid-1800s, agricultural practices had changed little for centuries. The raising of plants and animals had gradually spread to all continents. For the majority of their energy needs, the peoples of each culture depended on a native grain (wheat in the Mediterranean region, rice in Asia, oats in the British Isles, corn in the Americas) or a starchy root crop (potatoes in South America, cassava in Africa, taro in Polynesia).[6,13] They supplemented their diet with fruits, vegetables, and small quantities of meat and/or dairy products. The amount of land that could be cultivated was limited by people's capacity to do physical labor.

Industrial Society

The explosion of scientific and technological advances since the beginning of the Industrial Revolution has given rise to major changes in lifestyles, agricultural practices, and food processing techniques. Some of these advances have increased crop yield, storage time, and shelf life, thereby adding variety to our diet. As we will see throughout the text, however, not all of the changes brought about by industrialization have been positive. In fact, some of modern techniques used to grow and process food have resulted in an increased incidence of human and environmental ills.[8,11]

Over time, the physically demanding existence of hunter-gatherers and early farmers has given way to a lifestyle that for most people today is mentally taxing but physically undemanding. Two results of this shift are obesity and poor physical conditioning—both of which can lead to a variety of physical ills. *Epidemiologists* suspect that the shift from a diet based primarily on natural, unrefined foods to one that includes many processed items (which are typically high in fat, sugar, salt, and preservatives) may be responsible for the high incidence of cardiovascular disease, obesity, diabetes, and certain cancers seen in industrialized nations.[8]

Chemical fertilizers and pesticides may ensure a good harvest, but they also can pollute the environment. This problem is compounded by the use of fossil fuels to power farm machinery and food transport vehicles, and to synthesize plastics for food packaging. The end result is environmental illnesses such as acid rain, the greenhouse effect, and the near extinction of chemically sensitive species. With the benefit of hindsight, scientists and health care professionals are examining how modern agricultural and dietary practices affect our personal well-being and the well-being of our planet. Many agree that significant changes must be made, and made soon, if humankind and the Earth are to survive and flourish.[5,11]

Personal Culture

In addition to the prevailing contemporary culture, all of us are influenced by our own personal culture, which is a blend of ethnic traditions, religious beliefs, and family habits. In the United States, the custom of Thanksgiving dinner is a perfect example of how national, regional, and personal culture affect our diet. The meal traditionally features roast turkey with bread dressing, cranberry sauce, yams, a vegetable dish, and pumpkin pie. In reality, the dinner may have some regional variations to incorporate favorite local foods. For example, New Englanders often add oysters to the dressing or serve them as a side dish. Maple syrup, an-

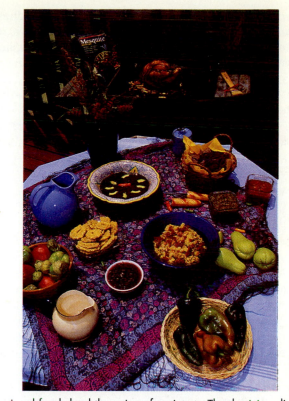

Regional foods lend the spice of variety to Thanksgiving dinner.

other local product, is frequently used to sweeten the yam dish or the pumpkin pie. In the South, cornbread and sausage are key ingredients in dressing, the pumpkin pie is often replaced by a pecan or sweet potato pie, and biscuits and gravy are staples. Southwesterners may enliven their turkey dinner with spicy flavorings common to that region. Visitors to the sunbelt states of Florida, Arizona, and California may be surprised to find turkey roasting on the barbecue instead of in the oven.

Each ethnic group also brings its own interpretation to the dinner. A sampling of California college students revealed these trends: Asian-American families may begin the meal with a traditional soup and serve Asian-inspired vegetable dishes and rice instead of stuffing and/or yams. Pasta often finds its way into Thanksgiving dinner in Italian-American households, as a side dish or in soup. Creamed onions and cranberry-orange relish are staples in German and Scandinavian households. Many African-Americans enliven their Thanksgiving meal with foods from the South: sweet potato

epidemiologists (ep-i-DEEM-ee-OLL-i-jists) scientists who study trends in disease within populations

pie, cornbread, and greens. Jewish families who adhere to religious dietary restrictions use kosher turkeys, do not eat pork-based sausage or shellfish dressings, and serve no sauces made with milk, cream, or cheese.

Economics

"No one can love his neighbor on an empty stomach."

— Woodrow Wilson, 1912

The availability of specific foods varies widely from one country to another. Economic conditions influence the foods a person can buy as well as which foods are raised and which are imported. Wealth is no guarantee of nutritional health, but it certainly enables people to purchase adequate amounts of food. Poverty, on the other hand, has long been linked to malnutrition. In developing countries, the drive to produce cash crops, such as exotic fruits and spices, tobacco, rubber, and beef, has had disastrous social and environmental effects. Wealthy persons have displaced poorer ones from fertile soil and have hired poor laborers to raise exportable cash crops rather than food to feed the country's people. Precious rain forests have been converted into fallow acreage for use as grazing land.[14]

Generally, the wealthier the nation, the greater the availability and variety of food. An abundance of food leads to an entirely different set of economic considerations than does food scarcity. Governments of industrialized nations attempt to stabilize food supply and demand by offering cash incentives for raising certain crops and, odd as it may seem, for *not* raising others. They routinely buy surpluses of food both as a hedge against disaster and as a way to control prices. Governments also have developed a complex system of price supports for many agricultural commodities.[14]

Further, multimillion-dollar food manufacturing firms influence food availability and consumer perceptions of good nutrition by shaping government nutrition policies through lobbying and advertising campaigns. In addition to creating new marketing niches, these companies develop products in response to consumer concerns. For example, as more women have entered the work force, there has been an increased demand for and supply of convenience foods. Consumer concern over the salt, fat, and sugar content of foods has spurred manufacturers to create many products that contain reduced amounts of these ingredients. Similarly, Americans' obsession with their body weight has prompted manufacturers to develop low-calorie fat and sugar substitutes.

Advertising

Among the technological advances that accompanied industrialization was the development of an increasingly widespread and influential media network. Newspapers and magazines became widely available. The steady stream of printed material was joined first by radio and later by television. Food manufacturers were quick to make use of these new avenues for reaching customers. Messages from subtle to blatant urge consumers to spend their dollars and calories on a wide array of offerings: diet drinks and meals, frozen foods, super-supplements, economy meals, fast foods, ethnic specialties, and "gourmet" products.

How can I as a consumer avoid falling prey to food manufacturers' inflated claims? To make the best nutrition decisions, you need to educate yourself about food content and values. You also need to understand the kinds of strategies food manufacturers use to sell their products and to develop skills for separating propaganda from reality. The accurate nutrition information provided throughout this text and the specific consumer advice at the end of each chapter will help you make knowledgeable food choices. In the last chapter, Looking to the Future, you'll learn the appropriate scientific method for investigating and proving cause and effect relationships. Appendix G lists resources that will help you keep abreast of new trends in nutrition.

In the meantime, being alert to common advertising techniques can help you make better food choices. Advertisements capture the attention of particular segments of the population by appealing to their value systems. For instance, a product that promises a quick, economical, nutritious meal attracts the attention of a busy working mother. A physical fitness enthusiast is likely to be more interested in a product that is said to contain all natural ingredients or is claimed to enhance performance or reduce the risk of heart disease. Still other people are drawn to foods that promote youth, beauty, or sex appeal. You as a consumer need to be wary of testimonials and endorsements by celebrities, supposedly satisfied customers, or alleged nutrition experts. Ask yourself: would Shaquille O'Neal be endorsing Pepsi if it weren't for his multimillion-dollar contract? Is the "satisfied customer" really an actor? What are the "nutrition expert's" credentials? (See the Nutralert box.)

Emotions

The complex intellectual and emotional makeup of humans is unique in the animal kingdom. Rather than simply eating to live, many people live to eat. Some foods gain popularity as status symbols, others as health remedies; some comfort us; others are synonymous with celebration. Certain items that are consumed readily in some cultures are considered taboo in oth-

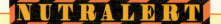

NUTRALERT

WHO CAN PROVIDE RELIABLE NUTRITION INFORMATION?

Anyone can call himself a "nutritionist." The only true nutrition experts are registered dietitians (RD) and/or people who have a graduate degree in nutrition (MS or PhD) from an accredited university. Registered dietitians are qualified professionals with 70 hours of undergraduate nutrition courses, a year-long internship, and a passing score on a qualifying exam administered by the American Dietetic Association. People with MS and PhD degrees in nutrition can become diplomates of the Certification Board for Nutrition Specialists (indicated by *CNS* after their title). This indicates that they have attended an accredited institution and demonstrated competency in the field of nutrition.

ers.[3] Given these powerful emotional connotations, it is little wonder that people often misuse food in societies where it is plentiful. As we will discover, the abuse of food can lead to a variety of physical problems.

Newer studies suggest that some of our emotional reactions to food may have a genetic basis. The predominant influence on our emotional reactions to a particular food is culture, but genetically governed taste preferences also play a role. For many years individual responses to a particular food were thought to be based largely on familiarity and positive associations. More recently, however, in comparing food preferences of identical twins, fraternal twins, siblings, and parents, researchers have observed genetic differences in **taste perception.**[4] Genetics has been found to influence the subjects' preference for orange juice, broccoli, cottage cheese, sweetened cereal, and hamburgers.

How does genetics influence food preferences?

Inherited differences in taste sensitivity, particularly with respect to bitter flavors, seems to shape food preferences. In general, the more sensitive one is to bitter flavors, the more food dislikes one has. The discovery of a biological basis for taste perception also suggests that there may be some validity to the concept of food-mood interactions.

Some researchers believe that emotions not only influence our food choices but also govern how our food is metabolized (see A Closer Look below).[15] This notion is based on the fact that the human body responds to stress as a physical threat, even when the stress is psychological rather than physical. The body initially produces the hormone **epinephrine** (adrenalin), which stimulates the release of stored fuel from the liver, raising blood sugar levels and priming the body for instant action. At this level, stress heightens awareness and may actually improve physical or intellectual performance. If the stress is prolonged, however, other, stronger hormones are produced that stimulate a heightened fear response and convert essential body tissues into fuel. The body cannot tolerate this level of stress indefinitely. A person who is subjected to long-term stress becomes less able to digest and absorb food, maintain a healthy body, and combat disease.[9]

A CLOSER LOOK

The Effect of Emotions on Food Absorption

The complex nature of the interaction between environmental influences and nutrition is clearly depicted in the results of a Swedish study conducted a generation ago. According to Dr. Walter Mertz, Director of the U.S. Department of Agriculture's Human Nutrition Research Center, researchers fed Swedes a diet of Thai food and Thais a diet of Swedish food. The Thai food was much spicier than the Swedes' relatively bland diet.

Surprisingly, the Swedes absorbed much less iron than usual while consuming Thai food. The same was true for the Thais eating Swedish food.

During the second phase of the experiment the meals were blenderized, and each group was fed its traditional diet in the form of an unappetizing *frappe* (a thick, milk shake–style drink). Iron absorption was lower in both groups when they drank these mixtures than when their native diet was served in an attractive manner. These findings demonstrate that how people feel about what they eat may be just as important to their nutritional well-being as which foods they eat. The research also suggests that stress affects nutritional status.

It is becoming increasingly clear that the golden rule for good health is the often repeated cliché "All things in moderation." To ensure good physical and emotional health, each of us needs to strike a balance between diet, exercise, work, and leisure.

NUTRI QUIZ What values are the manufacturers appealing to in these two ads?

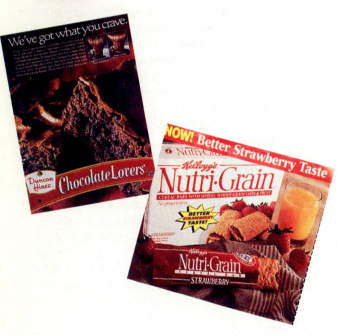

THE SCIENCE OF NUTRITION

The field of nutrition is relatively new. It has been just over 100 years since scientists first discovered that food contains substances that can prevent or cure specific diseases. These curative substances are called *nutrients*.

Nutrients

What exactly is a nutrient? A **nutrient** is defined as *any chemical substance present in food that provides the body with energy or with the building materials required for normal metabolic functioning.* All nutrients can be classified into six broad categories:

1. Water
2. Carbohydrates
3. Lipids (fats and oils)
4. Proteins
5. Vitamins
6. Minerals

Most nutrients must be provided by the diet. Such nutrients are said to be **essential** because insufficient amounts eventually will result in impaired health or metabolic functioning. Given enough building blocks, the body can make some nonessential nutrients. To date more than 40 essential nutrients have been identified for humans. They range from individual chemical **elements** to complex **compounds** (see A Closer Look on p. 7).

What is the significance of an organic nutrient? Carbon-based (organic) substances can be burned in the presence of oxygen to produce **energy** or, in scientific terms, **calories.** Undoubtedly you know that without oxygen you will die, but have you ever considered why? A practical example illustrates the importance of both carbon and oxygen to the maintenance of life: Suppose we want to cook with charcoal briquets in a kettle barbecue. Briquets are made from wood and contain mostly carbon. We light the briquets and let them burn down to white-hot coals. If we leave the kettle uncovered, the presence of oxygen will allow the coals to burn, releasing energy in the form of heat. If we cover the barbecue with a lid, however, and deprive the coals of oxygen, the fire will die.

Essentially the same reaction is continuously taking place on a minute scale in every cell of our bodies. Carbon obtained from the organic nutrients during digestion enters our cells along with oxygen from the air we breathe. Through a complex metabolic process known as **oxidation,** the carbon is "burned" to produce the energy that fuels our physical and metabolic activities. Some of the energy released during this process is given off as heat, which keeps us warm.

Although there are four classes of organic nutrients, one of these—vitamins—does not contribute any energy to the diet because the chemicals that regulate oxidation do not "recognize" the chemical structure of vitamins. So when scientists talk about sources of energy or calories in a diet, they consider only those supplied by protein, carbohydrate, lipid, and alcohol, if applicable. Although inorganic nutrients do not contribute to energy metabolism, they are vitally important to physical well-being, as we will discover in later chapters.

A CLOSER LOOK

What Are Chemical Elements?

Elements are the basic substances of which all matter is composed. Like primary numbers, elements cannot be reduced by ordinary means to a simpler form. Elements such as carbon, nitrogen, oxygen, calcium, and iron are the basic units making up the universe. As will be seen, they play significant roles in human nutrition as either elements or compounds.

Only one class of nutrients, the dietary minerals, is made up of individual elements. All the members of the five other classes of nutrients are made up of compounds, substances composed of two or more chemically bonded elements. For instance, water (H_2O) is made up of two hydrogen atoms, each bonded to one oxygen atom, whereas carbohydrates are made of carbon, hydrogen, and oxygen, chemically combined in various proportions.

These nutrient categories are further classified as organic or inorganic. In scientific terms, the word organic means a substance that contains the chemical element carbon (C). Four of the six nutrient classes—vitamins, proteins, carbohydrates, and lipids—contain carbon as part of their chemical structure and are considered to be organic. The remaining two classes of nutrients—water and minerals—do not contain carbon and are said to be inorganic (literally, without carbon).

NUTRI NUGGET

Is alcohol a nutrient? NO. It is unnecessary for human survival. It supplies calories but provides no other nutrients.

What is a calorie?   A calorie is a unit of measure for energy. Technically, a calorie is defined as "the amount of energy required to raise the temperature of 1 gram of water 1 degree centigrade." The amount of energy contained in food and expended by humans and animals is measured in **kilocalories** (that is, thousands of calories). The term *kilocalories* is sometimes abbreviated as **kcal,** pronounced "kay-cal." Like most people, nutritionists and other scientists tend to speak of energy units simply as "calories," but when writing they use the formal term "kcal" or sometimes "Calorie," spelled with a capital C. In this text we use *kcalorie(s)* in the narrative and the abbreviated form, *kcal*, in tables and figures.

Where do nutrients come from?   All living things, including the planet we live on, require nourishment to sustain their life force. Over millennia the Earth, its flora and fauna have developed an intricate and fragile ecology in which various species are dependent on one another for their survival. Rain nourishes the soil. Plants draw carbon dioxide from the air and moisture and minerals from the soil, and with the aid of sunlight convert these starting materials into carbohydrates, protein, fat, and vitamins. These nutrients are used for two purposes:

1. To form plant and animal tissues
2. To provide fuel for plants and animals

Plants have two possible fates. They grow until changes in their nutrient supply, the presence of disease, or the ravages of old age lead to their death. After death their tissues decompose, returning nutrients to the soil. Alternatively, plants are eaten by an insect or animal, in which case the plant's tissues and nutrient stores are used to synthesize and maintain the tissues of its predator. The plant's nutrients are returned to the soil in the feces of the animal that ate it or through decay of the animal's body after it dies. If the animal that consumed the plant in turn becomes the prey of another animal, the process of returning nutrients to the soil will take a little longer.

Human Nutrition Assessment

How are nutritional status and diet assessed?
Once scientists realized that certain nutrients cured or prevented specific diseases, they became interested in quantifying how much of a given nutrient was required to do the job. The result was standards of nutrient intake such as the ***Recommended Dietary Allowances (RDA).*** Next scientists focused on developing ways to determine the adequacy of a person's diet. The system they created, known as the ABCD's of nutrition assessment, consists of **a**nthropometric, **b**iochemical, and **c**linical evaluations (physical exam), along with a **d**iet history.[1]

What can be learned during a physical exam?   A physical exam reveals how well a person's reported food intake is meeting his/her physiological needs and whether any underlying metabolic disorders are interfering with nutrient metabolism.

RDA   Standards of nutrient intake developed by the Food Nutrition Board of the National Academy of Sciences

Anthropometrics

Anthropometric measurements (height, weight, skinfold thickness, and head circumference) supply valuable information about a person's nutritional status. Such measurements can indicate general conditions of over- or undernutrition as well as specific problems, such as bone loss induced by calcium deficiency.

Biochemical

A physician also can order a variety of laboratory tests that can pinpoint specific nutrition-related health problems. Such problems may be indicated by the presence of sugar or protein in urine or by an abnormal number and/or size of red blood cells.

Clinical

During a thorough physical exam, a competent physician or dietitian can detect some nutrient deficiency symptoms, such as the pallor of iron deficiency or the presence of a developing goiter (a sign of possible iodine deficiency).

Diet History

What can be learned by looking at food intake information?   Nutritionists determine the identities and quantities of specific nutrients in a person's diet by analyzing his or her diet history or diary. These records list the kinds and amounts of food consumed over a period of several days and often indicate when and where they were eaten. By analyzing diet records, nutritionists gain insight into a person's eating habits and nutritional status.[1]

NUTRI NUGGET Atwater and Woods published the first nutrient analysis of American foods in 1896. Approximately 2600 different food items were included in this reference.[2] Contemporary scientists continue in their footsteps, analyzing new products and refining existing data.

In theory, a thorough and accurate diet history will indicate a person's general eating patterns and nutrient intake over a longer period of time. In reality, however, the accuracy of diet records varies considerably, depending on the subject's memory and honesty, the skill and thoroughness of the record taker, and the method used to analyze the information. People often feel uncomfortable discussing their diet habits with a nutrition expert. Rather than revealing what they really eat, they tend to tell the interviewer what they think she or he wants to hear. Some people simply find it difficult to recall accurately how much of what foods they ate over a several-day period. If these same people are asked to keep a diary of everything they consume for several days, some of them may unintentionally distort the results. For instance, they may eat simple foods, like a hamburger or chicken breast, rather than the chili and casseroles they usually consume, so that they do not have to try to estimate how much of which ingredients these mixed items contained. A nutritionist who is a skilled interviewer sometimes can obtain more accurate information during a follow-up interview.

How do we know what nutrients are provided by each food?   Once a diet history has been taken, its nutrient content must be analyzed. This previously was a manual task that involved the use of printed food composition tables. Today diet histories are usually analyzed by computer.

What factors influence the accuracy of food composition data?   **Food composition tables** (see Appendix A), which are used to create computer databases, list the nutrient content of foods that has been obtained during repeated chemical anaylsis. Analyses for some nutrients are extremely accurate; others are less specific. Computerized databases cannot take into account seasonal variations in the nutrient content of foods, the effect of various food storage and preparation techniques on nutrient content, variations in the bioavailability (absorbability) of nutrients obtained

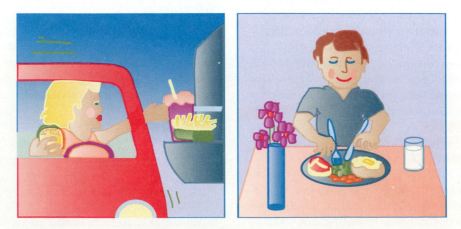

What's your style: grab 'n' go or sit and savor?

from different food sources, variations in nutrient content caused by genetic differences among strains of a particular food, and the mineral composition of water from different sources. In addition, it is difficult to estimate the composition of mixed foods, such as casseroles. Although the food composition databank is not perfect, its completeness and accuracy are very good and improving all the time.[1]

What determines the accuracy of a computerized diet analysis? The accuracy of a computerized diet analysis depends on the accuracy of the diet history data and the completeness of the food composition data. There are a number of diet analysis programs with varying degrees of sophistication. Some programs are designed for use by the general public, some are used in schools for teaching purposes, and others are used by professionals who work with patients.

Nutritional Status and Health

Incredible as it may seem, the impact of nutrition on health begins before we are born and continues until death. Your mother's dietary habits during your gestation determined your nutritional status at birth. Your own eating habits affect your future nutritional state. Because many common nutrition-related illnesses, such as cardiovascular disease and osteoporosis, develop over decades, it is often difficult to convince people of the association between diet and health. Once people accept the connection, they usually ask:

Is there a perfect diet? The answer is yes—and no.

YES! Although humans can subsist on a wide variety of foods, some diets seem to be healthier than others. In general, the best diet contains large amounts of unrefined plant products and small but nutritionally important quantities of animal-derived foods. Such a diet is naturally high in fiber and low in fat and cholesterol—three factors that are believed to decrease the risk of heart disease, certain cancers, diabetes, and obesity. This pattern of nutrient intake is much like that in many Asian countries, where the incidence of these so-called "diseases of affluence" is low. A low-fat, high-fiber diet is also believed to be quite similar to that consumed by our early hunter-gatherer ancestors.[8]

NO! Unlike many animals, which have very specific dietary requirements, human populations have been found living healthfully on diets ranging from almost purely vegetarian to nearly all animal based. Given health experts' beliefs about the role of diet in disease, many people have questioned how populations such as American Eskimos and the Masai tribe of Africa can subsist healthfully on diets high in fat and cholesterol-laden animal products. These populations' good health and their lack of diseases that are common in industrialized nations seem to be the result of strenuous physical activity and consequent low body fat content.

This illustrates an important aspect of the evolving science of nutrition: for many years nutrition was regarded as an isolated issue. It was believed that people could remain healthy simply by eating a good diet. Over the last 20 years, however, it has become increasingly apparent that diet cannot be separated from physical activity. Considering how early humans lived and how most people in developing nations still live, it is easy to see why this may be true.

People used to get a good physical workout simply in the process of obtaining food. This was certainly the case when hunter-gatherers wandered the Earth in search of food and in societies where people farmed the land by manual labor. Any weight gained during the seasons when food was abundant was readily lost during the winter. By contrast, many people living in industrialized nations spend most of their day in stationary pursuits earning money to buy food. Their lack of physical activity makes it easy for them to gain weight, and the year-round supply of food eliminates seasonal weight loss. Unless such people try to avoid unnecessary weight gain and purposefully pursue physical activity, they tend to grow heavier and less physically fit, making them prime candidates for many of the illnesses of modern living.

If exercise is the key to preventing diseases of modern living, why not tell people to eat whatever they want as long as they exercise? There are two reasons. First, we need a balanced diet to maintain optimal health. Second, a typical fitness program for other than elite athletes does not match the strenuous level of activity performed by people in unindustrialized nations. For this reason, and because of the abundance of food available to them, people in industrialized settings, even if they exercise regularly, often have higher levels of body fat than do their counterparts living in developing nations. Many scientists believe that body fat content may be an important factor in the development of certain diseases.[8]

Intake Standards

What should we eat? *People eat foods; cells eat nutrients.* Understanding this distinction is essential for understanding the field of nutrition. The recognition that many ancient illnesses such as scurvy (vitamin C deficiency disease) were actually nutrient deficiencies helped scientists understand that when people eat food they are actually feeding their cells nutrients. Scientists have been able to find the nutrients in foods that are necessary to life. They also have discovered how much

anthropometric (AN-throw-po-MEH-trik) *anthropo,* (resembling) man and *metric,* measure

of each of these nutrients is needed. These measures are reported in documents described in this text as **nutrient intake standards.**

Knowing which nutrients your body needs is important to your health, but you can't take a shopping list of nutrients to the grocery store. You don't eat individual nutrients; you eat foods that contain nutrients. To provide this information, other scientists have analyzed individual foods and calculated how much of which nutrients these foods contain. Through the efforts of both groups of scientists, **food intake standards** have been developed. As a result of these separate approaches to "nutrition," we use two different categories of standards: those that refer to nutrients and those that refer to foods. Table 1-1 lists some common standards in each of these two categories. We take an in-depth look at each standard in Chapter 2, Consumer Concerns.

These technical methods for assessing the adequacy of diets provide useful information and alert consumers to specific problem areas—but they do not supply all the information we need to design a healthy diet. The principles outlined below provide some unifying concepts you can use to create your own "ideal" diet.

Remember that although certain foods are better for you than others, a diet is neither "good" nor "bad" based on the consumption of a single food, one meal, or even one day's or one week's worth of meals. Rather, your nutritional status and its effect on your health are the consequences of a lifetime of eating habits. So strive for a diet that is:

- *Moderate*—to prevent overindulgence in certain "luxury" foods, such as sugar, fat, and alcohol
- *Balanced*—so it does not supply either too little or too much of selected nutrients
- *Varied*—to ensure that you obtain all essential nutrients, to gain the benefits provided by each of the food groups, and to minimize the risk of overexposure to natural toxins or pesticide residues peculiar to a given crop
- *Adequate*—so you consume enough kcalories and food from each group to supply adequate amounts of all essential nutrients
- *High in nutrient density*—nutrient density measures the ratio of nutrients to kcalories. The more

nutrients per kcalorie, the greater the nutrient density. As a rule processed foods such as refined grains, vegetable oils, purified soy products, potato chips, and ice cream are lower in nutrient density than the whole foods from which they came. Figure 4-10 in Chapter 4, Carbohydrates, compares the nutrient content of whole wheat and refined white flours.

Digestion

How do the foods I eat become the nutrients my cells require?   Digestion is the process that converts foods into nutrients. It involves breaking down food into successively smaller pieces, until it is in a form that the body can absorb. For instance, water, minerals, and vitamins released from food during the digestive process are absorbed directly into the body. The energy-containing nutrients carbohydrate, protein, and fat, by contrast, are too big to be absorbed in their native state. They must first be broken down into their molecular building blocks.[7] A Closer Look on p. 11 provides an overview of the digestive process. More detailed information on digestion is presented in the In Between section of each nutrient chapter.

NUTRI NUGGET   **If it seems difficult to believe that the gastrointestinal tract is external to the body, consider the fact that bacteria capable of causing severe illness can live in the large intestine without infecting the rest of the body!**

Absorption

How does absorption differ from digestion?   Digestion breaks foods into nutrients. Absorption is the process whereby nutrients move across the cells that line the intestine and into the body's circulatory system. Nutrients entering the cells pass into body fluids and are then carried to all the cells that need them.

What becomes of the nutrients after digestion and absorption?   We will explore in detail the digestion, absorption, and utilization of each nutrient class in later chapters. As you explore these processes, you will see that, in general:

- **Water** cools and purifies the body tissues and participates in biochemical reactions.
- **Carbohydrates** provide **glucose** for fuel and glycogen synthesis.
- **Lipids** provide **fatty acids, glycerol,** and some **cholesterol.** Small amounts of these three substances are used to synthesize hormones and cell membranes. Fatty acids are also used for fuel. Any excess is stored as body fat for future energy needs.

TABLE 1-1 Intake Standards	
Foods	**Nutrients**
Dietary Guidelines	RDA
	NIH Fiber Recommendations
Food Guide Pyramid	% Daily Value (labels)
5-A-Day Program	
American Heart Association	Dietary Goals
American Cancer Society	
People eat foods.	***Cells eat nutrients.***

Where Does Digestion Occur?

Many people erroneously believe that digestion of food occurs in the stomach. It actually takes place in the gastrointestinal tract (GI tract), which is a continuous tube that runs through, but is external to, the body. To picture what the gastrointestinal tract looks like, imagine a garden hose running through the body starting at the mouth, traveling down the throat and esophagus, enlarging to form the stomach, contracting back into tight coils to form the small intestine, then enlarging once again to form the large intestine and finally terminating at the anus[4] (Fig. 1-1).

How is digestion accomplished?   Digestion requires the integrated action of three major systems:

- The physical structures that make up the gastrointestinal tract and perform the mechanical aspects of digestion
- The chemicals synthesized by the body for use in the digestive process
- Regulatory factors, hormones and nerve signals, that control the rate of digestion

Working in concert these systems perform a series of activities. The steps of digestion and absorption include:

- *Entrance of food* (we masticate and swallow a ball of food, called a bolus)
- *Mixing and lignification of food in the stomach* to form a watery substance, called chyme
- *Controlled passage of food* through the gastrointestinal tract by a series of muscles and *sphincters*
- *Breakdown of food to nutrients* by chemical and mechanical means
- *Absorption of nutrients* in the intestine
- *Resorption of water* in both small and large intestines
- *Excretion of wastes* (feces)

Many complex physical and chemical activities are involved in keeping the digestive process going at a reasonable speed. Diet composition, hormones, enzymes, messages from the nervous system, physical activity, emotions, illness, and medications all play a role.

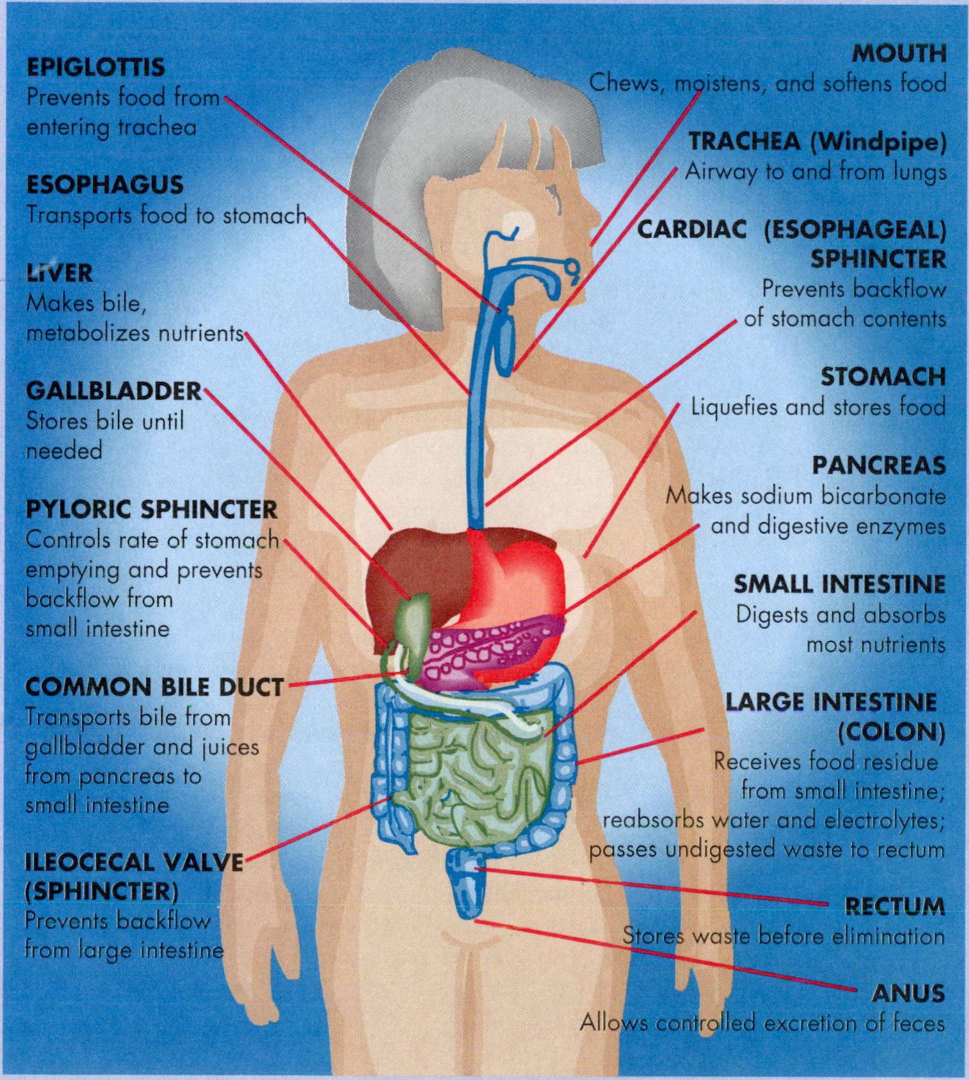

EPIGLOTTIS
Prevents food from entering trachea

ESOPHAGUS
Transports food to stomach

LIVER
Makes bile, metabolizes nutrients

GALLBLADDER
Stores bile until needed

PYLORIC SPHINCTER
Controls rate of stomach emptying and prevents backflow from small intestine

COMMON BILE DUCT
Transports bile from gallbladder and juices from pancreas to small intestine

ILEOCECAL VALVE (SPHINCTER)
Prevents backflow from large intestine

MOUTH
Chews, moistens, and softens food

TRACHEA (Windpipe)
Airway to and from lungs

CARDIAC (ESOPHAGEAL) SPHINCTER
Prevents backflow of stomach contents

STOMACH
Liquefies and stores food

PANCREAS
Makes sodium bicarbonate and digestive enzymes

SMALL INTESTINE
Digests and absorbs most nutrients

LARGE INTESTINE (COLON)
Receives food residue from small intestine; reabsorbs water and electrolytes; passes undigested waste to rectum

RECTUM
Stores waste before elimination

ANUS
Allows controlled excretion of feces

FIGURE 1-1 The human digestive system. Many organs work together to digest food, absorb nutrients, and eliminate waste products.

- **Proteins** provide **amino acids** from which structural and chemical components of the body are manufactured. During emergencies amino acids also may be used as fuel.
- The **vitamin** and **mineral** classes provide **cofactors** for the chemical reactions required to metabolize carbohydrates, proteins, and lipids. Some minerals also are involved in water metabolism.

Absorption marks the beginning of some of the most fascinating aspects of nutrition: the maintenance of nutrient balance (homeostasis) and nutrient utilization.

 If digestion occurs too fast it can lead to diarrhea. Too slow and constipation results. What effect, if any, do you suppose these conditions might have on digestion and absorption?

Maintaining Balance: Homeostasis

In earlier times scientists believed that tissue, once formed, stayed put. Today it is recognized that the entire body is in a continuous state of flux, with old tissues constantly being broken down and replaced with new ones. When any active system, including the body, achieves **homeostasis** by maintaining a balance between input and outflow, it is said to be in dynamic **equilibrium** (active balance).

How does the body maintain homeostasis? Through a series of metabolic checks and balances, known as **homeostatic mechanisms.** Nutritionists are interested in the impact on nutritional homeostasis of intake, absorption, storage, and excretion. The human body is genetically programmed to monitor and perform these functions—and many more. Depending on your dietary and physiological status, your body can either increase or decrease absorption or excretion of nutrients, as well as store any surplus for emergencies!

The only one of these functions that the body seems to lack control over is intake. Appropriately designed and executed studies have never been able to validate the common misconception that a food craving signifies a metabolic need for a particular nutrient or that people can instinctively choose healthy diets. Several studies have shown that, given a choice, laboratory animals and young children[2] automatically select a nutritionally balanced diet over an unbalanced one. However, subsequent experiments showed this is only true if the diets are equally **palatable.**[12] The palatability issue explains why many humans prefer sugar, salt, and fat-laden processed foods over healthier, natural ones.

Long-term consumption of a nutrient-poor diet taxes the body's ability to maintain homeostasis, resulting in various nutrient deficiency syndromes. Excesses of certain nutrients can be just as dangerous. Some nutrients if consumed in too high a dose overwhelm the body's homeostatic mechanisms and accumulate to toxic levels. Others, while safe from a toxicity standpoint, promote the development of chronic diseases.

Scientists are also interested in the impact of nutrient interactions on health. Some nutrients work alone; others collaborate. Calcium and phosphorus work together in forming strong bones and teeth. The electrolyte minerals (sodium, potassium, and chloride) have an interrelated effect on fluid balance. Such cooperative efforts depend on the body maintaining a balanced quantity of these nutrients since imbalances can have profound effects on metabolism. Imbalances occur when too much of a particular nutrient is added to an otherwise balanced and adequate diet, causing a relative deficiency of the nutrients with which it works. The remainder of the text will discuss nutrient utilization and how deficiencies, excesses, and imbalances of each of the 40 essential nutrients affect the body's ability to maintain homeostasis.

THE FOOD CHAIN IN THE ENVIRONMENT

Nutrition makes the world go round! The acquisition, consumption, and metabolism of foods are part of the vital cycle that drives life on Earth. The manner in which animals acquire food influences patterns of both plant and animal evolution. Herbivores eat plants. Some plants adapt to this threat by developing poisons to discourage their predators. Others come to rely on consumption by animals as a way to spread their seeds far and wide. Animals eat these "friendly" plants, then excrete their seeds in distant locales. Predators control populations of herbivores and other animals, ensuring that only the strong survive to reproduce. The dependence of one species on another in terms of predator/prey relationships is referred to as a food chain (Fig. 1-2). The seemingly one-way flow of nutrients in a food chain is supported by a series of elaborate nutrient recycling processes, which we will explore in later chapters. In essence, sunlight, water, and nutrients in the soil support plant growth, which in turn supports animal populations. Eventually, dead and decaying plant and animal matter return to the earth the nutrients they absorbed during life. New plants flourish, and the food chain begins again. Grasping the concept of a food chain and nutrient recycling systems will help you clarify some of the cause-and-effect relationships between food production and environmental issues that we will discuss in later chapters.

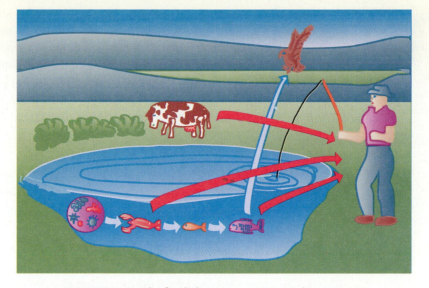

FIGURE 1-2 The food chain is nature's recycling process.

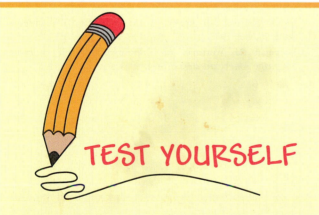

TEST YOURSELF

True or False. Put a **T** for true or an **F** for false in the space beside each question.

_F_ 1. There are five major classes of nutrients. six ✗
___ 2. Organic nutrients are those that contain oxygen. carbon
_F_ 3. The energy-providing nutrients are vitamins, carbohydrate, and lipid. fat, P, C

___ 4. Vitamins are inorganic nutrients.
___ 5. Religious beliefs, family eating patterns, peer pressure, economic status, and local customs all influence a person's food choices.
___ 6. Nutrition is the sum of the processes of eating, digesting, absorbing, and utilizing nutrients.
___ 7. Calories are the units we use to measure energy.
___ 8. A nutrient is a substance that provides the body with energy and/or the building materials that are required for normal metabolic functioning.

Short Answer

9. What does the _ABCD_ approach to clinical nutrition analysis stand for?
10. List three features of an ideal diet.
11. In one sentence describe what the process of digestion accomplishes.
12. In one sentence describe the significance of a food chain.

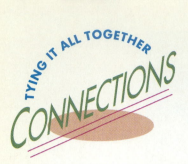

TYING IT ALL TOGETHER

CONNECTIONS

1. How do the foods served at an Asian restaurant compare with those served at an American restaurant?

2. How do both personal and social factors affect your food intake?

3. In a "family style" meal, dishes of food are placed on the table so that each person can help himself. What are the benefits and drawbacks of this service style compared with the common restaurant practice of serving each person's meal individually?

4. How can economic factors affect food choices?

5. How can emotions affect food intake?

6. How can you assess the nutritional adequacy of your diet?

7. Describe what must happen to an apple or a hamburger so that your cells can use its energy (kcalories).

8. Using the example in the Student Preface, draw a "cognitive map" of this chapter.

9. Compare your map with the expanded chapter outline in the table of contents.

   a. How are they similar?

   b. How are they different?

References

1. Assessment of nutritional status. In *American Dietetic Association manual of clinical dietetics*, Chicago, 1990, ADA.

2. Darby WJ, Jukes TH: *Founders of nutrition science*, vols 1 and 2, Rockville, Md, 1992, American Institute of Nutrition.

3. Darby WJ et al: *Food—the gift of Osiris*, vols 1 and 2, 1979, New York, Academic Press.

4. Falcigleu G et al: Evidence for a genetic influence on preference for some foods, *Journal of the American Dietetic Association* 94:154-158, 1992.

5. Gore A: *Earth in the balance: ecology and the human spirit*, Boston, 1992, Houghton Mifflin.

6. Grivetti LE: Nutrition past—nutrition today: prescientific origins of nutrition and dietetics, *Nutrition Today* Jan-Feb 13-24, 1991.

7. Johnson LR, ed: *Gastrointestinal physiology*, St Louis, 1991, Mosby-Year Book.

8. National Research Council report on diet and health: *Implications for reducing chronic disease risk*, Washington, DC, 1989, National Academy Press.

9. Sapolsky RM: *Why zebras don't get ulcers: a guide to stress, stress-related diseases, and coping*, New York, 1994, WH Freeman.

10. Scarre C: *Smithosonian time lines of the ancient world*, Washington, DC, 1993, Smithsonian Institution Press.

11. *Smithsonian* magazine, 20th Earth Day Issue, April 1990.

12. Storey M, Brown JE: Young children instictively know how to eat? The studies of Clara Davis revisited, *New England Journal of Medicine* 316:103-110, 1987.

13. Toussaint-Samat M: *History of food*, Cambridge, Mass, 1993, Blackwell Publishers.

14. United Nations 9th Annual World Food Day Teleconference Study Packet, 1992.

15. Wurtman RJ, Wurtman JJ: Carbohydrates and depression, *Scientific American* 260:68-75, 1989.

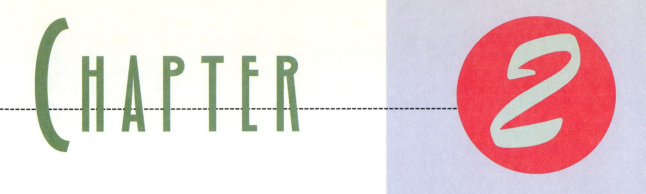

CHAPTER 2

CONSUMER CONCERNS
Tools for Healthy Choices

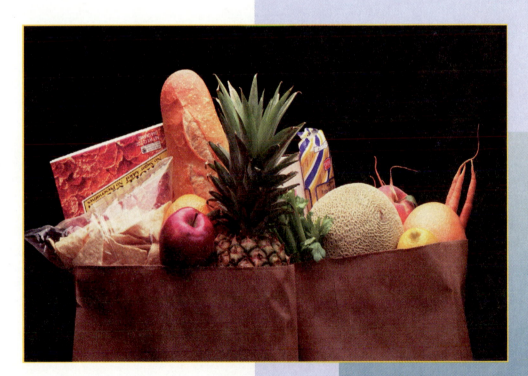

Seeing is deceiving.
It's eating that's
believing.
— *James Thurber*

Throughout the history of humankind, the major nutritional concern has been: "Is food available?" Thanks to modern technology, obtaining enough food is no longer a concern for most people in industrialized nations. Often, in fact, just the opposite is true: too much food is available for the amount of physical work most people perform.

Once there is enough dietary energy to run the human machine (about 1600 kcalories per day for women and 2200 for men), people's concerns turn to *nutritional adequacy* and *safety*. People ask: "What kinds of foods do I need"? "Do the foods I favor provide adequate nutrients"? and "Is the food supply safe"? In this chapter we will explore these questions from the consumer's viewpoint.

NUTRITIONAL ADEQUACY

Advice about diet and nutrition is not a phenomenon of the modern age. Writings from ancient cultures tell us that dietary recommendations existed in prehistoric times. These early works reflect the rudimentary understanding of science at the time they were written, and their advice is often colored by superstitions and religious beliefs. Yet they also contain a surprising number of the nutritional truths imparted in today's dietary advice. Contemporary intake standards (Table 2-1) incorporate sophisticated scientific knowledge of human nutrient requirements and of the nutrient composition of foods.

Food Intake Standards

Who uses food intake standards?   Standards of food intake have been developed to help consumers

TABLE 2-1   Intake Standards

Foods	Nutrients
Dietary Guidelines	RDA
	NIH Fiber Recommendations
Food Guide Pyramid	% Daily Value (labels)
5-A-Day Program	
American Heart Association	Dietary Goals
American Cancer Society	
People eat foods.	**Cells eat nutrients.**

BOX 2-1   1990 Dietary Guidelines for Americans

EAT A VARIETY OF FOODS DAILY

Include these foods every day: fruits and vegetables; whole-grain and enriched breads and cereals; milk and milk products; meats, fish, and poultry, and eggs, dried peas, and beans; 3 to 5 servings of vegetables; 2 to 4 servings of fruit; 6 to 11 servings of grains; 2 to 3 servings of dairy products; 2 to 3 servings of meat, fish, poultry, beans, peas, eggs, and nuts.

MAINTAIN A HEALTHY WEIGHT

Increase physical activity; reduce kcalories by eating fewer fatty foods and sweets and less sugar, and by using alcohol sparingly; lose weight gradually.

CHOOSE A DIET WITH PLENTY OF VEGETABLES, FRUITS, AND GRAIN PRODUCTS

Substitute starches for fats and sugars; select whole-grain breads and cereals, fruits and vegetables, dried beans and peas, and nuts to increase fiber and starch intake.

USE SUGARS IN MODERATION

Use less sugar, syrup, and honey; reduce concentrated sweets, like candy, soft drinks, cookies, and the like; select fresh fruits or fruits canned in light syrup or their own juices; read food labels (sucrose, glucose, dextrose, maltose, lactose, fructose, syrups, and honey are all sugars); eat sugar less often to reduce dental caries.

CHOOSE A DIET LOW IN TOTAL FAT, SATURATED FAT, AND CHOLESTEROL

Limit overall fat to 30% or less of total kcalories, with no more than 10% from saturated fat and no more than 10% from polyunsaturated fat. Choose low-fat protein sources such as lean meats, fish, poultry, dried peas, and beans; use eggs and organ meats in moderation; limit intake of fats on and in foods; trim fats from meats; broil, bake, or boil—don't fry; read food labels for fat content.

USE SALT AND SODIUM IN MODERATION

Reduce salt in cooking; add little or no salt at the table; limit intake of salty foods like potato chips, pretzels, salted nuts, popcorn, condiments, cheese, pickled foods, and cured meats; read food labels for sodium or salt content, especially in processed and snack foods.

IF YOU DRINK ALCOHOL, DO SO IN MODERATION

Limit consumption of alcoholic beverage (including wine, beer, liquors, and so on) to one or two drinks per day. *Note:* Use of alcoholic beverages during pregnancy can result in the development of birth defects and mental retardation (fetal alcohol syndrome).

From *Dietary Guidelines for Americans*, U.S. Department of Health and Human Services Home and Garden Bulletin #232, 1990.

convert nutrient intake information into a practical diet plan. For Americans, two key tools are the Dietary Guidelines and the Food Guide Pyramid.

Dietary Guidelines

In 1980 the U.S. Department of Agriculture (USDA) and the U.S. Department of Health and Human Services (USDHHS) issued a set of recommendations called the *Dietary Guidelines for Americans* (Box 2-1). These recommendations, updated in 1985 and again in 1990 to reflect new scientific data, are directed at healthy Americans 2 years of age and older. They are intended to provide guidance in selecting a diet that will promote health and reduce the risk of chronic diseases for which there is clear evidence of dietary involvement.[2]

The Food Guide Pyramid

The Food Guide Pyramid (Fig. 2-1), officially introduced in April 1992, serves two main purposes. It portrays the Dietary Guidelines in graphic form, and it replaces the Basic 4 Food Groups, which many of us learned in grade school, with a food intake standard that more accurately reflects contemporary nutrition knowledge.[16]

Personalizing the pyramid. How many servings of each food group do I need each day? The Food Guide Pyramid shows a range of servings for each major food group. The number of servings you need depends on how many kcalories you require. This in turn depends on your age, sex, size, activity level, and whether you are pregnant or breast-feeding.

Use Table 2-2 to determine how many servings of each food group you need and the maximum grams of fat to consume based on your kcalorie requirement. Note: your personal fat limit includes the fat in the foods you choose as well as any fat added during cooking or at the table.

Why was the pyramid shape chosen? USDA studies showed that, of all of the geometric shapes tested, the pyramid best conveyed the concepts of proportionality, variety, and moderation.

Proportionality. The ideal diet is composed of large amounts of grains, fruits, and vegetables with smaller but necessary quantities of foods from the meat and dairy groups. Food groups that appear at the same level of the Pyramid, such as the fruit and vegetable groups, supply similar kinds of nutrients.

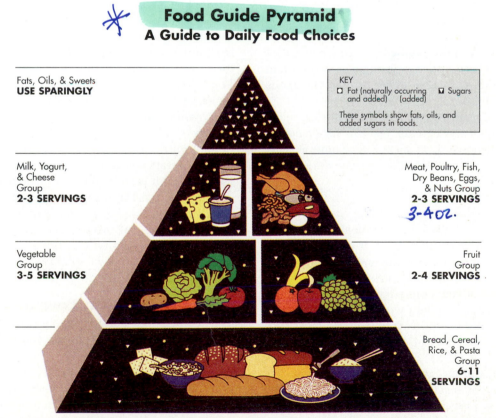

Food Guide Pyramid
A Guide to Daily Food Choices

Fats, Oils, & Sweets
USE SPARINGLY

KEY
□ Fat (naturally occurring and added)   ▨ Sugars (added)
These symbols show fats, oils, and added sugars in foods.

Milk, Yogurt, & Cheese Group
2-3 SERVINGS

Meat, Poultry, Fish, Dry Beans, Eggs, & Nuts Group
2-3 SERVINGS
3-4 oz.

Vegetable Group
3-5 SERVINGS

Fruit Group
2-4 SERVINGS

Bread, Cereal, Rice, & Pasta Group
6-11 SERVINGS

FIGURE 2-1 USDA's Food Guide Pyramid—A Guide to Daily Food Choices. This guide lists the food groups and the number of servings of each to consume. Note that for people under age 25, three servings should be chosen from the milk, yogurt, and cheese group.

TABLE 2-2 Recommended Servings from the Food Guide Pyramid

	Many Women, Older Adults	Children, Teen Girls, Active Women, Most Men	Teen Boys, Active Men
Kcal level*	1600	2200	2800
Bread group	6	9	11
Vegetable group	3	4	5
Fruit group	2	3	4
Milk group	2-3†	2-3†	2-3†
Meat group	2, totaling 5 oz	2, totaling 6 oz	3, totaling 7 oz
Total fat (grams)	53	73	93
Added sugar (teaspoons)	6	12	18

*These kcal levels are based on a diet that uses low-fat, lean foods from the five major food groups and uses fats, oils, and sweets sparingly.
†Women who are pregnant or breast-feeding, teenagers, and young adults to age 24 need three servings per day.

Variety. No one food or food group is superior to another. A variety of foods are needed for a healthy diet. Variety also minimizes exposure to natural toxins and/or chemical pesticides in food.

Moderation. Sweets and fats should be consumed in moderation.

According to the Food Guide Pyramid, which food group(s) should be the foundation of your diet?

Are all serving sizes equal?   No. The amount that constitutes a serving varies from one food group to the next. Serving sizes also differ among the foods within each food group.

To maximize the nutritional value of your diet, select whole-grain breads and cereals; use low-fat or nonfat dairy products; choose lean meats; consume at least one vitamin-C rich food each day and one dark green, leafy vegetable every other day.

Pyramid pitfalls. Does following the Food Guide Pyramid guarantee a healthy diet?   The Food Guide Pyramid can be a great meal planning aid for consumers, but it is not perfect. It makes no mention of the need for sufficient fluid, and it does not provide adequate information on controlling dietary fat intake. The lack of advice concerning appropriate fluid intake is a universal problem with food intake guidelines. This oversight is unfortunate because most people do not get enough water each day. The American Medical Association (AMA) believes strongly that inadequate and/or inappropriate fluid intake is a significant contributor to poor health. For this reason the AMA recommends that Americans make a New Year's health resolution to consume 6 to 10 glasses of water per day.

The major "pyramid pitfall" concerns its advice regarding dietary fat intake. First, like the Dietary Guide-

lines from which it was developed, the Pyramid recommends that fat constitute no more than 30% of total kcalorie intake. Most studies show, however, that for health benefits to be realized, a diet should derive only 20% to 25% of kcalories from fat. Second, the Pyramid specifies a low-fat diet but does not indicate which foods are leanest. For example, using the Food Guide Pyramid, you might choose a bran muffin for breakfast, an egg salad sandwich for lunch, and a grilled pork chop for dinner, without realizing that these choices are high in fat. The staff of *Eating Well* magazine put the Food Guide Pyramid to the test and found that less well-informed staffers had trouble picking the lean food alternatives.[15] To help clarify which foods fit the "lean" profile, you can use the Pyramid Food Choices chart in Appendix C and the information about fat content on food labels.

Pyramid pointers. The Food Guide Pyramid was designed to help healthy people age 2 years and older build a nutritious foundation diet. By restricting your intake of fats, oils, and sweets and combining the Pyramid with a guideline for produce consumption such as the 5-A-Day Program, you can meet 100% of your nutritional needs. Eating right is easy to do! Start by eating plenty of breads, cereal, rice, pasta, fruits, and vegetables. Add two to three servings of low-fat dairy products and two to three servings of low-fat choices from the meat group.

The National 5-A-Day Program

The National Research Council Food and Nutrition Board's 1989 report on diet and health recommends that people consume a variety of vegetables and fruits each day and include *cruciferous* vegetables to ensure that their diet provides ample fiber, vitamins, and minerals. The Council estimated that a minimum of five servings of produce a day are required for good health but noted that the average American eats only half that amount: approximately 2½ servings of produce daily.[11]

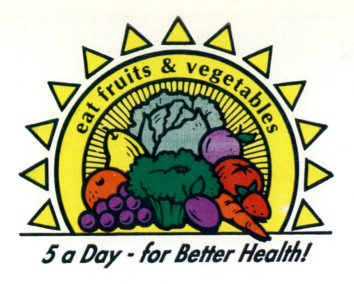

5 a Day - for Better Health!

To see whether a public education campaign could improve produce consumption, the state of California in 1990 launched the 5-A-Day Program on a pilot basis. In addition to recommending that people eat five servings of produce daily, the 5-A-Day Program specified classes of produce that people should eat. (See Chapter 7, Vitamins, for more details.) The success of California's pilot program convinced health professionals that all Americans could benefit from hearing the 5-A-Day message. Accordingly, a National 5-A-Day Program was launched in 1992.[8]

NUTRI NUGGET The National 5-A-Day Program is an excellent example of how a health message can be tailored to specific audiences. Adults are encouraged to remember the slogan Strive-For-5, whereas the children's version of the 5-A-Day Program promotes Give-Me-5 to get children to remember to include enough produce in their diets.

American Heart Association → Mid-Term

The American Heart Association's (AHA) dietary recommendations are aimed at controlling intake of both specific nutrients (fats and cholesterol) and whole foods (red meat, eggs) to reduce the risk of *cardiovascular disease*. Alcohol consumption also is discussed The AHA recommendations for persons over age 2 are[3]:

1. Reduce fat consumption to no more than 30% of total kcalorie intake.
2. Use fish or skinless turkey and chicken for most of your meat servings.
3. Trim all visible fat from red meats.
4. Limit intake of meat, fish, and poultry to 5 to 7 ounces per day (cooked weight).

5. Use no more than 5 to 8 teaspoons of vegetable oil in cooking, baking, and salads each day.
6. Eat no more than 100 milligrams (mg) of cholesterol per 1000 kcalories, up to a maximum of 300 mg of cholesterol per day.
7. Limit intake of shrimp, crab, and lobster.
8. Use no more than 4 egg yolks a week, including those added to baked goods, casseroles, etc. (a large egg yolk contains 225 mg of cholesterol).
9. Limit alcohol intake to no more than 2 ounces of ethanol per day (two 3 oz. glasses of wine, one 12 oz. beer, or 2 oz. of distilled liquor).

For optimal health people also need to eliminate other cardiovascular disease risk factors like tobacco use, excess body weight, stress, and lack of exercise.

American Cancer Society → Mid-term

Because recent evidence indicates that diet modification may be one of the most effective ways to reduce the risk of cancer, the American Cancer Society has published the following recommendations for healthier eating[12]:

1. Eat more low-fat, high-fiber foods. Specifically, eat more fruits, vegetables, legumes, and whole grains.
2. Decrease fat intake: select lean cuts of meat; trim all visible fat; bake or broil instead of frying. Choose low-fat or nonfat dairy products.
3. Use cruciferous and green leafy vegetables often.
4. To reduce *carcinogen* intake eat fewer char-broiled, salted, smoked, and pickled foods.
5. Decrease total fat.

Nutrient Intake Standards

How do scientists determine the amounts of nutrients healthy people need? Scientists have determined the nutrient needs of many species of animals and of humans by examining statistical relationships between nutrient intake and disease, conducting short- and long-term clinical studies, and studying cellular metabolism. The dietary recommendations of many nations, as well as those of the World Health Organization, are based on these research findings.

carcinogen (car-SIN-o-jin)   a substance that promotes cancer
cardiovascular   pertaining to the heart and blood vessels
cruciferous (crew-SIH-fer-us)   plants belonging to the cabbage family, such as turnips, broccoli, and bok choy, whose blossoms form a crosslike pattern

Who uses nutrient intake standards?   Nutrient intake standards were developed to help professionals determine precise dietary needs of animals, including humans. These standards then were used as the basis for the food intake recommendations provided to consumers. In the United States, nutrition and health professionals—who plan school lunch programs, design food assistance programs, assess the nutritional content of processed foods, and evaluate the nutritional adequacy of the nation's food supply—all rely on a nutrient intake standard known as the Recommended Dietary Allowances (RDA). Healthy diets also are planned using such guidelines as the Dietary Goals for the United States and the National Institute of Health (NIH) recommendations on fiber.

RDA

The federal government in 1941 convened a scientific committee to develop Recommended Dietary Allowances, or desirable **nutrient intake** levels, for *healthy* individuals. The committee established separate standards for men, women, infants, children, teenagers, young adults, and older adults because some nutrient requirements vary with age and gender. From age 11 on, separate RDA are given for males and females, reflecting the gender-linked changes in nutrient requirements that occur at puberty. In addition to providing for everyday needs, the RDA contain information about desired nutrient intake during special metabolic conditions such as pregnancy and lactation. The RDA are based on the best available scientific data. Because

new discoveries are constantly being made, the tables are updated approximately every 5 to 10 years. The latest version, published in 1989 and listed inside the front cover of this text, contains recommendations for consumption of energy (kcalories), protein, 13 vitamins, and 12 minerals.[10] The RDA do not give specific recommendations for carbohydrate or fat intake, on the assumption that people will consume adequate quantities of these nutrients in the process of meeting their energy needs.

How are the RDA established today?   Scientists on the RDA update committee review current research regarding the various nutrients. Because individuals' nutrient needs vary, the committee determines the *average* amount of a given nutrient required by healthy people in the specific age and gender categories mentioned above. A bell-shaped curve (Fig. 2-2) illustrates the variability in the actual nutrient needs of a population. Each dot under the curve represents one person. Note that the average requirement for nutrient "Z" is 50 units. Some persons need smaller amounts; others need more. This means that if the committee set the RDA for nutrient "Z" at 50 units, it would cover the needs of only half the population. Instead the RDA are set at a relatively high but safe level (meeting the needs of 95% of healthy persons) to ensure that they cover as many people as possible. Because of this built-in safety factor, consuming two thirds (67%) of the RDA of a given nutrient satisfies most people's needs. The only exception is the RDA for energy. Unlike the RDA for the other nutrients, the energy (kcalorie) RDA do not contain a safety factor because of the potential for creating widespread obesity. The RDA committee sets energy recommendations at the *mean* (the average amount needed by people in each category).

The RDA are recommendations, not requirements. They are designed to meet the needs of healthy persons

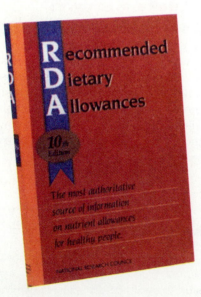

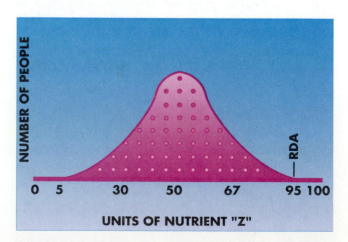

FIGURE 2-2 As this bell-shaped curve shows, the nutrient needs of a given population vary significantly. The RDA is set at a high but safe level.

who are eating a varied diet that includes ample amounts of whole (unrefined) foods, and they reflect the expected average intake of a given nutrient over a 3-day or longer time span. There are different RDA for each mineral and vitamin.

Dietary Goals

In response to the high incidence of diseases that are believed to be related to the high fat and cholesterol in the American diet, a Senate Select Committee developed *Dietary Goals for the United States* (Box 2-2).

The *Dietary Goals* are designed to show people how to moderate their fat and sugar intake. The distribution of kcalories in the average American diet currently is about 40% or more from fat, 12% to 16% from protein, 22% from complex carbohydrates (starches), and 24% from sugar. The *Dietary Goals* recommend that Americans consume no more than 30% of their total kcalories in the form of fat. Ideally these fat kcalories should be equally distributed among saturated, monounsaturated, and polyunsaturated sources of fat.[13]

NIH Recommendations for Fiber Intake

Prompted by mounting evidence that consuming greater amounts of insoluble as well as soluble fiber can reduce the incidence of colon cancer and decrease blood cholesterol levels, the **National Institutes of Health** (NIH) issued recommendations for fiber intake.[11] Americans currently consume an average of 13 g of fiber per day. While acknowledging that individuals require varying amounts of fiber to maintain good gastrointestinal function, most experts agree that Americans should strive to consume between 20 and 35 g of fiber each day from a variety of fruits, vegetables, and grains. Any program to increase dietary fiber intake should be undertaken gradually to prevent intestinal problems (see Chapter 4, Carbohydrates, for specific advice on dietary fiber).

What is the major difference between food intake and nutrient intake standards? Do they both provide the same basic information?

IN TODAY'S WORLD

Food safety became a public health concern in the United States as the economy shifted from agricultural to industrial. People moved from the farms, where they had known the entire history of their food, to cities, where they depended on marketed supplies for their food. **Why did people who grew their own food have fewer worries about food safety?** When people grew and gathered their own food, their primary defenses against food poisoning were knowing how to judge a food's freshness and being familiar with food preservation techniques such as salting, smoking, curing, fermenting, and drying. Today the first line of defense against consumption of harmful substances is a combination of knowledgeable consumerism and government regulations.

Food Safety Regulation[1]

Before the 1900s no federal regulations existed to set standards of food quality, quantity, or safety. Only two states had made an effort to regulate the growing food industry. In 1784 Massachusetts passed the first food law. Sixty-six years elapsed before California passed a pure food and drink law in 1850, soon after it became a state. In this legal vacuum the opportunist made his dollar! Dairies were filthy; meat packers chopped up anything that moved (including rats and finger pieces); dealers watered milk and adulterated coffee, cocoa, butter, and honey with extenders that might or might not be safe. Profits were high in this thriving and unregulated market.

In 1906, more than the San Francisco earthquake shook people up. That same year *The Jungle*, a serialized romance by Upton Sinclair, so clearly presented the horrible conditions in the Chicago meat packing plants that Congress passed the first national food laws, the Meat Inspection Act and the Food and Drug

---

BOX 2-2   Dietary Goals for the United States

1. To **avoid becoming overweight,** consume only as much energy (kcalories) as you expend. If overweight, decrease energy intake and increase energy expenditure.
2. **Increase consumption of complex carbohydrates** and "naturally occurring" sugars from about 28% to about 48% of energy intake.
3. **Reduce consumption of refined and processed sugars** by about 45% so they account for no more than 10% of total energy intake.
4. **Reduce overall fat consumption** from approximately 40% to about 30% of energy intake.
5. **Reduce saturated fat consumption** to about 10% of total energy intake, and balance that with polyunsaturated and monounsaturated fats, which should account for about 10% of energy intake each.
6. **Reduce cholesterol consumption** to about 300 mg a day.
7. **Limit sodium intake** by using no more than 5 grams (g) of salt a day.

From Senate Select Committee on Diet and Health, 1977.

Act. These regulations were followed by legislation requiring quantity information on packages. In 1927 the Food and Drug Administration was formed and charged with ensuring food quality and safety as well as verifying the validity of advertising claims.[5]

Seventy-two percent of shoppers believe food safety is a very important purchasing criterion; 82% have confidence in the safety of the U.S. food supply.[8]

Food Additives

In 1938 the Food, Drug and Cosmetic Act established exemptions and safe tolerances for substances that, while not desirable in food, were either necessary or unavoidable during production. This act also established the practice of food labeling. It required that food packages bear labels giving the manufacturer's name and address, the net weight of the contents, and ingredients (in order of descending quantity). Later amendments refined this act. Together the 1958 Food Additives Amendment and the 1960 Color Additives Amendment established two categories of food additives (intentional and incidental) and required food manufacturers to demonstrate the safety of any *new* intentional additive before it could be used in food production.[5]

Intentional additives are those that are purposefully added to a food. Box 2-3 lists examples of major categories of intentional additives. They are used to maintain or increase a food's nutritional value, enhance appearance or flavor, aid in processing, or act as a preservative. More than 2800 of these substances are currently approved by the FDA for use in foods.

In 1958 all intentional additives deemed safe for use in the United States were placed on the government's Generally Recognized As Safe (GRAS) list. Most of these additives never had been formally safety tested but continued to be used because of their long history in food production. All additives now in use have since been tested for safety. The Delaney Clause of the 1958 Food Additives Amendment states: "No additive shall be deemed safe if it is found to produce cancer when ingested by man or animals." Unfortunately, application of this provision has been somewhat uneven. Sodium cyclamate, a sweetener chemically similar to a bacterial mutagen, was banned, whereas saccharin, although shown to cause kidney cancer in male mice, was retained because of public outcry and because there was no evidence of damage to humans at the level consumed.

Incidental additives are substances such as packing material that sometimes unavoidably make their way into foods. More than 10,000 incidental additives have been identified in the food supply. Because they serve no useful purpose, they can be thought of as

BOX 2-3   **Intentional Additives**

NUTRIENTS

Iodide in some salt	Vitamins A and D

PROCESSING AIDS

Anticaking agents	Conditioners
Dough strengtheners	Drying agents
Emulsifiers	Enzymes
Firming agents	Flour treatments
Formulation aids	Leavening agents
Lubricants	Propellants
Solvents	Stabilizers
Surface agents	Surface finishing
Synergists	Texturizers
Thickening agents	

PRESERVATIVES

Antimicrobials	Antioxidants
Curing and pickling agents	Fumigants
Humectants	Sequesterants
Oxidizing and reducing agents	

APPEARANCE AND FLAVOR ENHANCERS

Color	Flavor enhancers
Flavoring agents	Nonnutritive sweeteners
Nutritive sweeteners	

contaminants. They enter foods during the production and preparation processes and through environmental contamination. Box 2-4 gives examples of incidental additives.

Which is the greater threat to your health: intentional additives or incidental additives? Why?

Like intentional additives, most incidental additives are regulated and must be closely monitored by food packaging companies. Incidental additives are allowed to enter the food supply so long as they can be proved to be harmless. Consumers report that food additives and chemical contaminants such as pesticide residues are their greatest food safety-related health concerns. In reality, microbial contamination (bacteria, molds, fungi, and viruses) is a much greater health threat. Over 90% of all food-related illnesses are the result of microbial contamination, most of it from bacteria. Food poisoning is so common that many physicians now believe that stomach flu is actually food poisoning. The reported incidence of food poisoning in the United States has risen over the last 2 decades. One reason is our in-

BOX 2-4   Incidental Additives

PRODUCTION CONTAMINANTS

Packaging materials (metal, plastic, paper)
Animal parts (for example, hairs, rodent and insect feces, bugs, worms, etc.)
Chemical toxins (for example, in moldy peanuts and poisonous mushrooms)

STORAGE AND PREPARATION CONTAMINANTS

Bacteria that thrive in foods (for example, salmonella, *Clostridium perfringens*, streptococcus, shigella, and listeria)
Bacterial toxins (such as those produced by staphylococcus and *Clostridium botulinum* that survive freezing and cooking)
Viral contamination (for example, infectious hepatitis from a human carrier or from shellfish harvested from polluted waters)
Parasites (like giardia from clear mountain streams, amoebic dysentery from contaminated food and water, trichinosis, and tapeworms)

ENVIRONMENTAL CONTAMINANTS

Chemical toxins (including algae "red tides," which contaminate shellfish, and heavy metals, such as lead and mercury)
Radiation (radioactive iodine contaminated the food supply of Europe after the Chernobyl disaster)

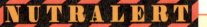

NUTRALERT

FOOD POISONING

About a third of all cases of food poisoning result from improper handling of food in the home.

creasing reliance on foods prepared outside the home. Additionally, scientists have broadened their understanding of the microbes and symptoms associated with food poisoning, so more cases are being identified and reported. Finally, some strains of bacteria, most notably salmonella, which is a problem in poultry products, appear to have become more virulent.

How does food poisoning affect my digestive tract?

Federal and state laws as well as safe food selection and preparation techniques are the consumer's first line of defense against food poisoning. The second line of defense against harmful substances entering the delicate cellular environment is the intestine, which is the transition zone between the body's internal and external environments. Intestinal defense mechanisms in-

clude vomiting and diarrhea, both of which encourage a swift exit of the noxious intruder. The third line of defense is the ability of the liver to detoxify and the kidneys to eliminate some toxins. (See Appendix E for details on the route of transmission and symptoms of the most common causes of food poisoning.)

NUTRALERT

BOTULISM

Botulism can literally "take your breath away." Whereas food poisoning is typically characterized by intestinal symptoms such as cramping, vomiting, and diarrhea, botulism toxin paralyzes the respiratory system. Survival depends on immediate medical attention.

Food Labels

How can I tell if the foods I buy are nutritious?

Food labels, both on products themselves and at the point of purchase, are the best way for you as a consumer to see if the foods you favor meet your nutritional needs. The food label is the place where food and nutrient intake standards merge. Next to advertising, food labels are the major way that consumers learn about a particular product.

In 1966 Congress passed the Fair Package Labeling Act and charged the Food and Drug Administration with its implementation. The law required that manufacturers provide clear information regarding package content. No terms like "Economy" or "Giant" could be used unless the precise weight or volume of the package contents was specified. This law also established the use of the U.S. RDA as a standard for providing nutrition information on food labels. Although this law provided consumers with useful information, it had a significant limitation: not all foods required a nutrition label. Nutrition content information was required on a label only if a nutritional claim was made (such as "low calorie") or if any nutrients were added ("enriched," "fortified"). The law did not apply to foods such as milk, eggs, meat, and poultry, which fell under USDA jurisdiction, or to fresh fish and raw produce, because they are sold in bulk form. Further, the law was somewhat liberal with respect to the kinds of information that could be printed on a label. Compounding these problems was the fact that the FDA was fairly lax about enforcing the labeling laws. As a result, food labels abounded with misleading health claims and nutrition information. Before 1994 the labels of all packaged foods had to list their ingredients. But only foods that contained an added nutrient (for example, enriched wheat flour, vitamin-fortified milk and cereals) or whose label made specific nutritional claims were required to carry nutritional analysis information. For all other foods, displaying such information was optional. You can easily see why frustrated consumers and health care lobbyists finally forced the government to implement significant changes in the labeling laws.

If you are among the 64% of Americans who routinely read food labels, you've undoubtedly noticed that they have a new look. Perhaps you've wondered where all this extra information came from and what it's doing on the label. The new label look is the result of the 1990 Nutrition Labeling and Education Act (NLEA). Beginning in mid-1994, this law requires that all packaged foods, except *fresh* meat, fish, poultry, milk, eggs, and produce, carry specific nutrition information on their labels.[1,5,6,17] Box 2-5 lists exceptions and exemptions to the NLEA.

How is the NLEA different from the previous laws?

As before, the ingredients in all packaged foods must be listed on the label in declining order of their proportion of the whole. A significant new feature of the law is that, with the exceptions noted above for fresh foods, labels on all packaged foods must provide nutritional analysis information. The key differences introduced by the Nutrition Labeling and Education Act are:

- Packaged foods must carry detailed nutrient content information on their labels.
- Health claims (such as "fiber reduces the risk of colon cancer") can be made only if they can be backed up by legitimate scientific research.

- Only 11 categories of nutrient claims (free, low, lean, extra lean, high, good source, reduced, less, light fewer, and more) that result in a variety of strictly defined terms, such as "lite," "low-sodium," and "fat-free" are allowed to describe the nutritional attributes of a food. (See Box 2-6.)
- Serving sizes are standardized so that manufacturers can no longer choose one that makes their product look good.
- For the first time, packages of vitamins, minerals, and other dietary supplements must comply with the current labeling laws. This means that only health claims sanctioned by the FDA can appear on the label and only the approved descriptive terms can be used to explain the supplement's nutrient content.[4]
- Likewise, restaurant menus[19] and food advertisements[20] that contain claims about the health-giving properties or nutrient content of certain foods must comply with the labeling laws regarding health claims and descriptive terms.

Why were certain fresh products exempted from the new labeling laws?

Fresh fish, meat, poultry, and produce are regulated by the Food and Drug Administration, but they do not require individual labels. Labeling would add greatly to the cost of these products, because many of them are sold in bulk form. To address this concern, the FDA has stated that grocery stores should voluntarily provide nutrition information at point of purchase for the 20 most commonly purchased fish and produce items and the 45 most of-

---

BOX 2-5   NLEA Exceptions and Exemptions

Special provisions were needed to deal with food labeling complications that arose for some products.

EXCEPTIONS

- Food packages with less than 12 square inches of space for labeling do not need to carry nutrition information, but they must provide the manufacturer's phone number and address so that interested consumers can obtain this information.
- Food packages with less than 40 square inches of labeling space may use an abbreviated version of the Nutrition Facts label format.
- Dairy milk and products made from it must provide the Nutrition Facts information required on other packaged foods. Milk and milk products may continue to use the terms "low-fat," "1% milk fat," and "2% milk fat" even though the dairy industry's definition of these terms is different from that specified under the NLEA. This decision was made to prevent confusion for consumers who have long been accustomed to purchasing these products.

EXEMPTIONS

The following foods are exempt from nutrition labeling requirements, but they may carry nutrition information so long as it meets the criteria specified by the NLEA.

- Foods produced by small businesses (defined by the FDA as an establishment with less than $50,000 of food sales each year).
- Foods served by restaurants, delis, cafeterias, airlines, and food service vendors like mall cookie and candy shops, bakeries, and vending machines, unless a nutritional claim is made for the product.
- Plain coffee and tea, food colorings, flavoring agents, and many spices, so long as these products do not contribute significant amounts of any nutrients.
- Medical foods (special diets obtained from a pharmacy by prescription)
- Alcohol

Additional categories of exemptions exist, but they apply to manufacturers, wholesalers, and retailers rather than to consumers.

ten purchased cuts of meat and poultry items. So look in the butcher and produce departments for permanent plaques or brochures carrying labeling information. You will find more detailed labeling information in the appropriate nutrient chapters.

What does the label term "Percent Daily Value" mean?

Percent Daily Value (% DV) information is intended to show consumers how much of a day's ideal intake of a particular nutrient they are eating (Fig. 2-3). It is similar in concept to the U.S. RDA that appeared on earlier food labels.

Does the Percent Daily Value apply to everyone?

Percent Daily Value (**% DV**) replaced the U.S. RDA in 1992. This new standard is actually composed of two sets of dietary standards: the Daily Reference Values (**DRV**) and the Reference Daily Intake (**RDI**). The DRV, which is based on a 2000 kcalorie a day diet, indicates what percentages of the daily intake of total fat, saturated fat, cholesterol, sodium, total carbohydrate, protein, and fiber are supplied by one serving of the food in question. This means that the macaroni and cheese dinner shown in Fig. 2-3 would supply higher percentages of fat, cholesterol, sodium, and carbohydrate than indicated for the many women who require only about 1600 kcalories per day. Conversely, it would supply lower percentages of these nutrients for people like active men and teen boys, who routinely consume more than 2000 kcalories per day. For the time being, the RDI data are really just the U.S. RDA renamed and limited to four nutrients: vitamins A and C and the minerals calcium and iron. The B-complex vitamins were dropped from the list to make room for information on carbohydrate, total fat, saturated fat, cholesterol, fiber, and sodium. Percent Daily Value data must, however, be supplied for any vitamins or minerals *added* to a product by enrichment or fortification.

If it is so general, how does the % DV apply to me?

The % DV can help you determine whether a food is a good or poor source of a particular nutrient. It is also useful when comparing different brands of similar products. A cereal whose label states it contains 50% of the DV for folate is sure to supply 50% *or more* of your folate requirement, because the % DV use the highest of adult RDA recommendations. If your need for folate is

---

BOX 2-6   FDA Definitions of Descriptive Terms

Following is a list of some common descriptive terms the FDA has defined and approved for use on food labels:

- **Free** can be used in reference to kcalories, sugar, sodium, salt, fat, saturated fat, and cholesterol: Less than 5 kcalories; fewer than 0.5 gram (g) of sugar; less than 5 milligrams (mg) of sodium; salt-free products must comply with definition of sodium free; 2 g or less of saturated fat per serving; less than 2 mg of cholesterol.

- **Unsalted, No salt added,** or **Without added salt** can all be used to describe products to which no salt is added during processing. This does not mean the product is free of sodium, since it may contain ingredients like milk that are natural sources of sodium.

- **No Sugar Added** or **No Added Sugar,** or **Without Added Sugar** means no sugar was added during processing; however, naturally occurring sugars may be present.

- **Low** can be used to describe kcalories, sodium, total fat, saturated fat, and cholesterol: Less than 40 kcalories; less than 140 mg of sodium; 3 g of fat or less per serving. 1 g or less of saturated fat; 20 mg or less of cholesterol (products low in cholesterol also must have 2 g or less of saturated fat).

- **High** or **Rich In** or **Excellent Source of:** Benefits the consumer by providing 20% or more of the amount recommended for daily consumption, as in "high fiber."

- **Source of** or **Good Source of:** Beneficial because it provides 10% to 19% of the nutrient's RDA.

- **Reduced** or **Less:** Both mean that the product contains at least 25% less sodium, fat, saturated fat, or cholesterol than the original product.

- **Lean:** A 100-g (roughly 3.5 oz) serving of meat, fish, or poultry that contains less than 10 g of total fat; less than 4 g of saturated fat, and less than 95 mg of cholesterol.

- **Extra Lean:** A 100-g (roughly 3.5 oz) serving of meat, fish, or poultry that contains less than 5 g of total fat, less than 2 g of saturated fat, and less than 95 mg of cholesterol.

- **Light** or **Lite:** If a product has more than 50% of its kcalories from fat, light means that there has been at least a 50% reduction in fat. If it has less than 50% of its kcalories from fat, the product can be described as light if it is either 50% reduced in fat or has a third less kcalories. A product can be light in sodium if the sodium content of the original product has been reduced by 50%.

- **More** or **Added** or **Enriched** or **Fortified:** The product contains at least 10% more of the DV than the comparison food.

Although not mandated by the 1990 NLEA, the FDA also has issued regulations regarding the use of the following terms:

- **Percent Fat Free:** The product must be "low fat" or "fat free," and its fat content must be expressed per 100 g (about 3.5 oz) of food. For example, 2.5 g of fat/100 g of food would be "95% fat free."

- **Healthy:** The product must be low in fat and saturated fat and must contain no more than 480 mg of sodium or 60 mg of cholesterol per serving.

- **Fresh:** Can only be used on products that have not been preserved, canned, frozen, or otherwise treated to extend their shelf life. The term "fresh frozen" is allowed.

From *Food Safety Notebook Labeling Update,* Dec 1992.

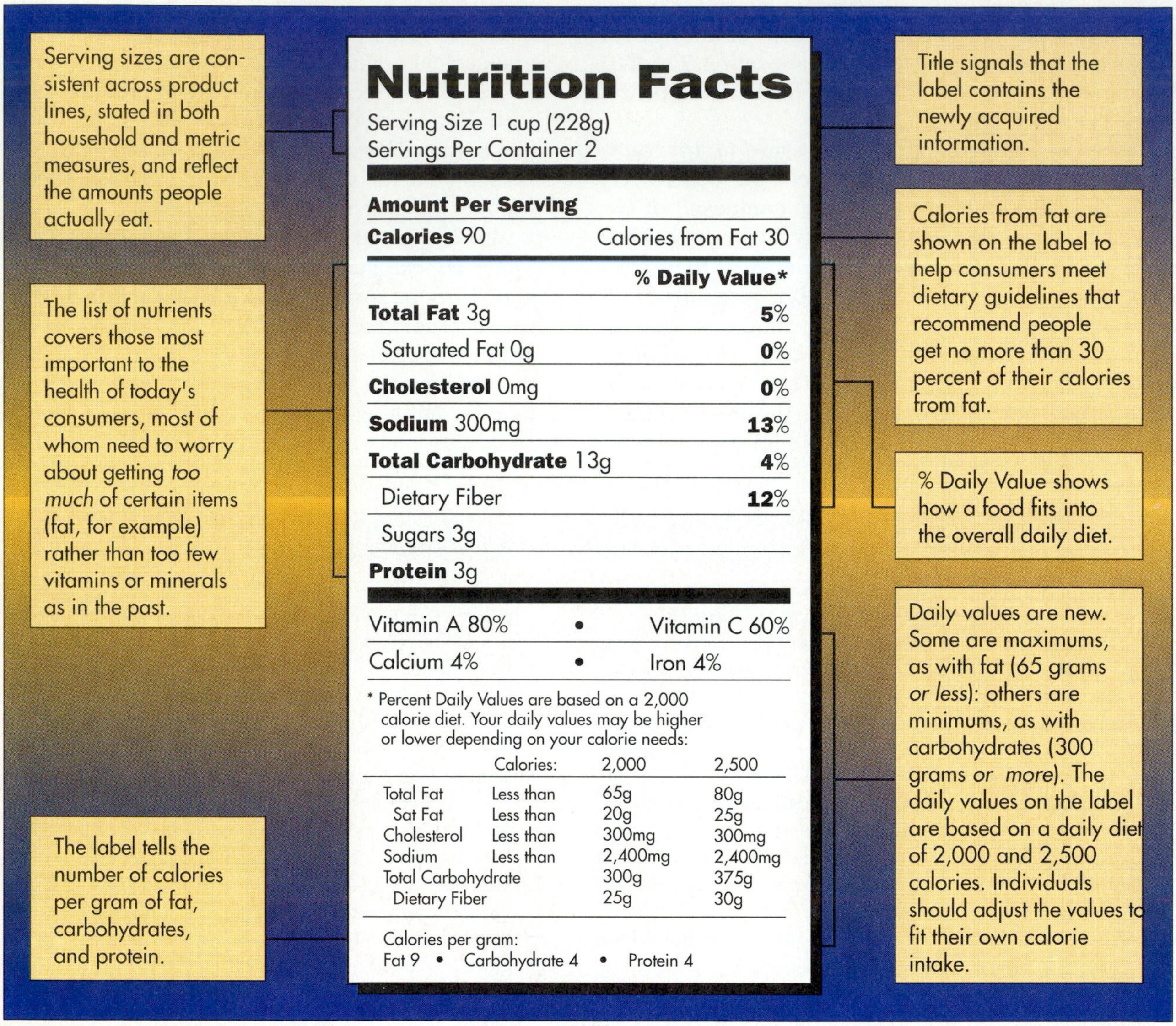

Serving sizes are consistent across product lines, stated in both household and metric measures, and reflect the amounts people actually eat.

The list of nutrients covers those most important to the health of today's consumers, most of whom need to worry about getting *too much* of certain items (fat, for example) rather than too few vitamins or minerals as in the past.

The label tells the number of calories per gram of fat, carbohydrates, and protein.

Nutrition Facts

Serving Size 1 cup (228g)
Servings Per Container 2

Amount Per Serving	
Calories 90	Calories from Fat 30

	% Daily Value*
Total Fat 3g	**5**%
Saturated Fat 0g	**0**%
Cholesterol 0mg	**0**%
Sodium 300mg	**13**%
Total Carbohydrate 13g	**4**%
Dietary Fiber	**12**%
Sugars 3g	
Protein 3g	

Vitamin A 80%	•	Vitamin C 60%
Calcium 4%	•	Iron 4%

* Percent Daily Values are based on a 2,000 calorie diet. Your daily values may be higher or lower depending on your calorie needs:

		Calories:	2,000	2,500
Total Fat	Less than		65g	80g
Sat Fat	Less than		20g	25g
Cholesterol	Less than		300mg	300mg
Sodium	Less than		2,400mg	2,400mg
Total Carbohydrate			300g	375g
Dietary Fiber			25g	30g

Calories per gram:
Fat 9 • Carbohydrate 4 • Protein 4

Title signals that the label contains the newly acquired information.

Calories from fat are shown on the label to help consumers meet dietary guidelines that recommend people get no more than 30 percent of their calories from fat.

% Daily Value shows how a food fits into the overall daily diet.

Daily values are new. Some are maximums, as with fat (65 grams *or less*): others are minimums, as with carbohydrates (300 grams *or more*). The daily values on the label are based on a daily diet of 2,000 and 2,500 calories. Individuals should adjust the values to fit their own calorie intake.

FIGURE 2-3 This nutrition label became the standard in mid-1994. % Daily Values replace U.S. RDAs as a standard for comparing nutrient intake from the product to generally agreed-on dietary standards. Other features make the label more consumer oriented.

different from the RDA, you can almost guarantee that it is lower. The same holds true for the other vitamins and minerals covered by the % DV.

The % DV for total fat, saturated fat, cholesterol, total carbohydrate, and fiber, however, are determined by how closely they match the recommended intake of these nutrients for a person consuming a 2000-kcalorie diet. This means you need to use caution interpreting the % DV data for these nutrients. You can personalize the % DV information by following the steps in Box 2-7. Specific information on how to interpret labeling information for each major nutrient class is given in the appropriate chapters.

What is the purpose of all of this information?

Beginning in May 1994 the labels on all packaged foods, with the exceptions noted earlier, must disclose how much total fat, saturated fat, cholesterol, sugar, fiber, and sodium they contain. This information is deemed vital for consumers who are trying to limit their risk of heart disease and certain cancers. It also may help people control their weight.

BOX 2-7   Personalizing the Food Label

STEP 1: FIND YOUR ACTIVITY LEVEL

Determine your current physical activity level.

Low Activity

You have a sit-down job or one that usually requires 4 hours or less of walking or standing each day. You do not participate in a regular exercise program. Recreational activities such as weekend golf or tennis, occasional jogging, swimming, or cycling do not count.

Moderate Activity

You participate in activities such as brisk walking, jogging, swimming, or cycling at least three times per week for 30 to 60 minutes each time.

High Activity

You exercise vigorously for 60 minutes or more at least 4 days per week.

STEP 2: FIND YOUR DAILY CALORIE LEVEL

Choose the correct chart for your gender. Find your age in the left column. Then use your activity level from Step 1 to find your approximate daily kcalorie needs.

Women

Age	Low Activity	Moderate Activity	High Activity
19-24	1800	2200	2600
24-50	1800	2200	2600
51+	1700	2000	2400

Men

Age	Low Activity	Moderate Activity	High Activity
19-24	2300	3000	3700
24-50	2300	3000	3800
51+	2000	2600	3200

Calorie levels derived from the *Recommended Dietary Allowances*, ed 10, National Research Council, 1989, pp. 29, 33.

STEP 3: FIND YOUR OWN NUTRIENT NEEDS

After finding your kcalorie level in Step 2, find that same level on the top of the chart below. Then read down the column to determine your own nutrient needs. If your daily kcalorie level is not listed, use the nutrient needs for the next lower kcalorie level.

Nutrient Needs for Different kcalorie Levels

Food Component	kcal 1600	2000	2200
Total Fat (g)	53	65	73
Saturated Fat (g)	18	20	24
Total Carbohydrate (g)	240	300	330
Dietary Fiber (g)	20	25	25
Protein (g)	46	50	55
Total % Daily Value for each of these nutrients can add up to:	80%	100%	110%

Food Component	kcal 2500	2800	3200
Total Fat (g)	80	93	107
Saturated Fat (g)	25	31	36
Total Carbohydrate (g)	375	420	480
Dietary Fiber (g)	30	32	37
Protein (g)	65	70	80
Total % Daily Value for each of these nutrients can add up to:	125%	140%	160%

My daily kcalorie level is: _____ kcal

My personal nutrient needs are:

Total fat	_____ grams or less
Saturated fat	_____ grams or less
Total carbohydrate	_____ grams or more
Dietary fiber	_____ grams or more
Protein	_____ grams

My total % Daily Value for *each* nutrient in all the foods I eat in one day can add up to:

_____ % Daily Value

You can use this information to make a card, like the one above, that you can refer to when you grocery shop. A more complicated but more accurate method for calculating your kcalorie requirement can be found in Chapter 10, Exercise.

IN MY DIET

One way to control the quality of the food you eat is to buy whole foods and prepare them at home. This means canning your own fruits and vegetables, grinding your own hamburger, and baking your own bread! A lucky few have the time and inclination to do so. Most of us must rely on knowledgeable consumerism and careful food handling techniques.[14]

Shoppers ranked nutrition second only to taste as the most important factor influencing food choices.[3]

At the Grocery Store

- If you have a lot of errands to run, remember to make the grocery store your last stop.
- Check all packages for evidence of damage, and read expiration dates. Don't buy products that are old or damaged.
- Select fresh, firm produce.
- Purchase nonperishable items first, followed by produce, dairy products, eggs, meats, and frozen foods.
- Make sure refrigerated and frozen foods are appropriately cold when you purchase them.
- Fish are very perishable. Avoid fish that have developed a "fishy" smell. If possible, purchase whole fish and be sure their scales are shiny and their eyes look clear.
- Meat, fish, and poultry are often contaminated with bacteria that live in the animal's digestive tract. Put these items into the plastic bags provided. Don't let their juices drip on other groceries!

What is the best way to store foods?

- Take groceries directly home. Store them promptly and appropriately in the reverse order in which they were purchased, that is, frozen goods first, shelf-stable ones last.
- If you have any produce that you are not going to be using within the next couple of days, store it in the refrigerator *unwashed.*
- Check the temperatures in your storage areas. Freezer *less than* 32° F, refrigerator *less than* 42° F. Make sure that dry goods storage areas *stay dry* and don't get excessively hot or cold.
- Rotate any shelf-stable items you purchased as you store them. Write the purchase date on the package and place newly purchased dry goods at the back of your food cabinets while moving older items to the front. Make a point of using dry goods within 6 months of purchase.
- Some shelf-stable items such as salad dressings must be refrigerated once they are open. Be sure to read and follow package directions in this regard.
- Make sure all stored items are well wrapped or sealed and keep foods properly stored (cold or sealed) until you are ready to use them. Defrost frozen foods in the microwave or refrigerator.[14]

In the Kitchen

Cleanliness, including hand washing, is extremely important in all types of food handling. Nothing is as unpleasant as seeing food handlers cough or sneeze on a meal or observing pets walking on kitchen counters and licking utensils used in food preparation. So keep your food preparation surfaces clean. Wash your hands and under your nails before handling food. And keep them out of your mouth while cooking.

- Don't taste a food with the spoon you are using to prepare it. Use a separate spoon and wash it between each sample.

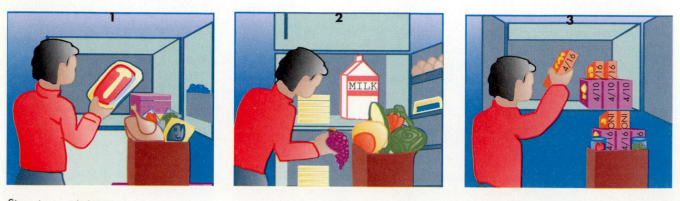

Steps to smart storage.

- Be extremely careful when handling raw animal products like meat, fish, poultry, and eggs; they are significant sources of bacterial contamination. (See the "In the Kitchen" of Chapter 6, Protein, for specifics on the best way to prepare these foods.)
- Use only containers intended for cooking and serving.
- Store leftover food in appropriate storage containers and refrigerate or freeze it immediately.
- Plastic storage containers that are intended for foods at room temperature may not be suitable for hot food storage because the plastic may break down and contaminate the food. Problems can arise even when using a container at the appropriate temperature. For example, bread wrappers turned inside out and used for storage may transmit harmful organisms picked up during production, shipping, and purchasing.
- Never leave foods sitting out for more than 2 hours. When you want to leave food out, keep hot foods hot: 140°F or hotter! And cold foods cold: 42°F or cooler.[7,14,18]

At the Table

Although for some of us it is acceptable to have a bite of a friend or relative's food, very few of us would choose to eat off a stranger's plate. To minimize the spread of germs, serving utensils should never touch an individual's food or plate. An individual diner's personal utensils should never be used as serving implements.

Eating Out

- Select restaurants with clean interiors.
- Make sure sneeze guards are in place on salad bars and in other areas where food is set out.
- Make sure that perishable items on the salad bar are sitting in ice.
- Washing hands at a restaurant is a good idea: just remember that the hand that turns on the faucet turns it off. Unless the sink is supplied with foot or knee controls, use a paper towel to turn off the faucet and to open the bathroom door as you exit.

TEST YOURSELF

Multiple Choice: Choose the one best answer

1. Which of the following statements best describes our relationship to food?
   a. Cells eat food, people eat nutrients.
   b. People eat food, cells eat nutrients.
   c. People eat food, cells, and nutrients.
2. According to the Food Guide Pyramid, how many servings of fruits and vegetables should people eat each day?
   a. Exactly five
   b. Five or more
   c. Five or less
   d. No more than 11
3. What percent of your total calorie intake should come from fat, according to the Dietary Goals for Americans?
   a. 30% or less
   b. 10 %
   c. 20% or less
   d. 40% or less
4. If you are running a lot of other errands, when should you do your grocery shopping?
   a. First
   b. Last
   c. It doesn't matter when
5. NLEA stands for:
   a. Nutrition Labeling Education Amendment
   b. Nutrient Loss Enrichment Act
   c. Nutrition Labeling and Education Act
6. NLEA made the food labeling laws
   a. Stricter
   b. More flexible
   c. About the same

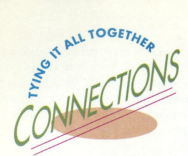

TYING IT ALL TOGETHER

CONNECTIONS

1. Plan one day's worth of meals for yourself that meet the recommendations of the Food Guide Pyramid for your activity level and gender.

2. Make a record of the foods you eat for 3 days and compare them to the Pyramid recommendations.

3. Identify two limitations of the Food Guide Pyramid.

4. List standards of food intake and standards of nutrient intake. What is the key difference between these two categories?

5. What would happen to the "average" person if s/he consumed only two thirds of the RDA for most nutrients?

6. Why is the phrase "Keep hot foods hot; keep cold foods cold" often used when training food service personnel?

7. What are the two categories of additives found in food? How do they differ?

8. What kinds of health claims are allowed on food labels, vitamin supplement packages, and restaurant menus?

References

1. Browne MB: *Label facts for healthful eating*, American Dietetic Association, ADA and National Food Processors Association in cooperation with USDA, 1993.

2. *Dietary guidelines for Americans*, U.S. Department of Health and Human Services Home and Garden Bulletin #232, 1990.

3. *Dietary guidelines for healthy American adults: A statement for physicians and health professionals*, American Heart Association, Dallas, 1991.

4. FDA press release, Dec 27, 1994.

5. Focus on food labeling: An FDA special report, *FDA Consumer*, 1993.

6. Food labeling update, *Food Safety Notebook* 3(12):110-115, 1992.

7. Food safety at home, patient information sheet, *Nutrition and the MD* 19(8):16, 1993.

8. For your information, *Journal of the American Dietetic Association* 1(2):1511, 1991.

9. Healthy people 2000: National health promotion and disease prevention objectives, U.S. Department of Health and Human Services, Public Health Service Bulletin #(PHS) 91-50212, 1990.

10. National Research Council *Recommended dietary allowances*, ed 10, Washington, DC, 1989, National Academy Press.

11. National Research Council Report on Diet and Health: *Implications for reducing chronic disease risk*, Washington, DC, 1989, National Academy Press.

12. Nixon DW: *Nutrition and cancer: American Cancer Society guidelines, programs, and initiatives*, Atlanta, 1990, American Cancer Society.

13. Senate Select Committee on Health, *The dietary goals for the United States*, ed 2, 1977.

14. Speurs MC, Vaden AG: *Quantity food sanitation in food service organizations: A managerial and systems approach*, New York, 1989, Macmillan.

15. Testing the Food Guide Pyramid, *Eating Well*, Jan 1993.

16. The Food Guide Pyramid, U.S. Department of Agriculture Home and Garden Bulletin #252, 1992.

17. The new food label, FDA Backgrounder, BG 92-4, 1992.

18. The safe food book: Your kitchen guide, U.S. Department of Agriculture Food Safety and Inspection Service Home & Garden Bulletin #241, 1985.

19. *University of California at Berkeley Wellness Letter*, p. 1, Jan 1994.

20. Food and Drug Administration Office of Food Label Technology, personal communication, June 13, 1994.

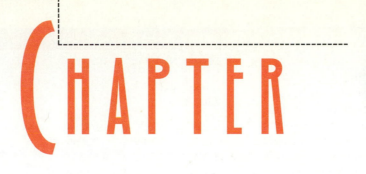

CHAPTER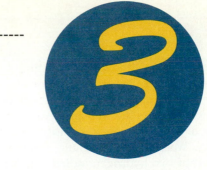

WATER
The Forgotten Nutrient

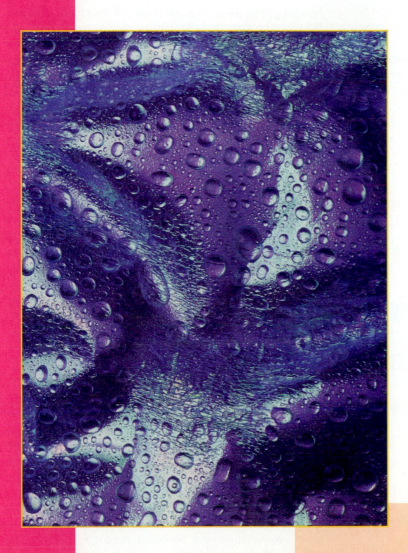

**Water,
taken in
moderation,
cannot
hurt
anyone.**
— Mark Twain

BLUE BEAUTY

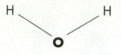 When people are asked to list the six major classes of nutrients, they often omit one of the most important nutrients: water. Water is the wellspring of life and is the nutrient needed in the greatest quantity and with the most frequency. Water is an inorganic, noncaloric nutrient composed of two hydrogen atoms bonded to one oxygen atom.

$$H \diagdown \qquad \diagup H$$
$$O$$

Seen from outer space, our planet Earth is distinctly blue because of the large bodies of water that cover its surface. The presence of water and its unique physical and chemical properties make life on Earth possible. Water has been central to every culture known on Earth. The Ganges River in India is a place where devout Hindus come to wash away their sins in the sacred water. The people of Egypt have long considered the Nile River holy. Since ancient times they have depended on its yearly floods to irrigate their fields and bring renewal of the land. The Tigris and Euphrates rivers in Iraq enclose the former garden spot of ancient civilization, the Fertile Crescent, where modern-day archaeologists have discovered the earliest records of agriculture and city life. Water has even influenced theories of creation. Whether you believe that life began by creation or by evolution, you will agree that life began in water.[10]

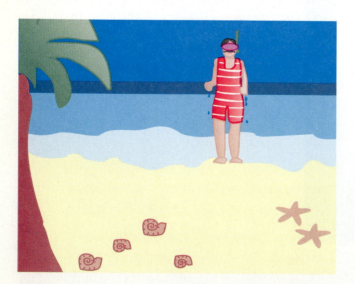

While a person can leave the water, the water never leaves a person.

TABLE 3–1	Preview
Dietary Nutrient:	**Water**
Building block	H_2O
Kcal content	0
Source	Beverages, foods
Intake standard	RDA, varies with age, temperature, activity, etc.
In the body	50% to 60% by weight; both mechanical and chemical
Deficiency	Dehydration
Excess	Electrolyte imbalance, water intoxication

Scientists have demonstrated that while the land masses and life forms left the sea, the sea never left them. Each new life begins as a single cell, bathed in a sea of life-sustaining fluid. Even after becoming a complex multicellular organism, every cell in a plant's or animal's body lives in a sea. In animals, rivers of blood flowing through the circulatory system replenish and cleanse this sea. In fact, water accounts for more than half (about 60%) of adult body mass. If you could remove all the moisture from a 75-kilogram adult (about 150 pounds), only 30 kilograms (about 60 pounds) of nonwater material would remain.

What purpose does water serve in the human body? A single cell floating in an ocean or pond has an endless supply of water with which to remove and dilute toxic waste. Multicellular organisms, on the other hand, must sacrifice some of their body water to excrete the cumulative waste produced by their numerous cells. Our kidneys accomplish this purification process for us by producing a minimum of 1 pint (2 cups) of urine per day. We must make this amount of urine, even in the absence of fluid intake, to keep from being poisoned by our own waste. As a result of this unavoidable fluid loss, adults in good general health can survive for 2 to 3 months without the nutrients contained in food, but can live only 3 to 4 days without water! Fatal deficiencies of water can occur rapidly in the absence of adequate replacement. Consequently, water is the nutrient that is most important to life.[11,12]

Since the advent of indoor plumbing some 100 years ago, Americans have been blithely turning on the tap, assuming that a clear, plentiful, and reasonable-tasting supply of water will be available. During the same period there has also been a massive increase in the production of beverages that are replacing water as the number one *thirst* quencher.

Fortunately, consumers are becoming aware of the value of water. The impact of technological advances on environmental and personal ecology is front-page news.[12] People are beginning to question how their lifestyles affect the availability and safety of the water supply. Researchers are investigating the health conse-

A CLOSER LOOK

Water Wisdom For All Seasons

You probably know you need to drink lots of cool water in hot and humid weather. According to the American Dietetic Association, however, keeping well hydrated isn't just a summertime thing; it's essential throughout the year, particularly in winter. When the furnace goes on, the air dries out, causing you to lose moisture through evaporation. Even if you don't feel thirsty, you need to replace that water. If you're coming in from the cold, drink warm beverages with water as the main ingredient.

Air travel also can upset your water balance. The dry, re-circulated air on the plane and the high altitude increase water loss through evaporation. The ADA advises you to drink one 8-ounce glass of water or juice for each hour of your flight; bring bottled water with you; and shun alcohol, caffeinated coffee, and tea, all of which increase your body's loss of water and may aggravate jet lag.

Data from the American Dietetic Association: *Water: the beverage for life,* Chicago, 1994, The Association.

---

quences of consuming endless soft drinks, punch, and coffee.[8,9,13] Many of us may need to revise both our personal and public water use policies.

IN THE DIET

How can I meet my daily water needs? Water relieves thirst, lubricates foods for easier swallowing, dissolves flavoring compounds—thereby enhancing the taste of some foods—and also dilutes noxious substances we may accidentally ingest. Water used in cooking softens foods and facilitates blending of ingredients. The water in raw food items maintains *turgor,* helping to give foods like celery a satisfying crunch.

Both beverages and foods provide dietary water. All beverages, regardless of their other constituents, contain water as their primary ingredient. Likewise, most foods (except sugar and oil) contain water. Water is also added to foods such as rice, bread, and oatmeal during the cooking process. And, naturally, water is available as the classic beverage.

Food Intake Standards

Which beverages are most healthful? We obtain about one third of our water requirement from the foods we eat. The remainder we consume in beverages. However, some beverages remove more fluid than they provide![5,13,14] Therefore we should strive to meet most of our fluid requirement by drinking plain water.

Thirst Quenching: All Beverages Are Not Equal

Remember drinking juice or a soda to quench your thirst and still feeling thirsty? Or avoiding coffee, tea, or caffeine-containing soft drinks before getting into a car for a long ride? Beverages like juice and soft drinks add fluid to the body, but they also add *solutes* (sugar, salt, various chemicals) that must be diluted as they en-ter the bloodstream. The sugars in fruit juices, the salt in soups, and the sugar and salt in soft drinks increase the concentration of these solutes in your blood. Your body first responds by pulling fluid from the cells into the bloodstream to dilute the sugar and salt. You then lose the increased fluid in your bloodstream forever when you excrete it as urine. Secondarily, your body will respond to the increased solutes and decreased fluid content by once again triggering your thirst mechanism.

Caffeine and alcohol *dehydrate* the body by a slightly different mechanism. These chemicals affect the hormones that regulate your body's fluid balance, causing you to produce more urine. That cup of coffee in the morning may actually be dehydrating you rather than replenishing your body's fluid supply! So start your day off with a large glass of water. Adding a little lemon or other fruit juice to plain water will make it more palatable. If the weather is cold and ice water has no appeal, try warming the water before drinking it (pauper's tea). Many people do not drink water because they falsely believe that doing so leads to water retention. In fact, the opposite is true. Consuming too little water causes your body to retain water because it believes a fluid crisis exists. When your water intake is sufficient, your body will dispose of any excess as urine. If you suddenly increase your water intake you will temporarily increase the frequency with which you urinate. Your body will eventually adjust, causing you

---

dehydrate removing water from the body or a tissue

solute a substance dissolved in another substance

thirst conscious desire for water

turgor ridigity of form; structure (from Latin *turgere,* "to be swollen")

to excrete larger volumes of urine less frequently.

One of the best ways to visualize your need for water over other beverages is to think of it as laundering the inside of your body. Now imagine that you are about to remove the soap from some clothes you have just laundered. What would you want to rinse them with? How about cola? No? Why? Is the cola color a problem? Well, then, how about a transparent uncola? NO! Why? You say the sugar and other chemicals in the drink would leave a residue on your clothes? Oh, so you want to rinse your laundry in pure clean water. What, then, do you want to use to rinse the inside of your body?

 If you do not have at least one pale yellow urination during the day, you need to drink more water.[4]

Nutrient Intake Standards

Water is at once a food and a nutrient. In this respect it is unlike the other nutrients, such as carbohydrates, proteins, and fats, which are typically constituents of foods. *An animal's need for water depends on its age as well as its physical and metabolic environment.* This means that water requirements can vary widely within a given species and even, at various times, within an individual. At the very least, humans need a little over 1 quart of water each day just to replenish unavoidable losses in urine, feces, sweat, and expired air. Elevated body temperature, altered physiological conditions such as pregnancy, diabetes, and severe burns, and the foods and beverages people consume can significantly increase this need. Nutrient intake standards offer some guidelines for ensuring adequate water consumption, although no table can state the exact quantity of water needed.

RDA. 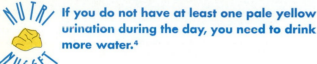 **How can I determine how much water is enough for me?** The authors of the Recommended Dietary Allowances (RDA) suggest that adults consume at least 1 milliliter (ml) of water for each kcalorie of energy they expend under normal conditions, or roughly 1 liter of water for every 1000 kcalories. They suggest that 1.5 ml per kcalorie may be a better goal to cover physiologic and environmental variations. Because few of us have accurately determined our kcalorie expenditure, this information is not very helpful.[8]

AMA. The American Medical Association Health Resolution for 1993 recommends that adults consume 6 to 8 glasses of *water* every day. Fruit juices and sodas just don't do it!

Sports trainers. A more useful estimate of water needs comes from researchers at the International Sports Training Center in Aspen, Colorado. This group recommends that inactive people consume 0.5 ounce of water per pound of body weight each day and that

physically active people increase daily intake to 0.67 ounce per pound. This equals eight to ten 8-ounce glasses of water daily for the average inactive woman or man. Active people should consume an additional couple of glasses each day. See Chapter 10, Exercise, for guidelines for water intake during exercise.

Age. **What factors influence the amount of water I need?** Elderly persons, infants, and children have special fluid requirements. Elderly people need to monitor water intake carefully to prevent dehydration because aging diminishes the sensation of thirst as well as the body's ability to conserve water. Infants and children, on the other hand, are at risk of dehydration for different reasons: (1) their bodies contain more water on a per-pound basis than do the bodies of adults; (2) the surface-to-volume ratio in children is larger than in adults, allowing for greater evaporation of fluid; and (3) they excrete more dilute urine and therefore more water than adults. Compounding these problems is the inability of very young children to communicate their sensation of thirst.[8,11,13]

Body Temperature. Because the body uses water as a coolant, any condition that increases body temperature, such as high environmental temperature, physical activity, or fever, simultaneously increases the need for water.

Metabolism. Natural physiological conditions, such as pregnancy and lactation, also increase the need for water. A pregnant woman needs extra water to maintain her increased maternal blood volume and to provide the amniotic fluid in which her fetus floats. Lactation demands increased fluid intake for the fluid in breast milk.

The chemicals contained in foods and drugs can alter the body's fluid needs. We are all familiar with the thirst-producing effects of salty foods. This occurs because the mineral sodium, which is part of salt, attracts water. Similarly, the body's water requirement is increased by the ingestion of many drugs, whether synthetic or natural (caffeine and alcohol) (see A Closer Look on p. 33).

NUTRI QUIZ
1. List three sources of body water.
2. List two mechanical functions of water.
3. List two types of chemical functions that use water.
4. What is the major excretory route of water?

IN BETWEEN: DIGESTION

Where is water digested? Water is not digested, but it is involved both mechanically and chemically in the entire process. It functions as a lubricant (ever try to swallow dry?), as a *solvent* in which the digestion of nutrients occurs, and as a *reactant* in chemical processes.

Absorption and transport. Water is freely absorbed, secreted, and reabsorbed in both the small and large intestines. Inability to resorb water due to infection, laxative abuse, or dietary protein deficiency results in loose, watery stools, called **diarrhea.** Once absorbed, water becomes part of both the blood *plasma* and the *lymph;* therefore water is the body's major transport system.

IN THE BODY

What sorts of things does my body do with water?

The 40 liters of water in an average human body perform many vital functions, which can be categorized as either mechanical or chemical in nature.

Mechanical Functions

Water plays many *mechanical* roles in the body *outside* of the cells.

Transport. The delivery of nutrients and products of metabolism to cells as well as the removal of metabolic waste is accomplished by the blood and lymph systems, which are composed mainly of water.

Temperature regulation. Water helps maintain a constant body temperature in two ways. Because water resists rapid changes in temperature, the body's high water content helps keep body temperature fairly stable. Water also helps cool the body. Moisture evaporating from the skin and respiratory tract cools the body by carrying off excess heat.

Cushioning. Water cushions delicate tissues in the body such as joints, the lens of the eye, the spinal cord, and a developing fetus.

Lubrication. Water moistens the mucous membranes in the joints and the gastrointestinal and respiratory tracts. Moist membranes facilitate movement as well as absorption of molecules, such as nutrients and oxygen, and the excretion of carbon dioxide.

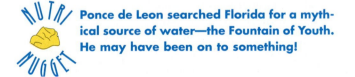

Ponce de Leon searched Florida for a mythical source of water—the Fountain of Youth. He may have been on to something!

Structure. Water is an important structural component of the body. It accounts for:
- 95% of a fertilized human egg
- 75% of a newborn infant's body
- 55% to 65% of an adult man's body
- 50% to 55% of an adult woman's body

The lower water content of women's as compared with men's bodies reflects their relatively smaller muscle mass. Similarly, water also makes up a smaller percentage of an obese person's body weight because of the presence of more water-free fat.

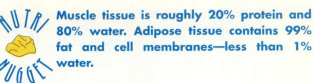

Muscle tissue is roughly 20% protein and 80% water. Adipose tissue contains 99% fat and cell membranes—less than 1% water.

Chemical Functions

Within cells, water participates in *chemical* reactions as both solvent and reactant. Many metabolic reactions cannot proceed without it. Acting as a solvent, water participates in vital metabolic processes like digestion and respiration, which can take place only in an aqueous medium. Other processes require water as part of the chemical reaction. For example, water is used as a reactant to separate the bonds between sugar molecules during digestion.

Balance—Intake and Output

Approximately two thirds of our daily water intake comes from beverages and the remaining one third from foods. A little bit of water is produced within the cells as a by-product of burning carbohydrate, protein, and fat for fuel. Average daily water loss varies greatly, depending on an individual's metabolic rate and activity level and the environmental temperature. The largest category of water loss (almost two thirds) is **urine,** excreted through the kidneys. Other routes of water loss are evaporation through the lungs and skin (about one third) and moisture in feces and sweat (may vary greatly).[11]

Maintaining Balance

Homeostasis, steady state, and *dynamic equilibrium* are alternate terms used by different scientific disciplines to describe balance. Maintaining water bal-

homeostasis (HOE-mee-o-STAY-sis) a state of physiological equilibrium produced by a balance of functions and of chemical composition within an organism (From Latin *homeo* "same"; *stasis* "state")

lymph transparent, slightly yellow opalescent liquid, about 95% water

metabolism (meh-TAB-uh-liz-um) chemical reactions that occur in the body, enabling cells to release energy from foods, convert one substance to another, and prepare end products for excretion

plasma the fluid portion of the blood in which blood cells are suspended

reactant a substance that enters into and is altered during a chemical reaction

solvent the liquid in which another substance (the solute) is dissolved to form a solution

urine a fluid that contains water, waste products, and excesses of some vitamins and minerals. It is produced and secreted by the kidneys, stored in the bladder, and voided by the urethra

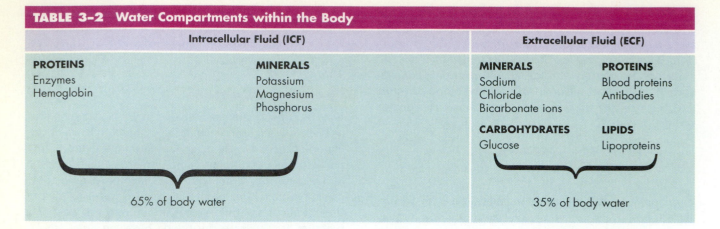

TABLE 3-2 Water Compartments within the Body

Intracellular Fluid (ICF)		Extracellular Fluid (ECF)	
PROTEINS Enzymes Hemoglobin	**MINERALS** Potassium Magnesium Phosphorus	**MINERALS** Sodium Chloride Bicarbonate ions **CARBOHYDRATES** Glucose	**PROTEINS** Blood proteins Antibodies **LIPIDS** Lipoproteins
65% of body water		35% of body water	

ance is extremely important because the body of an adult is approximately 60% water by weight.

How and where is water stored in the body?

Two separate water compartments exist in the body: the *intracellular fluid* and the *extracellular fluid* (Table 3-2). Intracellular fluid (ICF) accounts for about 65% of the body water and is where most of the metabolic work takes place. The remainder, extracellular fluid (ECF), is higher in salt content and transports nutrients and wastes throughout the body. It is found between the cells *(interstitial)* as blood plasma and lymph.

The body maintains the appropriate ratio and kind of fluid between the ICF and ECF compartments by "pumping iron"—well, actually by pumping minerals across the compartment membranes. A complex series of hormonal messages between the brain and the kidneys governs this movement of minerals. All minerals participate in the maintenance of fluid balance. Sodium, potassium, and chloride, collectively known as *electrolytes,* are the most intimately involved in this process. **Cations** are positively charged particles like sodium (Na^+); **anions** are negatively charged particles like chlorine (Cl^-).

Hormones such as antidiuretic hormone (ADH) and aldosterone affect fluid balance by regulating retention and excretion of water through the kidneys. Nutritional factors, such as mineral and protein intake, affect water balance indirectly and will be discussed in the chapters covering these nutrients. If minerals or other molecules become too concentrated in any one compart-

ment of the body, they will pull fluid from other compartments to dilute themselves. For example, when you eat pizza, you often find yourself feeling thirsty. The sodium from the table salt contained in the salty meats, sauces, and cheese accumulates in the ECF and pulls water from your cells. Sensors in the cells signal your brain of the danger of cellular dehydration, and you become thirsty. Whenever the minerals in one compartment become too concentrated, you will become thirsty and drink until they are appropriately diluted. If you drink more fluid than you need, the minerals will become too dilute. Your body will then signal the kidneys to make more urine by filtering the excess fluid out of the blood.

Why does water move between the two compartments?

Water passes across the membranes between the ICF and ECF compartments in response to changes in the mineral and protein composition of these two areas (Fig. 3-1). Minerals and proteins attract water. Sugar-rich molecules contained in a plant's root hairs attract ground water in much the same way. **Osmosis** is the process in which water flows across semipermeable membranes into an area of greater molecular density so that the concentration of molecules in solution on either side of the membrane becomes equal. (Semipermeable means some things pass through, others do not.) Osmotic pressure (the force that minerals, proteins, and other molecules exert on water) is powerful. If you have ever salted a snail, you have seen osmotic pressure in action. Remember watching the snail's body fluids fizz out to dilute the

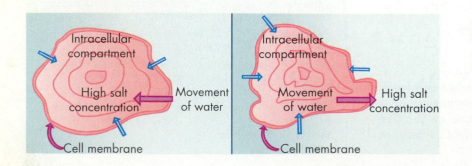

FIGURE 3-1 Water flows back and forth between the ICF and ECF compartments according to changes in mineral and protein concentration.

salt? Salt's ability to attract water is the reason it has been used to cleanse wounds and preserve meats: it kills bacteria by dehydrating them.

Thirst regulates water balance by affecting fluid intake. The primitive brain, the hypothalamus, is responsible for the basic drives, such as hunger and thirst, that help maintain life. Thirst can be triggered by decreased blood flow through the heart, excess blood glucose, some medications, or a decrease in either intracellular or extracellular water.

It is important to realize that thirst is not always a reliable signal of the need for water. Those who are very young or very old, participants in athletic competitions, and those who live in very hot, dry environments all need to drink water regularly whether or not they feel thirsty.

Imbalances: Edema

Typically the body maintains fluid homeostasis under a wide range of physical and environmental stresses. Severe illness and injuries, however, can lead to such extreme mineral loss that the normal control mechanisms are overwhelmed. Water then redistributes itself between the body compartments with disastrous results. (In Chapter 8, Minerals, we discuss this topic at greater length.) In **protein deficiency** the plasma protein content of blood plasma falls (the alpha, beta, gamma globulins, the *antibodies,* and the plasma *albumins*). Water from the blood plasma leaks out of the circulatory system and into the spaces between the cells (interstitial spaces). Sometimes the leakage is severe enough to cause a starving child to appear to develop a fat belly *(edema).* In reality, fluid, not fat, fills the interstitial spaces. This leak occurs because of the lack of proteins to promote water retention in the bloodstream.

Deficiencies

Dehydration, or excessive water loss, occurs in healthy people who are deprived of fluid or as a secondary effect of severe injury or illness, such as burns, fever, or gastrointestinal disease. Thirst is the first sign of dehydration. Clearly, then, each of us experiences mild dehydration on a daily basis. Additionally, most of us have experienced moderate dehydration in very warm weather, after physical exertion, or during a gastrointestinal illness. Usually we respond to our body's intensified thirst signals and rehydrate ourselves. Excessive physical exertion or prolonged gastrointestinal illness, however, can lead to severe dehydration. If not satisfied, thirst can progress rapidly to weakness, exhaustion, delirium, and death. Even if water balance is restored, people who have become significantly dehydrated may experience kidney damage because of the metabolic wastes that accumulated during their bout of dehydration.

Excesses

Water intoxication is a condition of excessive body water content. It usually results from metabolic disturbances that allow the body to accumulate too much water. In very rare instances, emotionally disturbed people have developed water intoxication by drinking such an incredible amount of water that it exceeds their body's capacity to excrete it. Whatever the cause, if left untreated, water intoxication can result in death.[11,13]

"Lose 20% of your body's water, and you're a goner. Yet the medicos say you could lose 80% of your intestines, one lung, one kidney, every organ in the pelvic area, your spleen, and 75% of your liver, and still survive."[2]

1. What is the major message of this quote?
2. What questions would you ask to evaluate the reliability of the quote?
3. How could you verify the truth of the statement?

IN TODAY'S WORLD

The 1990s had barely begun when they were proclaimed "The Earth Decade," reflecting growing concern regarding the impact of human technological advancement on ecology. The two major environmental issues regarding the water supply are pollution and conservation.

"You never miss the water till the well runs dry."

— *Rowland Howard*

Potable

A primary concern of people all over the world is to have a supply of water that is *potable.* The Earth's supply of water is limited. New water is *not* created; it is simply recycled through a continuous process of pre-

albumins (al-BUE-mins) a type of plasma protein

antibodies blood plasma proteins that provide immunity

edema (eh-DEE-mah) fluid in the interstitial spaces

electrolytes electrically charged particles

extracellular outside of the cell

interstitial (in-ter-STI-shuhl) between cells

intracellular within the cell

cipitation, percolation, and evaporation. Rain falling to the Earth carries with it minerals from the world's oceans. If you live where salt spray rusts the automobiles parked in the open, you already have seen the effects of airborne minerals. Rainwater is cleansed of these contaminants as it percolates through the layers of soil, eventually reaching subterranean rivers and lakes (aquifers) deep in the earth. This groundwater contains varying concentrations of naturally occurring minerals found in the area. Water is frequently described as being "soft" or "hard," based on its mineral content. Soft water has a low mineral content. It typically comes from sources deep in the ground and produces good soapsuds. Hard water, by contrast, comes from relatively shallow sources, is usually high in calcium and magnesium (though sulfur is present in some areas), reduces the sudsing action of soaps, and produces mineral deposits in pipes, tubs, and sinks and on clothes and dishware. Not surprisingly, soft water is preferable (from the consumer's perspective).

Pollution

In addition to the naturally occurring chemicals in water, some chemicals are by-products of human technological advances. Rainwater and irrigation leach pesticides, herbicides (weed killers), and fertilizers into the water supply. Water leaving the drains of urban homes empties into sewers that in turn transport it to community-operated purification plants. These plants treat used water to remove toxic waste before releasing it into major waterways or oceans. Likewise, manufacturing plants must treat waste water before returning it to the general supply. Overburdened municipal sewers and industrial water treatment facilities, however, add dangerous levels of potentially harmful microbes and/or chemicals to rivers and oceans. The legacy of human advancement is the declining populations of once abundant plant and animal species. This is becoming a major international concern as growing numbers of nations industrialize their economies with no impetus to respond to citizens' concerns for the quality of their environment.[12]

Safety

In rural areas many people still use well water, relying on the Earth's natural purification processes to keep it safe. Urban dwellers purchase water from municipal supplies and depend on technology to ensure its purity. Both populations may be living in a fool's paradise. As we have seen, the pollution accompanying human encroachment can overwhelm both natural and technological purification procedures, allowing harmful chemicals to remain in the water supply. You can take several courses of action to help ensure the safety of your water supply. If you use well water, have the water tested regularly to verify its continued purity. If

you use municipal water, contact your local water district for information about the chemical content of your water and the district's purification procedures. In either case, having tap water tested is a good way to make sure that impurities have not entered the water between the supply source and your kitchen faucet.

Public Health Issues

Chlorine. Municipal water systems use a variety of chemicals to improve the health properties of their water supply. The most common addition is a small amount of the mineral chlorine to kill microbes. Though it is harmless to humans in dilute concentrations, many people find the taste of chlorinated water unpleasant. If you are such a person, you can remove the chlorine from your water by boiling it or filling a large container with water and allowing it to stand uncovered overnight. In both cases the chlorine will evaporate, taking its characteristic flavor with it. See Chapter 8, Minerals, for a more complete discussion of the risks and benefits of chlorine.[3]

Fluoride. In some areas of the country, groundwater contains a natural supply of the mineral fluoride. In other areas fluoride is added to the water supply at the level of 1 ppm (part per million) because it strengthens teeth, thereby decreasing the incidence of dental *caries.* The federal Centers for Disease Control and Prevention sets standards for fluoride in water at 0.9 to 1.2 ppm.

In 1945 Grand Rapids, Michigan, became the first city to purposefully add fluoride to drinking water. Not all communities, however, believe in the benefits of fluoridation. Some have rejected fluoridation because many of their citizens believe it may have long-term, negative health consequences, although to date no adverse effects of fluoridation have been found at the recommended level of supplementation—1 ppm.[12]

Fluorosis or **fluoride toxicity,** a condition characterized by mottling (spotting) and excessive hardening of the teeth, has been observed in areas with naturally occurring excesses (2 to 8 ppm) of fluoride in the water.[8]

Aluminum. Some unpurified water contains aluminum. Many water districts add aluminum to the drinking water in the form of aluminum sulfate (alum) to precipitate matter. Nobody thought much about this practice until a British study correlated naturally high levels of aluminum in drinking water with an increased incidence of *Alzheimer's* disease.[6] This finding raised concerns that alum used in water treatment may contribute to this illness. The fear has proved groundless. According to Jean Pennington, a nutritionist with the Center for Food Safety and Applied Nutrition at the Food and Drug Administration, there is no evidence that dietary aluminum is in any way responsible for the elevated levels of aluminum found in the brains of Alzheimer's patients at autopsy. Furthermore, the Environmental Protection Agency guidelines have long required that aluminum containing precipitate be removed from water during the final filtration process. So even if aluminum were linked with Alzheimer's disease, purified water would not be a source.

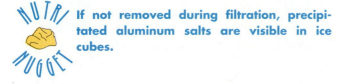

NUTRI NUGGET If not removed during filtration, precipitated aluminum salts are visible in ice cubes.

IN MY DIET

Water is the one nutrient you must have on a daily basis! Fortunately, your thirst mechanism will help remind you of this need.

At the Grocery Store

Distilled, purified, and mineral waters are available in your local grocery store. Is bottled water safer? Sometimes. Sometimes not! Reasons for purchasing

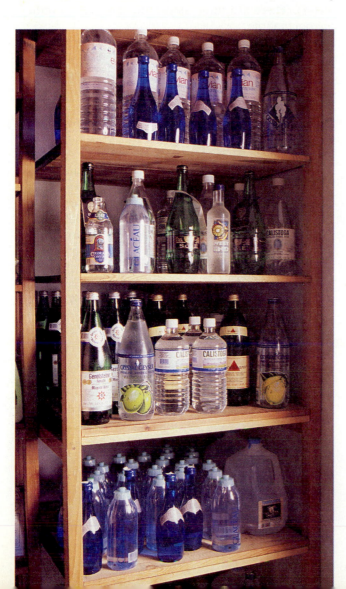

bottled water range from health concerns to personal taste preference. Discovering which product is "right" for you can be a challenging process. Some people on sodium-restricted diets elect to use distilled water. They should realize that it may contain a higher level of microbes than that found in tap water and is not intended to be used as drinking water. Distilled water, a mineral-free alternative to tap water, is really intended for use in steam irons or other appliances to minimize metallic deposits.

Purified bottled waters are the intended substitute for tap water. You may purchase these at your local grocery store or from a bottler for delivery directly to your home. Although some people purchase these waters because they taste better, many believe they are healthier. Tests conducted by the states of California and New York, however, found that purified bottled waters contained many of the same impurities present in tap water. Consumer groups and scientists alike have found bottles filled with the same tap water the consumers were trying to avoid. Additionally, water engineers caution that bottled water has a slightly higher microbial content than does tap water. Unless your public health department has recommended that you use bottled water, be aware that the only advantage of this product may be its taste. In states requiring source labeling, consumers can protect themselves by reading the label.

The North Carolina Department of Agriculture became the first government agency in the United States to take legal action against bottled water companies when it ordered eight brands removed from local store shelves because of false and deceptive labeling.[14] The federal government is currently developing the first set of bottled water regulations.[2]

Mineral Waters

Mineral waters, as their name implies, contain large quantities of naturally occurring metallic elements. Such waters exist worldwide, bubbling from springs and wells deep beneath the Earth's crust. Despite an absence of proof, mankind has long attributed powerful and sometimes miraculous healing properties to these waters. The current mineral water craze in America began in the 1970s with the international success of the French mineral water Perrier.[14]

Although seemingly a healthful alternative to sodas, mineral waters often contain potentially harmful met-

Alzheimer's (ALLS-high-mers)   a disease of progressive senility

caries   dental cavities

potable (POE-ta-bul)   fit to drink (From Latin *potare* "to drink")

als and large amounts of sodium. If you are a mineral-water enthusiast, stick to American or Canadian brands. These are less likely to contain heavy metals, such as cadmium and arsenic. Read labels of domestic brands carefully to find those lowest in sodium.

Flavors

If you prefer fruit-flavored mineral water, use those flavored with *fruit essence*. This way you can avoid the kcalorie and solute loads found in brands that contain sugary fruit juice concentrate.

Seltzer Water

If it's effervescence you crave, try seltzer water. Whether flavored or plain, it is simply sodium-free, carbonated water. Although lacking the "magical power"of minerals, it also lacks the risk of heavy-metal contamination.

In the Kitchen

The kitchen is an excellent place to start practicing nutritionally and ecologically sound water usage!

Encourage your family to drink more water by keeping a container of chilled water in the refrigerator, offering water rather than sodas as a beverage, and serving water with meals. Tempt children to drink water with water servers built into the refrigerator door or with a "sports-style" water bottle.

Pollution

As we have seen, the water from your tap contains more than just H$_2$O. In addition to chlorine and fluoride, water contains many naturally occurring minerals, potentially toxic heavy metals, and a variety of organic chemicals. Consumers often elect to alter the chemical characteristics of their water supply because of health concerns, taste preference, or ease of cleaning.

In response to consumer concerns regarding water pollution, numerous manufacturers have begun marketing home purification devices. The safety and reliability of these devices vary considerably. Several manufacturers market their product via door-to-door salespeople who promise a free water test. They then tell horror stories regarding the safety of the community water supply. Don't become a victim of mass hysteria. If you are concerned about the quality of your drinking water, have your local health department or an independent lab analyze it instead of succumbing to a slick sales pitch. If after testing you decide you need a purifier, purchase one approved by the National Sanitation Foundation (NSF).

It's a good idea to have your tap water tested for lead if you live in an older home. The water pipes in many older buildings were soldered with lead, which leaches into the water running through them (especially hot

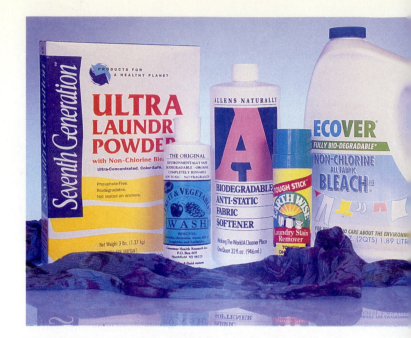

FIGURE 3-2 Do your part to protect the environment: use phosphate-free soaps and detergents.

water). There are three steps you can take to reduce contamination:

1. Run the water for 3 minutes after it has been standing in the pipes for 8 hours.
2. Use bottled drinking and cooking water.
3. Replace the pipes if you can afford to.

Also avoid contributing to water pollution. Don't dispose of toxic chemicals down drains. Use phosphate-free soaps and detergents (Fig. 3-2).

> **NUTRI NUGGET** If you can find it, use potassium chloride instead of sodium chloride in your water softener. It won't raise your blood pressure, and the potassium runoff will make plants grow nice and green.

Water Softeners

Many consumers who live in hard-water areas purchase water softeners. These devices replace the naturally occurring calcium, magnesium, and/or sulfur in hard water with sodium, creating soft water. Artificially softened water eliminates mineral deposits on plumbing fixtures and dishware and improves soap sudsing but adds blood pressure–elevating sodium chloride (salt).

Some studies have found that people who live in hard-water areas have lower blood pressure than those who live in areas with naturally soft water. Because naturally soft water contains little sodium, it appears that the minerals in hard water, not the absence of sodium, may help control blood pressure.

If you don't want to give up the advantages of softened water, hook it up only to the hot-water supply. Use the hot, softened water for bathing, dishwashing, and laundry; use the cold, hard water for drinking and cooking. Alternatively, connect the water softener to all of your household water but have a filter device installed in your kitchen to remove the sodium. Not only will your water taste better, but your cooking may improve as well. Very soft as well as very hard water can adversely affect the outcome of your cooking. If you are having difficulties with yeast breads, off-colored vegetables, or salty-tasting foods, try using bottled purified water for cooking. If your results improve, a kitchen-based water filter may be the answer.

Conservation

Don't waste water! People often mistakenly believe that they need to conserve water only during a drought. What they fail to realize is that, even in areas with ample rainfall, groundwater reserves (aquifers) are dwindling because people use wells to supply some of their water needs. As a result, groundwater that has taken hundreds of years to accumulate is being depleted relatively rapidly. We need to conserve water so that groundwater reserves will be available in the event of a drought.

You can take a number of simple steps to reduce water use. Some are highlighted in Box 3-1; others can be found in the excellent publication *50 Simple Things You Can Do To Save the Planet*, published by The Earth Works.[1]

BOX 3-1   Suggestions for Conserving Water

Don't leave the faucet running!
Install flow restrictors in your water faucets.
Minimize use of water-guzzling garbage disposals.
Heat only the amount of water needed on the stove or in a microwave.
Save water used to cook pasta or rinse produce for watering plants.
Wash dishes by hand or run the dishwasher only when filled to capacity.
Save the water that runs from the shower head while you wait for it to heat up or install a hot-water recycling unit for instant warmth.

NUTRALERT

ROAD SALT

Contrary to conventional wisdom, road salt is not washed away by spring rains and melting snow. Instead it accumulates in groundwater. Experts fear this will lead to a severe decline in water quality over the next 20 years.[12]

At the Table

Drinking water with meals has several health benefits. It helps us meet our daily water requirement; it provides some of the water needed for the digestive process; and it helps fill us up, reducing the likelihood of overeating.

Eating Out

Apply the same suggestions for incorporating water into your home health routine to eating out. As a conservation measure, restaurants in drought-stricken areas serve water only upon request. So don't forget to request a glass of this healthful beverage.

Menu Matrix

To ensure an adequate fluid intake, you should drink a *minimum* of four 8-oz glasses of water daily. This is in *addition* to any other beverages you consume. Gradually work your way up to drinking the six to eight glasses of water per day recommended by the American Medical Association. Spread your water intake over the entire day so that you hydrate yourself continually. Evaluate the thirst-quenching potential of the beverages you typically consume. Substitute decaffeinated beverages for at least half of the caffeine-containing ones you currently drink. Choose plain water, diluted fruit juice, or seltzer water instead of sodas. Remember to drink additional water when overheated, ill, pregnant, or lactating.

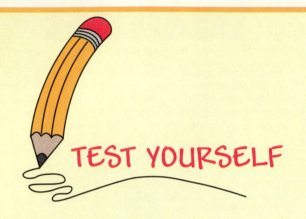

TEST YOURSELF

True or False. Put a **T** for true or an **F** for false in the space beside each question.

___ 1. Water is the most essential nutrient because a lack of water will kill you within days whereas a deficiency of any of the other 39 nutrients would take months or even years to prove fatal.

___ 2. There is a finite amount of water on Earth. New water is not made; the existing water is simply recycled.

T 3. No matter where you live in the United States, you should be careful not to waste water.

T 4. Water is classified as soft or hard depending on the amount and kinds of minerals that are dissolved in it.

___ 5. Some water districts add fluoride to drinking water to help prevent cavities.

___ 6. People with high blood pressure should not use artificially softened water.

Short Answer

7. List two mechanical and two chemical functions of water in the human body.
8. Approximately how much water do you need each day to stay healthy?
9. Identify at least two kinds of situations that increase your need for water.
10. Identify the major routes by which water is lost from the human body.
11. List three sources of water in the average person's diet.
12. List two kinds of beverages that can cause your body to lose water.

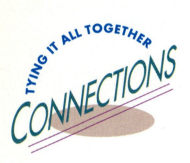

TYING IT ALL TOGETHER
CONNECTIONS

1. Evaluate the fluid intake record described below. Is this person getting enough of the proper types of fluid?

2. Suggest some ways that this person can improve his/her fluid status (bear in mind the fact that he or she dislikes water).

	Amount	Substance
Morning:	3	8-oz cups of caffeinated coffee
	1	6-oz cup of citrus fruit drink
Noon:	1	12-oz glass of iced tea or soft drink
Afternoon	1-2	6-oz cups of caffeinated coffee
and/or	1	12-oz can of soft drink
after work:	2-3	12-oz cans of beer
After dinner:	2	8-oz cups of decaffeinated coffee

References

1. *50 simple things you can do to save the planet*, 1991, The Earth Works.

2. FDA Press Office, personal communication, April 1994.

3. *Food safety notebook*, 4(3):33, 1993.

4. Health Tips, *The Johns Hopkins Medical Letter*, 5(3):8, 1993.

5. Klatskey AL et al: The relationships between alcoholic beverage use and other threats to blood pressure: a new Kaiser Permanante study, *Circulation* 73:628, 1986.

6. Martyn CN et al: Geographic relation between Alzheimer's disease and aluminum in drinking water, *Lancet* 8629(1):59-62, 1989.

7. Martyn CN: The epidemiology of Alzheimer's disease in relation to aluminum. Ciba Foundation Symposium, 1992, 169:69-79; discussion 79-86.

8. National Research Council: *Recommended dietary allowances*, ed 10, Washington, DC, 1989, National Academy Press.

9. Randal HT: Water, electrolyte and acid-base balance. In Shils ME, Young VR, eds: *Modern nutrition in health and disease*, Philadelphia, 1988, Lea & Febiger.

10. Scarre C: *Smithsonian time lines of the ancient world*, Washington, DC, 1993, Smithsonian Institution Press.

11. Vokes T: Water homeostasis, *Annual Review of Nutrition* 7:383, 1987.

12. Water—1993, Washington, DC, National Geographic Society.

13. Water. In *Present knowledge in nutrition*, ed 6, Washington, DC, 1990, International Life Sciences Institute, Nutrition Foundation.

14. *Time*, April 26, 1993.

CHAPTER 4

CARBOHYDRATES
The Staff of Life

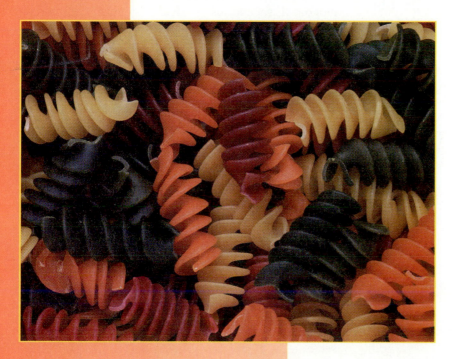

The trouble with eating Italian food is that five or six days later you're hungry again.
— *George Miller*

Bread is often called "the staff of life." Actually, this is an apt description of carbohydrates in general. Carbohydrates are obtained primarily from plants, which are the first link in the Earth's food chain. Without plants to convert raw materials into essential nutrients and oxygen for humans and animals alike, the Earth as we know it would be a very different place. Before the industrial revolution, carbohydrates were the major source of nutrients and kcalories for people the world over. From time immemorial, almost every culture has relied on a particular native starch or grain for a dietary staple[33]:

- **Rice** in Asia
- **Wheat** in the Mediterranean, Middle East, and northern Africa
- **Oats** and **barley** in the British Isles
- **Corn** and **potatoes** in the Americas
- **Taro root** (poi) in the Pacific Islands
- **Cassava root** in mid- and southern Africa

As exploration and transportation made the world "smaller," many of these carbohydrates were introduced to new areas, where they often became the preferred dietary staple. For example, if you asked people of Irish descent how long their ancestors had been eating potatoes, they would probably answer, "Forever." In reality, the potato was not introduced to Ireland until the mid-1600s. Yet it replaced the native carbohydrate source to such an extent that, when the Irish potato crop failed in the mid-1800s, thousands of people died of starvation and thousands of others left for America.[22]

Industrialization provided machinery for refining carbohydrates and led to significant changes in the pattern of consumption of this important class of nutrients. Machines cheaply and efficiently removed the fiber and nutrient-rich bran from whole grains so that white flour and white rice became the rage. Other machines extracted large quantities of table sugar from sugar cane and sugar beets.[2] Increasing reliance on these new products led people to shift from a high-fiber diet to one that was high in sugar and low in fiber. This trend marked the beginning of a rise in the incidence of obesity that some researchers attributed to the increased use of sugar. Perhaps because of this association between sugar and obesity, during the 1950s all carbohydrates were unfairly labeled as fattening.[30,38]

Carbohydrates have been liberated from this stigma in recent years; however, misconceptions still exist about their role in weight maintenance. Many people incorrectly identify starchy foods like bread, potatoes, and pasta as fattening instead of recognizing the true culprits: the high-fat extras like butter, sour cream, and cream sauces. Without these "enhancements," carbohydrate-rich foods are excellent, low-fat sources of both fiber and nutrients.

SUNSHINE'S SUGARS

What exactly is a carbohydrate? The term **carbohydrate** is Latin for hydrated (watered) carbon, and is a fitting description of the chemical structure of this class of nutrients. Carbohydrates are made up of building blocks called *monosaccharides* (single sugars: mono = 1, saccharide = sugar). The most common dietary monosaccharides are made up of six carbon atoms and six water molecules. Carbohydrates may contain as few as one or as many as several hundred saccharide molecules. The majority of dietary carbohydrates are made by the process of *photosynthesis* within the *chloroplasts* of green plants. Chloroplasts are essentially solar-powered "factories." These factories are staffed by enzymatic proteins that use the following raw materials:

- Ground water: sucked in through the roots
- Carbon dioxide: absorbed from the air
- Solar energy: absorbed by the pigment chlorophyll, is used to assemble the hydrated carbon ring known as a monosaccharide

In a nutshell, solar energy is responsible for sugar and starch production on planet Earth! The chloroplast factory also can produce disaccharides and polysaccharides by linking two or more monosaccharide units together. These starting materials are used to build the plant's roots, stems, stalks, leaves, flowers, fruits, and seeds.

Carbohydrates in the Carbon Cycle

Plants are an integral part of the Earth's ecosystem. They form the first link in the food chain by synthesizing from raw materials the nutrients essential for humans and animals. They maintain the oxygen content of our envi-

TABLE 4–1 Preview	
Dietary Nutrient:	**Carbohydrates**
Building block	Monosaccharides
Kcal content	4 kcal/gram
Source	Grains, fruits, vegetables, dairy products
Nutrient intake standard	Dietary Goals
Food intake standard	Dietary Guidelines, Food Guide Pyramid
In the body	Fuel (blood glucose), mucus, cell surface receptors
Deficiency	Gluconeogenesis (protein used for glucose), ketosis, constipation
Excess	Stored as glycogen, fat

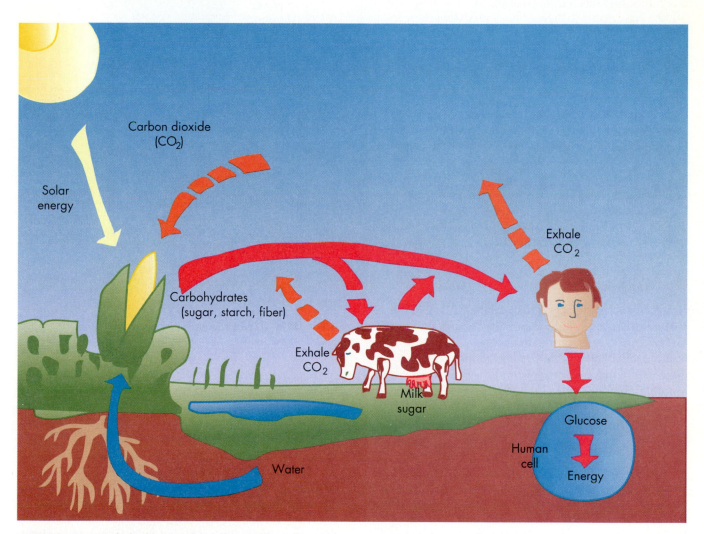

Carbon dioxide
(CO_2)

Solar
energy

Carbohydrates
(sugar, starch, fiber)

Exhale
CO_2

Exhale
CO_2

Milk
sugar

Water

Glucose

Human
cell

Energy

FIGURE 4-1 Carbohydrates in the carbon cycle.

ronment by converting the carbon dioxide breathed out by humans and animals back into free oxygen and carbon-to-carbon bonds (Fig. 4-1). Their roots prevent soil erosion by holding in place the nutrient rich topsoil so essential to plant growth. Animals eat these plants and digest them to monosaccharides, which are converted to glucose, then burned in the body's cells to produce energy.

Animals also make carbohydrates, but these are mostly for use in their own bodies. The exception is the

chloroplast   the part of the plant cell containing the pigment chlorophyll and the enzyme systems that are responsible for photosynthesis

monosaccharide   a single sugar molecule

photosynthesis   the formation of carbohydrates in the chloroplasts of plants from carbon dioxide and water under the influence of ultraviolet light

milk sugar **lactose,** which is found in dairy products as well as human milk. *Lactose is the only significant animal source of dietary carbohydrate.*

To keep track of the various forms of carbohydrate, scientists have developed both chemical and dietary classifications. Chemically speaking, carbohydrates are divided into four main categories, depending on the number of saccharide units they contain: **mono**saccharide (one), **di**saccharide (two), **oligo**saccharide (a few), and **poly**saccharide (many).

Monosaccharides

The **monosaccharides** (single sugars) are the major building blocks of dietary sugars, starches, and fiber. The most common monosaccharides in our diet are glucose (Fig. 4-2), fructose, and galactose. All three of these sugars contain the same ratio of carbon atoms to water molecules, but placement of their chemical bonds differs slightly. As a result they differ slightly in both shape and taste.[2,38]

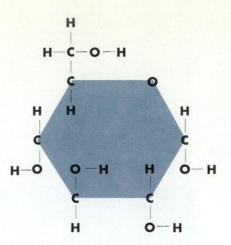

FIGURE 4-2 The chemical structure of glucose, shown here, is similar to that of other dietary monosaccharides.

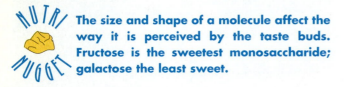

The size and shape of a molecule affect the way it is perceived by the taste buds. Fructose is the sweetest monosaccharide; galactose the least sweet.

Glucose ——— Glucose   Glucose ——— Fructose

Maltose   Sucrose

Glucose ——— Galactose

Lactose

FIGURE 4-3 Two monosaccharides combine to form each disaccharide: sucrose, lactose, and maltose.

Disaccharides

Which disaccharide is most common in the diet?
Disaccharides (double sugars) are made by combining two monosaccharide molecules. All of the commonly occurring disaccharides contain at least one molecule of glucose; consequently, there are only three possible combinations (Fig. 4-3). Sucrose, also known as table sugar, is the most common disaccharide in the American diet.

Oligosaccharides

The **oligosaccharides** are a special type of sugar, slightly larger than the disaccharides. They are composed of chains of a few monosaccharide units. These unusual sugars are found primarily in members of the legume family (beans and lentils). The oligosaccharides are not absorbable and pass on through the large intestine. They are easily metabolized by the bacteria in the gastrointestinal tract; it is the gaseous end products that give beans their reputation as flatulence producers.[30,38]

Polysaccharides

Both plants and animals link surplus glucose molecules together to create polysaccharides, which serve as sources of stored energy. In plants this energy reserve is formed of either straight or branching chains of glucose molecules and is called **starch. Glycogen,** the animal counterpart of starch, is formed in the livers of an-

imals when glucose molecules link together in a distinctive branching pattern.

Polysaccharides are further designated as **digestible** (starches) or **indigestible** (fibers).[38] Plants also use polysaccharides to make an indigestible building material known as fiber. **Fiber** is found exclusively in plants, where it performs a function comparable to that of bones in animals. Both animals and plants are made of cells. Animals have skeletons that form the framework that supports their cells. Plants do not have skeletons to hold them up, but they do have box-shaped walls around each cell that thicken and harden with age, providing a sturdy, stackable framework. This cell wall material contains various polysaccharide fibers and a noncarbohydrate substance, **lignin.** Like starch, fiber is made of repeating monosaccharide units (Fig. 4-4). However, the chemical links between the monosaccharide molecules of fiber are joined in such a way that they cannot be separated by human digestive enzymes. For this reason, fiber passes through our small intestine virtually intact. Dietary fiber is classified as soluble or insoluble depending on how it reacts with water.

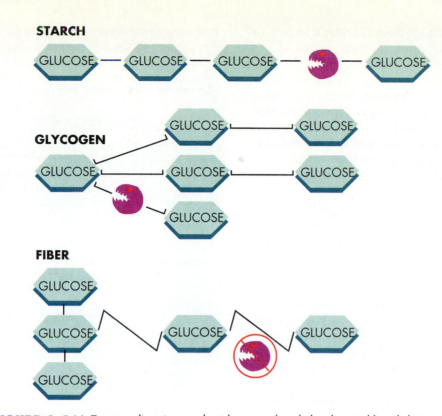

STARCH

GLYCOGEN

FIBER

FIGURE 4-4 N. Zyme, a digestive saccharidase, can break the chemical bonds between glucose molecules in starch and glycogen, but not in fiber.

Bacteria found in the stomachs of ruminant animals (cattle, sheep, and others with cuds) are able to digest the bonds connecting the sugars that make up fiber and release the nutrients for use by the host animal. The carbohydrate-digesting enzymes found in the human small intestine are unable to break these bonds. Bacteria in the colon of humans, however, are able to digest the bonds in soluble fibers. Because the sugars are now past the small intestine absorption sites, only the bacteria benefit from the kcalories released.

Insoluble fiber comes mainly from seeds, the protective bran layer on whole grains, and the stringy material in vegetables such as celery. Bacteria will not digest insoluble fiber. This type of fiber provides bulk by absorbing water.

Soluble fiber is gummy rather than stringy. It forms a gel when dissolved in water. Soluble fiber is found in legumes, oat bran, barley, vegetables, and fruit pulp. Soluble fibers such as pectin, guar gum, and carrageenan are often used as thickening agents in cooking and during food processing.[1,38] Anyone who has made marmalade, jam, or jelly has probably used the soluble fiber pectin as a thickening agent. Bacteria,

which flourish in the large intestine, can partially digest soluble fiber and use the resulting sugars for food. This allows them to reproduce rapidly, creating increased fecal bulk.

IN THE DIET

What foods supply most of the world's carbohydrate?
The major dietary carbohydrates are found in fruits, grains, root crops (like potatoes and cassava), and legumes (such as peas, beans, and lentils). Small amounts are supplied by vegetables. These foods serve many important functions in the diet. They add sweetness (sugars), thickening power (starches), and texture (fiber).[38] Climate, native species, local custom, and commerical value influence which carbohydrate-rich crops are produced in different parts of the world. Culture, economics, and politics in turn influence which crops people consume.[11]

Nutritionally, a scientist would describe dietary carbohydrates as being either **simple** (mono- and disaccharides) or **complex** (polysaccharides). Nonscientists categorize the carbohydrates they eat according to dietary functions, such as:

- **Sugars** (mono- and disaccharides): sweeteners
- **Starches** (digestible polysaccharides): thickeners

- **Fibers** (indigestible polysaccharides): chewy or gummy materials

Sugars

Almost everyone can identify sugar as the ingredient that makes foods sweet. Not as many people know that there are a number of dietary sugars and that their sweetness varies. Table 4-2 shows how the sweetness of various sugars and sugar substitutes compares with that of sucrose (table sugar), which, as the reference standard, is given a sweetness value of 100.

At one time the major sources of sugar in people's diets were fruits, vegetables, and small amounts of raw honey. These natural sugars are a combination of the disaccharide sucrose and the free monosaccharides fructose and glucose. Table 4-3 lists naturally occurring food sources of these sugars. Then industrialization led to the large-scale refining of sugarcane and cornstarch to produce sucrose (table sugar) and high-fructose corn syrup, respectively. Now sugar is present in a wide array of processed foods, including cereal, canned products, candy, and baked goods.[2,38]

 Fruits and honey taste very sweet. What do you suppose accounts for the sweetness of these foods?

Most people are surprised to learn that sugar acts as a natural preservative. In this regard it functions much as salt does, by pulling water from cells and disabling bacteria. Before the days of refrigeration, it was this preservative property of sugar that gave syrups and fruit preserves their long shelf life.

TABLE 4-2	The Sweetness of Sugars and Sugar Substitutes	
Type of Sweetener	**Relative Sweetness*** (Sucrose = 1.0)	**Typical Sources**
SUGARS		
Lactose	0.2	Dairy products
Maltose	0.4	Sprouted seeds
Glucose	0.7	Corn syrup
Sucrose	1.0	Table sugar, most sweets
Invert sugar†	1.3	Some candies, honey
Fructose	1.2-1.8	Fruit, honey, some soft drinks
SUGAR ALCOHOLS		
Sorbitol	0.6	Dietetic candies, sugarless gum
Mannitol	0.7	Dietetic candies
Xylitol	0.9	Sugarless gum
SUGAR SUBSTITUTES		
Cyclamate	30	Not in use in the United States
Aspartame	200	Diet soft drinks, diet fruit drinks, sugarless gum, powdered diet sweetener, pudding, gelatin, yogurt
Acesulfame-K	200	Sugarless gum, diet drink mixes, powdered diet sweetener, puddings, gelatin, yogurt
Saccharin (sodium salt)	300	Diet soft drinks

Adapted from American Dietetic Association, 1993.
*On a per gram basis.
†Sucrose broken down into glucose and fructose.

TABLE 4-3	Naturally Occurring Sources of Carbohydrates	
Carbohydrate Type	**Common Names**	**Naturally Occurring Food Sources**
MONOSACCHARIDES		
Glucose	Blood sugar	Fruits, sweeteners
Fructose	Fruit sugar	Fruits, honey, syrups, vegetables
Galactose	—	Part of lactose, found in milk
DISACCHARIDES		
Sucrose (glucose + fructose)	Table surgar	Sugar cane, sugar beets, fruits, vegetables
Lactose (glucose + galactose)	Milk sugar	Milk and milk products
Maltose (glucose + glucose)	Malt sugar	Germinating grains
OLIGOSACCHARIDES	—	Legumes, gas-producing vegetables
POLYSACCHARIDES		
Starches	Complex carbohydrates	Grains, legumes, potatoes
Dietary fiber	Roughage	Legumes, whole grains, fruits, vegetables

COMPARISON OF NUTRIENT CONTENT OF COMMON SWEETENERS

Nutrient	Blackstrap Molasses (1 T)	Honey (1 T)	Brown Sugar (1 T)	White Sugar (1 T)
Kcal	43	64	33	46
H₂O (g)	4.8	3.6	trace	0.1
Weight (g)	20	21	9	12
Protein (g)	0	0.1	trace	0
Carbohydrate (g)	11.0	17.3	8.7	11.9
Vitamins				
B₁ (mg)	0.02	0	trace	0
B₂ (mg)	0.04	0.01	trace	0
Niacin (mg)	0.4	0.1	0.02	0
Minerals				
Sodium	19	1	2.8	0
Potassium (mg)	585	11	31.2	0
Calcium (mg)	137	1	7.7	0
Phosphorus (mg)	17	1	1.8	0
Iron (mg)	3.20	0.10	0.31	0

Adapted from Pennington JAT: *Bowes and Church's food values of portions commonly used*, ed 16, Philadelphia, 1994, JB Lippincott.

a. What is the most significant contribution these sugars make to the diet?
b. How many kcalories per gram (g) of carbohydrate does each contain?
c. Compared to blackstrap molasses, is there a significant difference in either the vitamin or mineral content of the other three sweeteners?

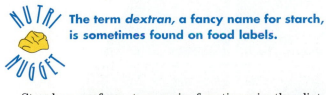
Unprocessed honey and fruit contain enzymes that break sucrose into free fructose and glucose. Free fructose tends to attract moisture that in turn liquefies the honey.

Starches

Which foods are the most common sources of dietary starch? Although they are made of sugar building blocks, starches do not taste particularly sweet. Small amounts of starch are found in many different types of plant cells. The majority, however, are concentrated in seeds (grains, legumes) and tubers (potatoes) to ensure a source of energy for the growth of a new plant. Starches are excellent sources of quick energy because they are readily broken down by human digestive enzymes into individual glucose molecules.

The term *dextran*, a fancy name for starch, is sometimes found on food labels.

Starches perform two main functions in the diet. First, they provide satiety (a feeling of fullness), on at least a short-term basis. If you have ever filled up on chow mein only to become hungry an hour later, you are familiar with this phenomenon. Second, purified starches, such as arrowroot and cornstarch, are often used as thickening agents in sauces and gravies and in ethnic and processed foods.

Fibers

Fibers add a satisfying chewy or crunchy texture to many foods. Because they are indigestible they help provide a feeling of satiety. Whole, unprocessed foods tend to be good sources of fiber. Table 4-4 lists common types of dietary fiber.

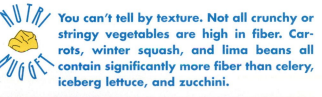
You can't tell by texture. Not all crunchy or stringy vegetables are high in fiber. Carrots, winter squash, and lima beans all contain significantly more fiber than celery, iceberg lettuce, and zucchini.

TABLE 4-4 Examples of Dietary Fiber

Fiber-Rich Foods	Purified Fibers
Barley	Bran
Brown rice	Carob bean gum
Oats	Carrageenan
Whole wheat	Cellulose
Fruits	Guar gum
Vegetables	Pectin

Food Intake Standards

How much carbohydrate do I need?   Whole, unprocessed foods provide a healthy array of carbohydrates, as shown in Table 4-3.

Dietary Guidelines

The *Dietary Guidelines for Americans* are directed at healthy people ages 2 years and older. They give the general public guidance in selecting a diet that will promote health and reduce the risk of chronic diseases for which there is clear evidence of dietary involvement. Below is an abbreviated list of these guidelines with the sugar, starch, and fiber recommendations emphasized.[13,14]

- **Choose a diet with plenty of vegetables, fruits, and grain products.** Substitute starches for fats and sugars; select whole-grain breads and cereals, fruits and vegetables, dried beans and peas, and nuts to increase fiber and starch intake.
- **Use sugars only in moderation.** Use less sugar, syrup, and honey; reduce concentrated sweets, like candy, soft drinks, cookies, and the like; select fresh fruits or fruits canned in light syrup or their own juices; read food labels—sucrose, glucose, dextrose, maltose, lactose, fructose, syrups, and honey are all sugars; eat sugar less often to reduce dental caries (tooth decay).

 Oat breads are not necessarily high in fiber. Most of the flour in oat bread is white flour. Except for a small amount of rolled oats or oat bran, they contain the same amount of fiber as any white bread.

Food Guide Pyramid

The Food Guide Pyramid visually depicts much of the information in the 1990 *Dietary Guidelines*. A key feature of this intake standard is the emphasis it places on dietary carbohydrate. Note that the majority of the Pyramid is composed of carbohydrate-rich foods, such as vegetables, fruits, breads, and pastas. The tip of the Pyramid includes a food group for sweets. It also uses a graphic to alert consumers to sugar hiding in other food groups. You can see this symbol in the key to the Pyramid. Figure 4-5 highlights recommended sources of sugars, starches, and fibers in the Pyramid.

Sugar is one carbohydrate that most people should consume sparingly. People who eat large amounts of sugar-rich foods often use them in place of more nutritious foods. For example, they drink sodas rather than milk and eat candies and other sweet snacks instead of fruit. Unless you have trouble getting enough kcalories even when consuming a balanced diet, only 18% to 20% of your daily kcalorie intake should come from sugar.

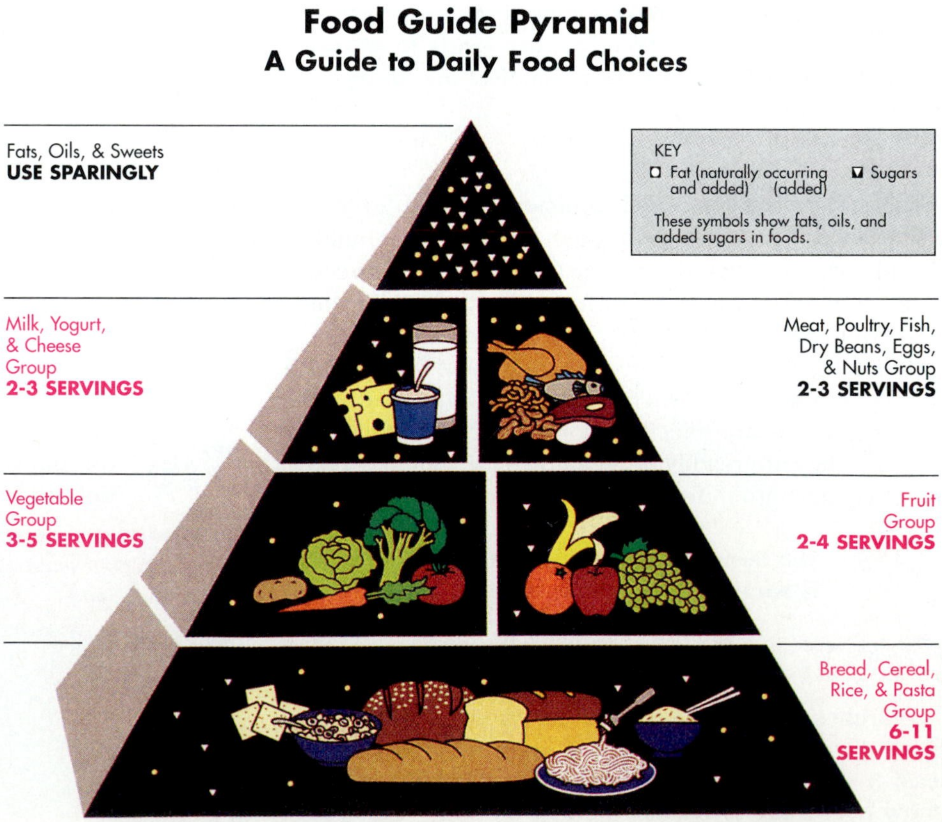

FIGURE 4-5 This illustration of the USDA Food Guide Pyramid highlights the food groups that are sources of carbohydrates.

Food Guide Pyramid
A Guide to Daily Food Choices

Fats, Oils, & Sweets
USE SPARINGLY

KEY
☐ Fat (naturally occurring   ☑ Sugars
and added)   (added)

These symbols show fats, oils, and added sugars in foods.

Milk, Yogurt, & Cheese Group
2-3 SERVINGS

Meat, Poultry, Fish, Dry Beans, Eggs, & Nuts Group
2-3 SERVINGS

Vegetable Group
3-5 SERVINGS

Fruit Group
2-4 SERVINGS

Bread, Cereal, Rice, & Pasta Group
6-11 SERVINGS

TABLE 4-5 Intake Standards	
Foods	**Nutrients**
Dietary Guidelines	RDA
	NIH Fiber Recommendations
Food Guide Pyramid	% Daily Value (labels)
5-A-Day Program	
American Heart Association	**Dietary Goals**
American Cancer Society	
People eat foods.	***Cells eat nutrients.***

This amount includes the sugar present in processed foods and jams, jellies, and preserves; any sugar you add to foods and beverages; and the sugars that occur naturally in fruits and vegetables. The milk sugar lactose is not considered in this estimate.

How much sugar can I add to my diet? Only 10% to 15% of your sugar intake should be from so-called added sugars: sweeteners, soft drinks, and candies. See the Personalizing the Pyramid section of Chapter 2 for details.[39]

Nutrient Intake Standards

Students of nutrition are often surprised to learn that there is no RDA for carbohydrates. There are two reasons for this. First, the major role of carbohydrates is to provide our bodies with energy. Because we also can derive energy from other food sources, such as fat and protein, it is difficult to pinpoint exactly how much we should obtain from carbohydrates. Second, when the original RDA were formulated, there were no known disease states that could be attributed to a lack of dietary carbohydrate.[27] More recent research suggests that inadequate fiber intake may contribute to constipation,[9] colon cancer, high blood cholesterol levels,[28] and **diverticulosis**.[36]

NIH Recommendations—Fiber

While acknowledging that not everyone needs the same amount of fiber to maintain good gastrointestinal function, most experts agree that Americans should try to consume 20 to 35 grams of fiber each day from a variety of fruits, vegetables, and grains. Any effort to increase dietary fiber intake should be undertaken gradually. Rapid increases in dietary fiber are often accompanied by cramping, bloating, gas, and diarrhea because the intestines and their bacteria take time to adjust to the increased residue. The optimal level of fiber intake varies by individual. We need to consume enough fiber to prevent constipation but less than an amount that produces diarrhea.[28]

Dietary Goals

The *Dietary Goals for the United States* recommend that carbohydrates provide more of our total kcalories; we are encouraged to increase consumption of com-

plex carbohydrates and naturally occurring sugars from about 28% to about 48% of energy intake and to reduce consumption of refined and other processed sugars to about 10% to 15% of our total energy intake.

The Food Guide Pyramid in Fig. 4-5 highlights most common dietary carbohydrate sources. Legumes and nuts are not highlighted, even though they contain some starch and fiber.
a. Which of the food groups do legumes and nuts belong in? Why?
b. Why is the meat group, as a whole, not highlighted here?

IN BETWEEN: DIGESTION AND ABSORPTION

To digest carbohydrates, our bodies perform a sequence of several steps and use a number of substances to aid in the process.

Sugars and Starches

Chemical digestion of carbohydrates begins in the mouth, where **salivary amylase** converts dietary starch to glucose (Fig. 4-6). Carbohydrate digestion resumes in the small intestine, where powerful **pancreatic amylases** dismantle starches, one glucose unit at a time.

Disaccharides present in food are not affected by pancreatic amylase. Instead they are split into their respective monosaccharides (glucose, galactose, and fructose) by special enzymes known as disaccharidases, which are present on the surface of the intestinal cells. The monosaccharides released from starch or disaccharides are rapidly absorbed by the intestinal lining and pass into the bloodstream. Some people have difficulty digesting certain carbohydrates, for instance, dairy products. A Closer Look on p. 53 focuses on two of these disorders.

Blood leaving the gastrointestinal tract is carried directly to the liver, where most of the fructose and galactose is converted into glucose before being released into the general circulation. Cells absorb glucose from the blood as needed and burn it for fuel, obtaining 4 kcalories of energy from every gram.

Dental Caries and Periodontal Disease

What happens if I eat too much sugar? Excessive sugar intake has been blamed for obesity, tooth decay, cardiovascular disease, diabetes, hyperactivity, and even violent criminal behavior. Over the years, however, scientists have disproved sugar's association with all of these health problems except caries (cavities),

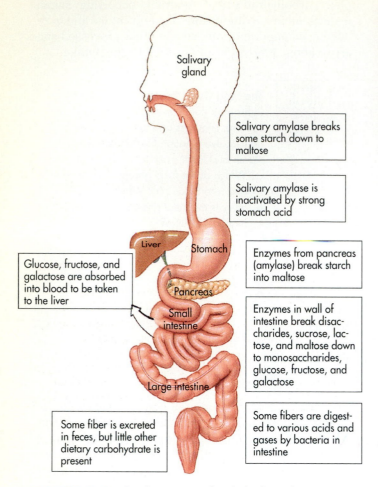

FIGURE 4-6 A brief summary of carbohydrate digestion.

Salivary gland

Salivary amylase breaks some starch down to maltose

Salivary amylase is inactivated by strong stomach acid

Liver   Stomach

Glucose, fructose, and galactose are absorbed into blood to be taken to the liver

Pancreas

Small intestine

Enzymes from pancreas (amylase) break starch into maltose

Enzymes in wall of intestine break disaccharides, sucrose, lactose, and maltose down to monosaccharides, glucose, fructose, and galactose

Large intestine

Some fiber is excreted in feces, but little other dietary carbohydrate is present

Some fibers are digested to various acids and gases by bacteria in intestine

Fuel Value of Nutrients	
	kcal per gram
Proteins	4
Carbohydrates	
Sugar	4
Starch	4
Fiber	0
Lipids	9

mouthwashes, and drinking water together with regular fluoride treatments and dental checkups are highly effective ways to reduce caries.[4]

Tooth decay results from the action of oral bacteria on dietary sugars. Colonies of bacteria living in the mouth form a sticky substance called plaque, which adheres to the surface of teeth. The bacteria use the simple sugars in food to meet their own energy needs. Acid, a by-product of bacterial digestion of sugar, erodes the enamel surface of teeth, forming caries (cavities; Fig. 4-7).[26]

Like dental caries, **periodontal** disease (which affects the tissues that surround the teeth) results from bacterial degradation of dietary carbohydrate residue. It is caused by bacteria that thrive under the gum line in the absence of oxygen. Once established, these bacteria will chew up the supporting bone structure. When the bone goes, the teeth wobble and eventually fall out. The best prevention is good oral hygiene. Mechanical means, like brushing or flossing, physically remove the trapped food particles and the bacteria colonies. Mouthwashes and toothpaste kill by direct attack, by either neutralizing the acid or dehydrating the bacteria.

and even this connection appears to be in question. For many years health care professionals have taught us that sticky and sugary foods are responsible for dental caries. Recent research, however, has shown the following:

1. The amount of sugar in a food is not directly related to its cavity-causing potential.

2. All sugars, not just sucrose, can cause cavities. Cooked starches also can promote cavity formatioin.

3. Ninety percent of all snack foods contain sugar or cooked starch.

4. The cavity-causing potential of a food is determined by the food's chemical makeup and the amount of time the food particles remain in the mouth. This means that sticky foods that are cleared from the mouth within a few minutes are less harmful than trapped particles of cooked starch that stay in the mouth for hours.

5. Routine use of fluoride-containing toothpastes,

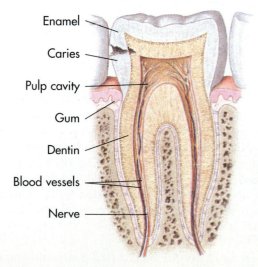

Enamel

Caries

Pulp cavity

Gum

Dentin

Blood vessels

Nerve

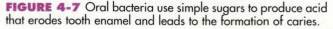

FIGURE 4-7 Oral bacteria use simple sugars to produce acid that erodes tooth enamel and leads to the formation of caries.

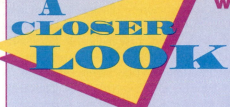

What If You Can't Digest Carbohydrates?

LACTOSE INTOLERANCE

One of the more common nutrient metabolizing disorders of the gastrointestinal tract is **lactose intolerance.** Once they are past childhood, the gastrointestinal tracts of many people, particularly those of African, Asian, Jewish, and Mediterranean descent, spontaneously decrease production of the enzyme lactase. This enzyme is required to split the disaccharide lactose, found in milk and milk products, into its constituent monosaccharides, glucose and galactose. Without lactase, the lactose in dairy products cannot be digested and absorbed. It accumulates in the large intestine, where it is fermented by the endogenous bacteria there to by-products, which result in cramping, bloating, gas, diarrhea, and sometimes nausea.

The most popular explanation of this phenomenon is that nature never continues to make what nature cannot use. In other words, "use it or lose it." Scientists who have studied lactose intolerance believe that it is natural for people to lose the ability to make this enzyme once they are past the milk-consuming stage of early childhood. These researchers theorize that the ability to make lactase well into adulthood is an adaptation seen only in people from ethnic groups that for generations have relied on dairy products as a major source of nourishment.

People vary considerably with respect to their degree of lactose intolerance. Further, there are many excellent ways to obtain dairy products that either contain significantly reduced amounts of lactose or are free of it altogether. (See the Dairy Decisions section of In the Grocery Store.)

CELIAC DISEASE OR GLUTEN-SENSITIVE ENTEROPATHY

Celiac disease is an older term for a disorder now known as gluten-sensitive enteropathy. The gastrointestinal tracts of persons with this disorder exhibit a toxic reaction to the protein gluten, found in wheat, rye, barley, and oats. Symptoms include diarrhea, atrophy of the intestinal lining, weight loss, and in children, growth retardation. The first signs of this disorder usually appear during infancy, when grain-based foods such as cereals and crackers are first added to the diet. However, some people show no symptoms until they reach their twenties. Treatment involves avoidance of all foods containing the protein gluten. Some of these, such as bread, cereal, and pasta, are obvious. But gluten may also be hiding in prepared meats, salad dressings, gravies, ice cream, and candies. Affected persons are able to consume cornmeal as well as flours made from rice, arrowroot, millet, and soy protein.

NUTRI NUGGET Ideally you should brush your teeth after every meal. Realistically this is not always possible, so the American Dental Association suggests chewing sugar-free gum for 15 to 20 minutes after a meal to remove trapped food particles.

Fibers

The major effect of dietary fiber on our bodies is seen in the gastrointestinal tract. Fiber is not digested by human enzymes, so it passes into the colon intact. Bacteria in the colon digest some of the fiber; the remainder is expelled in the feces. Except for its long recognized role in relieving constipation, fiber historically was considered unimportant nutritionally because its sugar units could not be used by humans for energy (kcalories). Researchers challenged this concept in the 1970s and reported that high-fiber diets prevent some health problems.[9] Although the initial research ignored several important considerations, such as levels of other major nutrients in the diet, it did stimulate interest and research in the area. Today scientists recognize that there are two types of fiber—insoluble and soluble—and that they play different roles in the prevention of disease.[1,15,28,29]

Insoluble Fiber

Insoluble fiber (like cellulose) is valued for its ability to prevent or relieve constipation. It absorbs water and causes an increase in bulk and fluid content in the intestine. This bulk puts pressure on the intestinal walls, which respond with muscle contractions, hastening the passage of material through the gastrointestinal tract. The associated water softens the stools, which makes for easier elimination.

Soluble Fiber

The gelatinous substance formed when **soluble fiber** mixes with intestinal fluid has the opposite effect. It slows emptying of the stomach and small intestine, which is why home remedies for diarrhea often included eating fruits rich in the soluble fiber pectin, such as apples and pears. Pharmaceutical manufacturers also add pectin to antidiarrhea medications. More recently, soluble fiber has been touted as a treatment for **hypercholesterolemia** (a high blood cholesterol level).[29] More research is needed before conclusive recommendations can be made. Perhaps scientists will find that there is truth to the old folk saying, "An apple a day keeps the doctor away."

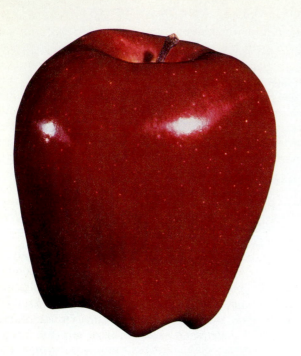

Clinical studies have shown that ample amounts of both soluble and insoluble fiber in the diet are useful for treating obesity and diabetes. The extra volume of a high-fiber diet helps keep weight watchers satisfyingly full without adding extra kcalories. Both kinds of fiber slow the release and subsequent absorption of glucose during digestion, which helps keep blood sugar levels stable for a longer period of time. Stable blood sugar improves people's weight control efforts because their brains aren't crying out for more food to turn into glucose. It also reduces the amount of insulin needed by persons with diabetes.[1]

What happens if I don't have enough fiber in my diet?   The task of interpreting fiber research is complicated by the fact that diets that are naturally high in fiber tend to be associated with other nutritional changes, such as a reduction in fat and sugar. It is not clear that dietary fiber is the only factor involved in prevention of the diseases mentioned below. The 1989 RDA say that people who want the benefits of a high-fiber diet should consume whole, unprocessed foods rather than refined fiber supplements or concentrates.[27]

NUTRI NUGGET Chemistry, not fiber, makes prunes a good laxative. At 3 g per serving, prunes are a good source of fiber; however, this amount is insufficient to account for their laxative property, which they owe to a naturally occurring chemical.

Deficiencies

Although there is no "deficiency disease" as such, a lack of adequate insoluble fiber appears to increase the risk of certain conditions.[6] Because insoluble fiber softens the stool and increases bulk, it effectively prevents constipation, which appears to play a role in the development of colon cancer and diverticulosis. Theoretically, the longer potentially carcinogenic substances contained in feces remain in the colon, the more opportunity they have to damage the intestinal lining.[6] Diverticulosis is a condition in which the muscles of the colon weaken, forming small pouches that can become painfully inflamed (diverticulitis) if food residue gets trapped within them. It often occurs in people who are chronically constipated. Researchers believe the exercise involved in moving bulky fiber residue along the gastrointestinal tract keeps it in good shape.[36] The jury is still out, however, with respect to how much fiber is needed to prevent these diseases and what, if any, other dietary factors may be involved. No disease has been associated with a dietary deficiency of soluble fiber.

NUTRI NUGGET Refined fiber? Yes! Bran, for example, is refined from the whole grain and is therefore missing nutrients contained in the whole grain.

Excesses

What happens if I take fiber supplements?   Clearly, there are health benefits associated with consuming moderate quantities of fiber. However, you should use fiber supplements only under medical supervision, because excesses of dietary fiber have been found to decrease mineral absorption, and too much insoluble fiber can cause diarrhea.

IN THE BODY: GLUCOSE AS FUEL

Why does my body need glucose? What does it do for me?   The primary function of carbohydrate is to provide the cells with their preferred fuel, glucose. The absence of glucose sends a general alarm to the body, signaling an energy crisis. Because both protein and lipid are fuel sources, this may seem to be an exaggerated response. The reason for the urgency is that glucose is essential for some tissues and nothing else will do.

A small amount of glucose is stored in the liver as glycogen. This provides a readily available source of blood glucose for the entire body. By contrast, the small amount of glycogen stored in muscle tissue is available only to the cell in which it is stored. Together these glycogen stores amount to about 400 g, or 1600 kcalories of potential energy.

NUTRI NUGGET

Seven tissues that absolutely require glucose:
1. **Pancreatic beta cells, which produce insulin**
2. **Red blood cells**
3. **Mucosa of the small intestine**
4. **Kidney tubules**
5. **Nervous tissue neurons**
6. **Retina**
7. **Skeletal muscle, working *anaerobically***

Deficiencies

What happens if I don't have enough blood glucose?

Because both too little and too much glucose are harmful, blood levels are maintained within a narrow range through the opposing action of the hormones *insulin* and **glucagon.** Insulin, which is released from the pancreas when blood glucose levels are high, helps the cells absorb glucose, thereby lowering the blood glucose level. When blood glucose levels fall beneath the acceptable limit **(hypoglycemia),** the pancreas releases glucagon, which stimulates degradation of liver glycogen to glucose. If the fuel crisis persists and the glycogen supply has been depleted, the body will begin to form glucose from protein and glycerol by a process known as *gluconeogenesis.* Either dietary or *endogenous* sources can supply the protein and glycerol used to make glucose.

How does my body decide whether it should make glucose from dietary or endogenous sources?

The human body requires about 100 g of carbohydrates each day for glucose production. If carbohydrate intake falls below this level, your body will first try to use dietary protein and fat to meet its energy needs. If none is present, your body will then use its own tissues for energy. Soluble body proteins, such as plasma proteins, enzymes, and antibodies, are the most vulnerable in this regard. If the glucose shortage is prolonged, your body will eventually metabolize muscle and organ proteins as well. Because protein is not used to produce glucose when carbohydrate is available, it is often said that "carbohydrate spares protein."

Ketosis and Reactive Hypoglycemia

Unlike protein, fat is intended to be used as an energy source. In the absence of carbohydrates, however, fat is not an efficient fuel. Of the 50-some carbons in the typical fat molecule, only three (glycerol) can be used to regenerate glucose; the remaining carbons (all fatty acids) yield energy but no glucose. Without a source of carbohydrate, however, these remaining fatty acids are an inefficient source of energy. This is because they cannot be completely burned (oxidized) without some carbohydrates to kindle the cell's fuel burning process. Instead intermediary products, known as **ketone bodies** or ***ketones,*** accumulate in the blood, producing a condition called **ketosis.** Ketosis occurs whenever cells are starved for carbohydrates. Consequently, this condition has been observed in untreated diabetes (without insulin, cells lack adequate glucose), during starvation, and in people who consume diets very low in carbohydrates.

Symptoms of ketosis include fruity-smelling breath, decreased appetite, increased urination, and thirst. Over the years a number of carbohydrate-free diets have been designed to take advantage of the possible capacity of ketosis to suppress appetite. The body's attempt to cleanse itself by excreting the ketones in urine, however, can lead to involuntary dehydration.[23] Adults can survive in a ketotic state for prolonged periods of time, but it is a dangerous metabolic condition for young infants and children. High levels of ketones can damage young brains. If it occurs during pregnancy, ketosis can irreversibly damage the fetal brain.

How do people know whether they have hypoglycemia?

Hypoglycemia has been a popular—and misused—term for many years. People often diagnose themselves as being hypoglycemic if they feel tired and lightheaded. It is important to realize that hypoglycemia (low blood sugar) is a symptom, not a disease. At one time or another, all of us have experienced the effects of hypoglycemia (dizziness, headache, muscle weakness, and tremors). These symptoms often occur when a person is not eating properly and his/her body is already taxed by lack of rest, overwork, emotional stress, or a mild illness. Hypoglycemia typically can be "cured" by eating, and future episodes can be prevented by learning to eat regularly timed, well-balanced meals. Many health experts believe that breakfast is the most important meal in this regard (Fig. 4-8). This is because the liver glycogen used to maintain blood glucose levels during sleep is nearly gone by morning, causing blood glucose to fall to the low end of its normal range. Eating a good breakfast provides a quick

---

endogenous produced or caused by factors within the body

gluconeogenesis the synthesis of glucose from noncarbohydrate sources

ketones a breakdown product of fatty acid catabolism

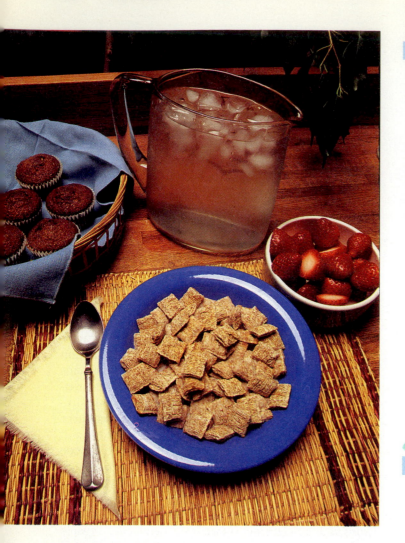

FIGURE 4-8 Start your day off right with a healthy breakfast.

source of energy and replenishes glycogen stores. People who get up and get going without eating breakfast are running on an empty fuel tank. Not surprisingly, they report a high incidence of hypoglycemic symptoms by midday. This transient and treatable condition is referred to as **reactive hypoglycemia** because it occurs as a reaction to insufficient food. In rare instances people develop a serious condition known as **spontaneous hypoglycemia.**[23] (For more details, see the Errors in Carbohydrate Metabolism section of the chapter.)

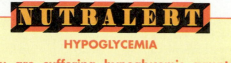

NUTRALERT

HYPOGLYCEMIA

If you are suffering hypoglycemic symptoms that are not cured by eating, seek immediate medical attention!

Excesses

What about a high blood sugar level?
Simply eating a lot of sugar or starch won't lead to dangerously high blood sugar levels. Hormones maintain a fairly constant blood sugar level by moving excess glucose into cells for storage as glycogen or fat. A chronically elevated blood sugar (glucose) level, such as occurs in diabetes, signals a serious metabolic problem.

Recent research points to an association between a high ratio of refined to unrefined carbohydrates and the development of health problems such as obesity, non-insulin-dependent diabetes, and cardiovascular disease.[13] However, other factors such as dietary fat intake, heredity, and stress also must be considered when analyzing the cause of these diseases.

Errors in Carbohydrate Metabolism

Some people are born with genetic abnormalities of carbohydrate metabolism. These conditions are diagnosed by medical professionals and typically require dietary adjustments. Recall from the section on digestion that the pancreas produces the hormones insulin and glucagon as well as a variety of digestive enzymes. Consequently, any disease or dysfunction of this organ has profound effects on carbohydrate metabolism.

Diabetes

What is diabetes?
Diabetes, or more properly **diabetes mellitus,** is a disorder of blood glucose regulation. It is caused by inadequacy or ineffectiveness of insulin. There are two major types of diabetes. **Insulin-dependent (Type 1) diabetes** is an *auto-immune* disease in which the body stops making insulin. It occurs more frequently in children and young adults, affecting 1 in every 200 people in this age bracket. People with Type 1 diabetes require daily insulin injections for life along with a carefully monitored diet and exercise program. **Noninsulin-dependent (Type 2) diabetes,** the more common form of the disease (accounting for 90% of all cases), is a metabolic disorder that results from the body's inability to make sufficient insulin and/or to use properly the insulin it does make. Weight loss, diet, and exercise are often the only treatment required. Some people may need oral antihyperglycemic drugs (medications that lower blood sugar) or insulin injections to get their symptoms under control. Type 2 symptoms often disappear once the patient loses weight. A normal blood sugar level, however, does not mean the disease is cured—only that it is in remission. Persons with Type 2 diabetes must be vigilant about keeping off extra pounds to prevent a recurrence of symptoms.[10,23]

Who is at risk?
Anyone who is over age 30 and overweight and/or has a family history of diabetes is at risk for developing the condition. Other risk categories

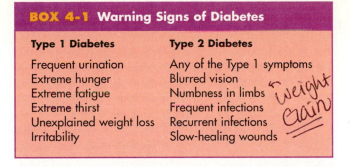

BOX 4-1 Warning Signs of Diabetes

Type 1 Diabetes	Type 2 Diabetes
Frequent urination	Any of the Type 1 symptoms
Extreme hunger	Blurred vision
Extreme fatigue	Numbness in limbs
Extreme thirst	Frequent infections
Unexplained weight loss	Recurrent infections
Irritability	Slow-healing wounds

Weight Gain [handwritten annotation]

include women who have had a baby weighing more than 9 pounds at birth, African-American heritage (risk is 1.6 times greater than general population), Hispanic heritage[31] (more than twice the risk), and Native American heritage (2.7 times the risk). According to the American Diabetes Association, as of 1993 more than 13 million Americans have diabetes but over half of them are unaware of it.[41] If you have any of the warning signs of diabetes (Box 4-1), check with your physician or student health center.

How can diabetes be controlled through diet?

The key to treating diabetes is to keep blood glucose at a constant and moderate level using a carefully planned diet and, if necessary, medication. Using a menu planning guide known as the Diabetic Exchange Lists, dietitians help clients with diabetes develop a meal plan that specifies how much of which types of food (exchanges) can be eaten at each meal and snack.

When the Diabetic Exchange Lists were first developed, diabetes was believed to be a disease of carbohydrate metabolism, so they emphasized controlling the intake of all carbohydrate-rich foods. Today health experts know that diabetes is a disease of energy metabolism in general and that a diet rich in complex carbohydrates but with small amounts of sugar is the key to controlling blood glucose levels.[18,28]

The most recent version of the Diabetic Exchange Lists separates individual foods into six lists: milk, vegetable, fruit, bread, meat, and fat. The milk, starch, and meat lists are further divided to identify high-, medium-, and low-fat food choices. The reason for dividing foods into these lists is that food items vary with respect to their carbohydrate, protein, fat, and kcalorie content. The foods in each Exchange List have roughly the same amounts of nutrients and kcalories, which makes it easy to exchange one food for another within a given list (Table 4-6 and Appendix C). For example, one slice of bread and ½ cup of cooked rice are considered to be nutritionally equivalent. Because each Exchange List contains a wide variety of foods, people with diabetes have considerable leeway in developing their own menus. The Exchange Lists concept has proved so successful in treating diabetes that versions have been developed for losing weight and treating kidney disease.[5]

Spontaneous Hypoglycemia

As with diabetes, the primary symptom of hypoglycemia is an error of glucose metabolism. However, this condition differs from diabetes in two important ways. First, blood sugar levels of persons with hypoglycemia are too low rather than too high, as in diabetes. Second, unlike diabetes, hypoglycemia is not a disease itself but a manifestation of other diseases or conditions. In rare instances people develop a severe form of hypoglycemia known as **spontaneous** or **fasting hypoglycemia.** This condition results from an underlying disease state, such as stimulation of excessive insulin production by a pancreatic tumor. No matter how much people with spontaneous hypoglycemia eat, their blood sugar remains too low. If they go for a long period without food, their blood sugar may drop so low that their energy-starved brain loses consciousness. Clearly this is a life-threatening condition that requires immediate medical treatment.

Carbohydrate recap. Table 4-7 reviews the body's handling of dietary carbohydrates. In the digestive tract, starches and sugars are broken down to their monosaccharide "building blocks." The liberated monosaccharides are then absorbed and transported to

---

autoimmune any of a number of diseases in which the body's immune system attacks body tissues

insulin hormones produced by specialized pancreatic cells and required for conversion of food to energy

---

TABLE 4–6 Exchange Lists					
List	Serving Size	g Carbohydrate	g Protein	g Fat	kcal
Starch/bread	½ cup, 1 slice	**15**	3	trace	80
Fruit	Varies	**15**	trace	trace	60
Milk	8 oz nonfat	**12**	8	trace	90
Vegetable	½ cup cooked	**5**	2	trace	25
Meat*	1 oz lean	0	7	3	55
Fat	1 tsp	0	0	5	45

TABLE 4–7   Review of Carbohydrate Digestion, Absorption, and Utilization

Structure	Carbohydrate
Mouth	Teeth crush fibers; salivary amylase digests starches.
Stomach	Hydrochloric acid stops amylase.
Small intestine	Pancreatic amylases digest starch to disaccharides; intestinal disaccharidases produce monosaccharides.
	Absorbed: **glucose, galactose, fructose**
Circulatory system	Portal vein carries blood and absorbed nutrients from intestinal wall to liver.
Liver	Enzymes change fructose and galactose to **glucose;** stores glycogen.
Cells	Burn (oxidize) glucose to carbon dioxide and water, producing ATP and heat; muscle cells store some glycogen; adipose cells store remainder as fat (triglycerides).
Large intestine	Bacteria ferment most soluble fiber; excretes undigested material.

the liver, where they are transformed into glucose and released into the general circulation. Glucose is used primarily to supply the body with fuel. It also may be synthesized into glycogen or fat.[23]

IN TODAY'S WORLD

Humankind's success at harnessing solar power (photosynthesis) through agriculture is believed to have been a key to the development of organized civilization. Agricultural practices, however, have not always been wise.[21] New insights into the interdependence of animals and plants and how to maintain the "cycling of minerals, water, and the flow of energy through the food chain"[32] provide substantial promise of reclaiming manmade deserts, preserving existing arable land, and preventing further destruction of native plant life.

Processing

How does processing affect carbohydrates?   Processing tends to reduce the **nutrient density** of carbohydrate-rich foods. Decreasing a food's nutrient density, however, does not always involve removing nutrients. Adding "empty calories" to a food produces the same results by diluting existing nutrients. For example, adding sugar to canned fruit or using oil to turn an ordinary potato into potato chips increases the food's kcalorie content, yet the nutrient level remains the same. Thus the ratio of nutrients to kcalories (the nutrient density) decreases.

Refining (*re*-fine = *re*-move)

Sugar is extracted from sugarcane and sugar beets through a process that purifies the sucrose molecule.

This is accomplished by removing all of the starch, fiber, minerals, and vitamins. Not surprisingly, the resulting refined sugar is considered "empty calories." Using a similar process, starch is refined from a variety of carbohydrates, including wheat, corn, soy, and arrowroot, for use as a thickening agent in processed foods. Each type of starch has different thickening properties. Some cook with minimal heat, which is nice for delicate dishes; some become clear when cooked, which gives fruit dishes an appealing glossy appearance; others freeze well. Cooking courses and cookbooks provide the home chef detailed information on the use of the various starches. Recently food manufacturers have begun to use chemically modified food starches as fat substitutes in a variety of processed foods. These products provide the moisture and smooth feel usually achieved with fat.

a. Which of the nutrients in Fig. 4-9 are carbohydrates?

b. The fat-soluble vitamins E and K are found in the germ of the wheat grain. What happens to the germ during refining?

c. Which vitamins are significantly (two thirds) lower in refined *enriched* flour?

d. Which minerals are significantly lower in refined *enriched* flour?

Like sugar and starch, whole grains are refined to make white flour. This process, which removes the fiber-rich **bran** and the vitamin-rich **germ,** leaves mainly the powdery, white starch of the **endosperm.**

To combat the deficiency diseases that occurred when people ate nutrient-poor refined white flour products, Congress passed the Enrichment Act in 1942.[16] It requires the manufacturers of any flour or flour product that crosses state lines to add back three of the B-complex vitamins (niacin, thiamin, and riboflavin) plus the mineral iron at the same levels in which they were present before refining. Not replaced, however, are fiber

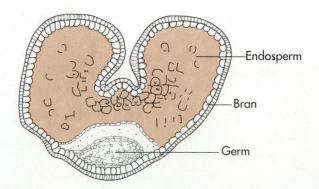

FIGURE 4-9 The refining process removes vitamins, nutrients, and dietary fiber from whole wheat.

and many other vitamins and minerals. The result is a major source of kcalories that is much lower in nutrient density than the whole grain from which it was derived (Fig. 4-10).

White rice, instant oatmeal, refined cornmeal, and instant mashed potatoes are additional examples of the many refined carbohydrates available to American consumers. Although these foods are refined, there is no standard for their enrichment. Because refining significantly decreases the nutrient density of carbohydrates, the Food Guide Pyramid recommends the use of whole-grain products whenever possible to fulfill the recommended daily servings of foods from the grain/cereal group.

Sugar Substitutes

Both synthetic and natural sugar substitutes are widely available. Synthetic sweeteners are produced in laboratories, using chemical reactions that would not typically occur. Natural sweeteners, on the other hand, are refined from foods.[2]

Synthetic sweeteners are used by people with diabetes and by people who want to eat sweets but not gain weight. These products are helpful for controlling diabetes but are of dubious value in weight control, as illustrated by the fact that consumption of sugar-free products is at an all-time high, as is the weight of the average American. Three synthetic sweeteners are currently in use in the United States: saccharin, aspartame, and acesulfame-K.

Saccharin is the oldest kcalorie-free synthetic sweetener. First introduced in the 1890s, it has survived many challenges regarding its safety. It is used predominantly in soft drinks and as a substitute for sugar at the table (Sweet-n-Low®).

Aspartame (Equal® or Nutrasweet™), a relative newcomer, has replaced saccharin as the synthetic sweetener of choice. Several factors account for its popularity, the most significant being that it tastes almost like real sugar (sucrose). It is made of two amino acids commonly found in foods, which gives the impression that it is "natural." Because it is composed of

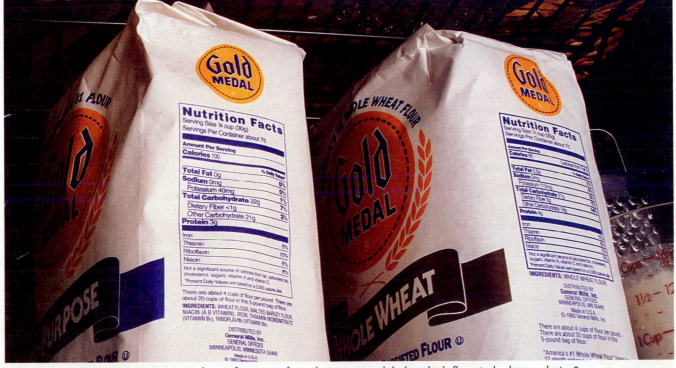

FIGURE 4-10 Based on information from their nutrition labels, which flour is the better choice?

amino acids, it contains 4 kcalories per gram, as would any protein. But because it is 200 times sweeter than sugar, a tiny amount goes a long way, adding up to big kcalorie savings. For example, a 12-ounce soft drink contains about 10 teaspoons or 160 kcalories of sugar, whereas the same drink sweetened with aspartame contains less than 2 kcalories.

Aspartame has only one drawback: it loses its sweetness when cooked at very high temperatures. However, aspartame's manufacturer has developed a way to slow this reaction at temperatures typically used in baking,[4,20] so you will soon see some new sugar-free products in the grocery store.

From a metabolic standpoint, aspartame appears to be relatively safe except for people who have phenylketouria (PKU), an inborn error of metabolism. Aspartame is made from phenylalanine, an essential amino acid, which they cannot metabolize.

Acesulfame-K (Sunette™), approved by the FDA in 1989, is the newest entry to the sweetener market. It is kcalorie-free and, unlike Nutrasweet, it can be used in cooking. It has been tested for 15 years in Europe and the United States and used for 5 years abroad.

The **sugar alcohols,** sorbitol, xylitol, and mannitol, are natural sugar substitutes. Tiny amounts of sugar al-

cohol occur naturally in fruits and vegetables as a result of **fermentation** of simple sugars. Large amounts are produced commercially for use in "dietetic" candies, confections, and "sugar-free" gum.

Like other carbohydrates, sugar alcohols contain 4 kcalories per gram. **Xylitol,** which is about half as sweet as sucrose, is used extensively in gum. **Sorbitol** and **mannitol,** which are even less sweet, are used more frequently in candies and confections. Unfortunately, the quantity required to sweeten these products makes a significant kcalorie contribution. The terms "dietetic" and "sugar-free", which were used to describe foods that contain sugar alcohols, were deceiving to most consumers, who tended to equate these statements with reduced-kcalorie foods. The major advantage of sugar alcohols is that bacteria cannot use them as a food source, so they reduce tooth decay. Other than the added kcalories, the major disadvantage of these sweeteners is that they cause many people to experience diarrhea. Understandably, this characteristic has limited their commercial value.[2] A Closer Look below reviews the safety of some sugar substitutes.

What general statement can be made about the nutrient density of artificial sweeteners?

A CLOSER LOOK

Sugar Substitutes: How Much Is Too Much?

Since their introduction to the American food supply, the use of sugar substitutes (also called nonnutritive sweeteners) has increased dramatically and is expected to continue growing rapidly well into the 1990s. Although they are widely used, many people question their safety. Just how much is too much is a common concern.

According to a report by the American Dietetic Association, the news on sugar substitutes is sweet music to the consumer's ears. Sugar substitutes, like other food additives, must undergo years of rigorous testing and meet strict FDA safety guidelines before they can be marketed. Beginning with aspartame (NutraSweet™) the FDA started to establish acceptable daily intake (ADI) levels for sugar substitutes. The ADI is defined as the amount of a food additive that can be safely consumed on a daily basis over a person's lifetime without adverse effects. It includes a 100-fold safety factor, so even if a person were to reach the ADI for a particular additive, s/he would still be well within the range of safe intake.

The ADI for aspartame is 50 mg/kg of body weight. To meet this level of intake, a 150-pound adult would need to consume 97 packets of aspartame-containing table-top sweetener or drink twelve 12-ounce cans of diet soft drinks. A 50-

pound child would need to drink seven cans of the same soft drink or use 32 packets of table-top sweetener. Aspartame appears to be very safe. No adverse effects have been observed with long-term consumption or in studies in which people were given three to four times this amount of aspartame all at once. Nonetheless, because aspartame is present in cereals, yogurt, fruit-flavored drinks, gelatin desserts, puddings, frozen yogurt, and so on, parents of very young children should make sure they are not consuming excessive amounts of this product.

The ADI for acesulfame-K (Sunette™) is 15 mg/kg body weight. A 150-pound person can consume 36 teaspoons without any ill effects. The ADI for sucralose is the same. An ADI was never established for saccharin, but at the time of its introduction in 1955 recommended consumption limits were 500 mg a day for children and 1000 mg a day for adults. Actual consumption was less than 100 mg a day (or 2½ packages of Sweet 'n' Low). At this level, saccharin is believed to be quite safe.

In general, sugar substitutes are safe to consume, but they should be used in moderation as part of a nutritious, well-balanced diet. Scientific monitoring of sugar substitute intake should continue to ensure that intake levels do not exceed acceptable limits as new types are introduced to the market and new uses are developed for existing products.

Data from the American Dietetic Association: Use of nutritive and nonnutritive sweeteners, *Journal of the American Dietetic Association* 93(7):816-821, 1993.

IN MY DIET

What diet meets my carbohydrate needs? The Dietary Guidelines recommend that you consume 6 to 11 servings of grain products and 5 to 11 servings of produce each day.[13,14] Because these serving sizes are relatively small, fitting these foods into your diet is easier than you might think.

At the Grocery Store

What should I shop for? Students of nutrition frequently ask: "If animals store glucose in their tissues as glycogen, why aren't meats a good source of dietary carbohydrate?" First of all, the amount of glycogen that animals, or for that matter humans, can store is relatively small. The entire body contains only a couple of hours' worth of energy in the form of glycogen. Second, any glycogen that was present in an animal's tissues is depleted when the animal is fasted or frightened before slaughter.

Dairy Decisions

Milk, on the other hand, provides a significant amount of dietary carbohydrate in the form of the milk sugar lactose. Unfortunately, once past childhood, many people and most animals lose the ability to digest lactose. As a result, much of the lactose in dairy products passes through the intestine undigested, causing cramping, gas, bloating, and diarrhea.

Some lactose-intolerant people find they can eat certain dairy products without taking any precautions. Others react adversely to even the tiny amounts of milk solids used in many processed foods. Often people with a relatively mild form of lactose intolerance can successfully drink a single glass of milk with meals. People with more severe cases of lactose intolerance who still wish to use dairy products as a source of calcium have several options.[7,25] They can:

1. Buy commercially prepared lactose-free milk and dairy products
2. Use hard cheese (most of the lactose is lost in the whey, discarded during cheese making) or yogurt made with live cultures (the bacteria that transform milk into yogurt digest the lactose)
3. Purchase lactase tablets and consume them with dairy products
4. Buy lactase in liquid form and add it to milk to predigest lactose

People who are highly sensitive to lactose may need to avoid milk products whenever possible. This means they must carefully scan the labels of prepared foods for evidence of milk or milk products. In addition to milk, some of the terms that signal the presence of lactose are whey, nonfat milk solids, casein, and sodium caseinate. To meet their daily calcium requirement, lactose-intolerant people can substitute fruit juices that have been fortified with highly absorbable calcium citrate, or they can use calcium supplements.

NUTRI QUIZ
a. Why do some people lose the ability to manufacture lactase?
b. Do lactose-intolerant people have to avoid all dairy products?

Pick of the Produce

Fruits and vegetables enhance the diet by adding natural sweetness, satisfying crunch, complex carbohydrates, and fiber. Eat a varied selection of produce daily and be sure to use the food label placards in the produce department to help you make the most of your fruit and vegetable choices.

Breads, Baked Goods, Cereals, and Grains

When shopping for baked goods, breads, cereals, grains, and snacks, whenever possible select whole-grain versions of these items. Improve your dessert selections by choosing oatmeal cookies, graham crackers, and whole wheat fruit Newtons. And before you take a product home, remember to *read the labels!* The tips in the next section will help you improve your carbohydrate shopping IQ.

Labels—Your License To Learn

Until recently, it took considerable detective work to confirm the presence of complex carbohydrates as well as ferret out fiber and sugars in processed foods. There is still no substitute for reading labels; thanks to the food label changes introduced in mid-1994, however, being a savvy carbohydrate consumer is easier than ever.

Federal law now requires food manufacturers to reveal how much of the total carbohydrate content of their foods is sugar. They also must clearly report their product's fiber content. There are strict limitations on the kinds of health and nutrition claims that can be made on the labels. Perhaps you have noticed that your favorite "healthy" cereal no longer proclaims its sugar-free status on the front of the package.[8,16,40]

Does this mean the manufacturer has changed the formulation? Probably not! Chances are that the sugar was always there, masquerading under a different name. Before May 1993, the FDA defined the term *sugar* as sucrose or table sugar. Now all sugars are considered to be sugar, regardless of their common name. Their presence must be noted on the label's nutrient content panel.

fermentation the enzymatic decomposition of organic material, especially carbohydrates

Claims like "no added sugar" also must be used more precisely. Traditionally, "no added sugar" meant that no *sucrose* was added. The food source itself, however, may have been naturally high in sugar, or it may have contained sugar-laden ingredients like dried fruits and concentrated fruit juices. Today "no sugar added" means just that: no sugar of any kind has been added.

What are these other sources of sugar? The six technical names you have already learned for sugar are not the only terms used to identify it on food labels. Sugar has many aliases but, as Shakespeare said about roses, a sugar by any name is still sweet. Box 4-2 lists alternative terms for sugar that are commonly found in the ingredient section of food labels.

Now that the sugar content of foods is easy to identify, you may want to see how much is in the foods you are currently consuming. Remember that sugar is added to many prepared foods for both its flavor and its preservative properties. This means consumers who need to lower their sugar intake must check every label, even for foods that do not taste sweet, like dill pickles, tomato sauce, canned vegetables, ketchup, and mustard. You undoubtedly will find sugar in some surprising places. See the Pyramid Food Choices Chart in Appendix D to get an idea of the foods in which sugar hides.

NUTRI QUIZ See how many foods you can find in your kitchen cabinets that contain sugar.

There was a time when the makers of foods that contained tiny amounts of fiber could get away with calling the products "fiber-rich." Thanks to the revised labeling laws, a food's fiber content must be clearly displayed, and only foods that supply 20% or more of an adult's daily fiber intake can be identified as "high fiber." To be promoted as a "source of fiber," a food must supply at least 10% of the recommended daily intake of fiber.

Laws help, but consumers still need to exercise good judgment. Just because a food contains fiber doesn't mean it is a nutritious product. During the 1980s, eating fiber-rich foods became a popular health fad. Manufacturers were quick to jump on the bandwagon, adding fiber to virtually everything. Many of these products are still being marketed, but the revised labeling laws can help consumers realize that they often get less fiber than they bargained for. In some instances the health benefits of the fiber are outweighed by hefty doses of sugar and fat. To get a true picture of a food's nutritional value, read the entire Nutrition Facts panel on the product package (Fig. 4-11).

BOX 4-2 Labeling Terms for Sugar

Syrup	Honey
Levulose (fructose)	Fructose
Dextrose (glucose)	Dried fruit
FruitSource™	Fruit juice concentrate
Sorbitol	Xylitol
	Glucose

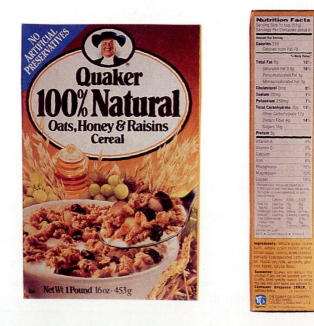

FIGURE 4-11 Healthful-sounding names, pictures that conjure up images of nutritious meals, and food coloring are just a few of the many ploys used by food manufacturers to make their products appear wholesome.

In the Kitchen

How important are cooking and preparation techniques? If potatoes, corn, toast, and brownies are the extent of your carbohydrate cookery, it is time to expand your repertoire with some quick-to-fix, fiber-rich foods. Many cooks shy away from preparing whole grains because of the time involved. They may be pleased to know that new technology has yielded a brown rice that can be cooked in 20 rather than 50 minutes, without sacrificing fiber content.

There are a host of other quick-fix, whole-grain products available. Among them are bulgur wheat pilaf, which can be fixed in 15 minutes, and whole-wheat couscous (Fig. 4-12), which cooks in 5 minutes. For variety, pilafs can be prepared with a mixture of brown rice, barley, and an exotic, ancient Peruvian grain, quinoa. Many of these grains are equally tasty served cold. Look for them in the health or gourmet food section of your grocery store. Box 4-3 lists the characteristics and uses of several kinds of grains.

Dried legumes still take time to prepare, but canned varieties are widely available and, like grains, can be served hot or cold. Many people avoid legumes because of their famed flatulence-producing quality. Cooks who invest the time in preparing legumes, however, can remove a significant amount of the oligosaccharides by using the recipe on p. 64.

A new product, Beano™, produced by the company that makes Lactaid™, has been developed to eliminate the gas-producing substances in beans as well as many vegetables and grains. The early response has been overwhelmingly positive, and preliminary studies indicate the product is effective.[37] A more thorough investigation is under way to confirm its effectiveness.

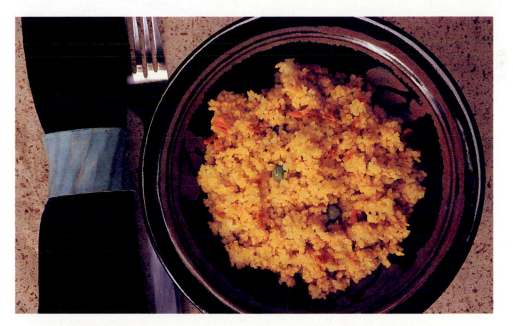

FIGURE 4-12 Whole-wheat couscous is a quick-to-fix, fiber-rich grain.

BOX 4-3 Getting To Know Grains

Grain	Color	Flavor	Uses
Amaranth	Golden	Cornlike	Porridge with maple syrup topping
Barley	Pearl	Nutty	Soups and salads
Buckwheat	Brown	Nutty	Porridge, flour
Bulgur	Golden	Nutty	Salads, pilaf
Couscous	Tan	Buttery	Bed for stews or salads
Kasha (roasted buckwheat)	Dark brown	Nutty	Pilaf
Millet	Ivory	Mild buttery	Bed for stews
Quinoa	Tan	Mild nutty	Use in place of rice

A ¾ cup serving of any of these grains contains about 150 kcalories, 1 g of fat, 4 g of protein, 30 g of carbohydrate, and less than 10 mg of sodium.
Bulgur and couscous are different forms of crushed wheat. Couscous is the finer ground of the two.

Polite Legumes

1. Place beans in a large pot.

2. Cover with water.

3. Heat to a rapid boil.

4. Turn off the heat and allow the beans to stand in the water for 20 minutes.

5. Discard the cooking water. (Do not save this water for soup.)

6. Repeat steps 1 through 5 two more times.

7. Finish cooking the beans according to the recipe of choice.

You can eliminate many of the gas-producing substances in legumes.

Banana Bread

BANANA BREAD
2 cups flour
³⁄₄ cup sugar
¹⁄₄ tsp salt
1 tsp baking soda
2 eggs
¹⁄₂ cup shortening
2 cups banana pulp
¹⁄₂ cup chopped nuts

SUBSTITUTE
1 cup each white and whole-wheat flour
¹⁄₂ cup honey

Sift dry ingredients together. Blend banana, eggs, and shortening. Gradually add dry ingredients to banana mixture, beating after each addition until smooth. Fold in chopped nuts. Turn into greased loaf pan. Bake at 350° F for 50 minutes or until a toothpick inserted in the center comes out dry. Cool 5 minutes before removing from pan.

You can use less sugar without altering the taste of the final product.

Recipe Revisions

Sugar content typically can be reduced by about 25% without appreciably affecting the taste of a baked product.

Another sugar-saving strategy is to replace table sugar with honey or granulated fructose (available in health food stores). Because both of these sugars are sweeter than sucrose, you can use less without altering the flavor of the finished product. By experimenting, you can replace all of the sugar in a recipe with honey, but you need to make some alterations:

- Reduce the amount of liquid in the recipe by $\frac{1}{4}$ cup for each cup of honey used.
- Add $\frac{1}{2}$ teaspoon of baking soda for each cup of honey used.
- Reduce oven temperature by 25° F.

Cookie and quick bread recipes can benefit further from replacement of half of the white flour with fiber-rich whole-wheat flour. Or you can look for recipes that use oatmeal in place of some of the white flour. The revised banana bread recipe shown on p. 64 illustrates how to put these principles into practice.

Healthful eating does not mean giving up dessert. Every-one deserves an occasional splurge. If you eat dessert routinely, you can improve its nutritional value by decreasing sugar and increasing fiber in many of your favorite recipes.

At the Table

The following suggestions can help you reduce sugar and boost fiber intake:

- Serve sugar-free breakfast cereals.
- Break the habit of adding sugar to foods before tasting them.
- Add only a tiny amount of sugar at a time.
- Envision your plate as a circle, two thirds of which is covered by complex carbohydrates and one third by animal-derived foods.
- Serve meat on top of or mixed with carbohydrates (for example, meatballs and spaghetti or turkey casserole)
- Serve whole-grain bread with meals.
- Take the old cliché of "an apple a day" one step further by adding a salad a day to your diet.
- Serve fresh fruit for snacks and desserts.
- Choose healthier baked products such as oatmeal cookies, whole-wheat fruit Newtons, or banana bread.

Eating Out

Sometimes Mom misses the mark! One old warning you no longer have to heed is, "Don't fill up on bread be-cause you won't have room for your dinner." Actually, eating unbuttered bread before dinner is a good way to take the edge off your appetite so you don't over-indulge. So the next time you are eating out, help yourself to the predinner bread—guilt free.

If the meal you select looks low in carbohydrates, add a salad or side order of vegetables, and don't be shy about asking to substitute a nutrient-rich baked potato for a less nutrient-dense carbohydrate, such as mashed potatoes or french fries. Remember to request whole-grain breads when ordering sandwiches or burgers.

Menu Matrix

Review the serving size information that accompanies the Food Guide Pyramid in Chapter 2. If you have not already done so, estimate how many servings of grain products and produce you are currently consuming and how much sugar you add to your diet. Compare what you are eating currently with what you should be eating using the Personalizing the Pyramid section of Chapter 2. Then turn to the Menu Matrix form (Appendix D) to help you organize your choices.

Before you get started, note that the matrix is for a week's worth of menus. There are two reasons for this. First, many dietary recommendations are given on a weekly rather than daily basis. The RDA, for instance, are an average of several days' intakes, not just one.

Second, we need to think about our long-term intake. Monotony, such as getting all our grain from six slices of bread every day of our life, can cause even the most dedicated of us to revert to poor eating habits.

When planning your diet, remember:

1. Starchy vegetables, such as potatoes, corn, or winter squashes can be substituted for grain.
2. About two thirds of each meal should be composed of carbohydrate-rich foods like grains, legumes, and produce.
3. High-fiber whole grains are better than enriched products.

If you are still having trouble fitting carbohydrates into your diet, consider planning your meals around the grain you intend to serve rather than around the meat dish, as most Americans do.

Two days of sample menus, which include plans for three main meals and at least two snacks per day, are presented in the NutriQuiz on p. 66. Note that people will choose various amounts of sweeteners, spreads, and salad dressings to increase kcalorie intake. Use these menus for inspiration when planning your own carbohydrate-rich meals.

a. Identify sources of carbohydrate in the Day 1 and Day 2 menus in the accompanying table.
b. Do these menus contain any legumes?
c. How many Food Guide Pyramid servings of grain products are included in each day's menu?
d. If you are trying to increase your carbohydrate consumption, should you drink more milk or eat more grains and produce? Why?

Day 1 Menu		**Day 2 Menu**
1 cup oatmeal 2 slices whole wheat toast Low-fat milk Melon	**Breakfast**	2 slices whole wheat toast Low-fat milk Hard boiled egg Orange juice
1 banana 1 whole wheat bagel with low-fat cream cheese	**Snack**	Nectarine Fat-free apple bran muffin
Peanut butter sandwich on 2 slices of whole wheat bread Carrot, pepper, celery sticks Apple Milk	**Lunch**	Vegetable soup with kidney beans Turkey sandwich with sprouts Tomato slices on whole wheat bread Milk Pear
2 whole wheat peach Newtons Low-fat milk	**Snack**	Oatmeal cookie, 4 dried apple rings, Low-fat milk
Spinach salad Carrots and zucchini Salmon Baby potatoes Dinner roll Mineral water Frozen nonfat yogurt with fresh fruit topping	**Dinner**	Mixed greens, carrot, and tomato salad Broccoli Breast of chicken 1 cup brown rice pilaf Bread sticks Mineral water Whole wheat banana bread

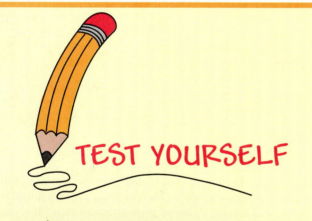

TEST YOURSELF

True or False. Put a **T** for true or an **F** for false in the space beside each question.

F 1. Fiber is an indigestible oligosaccharide.

T 2. Starch is made of chemically bonded glucose units.

F 3. Meat is an important source of glucose.

___ 4. Fructose, maltose, lipid, syrup, and concentrated fruit juice are all sources of sugar.

___ 5. The cells in your body use glucose for fuel.

___ 6. Many health experts think a good diet should get most of its kcalories from carbohydrates.

___ 7. Your body turns surplus sugars and starch into glycogen, which it stores in the liver and the muscle tissue.

___ 8. Eating a good breakfast helps your body replenish its glycogen stores.

Short Answer

___ 9. List the three common disaccharides in the American diet.

___10. Which food groups in the Food Guide Pyramid provide most of the carbohydrates in the American diet? Which foods should you eat more of to increase your fiber intake?

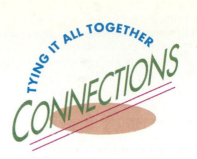

TYING IT ALL TOGETHER

CONNECTIONS

Ingredients: **whole barley, brown rice, wheat, oats, raisins, dates, fruit juice concentrate, brown sugar, almonds, corn, rice, salt, malt flavoring, rice bran**

CARBOHYDRATE INFORMATION:

Starch and related carbohydrates	17 g
Sucrose and other sugars	13 g
Dietary fiber	3 g
Total carbohydrate	33 g

1. Sample ingredient and carbohydrate content information panels from a commercially available cereal box appear below.

   a. How much sugar and starch does this product contain?

   b. Name the sources of sugar.

   c. How much fiber does this product contain?

   d. Which ingredients are good sources of soluble fiber?

   e. Which ingredients are good sources of insoluble fiber?

2. Below are the ingredients in three different brands of bread:

   Bread A: wheat flour, sugar, eggs, salt, and yeast

   Bread B: Unbleached enriched flour, honey, eggs, salt, and yeast

   Bread C: Whole wheat flour, sugar, eggs, salt, and yeast

   a. Which of these breads has the most sugar?

   b. Which has the most starch?

   c. Which has the most fiber?

   d. Which has the most vitamins and minerals? (See the In Today's World/Nutrient Density section.)

3. Which body stores and/or tissues are lost when dietary glucose is not available to the cells?

4. Which body tissue is gained when excessive amounts of dietary carbohydrate (glucose) are available?

5. What do you suppose would happen if the cells did not get glucose because of inadequate kcalorie intake (about 1000 to 1500 kcalories/day)?

REFERENCES

1. ADA Reports, Position of the American Dietetic Association: Health implications of dietary fiber, *Journal of the American Dietetic Association* 93(12):1446-1447, 1993.

2. ADA Reports, Position of the American Dietetic Association: Use of nutritive and nonnutritive sweeteners, *Journal of the American Dietetic Association* 93(7):816-821, 1993.

3. Anderson JW et al: Prospective, randomized, controlled comparison of the effects of low-fat and low-fat plus high-fiber diets on serum lipid concentrations, *American Journal of Clinical Nutrition* 56:887-894, 1992.

4. Aspartame update 1993, *Federal Register* 58:21097.

5. Diabetes mellitus. In *American Dietetic Association manual of clinical dietetics*, 387-413, 1990.

6. Bandaru SR et al: Effect of dietary fiber on colonic bacterial enzymes and bile acids in relation to colon cancer, *Gastroenterology* 102(5):1475-1482, 1992.

7. Brand JC: Reduced lactose milk curtails symptoms of lactose malabsorption, *American Journal of Clinical Nutrition* 54:148-154, 1991.

8. Browne MB: Label facts for healthful eating, American Dietetic Association, 1993, ADA & National Food Processors Association in cooperation with USDA.

9. Burkitt DH, Trowell HC: Refined carbohydrate foods and disease implications of dietary fiber, London, 1975, Academic Press.

10. Campbell PJ, Carlson MG: Impact of obesity on insulin action in NIDDM, *Diabetes* 42:405-410, 1993.

11. Colin CT: A study of diet, nutrition and disease in the People's Republic of China, Part 1, *Boletin-Asociacion Medica de Puerto Rico* 82(3):132-134, 1990.

12. Darby WJ, Jukes TH: *Founders of nutrition science*, vols 1 and 2, Rockville, Md, 1992, American Institute of Nutrition.

13. *Dietary guidelines for Americans*, 1990, U.S. Department of Health and Human Services, Home and Garden Bulletin #232.

14. Dietary guidelines for healthy American adults: A statement for physicians and health, Dallas, 1991, American Heart Association.

15. Evans MA, Shronts EP: Intestinal fuels: glutamine, short-chain fatty acids, and dietary fiber, *Journal of the American Dietetic Association* 92:1239-1246, 1992.

16. Focus on Food Labeling: an FDA Special Report, *FDA Consumer*, Rockville, Md, 1993.

17. Food labeling update: *Food Safety Notebook* 3(12):110-115, 1992.

18. Franz MJ: Avoiding sugar. Does research support traditional beliefs? *Diabetes Educator* 19:133-150, 1993.

19. How to get more fiber in your diet: patient information sheet, *Nutrition and the MD* 20(4), 1994.

20. For your information, *Journal of the American Dietetic Association*, 91(2):1511, 1991.

21. Gore A: Earth in the balance: ecology and the human spirit, Boston, 1991, Houghton Mifflin.

22. Gravetti L: Clash of cuisines: food patterns and medical-nutritional accounts from the new world 1492-1612, American Institute of Nutrition Annual Meeting, Anaheim, Calif, April 18, 1992.

23. Isselbacher KJ: *Harrison's Principles of Internal Medicine*, ed 12, New York, 1991, McGraw-Hill.

24. Healthy people 2000: National health promotion and disease prevention objectives, U.S. Department of Health and Human Services, Public Health Service Bulletin #91-50212, 1990.

25. Martini MC et al: Lactose digestion by yogurt B-lactosidose: influence of pH and microbial cell integrity, *American Journal of Clinical Nutrition* 45:432-430, 1987.

26. Moss S: Factors in caries formation (supplement), *Journal of the American Dietetic Association*, Oct 1992.

27. National Research Council: *Recommended Dietary Allowances*, ed 10, Washington, DC, 1989, National Academy Press.

28. National Research Council: *Report on diet and health: implications for reducing chronic disease risk*, Washington, DC, 1989, National Academy Press.

29. Poulter N et al: Oat bran and serum cholesterol revisited, *American Journal of Clinical Nutrition* 58:66-72, 1994.

30. Reiser S: Metabolic risk factors associated with heart disease and diabetes in carbohydrate-sensitive humans when consuming sucrose as compared with starch. In Reiser S, ed: *Metabolic effects of utilizable dietary carbohydrate*, New York, 1982, Marcel Dekker.

31. Royabal ER: Diabetes mellitus (NIDDM): an unrelenting but undeserved threat to the health of Hispanics, 1992, Select Committee on Aging, Committee Pub #102-844.

32. Savory A, quoted in Bingham S: Where animals save the land, *World Monitor*, Sept 1990, p. 38.

33. Scarre C: Smithosonian time lines of the ancient world, Washington, DC, 1993, Smithsonian Institution Press.

34. Senate Select Committee on Health: *The dietary goals for the United States*, ed 2, 1977.

35. Shaywitz BA et al: Aspartame, behavior, and cognitive function in children with attention deficit disorder, *Pediatrics* 93(1):70-75, 1994.

36. Snape WJ: Nutrition and chronic diverticular disease, *Nutrition and the MD* 20:1-3, 1994.

37. Solomens NW et al: Preliminary studies on the efficacy of Beano™, *American Journal of Clinical Nutrition* 53:12-28, 1991.

38. Szepesi B: Carbohydrates. In *Present knowledge in nutrition*, ed 6, Washington, DC, 1990, International Life Sciences Institute, Nutrition Foundation.

39. The Food Guide Pyramid, U.S. Department of Agriculture Home and Garden Bulletin #252, 1992.

40. The new food label, FDA backgrounder, BG 92-4, 1992.

41. The warning signs of diabetes, American Diabetic Association, 1993.

42. Wolraich ML et al: Effects of diets high in sucrose or aspartame on the behaviour and cognitive performance of children, *New England Journal of Medicine* 330(5):301, 1994.

CHAPTER 5

LIPIDS
Luxury and Necessity

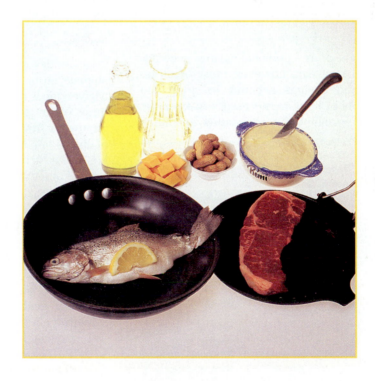

Never eat more than you can lift.

— *Miss Piggy*

Whereas carbohydrates are the staff of life, lipids (fats) may be thought of as the luxury of life. They have been considered kcalorie-rich treasures throughout much of history, especially when hunting, gathering, and growing food were difficult chores. Plants and animals make and store lipid only when excess energy is available. Just as surplus money can be stored in a savings account, so can lipid be stored in fat cells once all of the body's energy bills have been paid. The luxury of storing lipid has been recognized throughout history. In the past many societies equated plumpness with beauty because being fat signified that a person had enough money to afford the luxury of a consistent diet. Modern science further validated the luxury status of fat when it demonstrated that, gram for gram, lipid contains more than twice as much energy as either carbohydrate or protein.

How are the two nutrient classes shown in Table 5-1 alike? How are they different?

NATURE'S SAVINGS ACCOUNT

Lipid can be thought of as a personal savings account. Unlike a financial nest egg, however, most of us do not want our lipid savings account to grow too large. Tiny amounts of lipid are necessary to keep the body functioning normally. But consuming too much

"wealth" (eating too much fat), accumulating too much "wealth" (gaining too much weight), and investing in dangerous sources of "wealth" (eating too many saturated fats) can adversely affect health.

Where does this "wealth" come from?   Plants make fat from fragments of excess glucose molecules produced during photosynthesis. Animals make fat from surplus energy they obtain from dietary sources: carbohydrates, fat, and protein.

What exactly is lipid?   *Lipid* is a nutrient class more commonly known as *oil* if liquid or *fat* if solid. Lipid is a diverse group of chemical compounds that share an important characteristic: they are relatively insoluble in water.[2,9]

You will recall that most common dietary carbohydrates are composed of various combinations of saccharides. The structure of lipid is somewhat more complex. Lipids contained in dietary fats and oils as well as those found in the human body can be divided into three categories based on their chemical structure. The majority of lipid (more than 95%) in our diet and in our bodies is in the form of a molecule known as a *triglyceride*. Smaller amounts are present in the form of **phospholipids** and **cholesterol**.

Triglycerides

Triglycerides are the major form in which plants and animals store surplus fuel. As the name implies, a triglyceride is made of a single *glycerol* molecule with three other groups attached to it. The other three groups are *fatty acids* (Fig. 5-1). Fatty acids are made of chains of carbons ranging in length from 4 to 22 carbons. The carbons in these chains carry hydrogen and a small amount of oxygen. As we will see, any combination of fatty acids can be attached to a glycerol molecule: short chain, medium chain, or long chain, saturated or unsaturated.

Fatty Acids

Not surprisingly, then, when we discuss the properties of various lipids in our diet, we are really talking about the fatty acids attached to the glycerol molecule. Scientists classify these fatty acids according to:

1. the length of their carbon chains
2. the degree of saturation of the carbons in the chain (the number of hydrogens, and as a consequence, the number of double bonds between carbon atoms)
3. the position of these double bonds (omega number)

Chain length (number of carbons). Fatty acids are classified as short chain (4 to 6 carbons), medium chain (8 to 12 carbons), long chain (14 to 20 carbons), and very long chain (more than 20 carbons). The length of a fatty acid's chain affects its ability to dissolve in water. Short-chain fatty acids, such as those found in

TABLE 5-1	Review/Preview	
	Dietary Nutrient	
	Carbohydrates	**Lipids**
Building block	Monosaccharides	Glycerol and fatty acids
Kcal content	4 kcal/g	9 kcal/g
Source	Grains, etc.	Oils, fats
Nutrient intake standard	Exchange Lists	Dietary Goals
Food intake standard	Dietary Guidelines	Dietary Guidelines
In the body	Fuel (blood glucose), mucus	Cell membranes, fuel storage, hormone production
Deficiency	Ketosis, gluconeogenesis, constipation	(Unlikely); flaky dermatitis, decreased fat-soluble vitamin absorption
Excess	Stored as glycogen and fat	Obesity, cardiovascular disease, some cancers

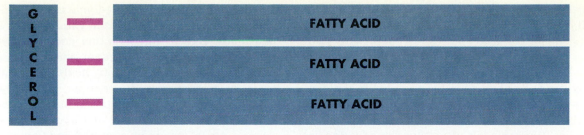
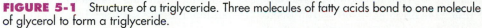

FIGURE 5-1 Structure of a triglyceride. Three molecules of fatty acids bond to one molecule of glycerol to form a triglyceride.

milk and milk products, are partially soluble in water; this is not the case for long-chain and very long-chain fatty acids, such as those found in plant oils and the fat of beef, lamb, and pork. The length of a fatty acid chain also affects the way it is absorbed from the digestive tract.

 What property of short-chain fatty acids explains why they are found in milk?

Saturation (number of hydrogens and double bonds). Carbons must form four bonds with neighboring chemicals to create stable molecules. Note that all of the carbons in the fatty acids depicted in Fig. 5-2, *A*, are bonded to four other atoms. Except for the carbons at either end of the fatty acid chains, every carbon is bonded to two other carbons and to two hydrogen atoms. These carbons are holding the maximum number of hydrogens and therefore are said to be **saturated.**

Occasionally a chemical reaction causes each of two neighboring carbons in a fatty acid to lose one hydrogen. These carbons then form a double bond between them so that they still have a total of four bonds. Such chains are called **unsaturated** because they are holding fewer than the maximum number of hydrogen atoms. If a fatty acid contains only one set of double bonds, it is said to be **monounsaturated** (Fig. 5-2, *B*). Fatty acids with two or more double bonds are termed **polyunsaturated** (Fig. 5-2, *C*). Single bonds between carbons result in a straight flexible chain that will pack into a hard fat. Double bonds between carbons result in a bend at the site of the double bonds that will not "pack" neatly, so they stay fluid.[2]

Omega number (placement of double bond). The **omega** number (omega is the last letter of the Greek alphabet) indicates the placement of the endmost double bond in an unsaturated fatty acid chain. Double bonds in naturally occurring fatty acids appear at the third, sixth, and ninth carbons from the methyl (nonoxygen) end.

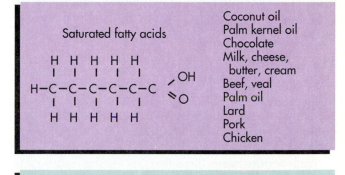

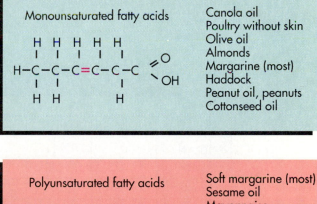

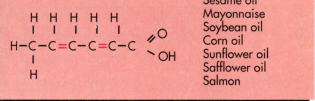

FIGURE 5-2 Unlike saturated fatty acids, unsaturated fatty acids contain one or more double bonds between carbon atoms. Sources of each fatty acid are shown.

fatty acids a lipid whose carbons are arranged in chains

glycerol a three-carbon compound that is part of all triglycerides

lipids a nutrient class commonly called *fats* and *oils;* a group of chemical compounds that are relatively insoluble in water

triglyceride a glycerol molecule with three fatty acids attached

What is an essential fatty acid?   We humans can make all the different kinds of saturated fatty acids our bodies need. We can also make all of the unsaturated fatty acids except two: omega-6 linoleic acid and omega-3 linolenic acid. Because these cannot be produced by the body, they must be provided in the diet and are termed *essential fatty acids* (EFA). Both of these polyunsaturated fatty acids are easy to obtain in a varied diet. Vegetable oils used in cooking tend to be good sources of omega-6 linoleic. Cold-water ocean fish like salmon and tuna are rich in omega-3 linolenic acid. The role of these essential fatty acids in human health is discussed in detail in the In The Body section of the chapter.

Fatty Acid Recap

Triglycerides differ in their fatty acid composition. Fatty acids in turn differ in the number of carbons in their chains, the number of double bonds (the more bonds, the softer at room temperature), and the omega number.

Triglycerides are classified as being saturated, monounsaturated, or polyunsaturated, depending on which kind of fatty acid predominates. Fig. 5-3 compares the kinds of fatty acids in various plant and animal lipids. Except for palm and coconut oil, triglycerides formed by plants contain mostly monounsaturated and polyunsaturated fatty acids, which are liquid at room temperature. In contrast, the triglycerides found in animal fat are composed mainly of saturated fatty acids, which are solid at room temperature. In general, plant fats are unsaturated and liquid, whereas animal fats are saturated and solid. If our body fat were mostly unsaturated it would be fluid at room temperature, and we would have trouble maintaining a constant shape as we moved about!

NUTRI QUIZ Note the difference in the carbon chains in Fig. 5-4. Identify which will be solid at room temperature. Hint: Saturated fats are solid at room temperature; mono- and polyunsaturated fats are liquid.

What about the other two categories of lipids? Small quantities of dietary lipid also are present as phospholipids (lecithin) and sterols (cholesterol).

Dietary fat	Cholesterol (mg/tbsp)	Breakdown of fatty acid content (normalized to 100%)			
Canola oil	0	6%	22%	10%	62%
Safflower oil	0	10%	77%	Trace-	13%
Sunflower oil	0	11%	69%		20%
Corn oil	0	13%	61%	1%-	25%
Olive oil	0	14%	8%	-1%	77%
Soybean oil	0	15%	54%	7%	24%
Margarine	0	17%	32%	-2%	49%
Peanut oil	0	18%	33%		49%
Vegetable shortening	0	28%	26%	-2%	44%
Palm oil	0	49%	9%		37%
Palm kernel oil	0	81%	2%-		11%
Coconut oil	0	87%	2%-		6%
Lard	12	41%	11%	-1%	47%
Beef fat	14	52%	3%-	-1%	44%
Butter fat	33	66%	2%-	-2%	30%

Polyunsaturated fat

■ Saturated fat   ■ Linoleic acid   ■ Monounsaturated fat

■ Alpha-linolenic acid

FIGURE 5-3 This chart compares dietary fats in terms of saturated fat, the most common unsaturated fats, and cholesterol content.

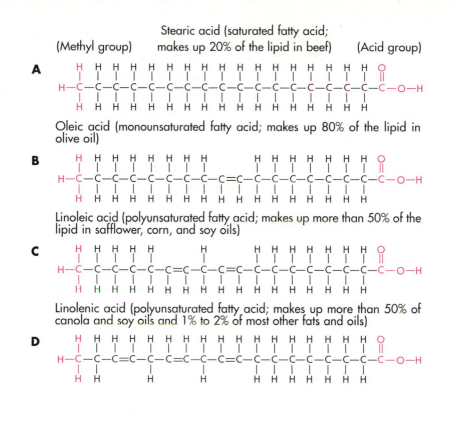

Stearic acid (saturated fatty acid; makes up 20% of the lipid in beef)

(Methyl group)   (Acid group)

A

Oleic acid (monounsaturated fatty acid; makes up 80% of the lipid in olive oil)

B

Linoleic acid (polyunsaturated fatty acid; makes up more than 50% of the lipid in safflower, corn, and soy oils)

C

Linolenic acid (polyunsaturated fatty acid; makes up more than 50% of canola and soy oils and 1% to 2% of most other fats and oils)

D

FIGURE 5-4 Structures of four fatty acids.

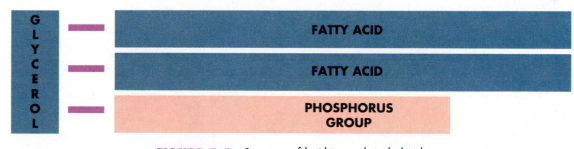

FIGURE 5-5 Structure of lecithin, a phospholipid.

Phospholipids

A **phospholipid** looks like a triglyceride that has a phosphorus-containing molecule attached in place of one of the fatty acids (Fig. 5-5). The phosphorus group is soluble in water, whereas the rest of the phospholipid remains soluble in fat. This property allows phospholipids to **emulsify** (hold together) molecules of fat and water that otherwise would separate. Phospholipids make up only a few percent of the total dietary

emulsify to disperse oil droplets in watery fluid

essential fatty acid a fatty acid that is not produced by the body and must be provided in the diet

phospholipid a compound similar to triglyceride but with a phosphorus-containing molecule replacing one of the fatty acids; they are natural emulsifiers

Fuel Value of Nutrients	
	kcal per gram
Proteins	4
Carbohydrates	4
Lipids	**9**

lipid intake. The most common dietary phospholipid is lecithin. It is found naturally in soybeans and egg yolk and is frequently added to salad dressings and baked goods to keep their ingredients from separating (Fig. 5-6). Health food consultants often advise people to take lecithin supplements to improve digestion and metabolism of fat. In reality this is not necessary; your body makes all the lecithin you need.[9,20]

Sterols (Cholesterol)

Sterols are lipids whose carbons form rings instead of chains. The best-known sterol is *cholesterol.* Although cholesterol has been portrayed as a villain, it plays many important roles in animal bodies. It is an essential component of animal—but not plant—cell membranes, and animals use it to synthesize a number of essential compounds.

Why don't plants make cholesterol?   Nature, being an expert conservationist, never makes something it cannot use. Plants have no need for cholesterol, so they do not make any. Animals do need it, so they synthesize it.

IN THE DIET

What value do lipids have in the diet?   Lipids are a concentrated source of energy. Selected lipids supply the fat-soluble vitamins A, D, E, and K and the essential fatty acids. For example, wheat germ oil is rich in both vitamin E and the essential fatty acid linoleic acid.

Fats and oils also enhance our enjoyment of the foods we eat and help satisfy our appetite (psychological desire to eat) and our hunger (physiological desire for food). Studies have shown that people almost always choose the product that has the most fat as being the best tasting. We have an innate preference for smooth, creamy textures—probaby to ensure that we eat enough high-kcalorie foods.[4] This was a great idea when the food supply was less stable, but it has been the undoing of many people in industrialized nations. Another factor in our preference for fat is that its aromatic (pleasant smelling) compounds make it easier for us to detect a food's flavor by carrying its scent to our nose. Further, high-fat foods slow digestion. The high kcalorie content of fat (remember, it has over twice as much energy per gram as either carbohydrate or protein) slows the rate at which our stomachs empty, causing us to feel full longer. Because fats satisfy hunger they are said to have a high *satiety* value.[9]

Food manufacturers are well aware of our inborn preference for fat. They add fat to enhance the flavor of many products and tout the rich, creamy, satisfying nature of their foods in advertisements to capture our interest. Because most of the fats added to processed foods are not visible, consumers are often unaware that they are eating a lipid-laden food.

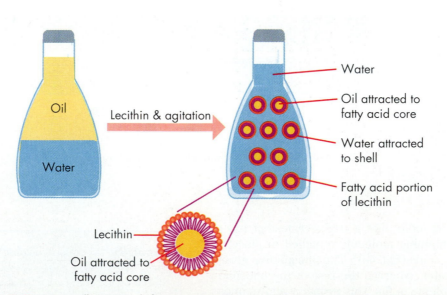

FIGURE 5-6   We've all seen emulsifiers in action! They are what keep many brands of salad dressings and other condiments from separating into layers of water and fat. Emulsifiers like lecithin are ball-shaped molecules. They hide their fatty acids inside and their water-friendly group on the outside. Add them to salad dressing, shake well, and like magic they hide the oil in the dressing in the center of their molecules and keep the water on the outside.

What are the major sources of fat consumed around the world? Societies differ with respect to how much fat they consume and which sources of fat are most common in their diet (Fig. 5-7). In general, citizens of industrialized nations consume more total lipid than those of developing countries. They also eat more animal protein rich in saturated fat and use more sources of refined animal fat like butter and cream. Oils refined from plants such as olives, peanuts, safflower, and coconut are the most popular sources of lipid in many developing nations. Regional exceptions exist, however. For instance, despite industrialization, olive oil is still the major source of dietary lipid in Italy.[11,36]

Food Intake Standards

The average American obtains 37% of his/her kcalories from fat, 12% to 16% from protein, 22% from complex carbohydrates (starches), and 20% to 24% from sugar. S/he also eats a little over 0.5 g of cholesterol each day.[7,8] Because this is considerably more fat than is needed to meet our essential fatty acid requirements, there is widespread concern among health experts about the dangers of consuming too much fat. The Dietary Guidelines, the Food Guide Pyramid, the American Heart Association, the American Cancer Society, and the Dietary Goals for Americans all advise us to cut consumption of fat, saturated fat, and cholesterol (Table 5-2).

Why the emphasis on reducing dietary fat? The major reason to reduce dietary fat, particularly saturated fat, is to decrease the risk of **cardiovascular** disease (CVD). CVD, which affects one out of every four people, is the number one killer of Americans over age 40. The first sign of CVD often is death—a fatal heart attack or stroke. Given this unpleasant reality, it

TABLE 5-2 Intake Standards	
Foods	**Nutrients**
Dietary Guidelines	RDA
Food Guide Pyramid	**% Daily Value (labels)**
American Heart	**Dietary Goals**
Association	
American Cancer Society	
5-A-Day Program	
People eat foods.	***Cells eat nutrients.***

seems wise to eliminate as many cardiovascular disease risk factors as possible. This approach also reduces the odds of contracting certain cancers, minimizes the symptoms associated with **autoimmune** diseases like multiple sclerosis, and facilitates weight control.[6,14,16,21,24] This does not mean we have to give up all of our favorite high-fat foods. We simply need to learn to enjoy them in moderation. You will find a more detailed discussion of how high-fat diets lead to health problems in the In The Body section of the chapter.

Dietary Guidelines—1990 USDA, USDHHS, and Food Guide Pyramid

The Dietary Guideline that relates directly to fats is shown in Box 5-1 on p. 76. It provides specific advice about how much fat and saturated fat we should eat and gives examples of high-fat foods.[7,8] The complete text of the Guidelines is in Chapter 2. The Food Guide Pyramid illustrates these recommendations.

How do I find hidden fat in foods? The first step is to become aware of the whole foods in which it hides. The second step is identifying fat in processed food. Reading the labels on packaged foods is one of your best defenses against eating too much fat. Once you start inspecting labels, you will find that fat is everywhere—from frozen dinners to baked goods to condiments to snack foods. It even shows up in some surprising places—like diet foods!

The Food Guide Pyramid will help you identify fat in two ways.[28] The top of the Pyramid has a food group for fats (such as those added during cooking, at the table,

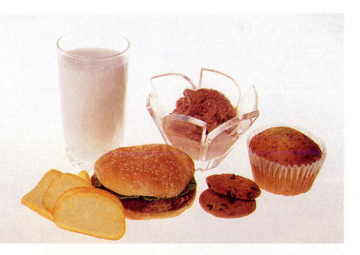

FIGURE 5-7 Check out the fat content of these all-American favorite foods. Ten Pringle's chips: 1½ tsp fat. McDLT: 9 tsp fat (15 tsp with cheese). Two Chips Ahoy cookies: 1¼ tsp fat. 8-oz glass of whole milk: 1⅔ tsp fat. 1½ cups of ice cream: 4-5 tsp fat. Cupcake size banana nut muffin: 3 tsp fat.

autoimmune pertaining to the development of an immune response against one's own body tissues

cardiovascular pertaining to the heart and blood vessels

cholesterol a waxy, fatlike substance found in animal tissue

satiety (sa-TIE-ity) the full satisfaction of hunger

sterol a lipid whose carbons are arranged in rings, for example, cholesterol

BOX 5-1   Dietary Guidelines for Fat Consumption

Choose a diet low in fat, saturated fat, and cholesterol. Thirty percent or less of the kcalories in the diet should come from fat, and saturated fat should be no more than one third of total fat intake (10% or less of total kcalories).

Limit cholesterol to 300 mg per day or less. Use small amounts of salad dressing and spreads, such as butter, margarine, and mayonnaise; choose liquid vegetable oils most of the time; check labels for the amount of fat and unsaturated fat in foods.

Eat only 6 ounces of meat, fish, and poultry daily; trim all fat from meat and remove skin from poultry; broil, bake, or boil instead of frying; occasionally substitute cooked, dried beans, peas, and lentils for meat; use egg yolks and organ

meats in moderation. Choose skim (nonfat) and low-fat dairy products to fulfill your daily milk requirement.

Adults over age 20 should have their blood cholesterol level checked routinely and, if it is above 5.2 millimole/ liter or 200 mg/deciliter, follow the advice of health professionals regarding diet, exercise, and, if necessary, medication to reduce it. (Note: if you have a family history of heart disease, or other chronic health problems, cholesterol testing may need to begin during childhood.)

From National Cholesterol Education Program: *Report of the expert panel on blood cholesterol levels in children and adolescents*, U.S. Department of Health and Human Services, Washington, DC, 1991.

and hidden in sweets); it also uses a graphic to alert consumers to fat hiding in other food groups. (You can see this symbol in the key to the Pyramid at top right.) Fig. 5-8 highlights common fat-containing foods in each of the Pyramid food groups. (See Table 2-4 in the Personalizing the Pyramid section of Chapter 2 for information on the fat content of individual items.)

The third step for fat savvy shoppers and cooks is learning to select foods low in cholesterol and cholesterol-forming saturated fat. For processed foods this information is on the label. For whole foods, you need to know where saturated fat and cholesterol hide.

If I trim the fat from my diet, I trim the cholesterol, right?   Not necessarily. This works with milk

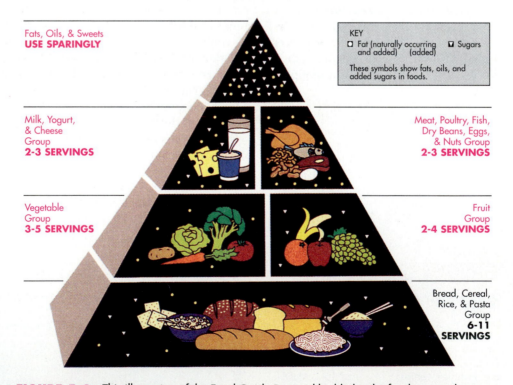

Food Guide Pyramid
A Guide to Daily Food Choices

Fats, Oils, & Sweets
USE SPARINGLY

KEY
□ Fat (naturally occurring and added)   ☑ Sugars (added)
These symbols show fats, oils, and added sugars in foods.

Milk, Yogurt, & Cheese Group
2-3 SERVINGS

Meat, Poultry, Fish, Dry Beans, Eggs, & Nuts Group
2-3 SERVINGS

Vegetable Group
3-5 SERVINGS

Fruit Group
2-4 SERVINGS

Bread, Cereal, Rice, & Pasta Group
6-11 SERVINGS

FIGURE 5-8   This illustration of the Food Guide Pyramid highlights the food groups that contain fat. Are you surprised to see the vegetable and fruit groups highlighted? An avocado contains about 40 grams of fat—and check out the labels on a jar of olives and on bottles of vegetable and coconut oils.

because the cholesterol in milk is associated with fat droplets. But cholesterol hides in other foods in unique ways! It is part of the membrane structure in all animal cells, so removing visible fat from meats, fish, and poultry will not eliminate significant amounts of cholesterol. Decreasing your intake of these foods and egg yolks, however, will automatically decrease your cholesterol intake.

Unfortunately, decreasing dietary cholesterol is not the final answer to lowering blood cholesterol because the liver makes cholesterol from saturated fat. High levels of saturated fat in the diet tend to increase cholesterol production in the liver and also appear to inhibit the body's ability to break down and dispose of cholesterol. This means you need to concentrate on restricting your use of saturated fats as well as your intake of cholesterol.[14] Table 5-3 lists some fat-containing ingredients commonly used by home cooks and found in many prepared foods. The cholesterol content of specific foods is listed in Table 5-4.

 NUTRI QUIZ Which kingdom, animal or plant, produces cholesterol?

Nutrient Intake Standards
The RDA

There is no RDA for fat, but scientists estimate that 1% to 2% of our total daily kcalorie intake should be in the form of essential fatty acids. One tablespoon of vegetable oil per day will supply all of the essential fatty acids you need.[20]

Dietary Goals: % Kcalories

As noted earlier, the Dietary Goals recommend that no more than 30% of our total kcalories be in the form of fat.[24] Some scientists say a 30% fat diet may not be low enough. Long-term studies from China suggest a 20% fat diet may be even healthier.[14] See A Closer Look on p. 78 to learn the views of some experts who favor the lower-fat diet.

Why the emphasis on SFA, PUFA, and MUFA?

For many years all fats were treated as dietarily equivalent. During the 1950s it became clear that consuming a large amount of saturated fat increases the risk of heart disease, so health practitioners began advising people to substitute polyunsaturated fat for saturated fat. On the basis of more recent evidence, scientists now believe that each type of fatty acid performs very specific and specialized functions in the human body. To restrict saturated fat intake as well as to ensure that we have adequate amounts of the various types of fatty acids, we are now advised to divide our fatty intake equally among saturated, polyunsaturated, and monounsaturated fats.[7,8] Health experts also recommend that we consume at least two servings per week of cold-water ocean fish such as salmon or tuna; they are rich in the omega-3 polyunsaturated fatty acids that appear to

TABLE 5-3 Predominant Fat Source in Selected Foods

(C) indicates that food contains cholesterol.

Saturated Fat	Monounsaturated Fat	Polyunsaturated Fat
PLANT		
Chocolate, cocoa butter	Olive	Vegetable and nut oils
Coconut	Canola (rapeseed)	Nut butters
Palm oil, palm kernel oil	Avacado	
Partially hydrogenated vegetable oil		
Vegetable shortening		
ANIMAL		
Any animal product (except nonfat milk and nonfat milk products) (C)	Poultry without skin (C)	Cold-water ocean fish rich in omega-3-fatty acids: salmon (C) and tuna (C)
Butter, butter oil (C)	Flounder (C)	
Chicken fat (C), lard (C), tallow (C)	Haddock (C)	

TABLE 5-4 Cholesterol Content of Selected Foods

Food Item	mg Cholesterol/Serving	Food Item	mg Cholesterol/Serving
Organ meats	400/3.5 oz.	Clams and scallops	20/3 oz.
Eggs	225/large egg yolk	Hard cheese, varies	33/oz.
Meat and poultry	80 to 100/3 oz.	Cream cheese	28/oz.
Fish	60 to 70/3 oz.	Butter	33/tbsp.
Lobster	81/3 oz.	Cream	21/tbsp.
Oysters	4.6/3 oz.	Whole milk	35/8 oz.
Crab	76/3 oz.	Low-fat (2%) milk	18/8 oz.
Shrimp and crayfish	150/3 oz.	Nonfat milk	5/8 oz.

A CLOSER LOOK

Dietary Fat: How Low Can You Go?

A diet that obtains 30% of its kcalories from fat is considered by most health professionals to be both healthful and reasonable for Americans. A few experts, however, including self-styled heart disease rehabilitation specialist Dean Ornish, MD, believe that the maximum health and weight control benefits can be achieved only with a diet that gets 10% or less of its kcalories from fat.

Critics of this stance, including obesity specialists Wayne Calloway, PhD, of George Washington University and Johanna Dwyer, PhD, of the New England Medical Center Nutrition Clinic, believe a diet this low in fat is bound to create nutritional deficiencies. They acknowledge that much of the world's population subsists on a 10% fat diet. They are quick to point out, however, that while people on very low-fat diets are not dying of heart disease and cancer, they are not necessarily enjoying optimal health. It is possible to eat a nutritionally adequate 10% fat diet, but most Americans would require special training and high motivation to stick to it.

A very low-fat diet is by definition very high in carbohydrates. Such a diet may not provide enough energy for people under age 20, who need extra calories to grow properly. It could also be dangerous for the approximately 10% of the population who are carbohydrate sensitive. These people develop high levels of fat in their blood after eating large amounts of carbohydrates.

Even if a 10% fat diet proved to be healthful, Ornish's critics believe few people would be willing to adhere to it. Such a diet would exclude the traditional processed foods found in the American diet and would contain very small amounts of animal protein. The mainstays of Ornish's regimen, for instance, are large servings of legumes, grains, and produce supplemented with small amounts of nonfat milk products. Meat, fish, and poultry are excluded.

According to Dr. Marion Nestle of New York University, people need a diet that is comfortable, convenient, pleasant, and easy to adhere to. She and many other authorities believe that a diet that contains 20% to 30% fat can give you the health benefits you desire, along with the taste you appreciate and the convenience essential for your busy lifestyle.

Adapted from Burros M: Eating well—low-fat diets: just how low can you go? *New York Times*, Jan 12, 1994.

---

improve cardiovascular health. Use Table 5-3 to help you choose foods that provide a balanced fat intake.

Exactly how much fat can I eat? You already may have estimated your fat intake goal in the Personalizing the Pyramid section of Chapter 2. You can use this rough estimate, or you can get a more precise answer. Follow the instructions for determining your personal kcalorie needs on p. 27 of Chapter 2. Next, multiply your suggested kcalorie intake by 0.3. Finally, divide the result by 9 (because fat supplies 9 kcalories per gram), as shown in Table 5-5.

TABLE 5-5 Recommended Fat Intake at Various kcal Intakes

	Teenage Boy	Active Adult Woman
kcal from RDA 30% of kcal	3000 kcal ×0.3	2200 kcal ×0.3
Amount of kcal from fat	900 kcal	660 kcal
9 kcal/g fat	900 kcal ÷ 9 kcal/g fat	660 kcal ÷ 9 kcal/g fat
Fat intake maximum	100 g of fat	73 g of fat

What do these numbers mean in terms of actual food intake? There are two ways to go about meeting your fat intake goal. One is to carry around a food composition book and a calculator. The other is to learn to "eat lean" by following the tips detailed toward the end of the chapter. For most people the recommended changes are not drastic. You won't necessarily be changing the kinds or quantities of food you eat; many people can reduce fat intake simply by eating lower kcalorie versions of their favorite foods. This seemingly small change can add up to big savings. If you are moderately overweight, cutting your fat intake can effectively reduce your waistline. If you are of normal weight, you can actually eat more food by replacing the lost fat with extra servings of low-fat and nonfat foods.[17]

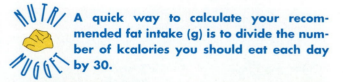 **NUTRI NUGGET** A quick way to calculate your recommended fat intake (g) is to divide the number of kcalories you should eat each day by 30.

 NUTRI QUIZ Can you estimate how many grams of saturated fat you should eat? Hint: multiply your kcalorie intake by 0.1.

IN BETWEEN: DIGESTION AND ABSORPTION

Lipid digestion starts with the warming of fats in the mouth. Chemical digestion, however, does not begin until lipid enters the small intestine, where specialized cells sense its presence and release the hormone cholycystokinin (CCK). CCK in turn stimulates the release of *bile* from the gallbladder and lipase, a lipid-digesting enzyme, from the pancreas. The liver synthesizes bile from a chemical made from cholesterol. Bile emulsifies lipid by breaking it into small pieces and blending it with the water secretions of the gastrointestinal tract. Once the lipid is emulsified, pancreatic lipase begins to dismantle it, one fatty acid at a time. The end products of this process are cholesterol, monoglycerides, fatty acids, and glycerol.

Errors in Lipid Digestion

Problems with lipid utilization sometimes begin in the intestinal tract, as is the case with gallbladder disease and cystic fibrosis. Gallstones develop spontaneously in some people from a combination of bile salts and cholesterol. The stones can irritate the lining of the gallbladder and block the bile duct. In addition to causing acute pain, blockage prevents bile from reaching the digestive tract, so fats pass through the intestine largely undigested. This condition is seen most often in females, particularly middle-aged, overweight women who have had more than one child. Gender, heredity, and diabetes all have been implicated in the development of gallstones. Depending on the severity of the condition, therapy may include drugs, surgery, and a change in diet.[6] Persons with cystic fibrosis cannot produce enough lipase to digest fat, so they must consume digestive enzyme supplements with their meals. Intestinal disorders that interfere with fat digestion or absorption also impair the absorption of fat-soluble vitamins.

IN THE BODY

Lipoproteins

How do lipids circulate in the blood? Lipids are not water soluble, so in their native state they cannot circulate freely in the fluid portion of the blood. Nature met this challenge by developing specialized molecules (lipoproteins) that are soluble in both lipid and water. The outer portion of a lipoprotein is made of a water-soluble coat of emulsifying phospholipid (remember lecithin, which can hold fat and water together) and some protein molecules. Inside this coat, protected from the blood, are triglycerides, cholesterol, and fat-soluble vitamins. Thus packaged, fats and fat-soluble metabolites travel safely throughout the human body. Cells extracts lipids from the lipoproteins as needed. Some of the lipid is used for energy; some to build cell membranes or to convert into other metabolites such as cholesterol. Any excess is stored in *adipose* (fat) tissue.

Several different kinds of lipoproteins occur in blood plasma. The relative proportion of each is influenced by diet and in turn affects cardiovascular health. *Chylomicrons* are the lipoproteins that transport lipids and cholesterol from the gastrointestinal tract into the body. Chylomicrons circulate through the blood until they reach the liver, where any lipids not yet picked up and used by cells are repackaged in new lipoprotein particles called *low-density lipoproteins (LDL)* and *very-low-density lipoproteins (VLDL)*. Triglycerides released from adipose tissue travel through the blood packaged in particles known as *high-density lipoproteins (HDL)*.

Both LDL and HDL contain cholesterol. LDL cholesterol circulates in the blood, dropping off lipid and cholesterol wherever they are needed for cell building and metabolizing activities, and leaving cholesterol residue on the interior walls of the blood vessels. Because LDL is the major route by which dietary cholesterol travels in the blood, LDL cholesterol is called "bad" cholesterol. Conversely, HDL is called "good" cholesterol because as it travels through the blood it picks up any free cholesterol and carries it to the liver for processing and excretion. High levels of LDL are correlated with cardiovascular disease, whereas high levels of some types of HDL seem to have a protective function (Table 5-6 on p. 80). (See the section on blood disorders in Errors in Lipid Metabolism later in the chapter for an explanation of how the quantity and types of dietary lipid in addition to exercise habits affect the amounts of each lipoprotein in plasma.)

---

adipose a tissue composed of fat cells

bile a substance made by the liver and stored in the gallbladder; it is released into the intestine to aid in fat digestion and absorption

chylomicron (ki-lo-MI-cron) a lipoprotein that contains mostly dietary triglycerides

high-density lipoprotein a lipoprotein made up of half protein, half lipid; 20% to 30% of total plasma cholesterol

low-density lipoprotein a lipoprotein that contains mostly cholesterol; 60% to 70% of total plasma cholesterol

very-low-density lipoprotein (VLDL) a lipoprotein that contains mostly endogenous triglycerides; 10% to 15% of total plasma cholesterol

TABLE 5-6	Plasma Cholesterol Levels and Cardiovascular Disease Risk		
	Low	Medium	High
Total cholesterol	<200 mg/day	200-239 mg/day	≥240 mg/day
LDL	<130 mg/day	130-159 mg/day	≥160 mg/day
HDL	>60 mg/day	60-34 mg/day	≤35 mg/day

Lipids in the Body

Why does my body need lipid? What does it do?
Lipid performs both structural and functional roles in the body. Triglycerides stored in adipose tissue form the body's largest fuel reserve and provide vital insulation. Having fat stored in adipose cells is like having your own personal oil well: your body can draw on it during an energy crisis. Adipose tissue acts like a blanket, insulating your body from the cold. It also serves as a shock absorber, cushioning delicate organs, most notably the kidneys, from a moderate amount of traumatic injury.

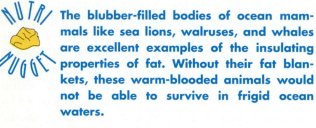 **The blubber-filled bodies of ocean mammals like sea lions, walruses, and whales are excellent examples of the insulating properties of fat. Without their fat blankets, these warm-blooded animals would not be able to survive in frigid ocean waters.**

When the body needs energy it dismantles the fatty acids in triglycerides two carbons at a time. The two-carbon units are then used to provide energy (fuel) for body functions, such as heat production and work. Fatty acids also supply materials for the production of cell membranes, hormones, and cholesterol. For example, *omega-6 linoleic acid* is required to make many kinds of cell membranes, including those of skin cells; whereas *omega-3 linolenic acid* is needed to make nerve and brain cell membranes. These essential fatty acids are also used to make different hormonelike compounds that regulate blood pressure, blood clot formation, the immune response, the inflammatory response to injury or infection, and many other vital body functions.[14]

Linolenic acid (omega-3) has received considerable attention in scientific journals and in the popular press during the last decade because of its reputation as an anticardiovascular disease nutrient. It seems odd to think of a fat as a heart-friendly nutrient, but here is how it works. Our bodies are always forming and destroying tiny blood clots. The body uses omega-3 linolenic acid to make substances that reduce blood clot formation. This helps keep our blood "thin" and flowing smoothly, lessening the risk of a heart attack or stroke. In contrast, compounds produced from omega-6 linoleic acid counterbalance those made by omega-3 linolenic by increasing blood clot formation and blood pressure.

Saturated fatty acids are used to synthesize cholesterol. Cholesterol in turn is used to make cell membranes, bile, and steroid hormones.

a. What foods contain cholesterol?
b. About how much cholesterol do most Americans eat each day?
c. Why does your body make cholesterol?

Lipid Deficiencies

A dietary deficiency of lipid is rare. However, deficiencies have been observed in newborns (because lipid is not easily transported from mother to fetus), in people who have gone on overly rigid reducing diets, and in people who are unable to absorb lipids in their intestines. The major symptom of dietary fat deficiency is a flaky dermatitis (skin inflammation). Fat deficiency also can lead to a decreased growth rate or arrested growth rate in young animals and children and can cause fat-soluble vitamin deficiencies.[20]

Why do these symptoms accompany fat deficiency? Remember that fat is required for the synthesis of new cell membranes. Because growth is accomplished by synthesis of new cells, growth ceases when the formation of new cells ceases. Likewise, fat is needed for the repair and replacement of cells in mature animals. When fat is lacking, cells are not replaced promptly and the outermost layer of the skin (the epidermis) becomes dry. For some time only omega-6 linoleic acid was recognized as being essential, since signs of fat deficiency disappeared if small amounts of it (less than 2% of total daily kcalorie intake) were added to the diet. Recently omega-3 linolenic acid was also recognized as being essential in the diet for laboratory animals and infant humans. No RDA are currently given for specific fatty acids, despite their recognized role in health maintenance.

Lipid Excesses

What happens if I have too much fat in my diet?
People can be divided into two categories with respect to excessive fat intake. One group is genetically predisposed to accumulating high levels of fat and/or cholesterol in their blood. These persons must rigorously re-

strict their dietary fat and cholesterol intake. If diet modification alone is not effective, a combination of drug and diet therapy will be instituted (see Errors in Lipid Metabolism later in the chapter for a more complete review of cardiovascular disease). The second and larger group is composed of those of us who simply overdo it. Following are the effects of excessive fat intake in the general population.

Total Fat

Although fat deficiency is rare, excessive total fat intake (over 30% of total kcalorie from fat) is relatively common and is known to contribute to obesity, gallstones, cardiovascular disease, hypertension, some cancers, and possibly the worsening of the symptoms of autoimmune diseases such as multiple sclerosis.[21]

Saturated Fatty Acids

Saturated fatty acids, commonly found in animal-derived foods and coconut and palm oils, tend to raise blood cholesterol levels and are positively correlated with an increased risk of cardiovascular disease, hypertension, and colon cancer. Recent research, however, suggests that not all saturated fatty acids are equally harmful. For example, SFA containing 12 or fewer carbons and 18-carbon stearic acid (found in animal fats, especially beef tallow) did not increase cholesterol levels when fed to laboratory animals or humans as the sole source of dietary fat. It is unclear, however, what effect these fatty acids have when fed as part of a mixture of fats.[33]

Monounsaturated Fatty Acids

MUFAs thus far have not been associated with the development of any health problems. In fact, just the opposite seems to be true: research suggests that a diet rich in monounsaturated fatty acids may reduce the risk of cardiovascular disease by lowering LDL cholesterol.

Polyunsaturated Fatty Acids

PUFAs are found in vegetable oils. In animal studies they have been positively correlated with the development of certain reproductive organ cancers. People who consume excessive amounts of the PUFA omega-6 fatty acids may be at increased risk for high blood pressure and cardiovascular disease. People who consume too much of omega-3 fatty acids may be vulnerable to hemorrhaging if they are injured because of suppression of their body's natural clotting mechanism.

Cholesterol

Excessive intake of cholesterol-rich foods has been associated with the development of cardiovascular disease because it promotes buildup of fatty deposits (plaque) on arteries in genetically sensitive people.

Errors of Lipid Metabolism

Some disorders of lipid metabolism are congenital (present at birth). Others develop over time in genetically susceptible persons who live unhealthy lifestyles.

Atherosclerosis

Atherosclerosis typically begins when some of the fat and cholesterol circulating in the blood accumulate in the inner wall of the arteries, forming deposits called **plaque** (Fig. 5-9 on p. 82). Gradually plaque enlarges and hardens, causing the arteries to lose their natural elasticity **(arteriosclerosis).** The combination of clogged and constricted arteries causes blood pressure to rise (hypertension), which in turn promotes formation of additional plaque. Over time plaque can grow so large that it severely restricts blood flow to the heart or other tissues, causing them to die slowly. People with cardiovascular disease usually have warning symptoms, such as pain in their chests or extremities caused by the inadequate blood flow. But cardiovascular disease also can be a swift and silent killer. Sometimes the first "warning" is a fatal heart attack or stroke. The presence of plaque also has been shown to increase the risk of blood clot formation, which in turn can cause heart attacks and strokes. Heredity, diet, and lifestyle are all known to play a role in the development of CVD. Some people have a greater risk than others of developing CVD because they have a genetic tendency toward high levels of fat and cholesterol in their blood.[25]

What is the role of dietary fat and cholesterol in the development of cardiovascular disease? Health experts agree that high levels of fat and cholesterol in the blood, especially LDL (low-density lipoprotein) cholesterol, correlate with an increased risk of cardiovascular disease. What the experts disagree about is:

1. Whether diet affects blood cholesterol levels[3]
2. Whether reducing blood cholesterol levels decreases the risk of cardiovascular disease
3. Even if the diet–blood cholesterol–cardiovascular disease link is valid, should so much emphasis be put on dietary fat and cholesterol given that they are only two of many risk factors for cardiovascular disease?[6,21]

---

atherosclerosis (athero-skler-OH-sis)   the formation of deposits **(plaque)** composed of fat and cholesterol on the internal lining of the blood vessels

omega-6 linoleic acid   a long-chain fatty acid the body needs to make cell membranes; increases blood pressure and blood clot formation

omega-3 linolenic acid   a long-chain fatty acid the body needs to make nerve and brain cells; helps make substances that reduce blood clot formation

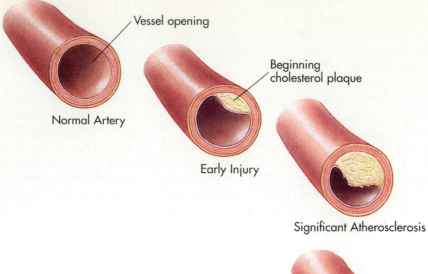

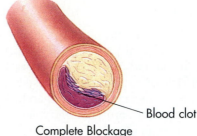

FIGURE 5-9 This illustration shows what happens when a normal artery becomes progressively clogged with fat and cholesterol.

The Cholesterol Controversy

Many respected scientists believe there is little evidence that a diet high in saturated fat and cholesterol is responsible for high blood cholesterol levels. They note that studies exploring the role of diet in cardiovascular disease have not conclusively shown that lowering fat and cholesterol intake reduces the incidence of cardiovascular disease. Nor have these studies proved that everyone is equally susceptible to cardiovascular disease, given a high-fat, high-cholesterol diet.

Scientists who doubt the diet–cardiovascular disease link believe that heredity and other risk factors, such as stress and smoking, play a more significant role in the development of cardiovascular disease. They observe that a simple change in diet is not sufficient to control genetically based high blood cholesterol and high blood fat levels.

The National Institutes of Health (NIH) and the American Heart Association (AHA) take the opposite point of view. They currently support the link among diet, blood cholesterol levels, and cardiovascular disease.[8,21] They cite a study that compared the blood cholesterol levels of Japanese men living in Tokyo, Honolulu, and San Francisco. The results demonstrated that the typical high-saturated fat, high-cholesterol American diet correlated with an increase in serum cholesterol and cardiovascular disease.

NUTRI NUGGET One piece of cheesecake won't kill you—or will it? Most heart attacks occur in the early morning. Researchers may be one step closer to understanding why. Two studies reported at the 1993 American Heart Association's Science Writer Meeting claim that high-fat dinners significantly increase a person's risk of heart attack by increasing the blood's tendency to form artery-clogging clots 6 to 8 hours later. So if you want to indulge, do so early in the day and exercise off the fat kcalories.[29]

NUTRI QUIZ How can exercise reduce a person's risk of cardiovascular disease?

Who is right?   Only time will tell. The most rational point of view is expressed by researchers who acknowledge that diet is a risk factor for cardiovascular disease but believe that it is just one of many variables. These experts also point out that diets low in fat, cholesterol, and sodium tend to be high in other nutrients, such as complex carbohydrates, fiber, and certain vitamins and minerals, all of which have been shown to provide protection against cardiovascular disease. It may be the presence of such nutrients, rather than the absence of fat and cholesterol, that makes these diets heart healthy.

How do maintaining a healthy body weight and a regular exercise program lower blood pressure?
(Hint: See Consequences of Obesity in Chapter 10 and Physiological Benefits of Exercise in Chapter 11.)

While the experts debate, what should the average person do with respect to dietary fat, cholesterol, and sodium intake? It is believed that by age 30 all Americans will have developed some degree of atherosclerotic plaque. Statistics show that 25% of the U.S. population eventually will suffer from cardiovascular disease, but currently there is no way to determine who will be affected. Because diet is only one of the many risk factors associated with cardiovascular disease, the safest course of action is to strive for a balanced and moderate lifestyle. This includes the following:

- Consuming the so-called heart-safe diet (low in fat, cholesterol, and sodium; high in complex carbohydrates and fiber)
- Maintaining a healthy body weight (see Chapter 9, Energy)
- Avoiding tobacco (both smoking and chewing varieties)
- Participating in a regular exercise program
- Reducing stress throughout adulthood

In assessing your chances of developing cardiovascular disease, you also must consider other risk factors: age (over 45 for men and 55 for women the risk increases); a family history of premature cardiovascular disease (a father with cardiovascular disease before age 55 or a mother before age 65); and gender (males are at higher risk earlier in life than females).[30]

Lipid Recap

Table 5-7 will help you visualize what happens to the fats you eat. The plant or animal fats contained in foods are digested to fatty acids, cholesterol, and glycerol, then reassembled into triglycerides and packaged in a special lipoprotein, known as a chylomicron, within the cells that line the digestive tract. The chylomicrons then carry the fat through the bloodstream. Upon reaching the liver, some of the chylomicrons are converted to other types of lipoproteins, which are then re-released into the bloodstream. The lipoproteins in the blood can transfer the triglycerides they contain to any cell in the body that requires fat. The fat is then used for fuel and to make cell membranes, hormones, or other substances. Any excess is stored in adipose tissue.

IN TODAY'S WORLD

What kinds of environmental concerns are linked to fat? Plants and animals absorb fat-soluble chemicals, such as pesticides. If these chemicals cannot be excreted or metabolized into nontoxic compounds, they are stored in fat and oil. People who use these plants and animals as food absorb some of the stored chemicals. As people eat additional quantities of contaminated food, more and more of the chemical will accumulate in their adipose tissue.

Fat-Soluble Chemicals

Eventually these stored toxins may produce severe health problems, such as birth defects and cancer. Such problems were seen with the banned pesticide DDT. After many years of widespread use in the United States, DDT began to appear in high concentrations in the body fat of animals. It showed up in creatures all along the food chain, from fish to humans, and nearly led to the extinction of the American eagle.[14]

TABLE 5-7	Review of Lipid Digestion, Absorption, and Utilization
Structure	**Lipid**
Mouth	Fats warmed
Stomach	
Small intestine	Emulsified by bile; digested by pancreatic lipases
	Absorbed as glycerol, fatty acids, triglycerides, some cholesterol; synthesizes chylomicrons
Circulatory system	Portal for short-chain fatty acids and glycerol; lymph for most medium- and long-chain fatty acids
Liver	Recycles and makes cholesterol; repackages dietary lipids found in chylomicrons as VLDL and LDL
Cells	Take lipids from chylomicrons, VLDL, and LDL; use lipid to make membranes and hormones; burn lipid (oxidize) to carbon dioxide and water, producing ATP and heat; store excess in adipose cells (triglycerides). Release stored triglycerides into bloodstream packaged as HDL
Large intestine	Excretes undigested material

Processing
Refining (*re*-fine = *re*-move)

How does processing affect lipids?   Refining the oil from corn, cottonseed, soy, and other lipid-rich plants produces a very pure product (Fig. 5-10). All fat-soluble and water-soluble impurities, including valuable vitamins, are removed by steam distillation. The result is a kcalorie-dense product with low nutrient density. Some plant oils undergo additional refining to yield lecithin, monoglycerides, and diglycerides. These products then are used as emulsifiers in a variety of processed foods.

Hydrogenation

In other cases plant oils are solidified to produce substitutes for more expensive animal fats, such as lard or butter, by adding hydrogen to the polyunsaturated fatty acids. This process of artificial saturation is known as **hydrogenation.** Procter and Gamble introduced Crisco,™ the first hydrogenated vegetable oil product, in 1911. Before then, cooks who needed a solid fat for their pie crust had three choices: butter, lard (pig fat), or beef tallow.

During hydrogenation, the bent double bonds of vegetable oils are "straightened" by saturating their double-bonded carbons with more hydrogens (Fig. 5-11). The resulting margarines and vegetable shortenings typically contain a mixture of saturated, monounsaturated, and polyunsaturated fats. The more saturated fat the product contains, the more solid it is at room temperature. In addition to the health problems already discussed with respect to saturated fat, recent epidemiological studies have shown that artificial saturation has other health pitfalls.[10]

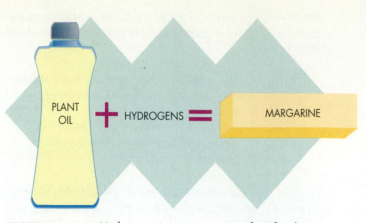

FIGURE 5-11 Hydrogenation is a process of artificial saturation.

The cis-trans controversy. Fatty acids exist in two forms: *cis* and *trans*. Most fatty acids in natural foods are in the *cis* form, but margarine and vegetable shortenings, which have been touted as heart-healthy alternatives to butter and lard, contain high concentrations of *trans* fatty acids. Recently some researchers who are studying the effects of different types of fats on metabolism found that consumption of fats with *trans* bonds is associated with elevated cholesterol levels. It seems that when oils are saturated to form margarine or shortening, a certain proportion of the unsaturated bonds remaining in the finished product are altered so that, instead of bending in the same direction from the double-bond location *(cis)*, the molecule twists in opposite directions *(trans)*. Trans bonds are present in very small amounts in natural foods. Whether natural or artificial, trans bonds tend to act like saturated fat in the body.[32,37] Before deciding that avoiding high levels of trans bonds in hydrogenated spreads is the perfect excuse for eating butter, bear in mind that the jury is still out with respect to this finding. What to do? See Dairy Decisions later in the chapter for particulars.

Fish Oil Capsules

To get more of the beneficial omega-3 fatty acids into their diets, many people take fish oil capsules. These supplements, which are produced by extracting oil from fish livers, seem to do more harm than good. Side effects include hemorrhaging and symptoms of fat-soluble vitamin toxicity.[33]

Fat Substitutes

Because we humans so love the taste of fat and so dislike the effects of fat on both our appearance and our health, technology has been searching for the "perfect" fat—one that will taste wonderful yet contain few

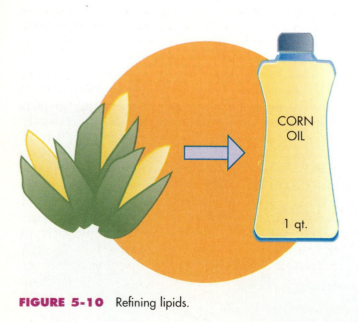

FIGURE 5-10 Refining lipids.

kcalories. The size and shape of its molecule are what give fat its creamy texture. Using this information, manufacturers have developed several substitutes.[1,27]

Simplesse® is a combination of milk protein and water, processed to form particles that duplicate the texture and taste of fat. Simplesse® replaces 3 grams of fat, worth 27 kcalories, with 2 grams of water and 1 gram of protein, worth 4 kcalories. It looks like mayonnaise and tastes like fat. It jells when heated, so it is not suitable for cooking. Food applications include ice cream, frozen yogurt, and salad dressings.

Olestra®, a potential competitor of Simplesse®, has somewhat different characteristics. It combines sugar with oil into a nondigestible, heat-stable compound that tastes and cooks like oil. But . . . BINGO: NO KCALORIES! If this product is approved by the FDA, it will be an ingredient in the oils sold in grocery stores and used in restaurants as well as in processed foods such as salad dressings.

Numerous other fat substitutes are in various stages of development. Many are made of modified food starches and therefore do not need FDA approval. One such product, known as Stellar®, is expected to be used in baked goods, margarine, salad dressings, sour cream, ice cream, dairy and cheese products, soups, gravies, and sauces. It contains a scant 1 kcalorie per gram and is heat stable, so it can be used in a variety of cooked foods.

Although fat substitutes now are used in only a few foods, we can expect a flood of new or altered food items containing these products. Fat substitutes will be a boon to those who must restrict their fat intake for medical reasons. But their use is not expected to have any significant impact on the nation's health problems. Like sugar substitutes, fat substitutes probably will do little more than make us feel better about eating empty calories.

IN MY DIET

How can I plan a diet that is not too high in fat?
We have seen that eating too few fiber-rich complex carbohydrates and too much fat, particularly cholesterol-producing saturated fat, are major nutritional concerns for people who live in industrialized nations. Changing these well-established dietary patterns requires that we be able to:[17]

1. Recognize sources of fat and cholesterol in the food supply
2. Differentiate among saturated, monounsaturated, and polyunsaturated fats
3. Become familiar with low-fat cooking techniques

At the Grocery Store—Avoiding the Fat Lane

If you are in the habit of buying the same old thing, make a point of exploring the new food options available at your local grocery store.

Butchering the Fat

Butcher departments are changing their product lines in response to consumer demand. Many meat departments now carry lower-fat strains of beef and pork. Trim additional fat from your diet by selecting low-fat cuts like flank steak, pork loin, and pork cutlet. Remember the acronym FiRST (*F*lank, *R*ound, *S*irloin, *T*enderloin) to help you select the leanest cuts of red meat and pork. Use as little ground beef as possible.

Replace at least part of the red meat you consume each week with its leaner cousin, poultry. When a recipe requires ground beef or pork, substitute skinless ground chicken or turkey meat. This will reduce your fat intake by nearly one third compared with even the leanest ground beef. Similarly, turkey and chicken are excellent substitutes for beef in stir-fry dishes, fajitas, grilled sandwiches, and in gourmet recipes, such as veal piccata and veal scallopini. In the poultry department, stick to *terrestrial* (land) birds like turkey, chicken, Cornish game hen, quail, and pheasant. Such animals carry most of their fat in and directly under their skin, unlike mammals and *aquatic* birds, which have much of their fat dispersed throughout their meat. If you have a yen for aquatic birds, such as duck and goose, substitute a serving of either for one serving of red meat.

Remember to stop at the fish counter. Fish is an excellent low-fat alternative to red meats. As mentioned earlier, cold-water ocean fish are especially healthful because their oils are rich in heart-friendly omega-3 oils. Salmon, sea bass, tuna, and swordfish are all good choices. Shellfish have a somewhat undeserved reputation for being high in cholesterol. Newer methods of measuring cholesterol have led to the discovery that bivalve shellfish (those with two shells) like oysters, clams, and scallops were mistakenly identified as being high in cholesterol because they are high in plant sterols—harmless relatives of cholesterol. Even the single-shelled varieties, like shrimp, crab, and lobster, may not be as bad as once thought. Although they are high in cholesterol, they are low in fat, so if you broil or grill them, they can be part of your diet.

Sausages and luncheon meats also have received nutrition makeovers. Here again, it's essential to be a compulsive label reader. Some of these new products are truly low in fat. Others, although leaner than the original recipe, have a long way to go nutritionally. No matter what their fat content, sausages and luncheon meats tend to be full of salt, supplying about 25% of the daily sodium intake, so use them sparingly.

Better Baked Goods

Skip the giant muffins, which can have up to 500 calories—half in the form of fat. Choose pita bread, corn tortillas, and Italian, French, and sourdough breads, which typically have no added fat. Look for low-fat versions of your favorite snack foods and desserts. And *pay attention to serving size.* Although many of these products are fat free, they aren't kcalorie free. The desserts in particular tend to be concentrated sources of sugar but offer little else in the way of nutrients. Fig. 5-12 shows some products that are good candidates for careful label reading.

Dairy Decisions

Dairy products are excellent sources of calcium and protein—but they also can contribute considerable amounts of unnecessary fat to your diet (Fig. 5-13).

Cheese. Cheese, which is essentially concentrated whole milk, is high in kcalories, fat, and cholesterol. Cheese contains about 100 kcalories per ounce, versus 20 kcalories per ounce for whole milk and 40 to 50 kcalories per ounce for meat. In fact, 85% to 90% of the kcalories in cheese come from fat, much of which is saturated. One last, sad fact for cheese lovers: a 1-ounce serving of cheese contains approximately

10% (30 mg) of the recommended daily cholesterol intake. Fortunately, reduced-fat and nonfat varieties of cheese are widely available.

Unless advised to do so by your physician, you do not have to swear off cheese completely—just rethink the way you use it. Buy the leanest version of your favorite cheese. Use small quantities of full-fat cheeses as a flavor enhancer rather than as a main protein source. For example, replace a mild-flavored cheese like Parmesan with smaller amounts of stronger flavored cheeses like Romano and Asiago. On days when cheese is a major source of protein, make sure that the rest of day's diet is low in fat. For everyday meals, skip the extra cheese topping on pizza and have a plain hamburger instead of a cheeseburger.

Cream and butter. Cream and butter (made from churning cream) are little more than milk fat. Like other high-fat foods, they make a nice treat but should not be used on a daily basis. Fortunately, many good substitutes are available. Whipped butter contains less fat than stick butter. Frozen whipped toppings to use in place of whipped cream have been around for years. Evaporated nonfat milk can be substituted for cream in soups and sauces, and if whipped with one of the new ultra-high-speed, hand-held mixers, it can even replace whipped cream.

Margarine, as we have seen, contains saturated fat and some trans fatty acids, both of which have the po-

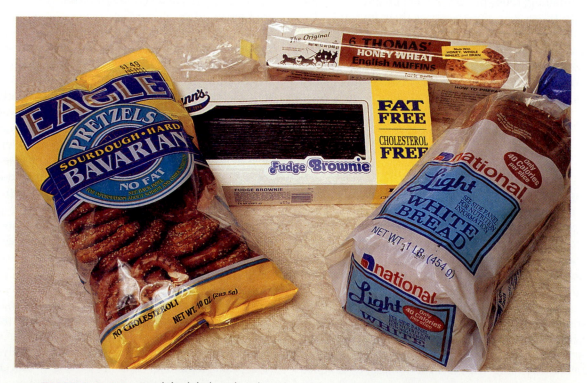

FIGURE 5-12 Read the labels rather than the advertising claims to find out the fat content of products like these.

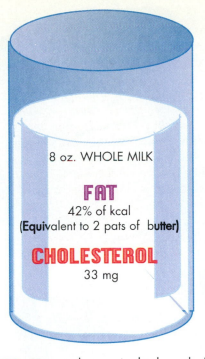

8 oz. WHOLE MILK

FAT
42% of kcal
(Equivalent to 2 pats of butter)

CHOLESTEROL
33 mg

FIGURE 5-13 You may be surprised to learn the fat content of a glass of whole milk.

Chestnuts are the exception to the rule that all nuts are high in fat. One ounce of dry roasted chestnuts contains a scant 1 gram of fat compared with 14 grams and 21 grams for dry roasted peanuts and macadamia nuts, respectively.[33]

Labels—Your License to Learn

In addition to the simple whole foods we have identified as common sources of dietary fat, almost all processed foods contain significant amounts of fat. Most processed foods contain a direct source of fat, like oil or butter. In some instances no direct sources of fat are listed on the label but the food contains ingredients, such as animal protein, nuts, coconut, or chocolate, that are themselves sources of fat and possibly cholesterol. Restrict your intake of processed foods, read labels, and select low-fat versions whenever possible.

Fortunately, food manufacturers are responding to consumer demand for leaner foods by offering reduced-fat crackers, chips, desserts, spaghetti sauces, frozen dinners, waffles, and even egg McMuffin-style breakfast foods. Read the Nutrition Facts portion of the labels on these foods to make sure you are not getting more lipid than you bargained for (Fig. 5-14).

Thanks to the Nutrition Labeling and Education Act, the labels of most packaged, processed foods clearly report their total fat, saturated fat, and cholesterol content. In addition, grocers supply this same information for the 20 most commonly consumed raw fruits, vegetables, and fish, as well as for the 45 most frequently used cuts of meat and poultry. This information may be displayed on signs or provided in brochures available at the point of purchase. To further assist consumers, standard definitions have been developed for descriptive terms used on food labels.[12,31] The definitions of these terms with respect to fat are shown in Box 5-2.

The use of health claims such as "reduces cholesterol" and "decreases the risk of heart disease" on food labels is now regulated by the federal government. Only claims for which there is compelling scientific evidence are allowed. Such claims are not allowed on foods that are low in one undesirable compound but high in another. For example, foods that are low in preformed cholesterol but high in cholesterol-forming saturated fats cannot claim on their labels that they are low in cholesterol.

Unfortunately, the Nutrition Labeling and Education Act did not rectify all the problems with food labels. There are shortcomings of the laws with respect to fat. The reference dietary fat intake information and % Daily Value for fat provided on food labels are too high for much of the population (for details, see pp. 25-27 in Chapter 2, Consumer Concerns). Also, the descriptive terms allowed on labels for milk and milk products are misleading.

tential to increase blood cholesterol levels. Consumers also may mistakenly assume that margarine is lower in kcalories than butter. Unfortunately, this is just wishful thinking. A gram of fat—whatever the source— supplies 9 kcalories of energy.

What is the confused consumer to do? First, reduce the amount of margarine or butter you use each day. Second, further decrease your fat intake by using diet butter or margarine. Finally, use soft spread or liquid margarine at the table; being less solid than stick margarine, they contain less saturated fat and trans fatty acids. Substitute vegetable oil for shortening in baked goods for the same reason.

Eggs. The American Heart Association recommends no more than four egg yolks per week, including those consumed in baked goods, custards, and so on.[8] If you have a significant blood cholesterol problem, use egg substitutes.

Pick of the Produce

With the exceptions noted below, produce is nearly fat free, so go ahead and indulge in plenty of fresh fruits and vegetables! Nuts, seeds like sunflower and sesame, avocados and the products made from them are high in fat, but rich in other nutrients. Olives and coconuts are high in fat, and not much else. The final word: No matter how many other healthful nutrients they contain, use these items sparingly in your cooking and snacking!

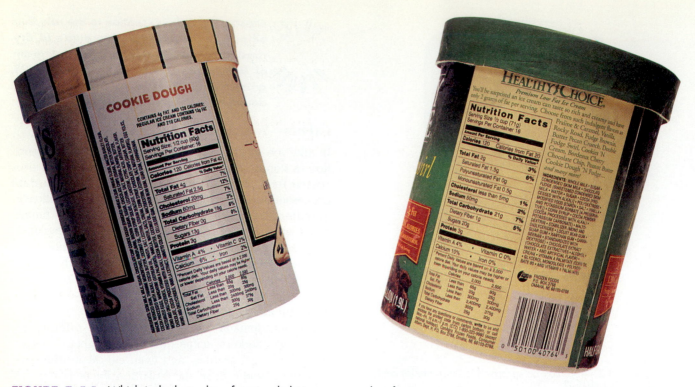

FIGURE 5-14 Which is the better buy, fat-wise: light ice cream or low-fat ice cream?

Fat-free: The product contains essentially no fat or cholesterol.

Lean and extra lean (to be used for fat content of meat and poultry): Lean products contain less than 10 grams of total fat, 4 grams of saturated fat, and 95 milligrams of cholesterol per serving. Extra lean products contain half the amount of fat but the same amount of cholesterol per serving.

Low fat: The product contains 3 grams of fat or less per serving.

Low saturated fat: The product contains 1 gram or less of saturated fat per serving.

Low cholesterol: The product contains less than 20 mg of cholesterol per serving.

Reduced: The product contains 25% less fat or cholesterol than the one it is being compared to.

Light: The product contains half as much fat as the one it is being compared with.

___ % fat free: The product must meet the definition for "low-fat" or "fat-free" shown above, and the percentage of fat must be expressed as grams of fat per 100 grams of food.

Healthy: The product must be low in fat and saturated fat and must contain 60 mg or less of cholesterol.

How can I interpret the % Daily Value? The best way to make sure you are not eating too much fat is to know how much you can safely consume each day, given your kcalorie intake. Food labels provide total and saturated fat content per serving, the % Daily Value for fat, and Reference Total Daily Fat Intake so you can determine how much of your fat budget one serving of the product will use (Fig. 5-15). "Great," you say. Hold your applause. The two reference diets cited on the label contain relatively large numbers of kcalories—2000 and 2500—so the amount of fat allowed in these diets is relatively generous. Many adult women consume considerably fewer kcalories than this. About 1600 to 1800 kcalories a day is typical for inactive females. Because their kcalorie intake is lower, their allowable fat intake is lower (54 and 60 grams, respectively). The label information can give women a false sense of security regarding the amount of fat they are consuming. See p. 27 in Chapter 2 for information on how to calculate your own % DV for fat and cholesterol.

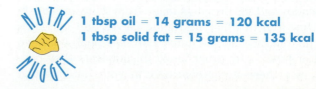

1 tbsp oil = 14 grams = 120 kcal
1 tbsp solid fat = 15 grams = 135 kcal

Nutrition Facts

Serving Size: 1/2 cup (114g)
Servings Per Container: 4

Amount per serving

Calories 260
Calories from Fat 120

	% Daily Value*
Total Fat 13g	20%
Saturated Fat 5g	25%
Cholesterol 30mg	10%
Sodium 660mg	28%
Total Carbohydrate 31g	11%
Sugars 5g	
Dietary Fiber 0g	0%
Protein 5g	

Vitamin A 4% • Vitamin C 1% •
Calcium 15% • Iron 4%

*Percents (%) of a Daily Value are based on a
2,000 calorie diet. Your Daily Values may
vary higher or lower depending on your calorie
needs:

Nutrient	2,000 calories	2500 calories
Total Fat	<65g	80g
Saturated Fat	<20g	25g
Cholesterol	<300mg	300mg
Sodium	<2,400mg	2,400mg
Total Carbohydrate	300g	375g
Fiber	25g	30g

1g Fat = 9 calories
1g Carbohydrate = 4 calories
1g Protein = 4 calories

FIGURE 5-15 The revised food label contains valuable information about fat content.

Dairy Label Dilemmas

Why are the descriptive terms used on dairy products different from those on other foods? To avoid confusion in the dairy department, the FDA allowed milk companies to use the same descriptive terms that have appeared on their products for many years. Historically the fat in milk and milk products like yogurt has been expressed as a percent of fat by weight rather than a percent of kcalories from fat, as is customary on food labels today.

Similarly, the term *low fat* has traditionally been used to designate milk products that have had part of their milk fat removed, regardless of the finished product's fat content. This practice is at odds with the revised labeling laws. For a product to be termed low fat according to today's regulations it must contain no more than 3 grams of fat per serving. At 5 grams of fat per serving, 2% low-fat milk does not meet the new low-fat criterion. We can expect to see changes in milk product labels in the future, but for now consumers need to know how to deal with this inconsistency.

By now you have it firmly ingrained in your mind that fat should make up no more than 30% of your daily kcalorie intake. While shopping, you notice that the milk carton label (Fig. 5-16) states that it contains 2% fat. It seems you have found the perfect food. *WRONG!* By convention, makers of milk products are allowed to express their fat content as a percent of weight rather than as a percent of kcalories. As a result, "2% milk" means that 2% of the *weight* of an 8-ounce serving of milk (roughly 0.16 ounce or 4.7 grams) is fat. What percent of the kcalories are contributed by fat? We can calculate this information if we know the total kcalories and the total grams of fat per serving. The nutrient panel states that one 8-ounce serving of low-fat milk contains 140 kcalories and 5 grams of fat. First we need to determine how many kcalories of fat are in 5 grams.

5 grams of fat × 9 kcalories per gram of fat
= 45 kcalories of fat

Next we must calculate what percent of the total kcalorie content is equal to 45 kcalories.

45 kcalories of fat / 140 total kcalories = 0.32 fat
0.32 fat × 100 = 32% fat

You can see that one 8-ounce serving of low-fat (2%) milk gets 32% of its kcalories from fat. Switching to nonfat (skim) milk will eliminate over 4 grams of fat, 13 grams of cholesterol, and 40 kcalories.

Remember: It is the nutrient content of your diet as a whole, not just one food, that makes or breaks your health. Nonetheless, knowing what pitfalls to look out for is an essential part of being a savvy shopper.

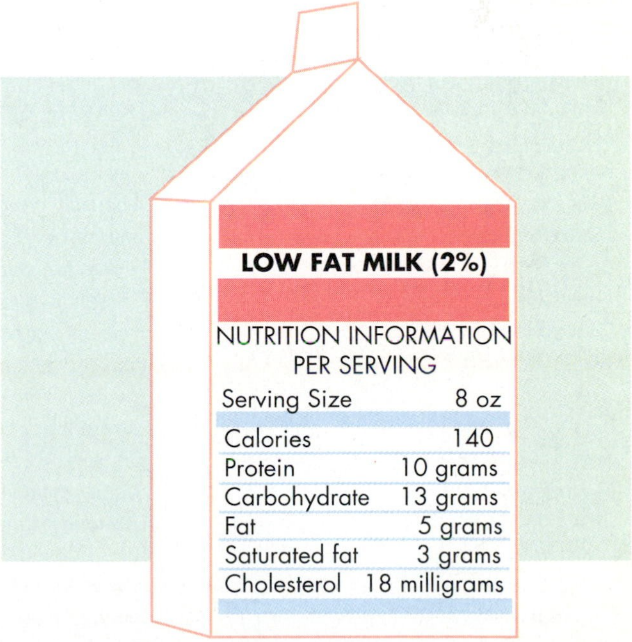

LOW FAT MILK (2%)

NUTRITION INFORMATION
PER SERVING

Serving Size	8 oz
Calories	140
Protein	10 grams
Carbohydrate	13 grams
Fat	5 grams
Saturated fat	3 grams
Cholesterol	18 milligrams

FIGURE 5-16 Is 2% milk really "low fat"?

In the Kitchen

Are cooking and preparation techniques important?

Do not destroy your good work at the grocery store by adding fat in the kitchen. Become proficient at low-fat cooking techniques: remove fat in the kitchen both by trimming any visible fat from the foods you have purchased and also by trimming fat from your recipes.[17]

1. Remove as much excess fat as possible from meats before cooking, unless the fat can be easily removed from the cooked dish. Trim fat from the edges of steaks and chops, and skin poultry before cooking. Roasted fowl is tastier and moister if it is cooked with the skin on. The skin can easily be removed at serving time, and little fat is added to the dish by cooking it this way.

2. Rethink your recipes. Simple substitutions can help you update your favorite dishes and treasured family recipes.

 To avoid large doses of saturated fat, look for vegetarian versions of prepared foods. These contain no animal fat. For example, vegetarian chili, baked beans, and tortillas are made with vegetable oil rather than lard or tallow.

3. Fry foods infrequently. Instead, broil, grill, bake, roast, poach, microwave, or steam. Sauté foods in small amounts of oil or vegetable spray. Stir fry food in tiny quantities of very hot oil.

4. With some recipes, additional fat can be removed even after the dish is cooked. For example, chilling soups and stews for several hours after cooking causes excess fat to float to the top and harden. It can be easily removed after the dish is reheated.

5. Invest in cookware and kitchen gadgets like nonstick cookware, vegetable steaming trays, and gravy skimmers (to remove fat from soup, stew, and gravy) that can help you eliminate fat as you cook.

 Store cooking oil and whole-grain flour in the refrigerator to prevent their fatty acids from getting rancid.

Butter-Wise Baking

Being fat conscious does not mean you must dispense with dessert altogether. An unexpected bonus of the health community's focus on fats has been the many ingenious methods food professionals have developed that allow people to literally "have their cake and eat it too." The American Dietetic Association suggests that home chefs can reduce the fat in baked items by 30% to 50% without affecting the quality of the final product.[17] To be a butter-wise baker, use the ingredient substitutions shown in Table 5-8 and the rules of thumb for fat reduction in Table 5-9.

If you are really daring, you can eliminate the fat in many recipes altogether by using pureed prunes or applesauce in place of shortening, butter, margarine, and

TABLE 5-8 Food and Ingredient Substitutions

Instead of	Try
Doughnuts, muffins, biscuits	Whole wheat, raisin cinnamon, English muffins, pancakes, waffles, or bagels
Wheat Thins	Ak Mak crackers, soda crackers, flavored rice cakes, bread sticks, pretzels
White flour tortillas	Vegetarian whole wheat or corn tortillas
French fries	Baked potato
Baked potato with sour cream and chives	Low-fat or nonfat sour cream substitute; plain, low-fat yogurt
8-oz rib steak	4-oz (raw weight) filet mignon
Sausage pizza	Cheese and vegetable pizza
Chili con carne; refried beans	Vegetarian chili; vegetarian refried beans
American style bacon	Canadian style bacon
Ground beef	Skinless ground turkey
Full-fat cheese	Reduced-fat cheese
Cream cheese	Low-fat cream cheese; low-fat margarine and jam, fruit butters
Butter	Margarine
Stick margarine	Soft spread, diet, or liquid margarine
Mayonnaise	Diet mayonnaise; mustard; salsa
Salad dressing	Low-fat dressing; seasoned vinegar, herbs
Chocolate, 1 oz	3 tbsp cocoa + 1 tbsp margarine
2 eggs	1 egg + 2 whites; egg substitutes
Ice cream	Nonfat frozen yogurt; sherbert; ice milk
Apple pie	Baked apple
Frosted cake	Angel food cake; commercial fat-free cake

TABLE 5-9   Healthy Baking Tips

Cakes and soft drop cookies	Use no more than 2 tablespoons of fat per cup of flour.
Muffins, quick breads, and biscuits	Use no more than 1-2 tablespoons of fat per cup of flour.
Pie crust	Use ½ cup margarine for 2 cups of flour.

BOX 5-3   7 Keys to a Low-Fat Diet

1. Eat more whole, unprocessed foods such as carbohydrate-rich grain products and produce.
2. Substitute low-fat versions of processed foods whenever possible.
3. Reduce the portion size of any meat you eat.
4. Switch to low-fat or nonfat dairy products.
5. Use low-fat cooking techniques.
6. Restrict use of the foods contained in the fat group of the Food Guide Pyramid, such as high-fat condiments and sweets.
7. Take advantage of published menus at school or work to help you with your menu matrix plans. Also, familiarize yourself with the food choices available at your favorite restaurants. Many eating establishments, including fast-food franchises, provide nutrition information to help patrons select a healthful diet.

oil. According to industry sources, both packaged baking mixes and from-scratch recipes can benefit from these substitutions. The numbers are certainly convincing. One half cup of oil contains 950 kcalories and 110 grams of fat. By contrast, an identical amount of pureed prunes supplies 270 kcalories and 0.5 gram of fat. The same amount of applesauce has a scant 55 kcalories and a mere trace of fat.

If you are eager to "prune" the fat in your baked goods, you can obtain recipes from prune and applesauce suppliers. Other manufacturers are coming up with equally healthy ideas.

At the Table

Stop before you take one bite! You are not home free yet. All of your good fat-fighting work can be undone if you use the wrong condiments. Many of these are fat traps. Consult Table 5-9 for appropriate substitutions.

Review the recipe shown below. Note all changes you would make to create a more "heart healthy" version of this dish. (You can check your nutritional savvy in Appendix A.)

PASTA a la PENNA

1 lb	Tubular pasta like penne or rigatoni
1	Yellow onion, coarsely diced
1	8-oz can tomato sauce
1	16-oz can plum tomatoes
¼ lb	Diced ham
1	Cup frozen peas, defrosted
1	Cup cream

Serve with grated Parmesan cheese

Eating Out

If you eat out more than once or twice a week, follow the 7 Keys to a Low-Fat Diet in Box 5-3. Ask to have all fat-filled sauces, dressings, and condiments served separately so that you can use them at your own discretion. Be careful at salad bars! Except for the plain vegetables, many of the offerings, such as ambrosia and pasta salad, are high in fat. Look for a diet dressing or use small quantities of an oil and vinegar dressing or plain lemon juice. Skip the dessert selections. If you must have dessert, share one or get a nonfat frozen yogurt on the way home.

Menu Matrix

Remember that much of the advice regarding reducing dietary fat consumption is on a weekly rather than daily basis. To translate this advice into action, you need to have a basic weekly meal plan rather than just grabbing the most convenient food whenever you are hungry. Because fat is typically hidden in or added to other foods, planning dietary fat changes is an excellent opportunity to practice integrating the other dietary recommendations presented thus far. The information on ferreting out the fat in foods that you learned on our imaginary trip through the grocery store, together with the following tips, will help you complete the menu matrix.

The key to cutting dietary fat is reducing consumption of meat, full-fat dairy products, and processed foods. Your menu matrix should already contain plenty of carbohydrate-rich foods. The next step is to count up your servings of meat and dairy products. The Dietary Guidelines suggest you eat a minimum of two servings of milk and a maximum of two servings of meat per day.

How do you apportion these servings so that you win the low-fat game?   Dairy is easy: just choose reduced-fat varieties. Meat takes a bit more know-how. Even if your number of servings is not excessive, the size of each serving may be (remember: one serving = 3 ounces of cooked meat). The American Dietetic Association suggests that you choose lean meats like poultry or fish (remember at least two of these fish servings should be varieties that are rich in omega-3 linolenic acid) more often than red meats, that you experiment with low-fat vegetarian dishes a couple of times each week, and that you eat no more than 3 ounces of high-fat meat per week.[17]

Why so little red meat?   One large-scale study found that women who ate red meat once a week or less frequently had a significantly lower rate of colon cancer than those who ate it more often.[26] Another study found that the more meat, eggs, and whole milk products men ate, the greater their risk of developing prostate cancer.[15]

Nutrition experts seem to agree that, when it comes to red meat, even lean cuts should be used sparingly. In a *Consumer Reports* survey of 94 nutrition professionals, including scientists, clinical dietitians, and educators, 60% of respondents believed red meat should be limited to three 3-ounce servings per week.[5] Also, the World Health Organization issued a Mediterranean diet food guide pyramid that emphasizes reducing red meat intake.[18]

If you are a vegetarian, don't rely too heavily on eggs, full-fat cheese, and other whole milk products to round out your protein intake. Instead make the appropriate combinations of plant proteins, as described in Chapter 6, the centerpiece of your diet. Limit egg yolks to four per week and use low-fat or nonfat milk products.

Whatever your eating style, once you have selected your foods, add up the approximate amount of fat used up by your meat and milk group choices (see the Personalizing the Pyramid section of Chapter 2 for details). Subtract it from the total fat budget you calculated on p. 27 of this chapter. Now figure out where you are going to spend the rest of your fat budget: processed foods, condiments, or desserts?

Remember, healthful eating allows room for occasional guilt-free splurging on high-fat foods!

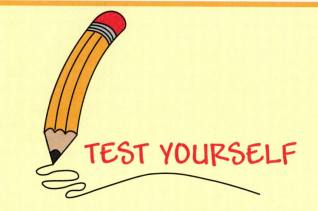

TEST YOURSELF

True or **False.** Put a **T** for true or an **F** for false in the space beside each question.

_____ 1. Lipids are classified as oils if they are liquid and fats if they are solid.

_____ 2. Fatty acids and glycerol are the building blocks of the most common dietary fats.

_____ 3. Bile is needed to emulsify fats so they can be digested.

_____ 4. Phospholipids and cholesterol contribute a significant quantity of kcalories to the American diet.

Short Answer

5. List three functions of fat in the human body.

6. Cholesterol is found in which food groups of the Food Guide Pyramid? Why?

7. If you melt butter or margarine, are their fatty acids still saturated? Explain.

8. List at least two things people can do to decrease their dietary fat intake.

9. The human body can make all the fatty acids it needs except _____ and _____ , which are found in _____ and _____ , respectively.

10. What are the major health risks associated with consuming too much fat?

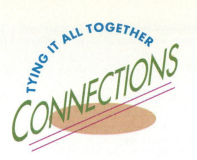

TYING IT ALL TOGETHER

CONNECTIONS

1. Read the ingredient content information from a popular butter substitute (on the left) and answer the questions as completely as possible.

   a. List all the types of fat molecules in this spread.

   b. Does this product contain any saturated fat?

   c. What, if any, are the sources or potential sources of saturated fat in this product?

   d. Does this product contain any cholesterol?

   e. What, if any, are the sources (or potential sources) of cholesterol in this product?

   f. Can you identify any source of an omega-3 fatty acid in this product?

   g. Can you identify any source of an omega-6 fatty acid in this product?

   h. Can you identify an emulsifier in this product? What is the function of an emulsifier?

2. Why do dietary fats keep people feeling full longer than carbohydrates?

3. Are fats organic? What does organic mean?

4. Are lipids good sources of energy? How much energy does a gram of fat provide?

5. Lipids are commonly found in foods as mixed triglycerides. Glycerol is always the same, so what is mixed?

Butter Substitute

CONTENTS: Soybean oil, partially hydrogenated corn oil, water, lecithin, salt, vegetable monoglycerides, and diglycerides.

REFERENCES

1. ADA Reports, Position of the American Dietetic Association: Fat replacements, *Journal of the American Dietetic Association* 91(1):1285-1288, 1991.

2. Atkins PW: Molecules, series: *Scientific American Library*, New York, 1987, WH Freeman.

3. Berner LA: Roundtable discussion on milkfat, dairy foods, and coronary heart disease risk, *Journal of Nutrition* 123(6):1175-1184, 1993.

4. Birch LL: Children's preference for high-fat foods, *Nutrition Reviews* 50:249-255, 1992.

5. *Consumer Reports*, Oct 1992, p 644.

6. Diet, nutrition, and the prevention of chronic diseases: A report of the WHO study group on diet, nutrition and prevention of noncommunicable diseases, *Nutrition Reviews* 49(10):291-301, 1991.

7. Dietary guidelines for Americans, 1990, U.S. Department of Health and Human Services, Home and Garden Bulletin #232.

8. Dietary guidelines for healthy American adults: A statement for physicians and health care professionals, Dallas, 1991, American Heart Association.

9. Dupont J: Lipids. In *Present knowledge in nutrition*, ed 6, Washington, DC, 1990, International Life Sciences Institute, Nutrition Foundation.

10. Emken EA: Trans fats—healthy or unhealthy? *Fat and Nutrition Update* 1(2):1-5, 1992.

11. FAO Agriculture Series #23, The state of food and agriculture 1990, Rome, 1991.

12. Focus of food labeling, an FDA special report, *FDA Consumer*, 1993.

13. Food labeling update, *Food Safety Notebook*, 3(12):110-115, 1992.

14. Fourteenth Marabou Symposium: The nutritional role of fat, part 1, *Nutrition Reviews* 50:1-71, 1992.

15. Giovannucci E et al: A prospective study of dietary fat and risk of prostate cancer, *Journal of the National Cancer Institute* 85(19):1571-1579, 1993.

16. Healthy people 2000: National health promotion and disease prevention objectives, U.S. Department of Health and Human Services, Public Health Service Bulletin #(PHS)91-50212, 1990.

17. Lean toward health, a publication of the National Center for Nutrition and Dietetics, Chicago, 1992, American Dietetic Association.

18. Burros M: The eating right pyramid faces some Mediterranean competition, *New York Times*, April 27, 1994.

19. National Cholesterol Education Program: Report of the expert panel on blood cholesterol levels in children and adolescents, U.S. Department of Health & Human Services, NIH Pub #91-2732, Sept 1991.

20. National Research Council: *Recommended dietary allowances*, ed 10, Washington, DC, 1989, National Academy Press.

21. National Research Council: *Diet and health: implications for reducing chronic disease risk*, Washington, DC, 1989, National Academy Press.

22. Nixon DW: *Nutrition and cancer: American Cancer Society guidelines, programs, and initiatives*, Atlanta, 1990, American Cancer Society.

23. Sabaté J et al: Effects of walnuts on serum lipid levels and blood pressure in normal men, *New England Journal of Medicine* 328(9):603-607, 1993.

24. Senate Select Committee on Health: *The dietary goals for the United States*, ed 2, 1977.

25. Smith RS: *Nutrition, hypertension and cardiovascular disease*, ed 2, Portland, Ore, 1989, Lyncean Press.

26. Stampfer MJ et al: Postmenopausal estrogen therapy and cardiovascular disease: ten-year follow-up from the Nurses' Health study, *New England Journal of Medicine* 325(11):756-762, 1991.

27. Stern J, Herman-Zaidens M: Fat replacements: a new strategy for dietary change, *Journal of the American Dietetic Association* 92(1):91-93, 1992.

28. The Food Guide Pyramid, U.S. Department of Agriculture, Home and Garden Bulletin #252, 1992.

29. The immediate benefits of low-fat eating, *University of California at Berkeley Wellness Letter* 9(7):1, 1993.

30. Health after 50: Nine strategies for cutting heart disease risk, *Johns Hopkins Medical Letter*, 4(12):4, 1993.

31. The new food label, FDA backgrounder, BG 92-4, 1992.

32. Troisi R et al: Cross-sectional study of trans fatty acid use in 700 male veterans, *American Journal of Clinical Nutrition* 56:101, 1992.

33. *University of California at Berkeley Wellness Letter* 9(7):1, 1993.

34. *University of California at Berkeley Wellness Letter* 9(5):3, 1993.

35. Wallingford JC, Yetley EA: Development of the health claims regulations: the case of omega-3 fatty acids and heart disease, *Nutrition Reviews* 49(11):323-331, 1991.

36. WHO: Report on the world use of fats and oils, 1989.

37. Willet W: Trans fatty acids and risk of coronary artery disease among women, *Lancet* 341(8845):581-586, 1993.

38. Willett WC et al: Relation of meat, fat, and fiber intake to the risk of colon cancer in a prospective study among women, *New England Journal of Medicine* 323:1664, 1990.

CHAPTER

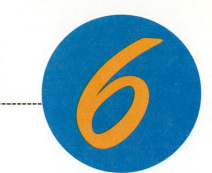

6

PROTEINS
The Body's Building Blocks

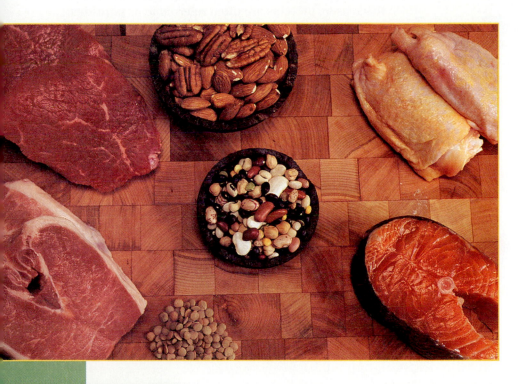

**To eat is human,
to digest divine.**

— Mark Twain

When scientists first identified protein about 150 years ago, they acknowledged the significant role it plays in sustaining life by giving it a name meaning *primary*—derived from the Greek word *proteios*. Protein, like carbohydrate and fat, is a potential source of fuel for the body.

Despite this similarity, protein has some important differences from the other nutrients shown in Table 6-1. Only protein is primarily a source of materials to build body tissues, such as organs, muscle, cartilage, and skin. All three nutrients contain carbon, hydrogen, and oxygen, but only protein also is a source of **nitrogen.** Protein is composed of these four elements arranged in building blocks known as **amino acids.**

THE NITROGEN CYCLE

Plants are the first step in the carbon cycle; they also are the first step in "fixing" nitrogen.

Nitrogen to Amino Acids

Where does the nitrogen in protein come from?
Nitrogen, like carbon and oxygen, is constantly cycling throughout the Earth's ecosystem (Fig. 6-1). Nitrogen

Fuel Value of Nutrients	
	kcal per gram
Carbohydrates	4
Proteins	4
Lipids	9

moves from the air to the soil, into plants, then into animals, and finally back into the soil. Plants make amino acids by combining nitrogen absorbed from the ground with carbon fragments that plants produce during photosynthesis. Then they link these amino acids together to form plant proteins, many of which are consumed by animals and converted into animal protein. We humans consume plant proteins directly or indirectly when we eat animal products. Nitrogen is returned to the soil via animal excrement and decaying plant and animal tissue. This nitrogen is part of the special building block of protein called *amino acid (AA).*

Amino Acids to Protein

How are proteins produced from amino acids?
Proteins form when the *amine* (nitrogen-containing) group of one amino acid bonds with the carboxylic acid (carbon and oxygen-containing) group of another, forming chains that range from a few to several hundred amino acids in length. The chemical link formed between amino acids is known as a **peptide bond.** For this reason, proteins are often referred to as **peptides.**

Interlocking Building Blocks

To date, about 20 structurally unique amino acids have been identified in edible proteins. Each amino acid has an identical chemically bonded backbone composed of a nitrogen-containing amine group, a carbon (C) group, and a carboxylic acid group, as shown in Fig. 6-2. They also have a distinctive side chain called a *radical* or *R group.* The chemical differences between R groups give each amino acid its unique shape and function.

TABLE 6-1   Review/Preview

	Dietary Nutrient		
	Carbohydrates	Lipids	Proteins
Building block	Monosaccharides	Triglycerides	Amino acid
Kcal content	4 kcal/g	9 kcal/g	4 kcal/g
Source	Grains, cereals	Oils, fats	Meat, fish, poultry, animal products, legumes, nuts, seeds, grains
Nutrient intake standard	Dietary Goals	Dietary Goals	RDA, 0.8 g per kg
Food intake standard	Dietary Guidelines	Dietary Guidelines	Dietary Guidelines
Use in the body	Fuel (blood glucose), mucus	Cell membranes, fuel storage, hormones	Structural proteins (organs, muscles) Functional proteins (enzymes, antibodies, plasma proteins)
Deficiency	Ketosis, gluconeogenesis	Flaky dermatitis (unlikely)	Decreased growth, anemia, edema, impaired immune function, tissue wastage
Excess	Stored as glycogen and fat	Obesity, CVD, some cancers	Excess nitrogen becomes urea; excess carbon, stored as fat

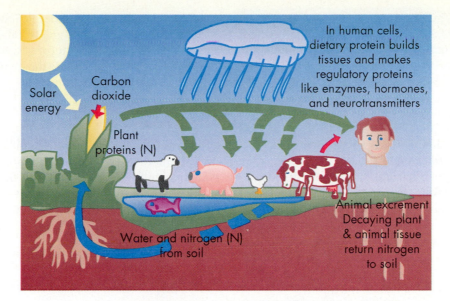

FIGURE 6-1 The nitrogen cycle.

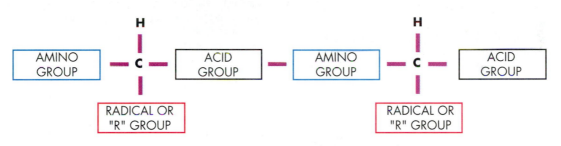

FIGURE 6-2 Structure of an amino acid.

Essential Amino Acids

The commonly occurring amino acids are divided into two groups—essential and nonessential—depending on the body's ability to *synthesize* them. **Essential amino acids** are those the body either cannot synthesize or can produce only in insufficient amounts. These amino acids must be provided by the diet. Table 6-2 lists the 10 essential amino acids for humans.

Nonessential Amino Acids

A **nonessential amino acid** (Table 6-2) can be formed within your cells from nitrogen and a carbon chain or from the similar essential amino acid. For example, your body can form tyrosine from phenylalanine, or cysteine from methionine.

IN THE DIET—QUANTITY

Global Sources

Not all cultures depend as heavily on animal sources of protein as do Americans. In many parts of the world, plant proteins are the major source of nitrogen.

TABLE 6-2 Essential and Nonessential Amino Acids

Essential	Nonessential
Phenylalanine	Glycine
Tryptophan	Alanine
Valine	Proline
Leucine	Tyrosine
Isoleucine	Serine
Methionine	Cysteine
Threonine	Aspartate
Lysine	Glutamate
Arginine	Asparagine
Histidine	Glutamine

amine an organic compound that contains nitrogen

amino acid an organic chemical compound composed of an amine group, a carbon group, and a carboxylic acid group

radical (R) group a group of atoms that forms a fundamental portion of a molecule

synthesize to produce new material by combining separate elements

What are the major food sources of protein around the world?   Meat, milk, eggs, fresh-water and marine fish, crustaceans, and aquatic animals are animal sources of protein. *Legumes,* peas, and beans are the richest plant sources of protein. Small but important amounts are also provided by *grains* (rice, wheat, oats, etc). Individual choices are determined by availability, culture, personal preferences, and sometimes allergies.[9] Animal-derived proteins provide the best array of essential amino acids (see the Protein Quality section), add a natural salty flavor to meals, and, because of the time required to digest them, help make a meal "satisfying." Plant-derived protein sources are lower in fat and digest less completely but more quickly than animal sources. Because individual plant proteins typically lack one or more of the essential amino acids, they must be eaten in the appropriate combinations to provide adequate nutrition.[2]

How much protein do I need each day?   Two issues are important when choosing dietary protein:

1. The *quantity* of protein (measured as nitrogen) in the diet
2. The *quality* of the protein (how much of each essential amino acid it contains)

The amino acid composition of a protein is just as important as the quantity consumed. Accordingly, nutri-

ent and food intake standards have been developed that address either the quality or quantity of protein (Table 6-3). It is important for you to be aware of these distinctions when you study the meal planning tools described later in the chapter.

Food Intake Standards—Food Guide Pyramid

How much of my diet should be protein-rich? Most Americans consume more protein than they need. This practice is expensive, both financially and physically.[21] Ounce for ounce, animal proteins tend to be more expensive than plant proteins; and, as we saw in

TABLE 6-3 Intake Standards	
Foods	**Nutrients**
Dietary Guidelines	**RDA**
Food Guide Pyramid	% Daily Value (labels)
5-A-Day Program	
American Heart Association	Dietary Goals
American Cancer Society	
People eat foods.	**Cells eat nutrients.**

Food Guide Pyramid
A Guide to Daily Food Choices

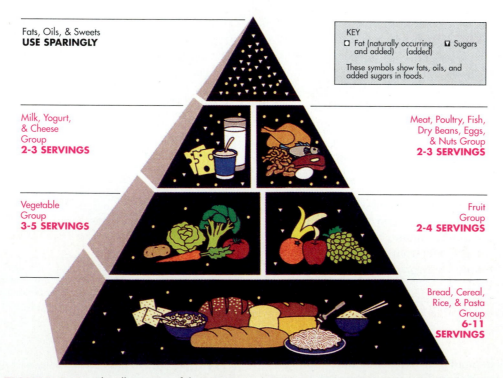

Fats, Oils, & Sweets
USE SPARINGLY

KEY
☐ Fat (naturally occurring and added)   ☑ Sugars (added)
These symbols show fats, oils, and added sugars in foods.

Milk, Yogurt, & Cheese Group
2-3 SERVINGS

Meat, Poultry, Fish, Dry Beans, Eggs, & Nuts Group
2-3 SERVINGS

Vegetable Group
3-5 SERVINGS

Fruit Group
2-4 SERVINGS

Bread, Cereal, Rice, & Pasta Group
6-11 SERVINGS

FIGURE 6-3   This illustration of the USDA Food Guide Pyramid highlights the food groups that are sources of protein. Only tiny amounts of protein are supplied by the fruit and vegetable groups. These are important sources of protein for vegans vegetarians, who eat no animal products.

Chapter 5, Lipids, they contain concentrated sources of health-threatening saturated fat and cholesterol. For these reasons the Dietary Guidelines[7] depicted in the Food Guide Pyramid[28] emphasize controlling animal protein intake. The Guidelines also suggest that we choose a vegetarian protein source, such as legumes, at least once a week. Protein is scattered throughout most of the food groups in the Food Guide Pyramid (Fig. 6-3). The milk and meat/meat substitute groups provide the most concentrated sources of protein for most Americans. Vegetarians also get a significant amount of their dietary protein from grains.

What do the positions of the milk and meat groups in the Food Guide Pyramid tell people about the recommended quantities of these foods in their diet?

Table 6-4 shows that with milk providing 8 g of protein per serving and meat an additional 14 to 21 g per serving, a person using this meal plan would consume a total of 70 to 127 g of protein daily. This will more than adequately meet protein needs (estimated to be 45 to 65 g per day).

NUTRI NUGGET Lentil, bean, and pea company officials are unhappy with their products' designation as meat substitutes in the new Food Guide Pyramid. True legumes are protein-rich foods that can take the place of meat. What industry officials are unhappy about is the fact that the meat category is dotted with numerous fat symbols. Although fat is a feature of the meat and cheese in this category, it does not apply to legumes. Moreover, the new categorization fails to tell consumers that, unlike animal proteins, legumes are good sources of dietary fiber.

Following the Food Guide Pyramid is an excellent way to control your protein intake. However, it is still easy to select a high-fat, high-cholesterol diet by choosing whole milk, eggs, cheese, pork, lamb, and beef. It is also possible to choose a vegetarian diet that is low in

both iron and zinc. This means you need to learn how to make the healthiest food choices from each food group. The Exchange Lists and Pyramid Food Choices Charts in Appendix C can help you identify low-fat protein choices.

Nutrient Intake Standards—RDA

The amount of protein a person needs is determined by how much protein s/he loses each day in urine, feces, sweat, mucus, lost hair and nails, and sloughed skin cells and how much, if any, s/he needs for growth. In healthy individuals, growth is the major metabolic function of protein during youth; maintenance is the primary function after maturity. Consequently, children need quite a bit more protein than adults[8] (see Chapter 12, Life Cycle, for details). The RDA for protein states that healthy adults should consume 0.8 g of protein per kg of healthy body weight each day.[20] Elite athletes[18] (see Chapter 10, Exercise and Nutrition) and people experiencing high levels of physical or emotional stress may require more.

Approximately how much protein does this work out to? The RDA for protein is 0.8 g per kg of healthy body weight. To interpret this RDA, you need to know that:

- Animal products are not 100% protein: animal flesh is at most 20% protein by weight, and milk is only about 5%.
- Healthy body weight means the weight of a person who is well muscled and has only a moderate amount of body fat.[1]
- A kilogram (kg) is a unit used to measure mass or weight in the metric system (Box 6-1).

grain the seed-bearing fruits of grasses; each kernel of grain contains a seed at its core; this seed is surrounded by a layer of starch (intended for use by the seed as it germinates into a plant); the starch is wrapped in a protective layer of bran (fiber) capped by an outermost inedible layer known as the hull

legume the seed of a plant belonging to the legume family; distinguished from other plants by pods containing a single row of seeds; peas, beans, and lentils are examples

TABLE 6-4	**Control Your Protein Intake Using the Food Guide Pyramid***			
Food Group	g Protein/Serving Size†	Number of Servings		Total Protein
Milk	8/(8 oz)	2-3	=	16-24 grams
Meat, eggs, legumes	21/(3-oz meat)	2-3	=	42-63 grams
Fruit and vegetables	0-2/(½ cup)	5-9	=	0-18 grams
Grains and cereals	2/(½ cup)	6-11	=	12-22 grams
Day Total				**70-127 grams**

*Daily protein needs are estimated to be 45 to 65 grams.
†The serving sizes for meat, cereals, and grain refer to cooked volumes or weights.

At a healthy body weight of 120 pounds (55 kg), a woman's RDA for protein would be 44 grams. If she gained 100 pounds (so that she weighed 220 pounds or 100 kg), her RDA for protein would remain at 44 grams. This is because the weight she gained would essentially be all fat. Fat tissue is not continually being replaced by protein; therefore she would need no additional protein.

How much food is equivalent to 44 g of protein?
We get protein from a variety of different food sources, none of which are pure protein. Meat is only about 20% protein, so 7.8 ounces of meat would provide about 44 g of protein.

> 55 kg × 0.8 g per kg = 44.0 g
> 44 g protein/0.20 = 220 g meat
> 220 g of meat/28 g per ounce = 7.8 oz of meat

IN THE DIET—QUALITY

Food Intake Standards

An easy way to ensure you are consuming the proper quality of protein is to categorize foods as either **complete** or **incomplete, complementary** or **supplementary,**[17] according to the following criteria.

Complete proteins contain all the essential amino acids in the needed proportions. The standard of comparison used is either the egg white protein, albumin, or the milk protein, casein. Animal sources of protein, except for gelatin, provide complete proteins.

Incomplete proteins, by comparison, are low in one or more of the essential amino acids. According to this criterion, gelatin and plants contain incomplete proteins.

Complementary proteins are two incomplete proteins that, when combined, form an amino acid pattern equal to that found in a complete protein. For instance, grains tend to be low in one essential amino acid, whereas legumes tend to be low in another. A combination of grains and legumes forms a more complete protein. The Menu Matrix section provides more information on complementary proteins and vegetarian meal planning.

Supplementary protein is a small amount of a high-quality protein added to a meal that is otherwise mar-

ginal in terms of protein quantity and/or quality. An example of supplementation is adding cheese or milk to a high-carbohydrate meal, as in preparing a macaroni and cheese casserole.

NUTRI QUIZ

How can you improve the protein quality of the following food items without adding meat, fish, or poultry?
1. Macaroni with butter
2. Bread and jam
3. Spanish rice

Nutrient Intake Standards

In the early 1900s, researchers found that the source of a protein affects its quality. If all other dietary factors are equal, proteins of animal origin are both better sources of essential amino acids for humans and are more completely digested than are proteins of plant origin. In the hierarchy of protein quality, animal proteins have greater nutritional value than legumes, and legumes are more nutritious than grains. Quiona (keen-wa), an ancient Peruvian grain known to the Incas, and soybean protein, a popular ingredient in Asian dishes, are the exceptions to the rule. Scientists were delighted to find that these foods provide an essential amino acid ratio very similar to that of animal protein.[15]

Measures of Protein Quality

In theory, the amino acid composition of a protein is just as important as the quantity of protein consumed because foods deficient in one or more of the essential amino acids will not support protein synthesis if used as the sole amino acid source in a diet. In reality, protein quality is of concern only in instances where the diet is energy-deficient and both the quantity and variety of protein-containing foods are limited. Because limitations of this type are common in many parts of the world, researchers have developed methods to determine protein quality[27] (see A Closer Look on p. 101).

The most important concept with respect to protein quality for those of us consuming a wide range of foods is that the nutritional value of any protein is usually enhanced by eating it as part of a balanced meal. This is because carbohydrate, fat, vitamins, and minerals, not just amino acids, are needed to facilitate protein use.

IN BETWEEN: DIGESTION

Mechanical digestion of protein occurs in the mouth, where teeth tear and shred animal and plant matter into smaller pieces. Chemical digestion begins in the stomach in the presence of hydrochloric acid. This strong acid environment:

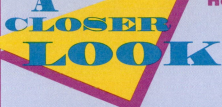

A CLOSER LOOK

How Do Scientists Measure Protein Quality?

CHEMICAL SCORE

Several methods can be used to measure the quality of a protein. Using the Chemical Score (CS) approach, scientists look up the essential amino acid composition of a given protein source in a reference book and compare it with the known EAA requirements of human beings. Proteins such as albumin (egg white protein) and casein (milk protein) are considered reference proteins and are assigned a chemical score of 100. Proteins from other single foods are then compared, EAA by EAA, with the reference proteins and assigned a chemical score reflecting how closely their amino acid composition approaches the established standard. Essential amino acids that are in short supply in a given protein are termed *limiting amino acids* because their absence limits the usefulness of the protein.

DIGESTIBILITY AND ENDOGENOUS SOURCES OF PROTEIN

A weakness of the CS rating system is that it fails to take into account both digestibility and efficiency of utilization. Plant sources of protein are less digestible than animal sources because of the fibrous cell walls that enclose the plant cells. Thus the nutritional value of a plant protein may be significantly lower than one would conclude on the basis of its chemical score. Conversely, protein wastes (cell parts and products) that are released in the digestive tract can be digested and reused along with the dietary protein source, providing for much better amino acid quality than would be expected on the basis of the CS alone.

PROTEIN EFFICIENCY RATIO

To compensate for the limitations in the CS, scientists use one of several methods that analyze the growth of animals fed a given food as the sole source of protein. The most widely used of these animal-based techniques is the Protein Efficiency Ratio (PER). This technique compares the growth of rats fed protein from single food sources, such as corn or wheat, with their growth when the animals are fed a nutritionally optimal diet using casein as the protein source. Although the animal-based techniques provide more information about the utilization of a protein than can be obtained from the CS method, these techniques are not without their shortcomings. Species differences exist with respect to amino acid requirements; therefore a major problem with animal studies is the need to extrapolate the data obtained from animals to human nutritional needs. For instance, using the PER technique, many proteins appear to be of lower quality than they really are because they do not meet the amino acid needs of rats as well as they do of humans. The PER owes its popularity to the fact that it is the method used to determine the quality of a protein for food labeling purposes. Depending on quality, the U.S. RDA recommends two different levels of protein consumption. Proteins that produce growth equivalent to the level obtained with casein are considered to be of high quality; proteins that produce less than the casein-based level of growth are considered to be of poorer quality. According to the U.S. RDA, healthy adults should consume 45 g of high-quality protein or 65 g of low-quality protein each day.

BIOLOGICAL VALUE AND NET PROTEIN UTILIZATION

Both of these technqiues measure nitrogen intake from a single food source and compare it to nitrogen loss (sloughed tissue and excrement). The bilogical value (BV) measure, which is possible to determine with humans, yields data regarding how much of the nitrogen in a consumed protein was retained in the body. The net protein utilization (NPU) operates on a similar principle. Rather than simply measuring the amount of protein consumed, however, it determines how much was digested, then compares the amount of nitrogen in the digested food with the amount lost from the body. With both techniques, the more nitrogen retained, the higher the quality of the protein tested.

- Denatures protein (changes its characteristic shape or nature)
- Breaks (hydrolyzes) some of the peptide bonds linking the amino acids
- Activates the protein-digesting enzyme **pepsin**

NUTRI NUGGET The peptide bonds in proteins are sensitive to both heat and pH (acid or base). When the bonding is disrupted by changes in either factor, the protein loses its characteristic shape or *nature*. We say that it has been *denatured*. Cooking an egg white denatures its protein, thereby changing its texture and fluidity.

Pepsin breaks peptide bonds in the amino acid chains of protein, forming polypeptides of various lengths. In the small intestine, pancreatic proteases digest the **polypeptides** to **tripeptides** and **dipeptides**.

dipeptide two amino acids joined by a peptide bond

polypeptide many amino acids joined by peptide bonds

tripeptide three amino acids joined by peptide bonds

Absorption and transport. The dipeptides and tripeptides are digested by special enzymes produced on the surface of the intestinal cells. Scientists believe these enzymes digest the final peptide bond while simultaneously throwing the resulting amino acids into the cell.

NUTRI NUGGET Supplements containing free amino acids were promoted as muscle-building agents until it was discovered that intestinal cells use dipeptides and tripeptides more readily. Now dipeptide and tripeptide supplements are sold!

IN THE BODY

Amino acids are absorbed through the intestinal cells and are carried through the blood to the liver. The liver cells may use the amino acids for protein synthesis or remove the amine group, using the carbon chain for fuel (4 kcalories per gram). The liver exerts quality control by maintaining a precise ratio of the 20 different amino acids in the bloodstream. If too much of one is consumed, the liver may convert it to a related amino acid before shipping it through the bloodstream to other cells, where it is synthesized into a variety of specialized proteins.

Flexibility of Form

Protein's capacity to assume diverse structures and functions results from the enormous number of different sequences in which 20 amino acids can be arranged. Suppose a jeweler has 20 different types of gemstones and draws as many different necklace designs as possible using all 20 stones. If the jeweler made a necklace from all 20 stones using each stone only once, there would be over 2.4 quintillion different sequences in which to string the stones. When you consider that in proteins, any given amino acid can be used more than once, the number of possibilities truly boggles the mind!

Limiting Amino Acids

Your body can produce all the proteins it needs, provided it has an adequate supply of essential amino acids. Suppose a wealthy admirer sent you a box of jewels (real ones, of course) to string into 25 necklaces, using the design pictured in Fig. 6-4. You received 25 emeralds (E), 200 diamonds (D), 25 rubies (R), and 50 sapphires (S). Each necklace is to contain 1 emerald, 2 rubies, 2 sapphires, and 8 diamonds. How many necklaces could you string to match this pattern? (No other necklace pattern is acceptable.)

You can make only 12 necklaces because you run out of rubies. You could take the partially finished thir-

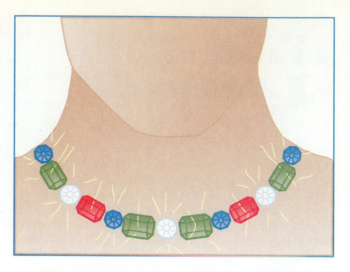

FIGURE 6-4 *Constructing an amino acid "necklace."*

teenth necklace apart and make some other piece of jewelry with it, or you could sell off the extra jewels. If the necklace had been protein made out of essential amino acids, you would have run out of lysine if your amino acids were from grains, or methionine if the source of amino acids were legumes. In these situations lysine and methionine are called **limiting amino acids.** Just as a shortage of rubies prevented full use of the gemstones, EAA deficiencies prevent the full use of dietary proteins. That is, the essential amino acid in smallest supply in a food or diet becomes the limiting factor because it limits the amount of protein the body can synthesize. Table 6-5 lists some foods, their limiting amino acid, and food combinations that yield complementary proteins.

Form and Function

How does a protein's shape affect how it functions in my body?   Proteins are more than straight chains of amino acids strung together with peptide bonds. The chains are able to assume many different shapes, which accounts for protein's ability to perform a wide variety of tasks. Proteins can be divided into two major categories, **structural** and **functional,** with respect to the tasks they perform in our bodies.

Structural Proteins

Some chains of amino acids tend to arrange themselves into bundles and form water-insoluble *fibrous* protein. Three triple strands of protein, like a strong rope, form the protein collagen. The body cells use this material to make structural parts such as skin, tendons, bone matrix, cartilage, and connective tissue. Other arrangements of fibrous protein form the muscles and organs.[27]

Functional Proteins

Whereas some proteins become structural parts of our bodies, others remain invisible, dissolved in body flu-

TABLE 6-5 Limiting Amino Acids in Plant Foods

Food	Limiting Amino Acids	Good Plant Source of the Limiting Amino Acids*	Traditional Uses of Complementary Proteins
Soybeans and other legumes	Methionine	Grains, nuts, and seeds	Tofu (soybean curd) and rice
Grains	Lysine, threonine	Legumes	Rice and red beans, lentil curry and rice
Nuts and seeds	Lysine	Legumes	Soybeans and ground sesame seeds (miso); peanuts, rice, and black-eyed peas; sunflower seeds; green peas
Vegetables	Methionine	Grains, nuts, and seeds	Green beans and almonds
Corn	Tryptophan, lysine	Legumes	Corn tortillas and pinto beans

From Wardlaw GM, Insel PM, Seyler MF: *Contemporary nutrition*, ed 2, St Louis, 1994, Mosby.
*Animal products in the diet serve the same purpose, such as when fish is consumed with rice.

ids. These invisible proteins are formed of chains of amino acids that twist and fold into a globular or functional protein. Functional proteins regulate activity within the body's fluid compartments. They also form certain hormones, enzymes, transport proteins (remember lipoproteins?), and chemical messengers known as neurotransmitters.[27]

Imagine what would happen to your body if all the structural proteins suddenly disappeared. Your hair, skin, nails, and organs (such as liver and heart), your muscles, and the collagen in your bones and between your cells would be all gone. What would remain? Humans are about 60% water by weight, 12% to 20% fat, and a few percent minerals. You would be a puddle of water plus fat and minerals!

Put all the structural proteins back in your body. Now imagine that you remove only the invisible, functional proteins. How would this affect your body? Loss of functional or globular proteins would erase: *blood proteins*, including hemoglobin, which carries oxygen to your cells and carries carbon dioxide waste away; *plasma proteins*, which help maintain fluid balance; *antibodies*, which help fight disease; *hormones* such as insulin and glucagon, which help maintain blood glucose levels; *enzymes* for breaking down metabolic reactions such as digestion; and *transport proteins*, which move nutrients throughout the body.

With all these proteins missing from your body, metabolism would come to a screeching halt! As you can see, functional (globular) proteins are essential to normal body processes.

NITROGEN BALANCE

Nitrogen balance in an adult means that the amount of nitrogen entering the body is equal to the amount the cells need to replace parts. Nitrogen enters the body (N_{in}) as food (dietary protein) and leaves the body (N_{out}) as urea, feces, sweat, mucus, sloughed skin, and lost hair and nails (Table 6-6).[27,30]

Positive nitrogen balance signifies that protein is being absorbed into the body and accumulating there. This process occurs during periods of growth, including pregnancy, and to a lesser extent during muscle building. Positive nitrogen balance also occurs during repair of tissue after surgery or injury. Conversely, negative nitrogen balance signifies a loss of body protein. This occurs during rapid weight loss, starvation, prolonged metabolic or emotional stress, and with protein-deficient diets.

Protein Deficiency

What happens if I don't get enough dietary protein?

Dietary protein deficiencies result in negative nitrogen

TABLE 6-6 Nitrogen Balance

Balance			
Balance	N_{in}	$=$	N_{out}
Positive balance	N_{in}	$>$	N_{out}
Negative balance	N_{in}	$<$	N_{out}

1. One third of the cells lining the digestive tract are replaced daily. What happens if you do not eat enough protein to renew the supply?
2. What happens to the production of antibodies, hemoglobin, and plasma protein under the same conditions?
3. What would happen to bone formation if you took lots of calcium supplements but ate very little protein?

balance. People also may show signs of protein deficiency when their diet contains an adequate quantity of protein but lacks adequate kcalories or contains a high amount of a poor-quality protein. In both cases the protein is burned for energy instead of being used to maintain nitrogen balance.

Symptoms of protein deficiency are first seen in the tissues that are replaced most often. The first to suffer are red blood cells and blood proteins, as well as cells lining the digestive tract and liver cells. This leads to *anemia,* lowered resistance to infection, and *edema.* Eventually the hair and nails become brittle and stop growing. The skin develops a dry and scaly appearance. Sores appear and do not heal, providing avenues for opportunistic infections to invade the body. The severity of symptoms intensifies during prolonged deficiency or starvation. Ultimately, refeeding a person is of little use. In such cases the body has stopped producing digestive enzymes in an effort to conserve protein. Likewise the body stops producing transport proteins for absorption of vitamins and minerals. Ultimately the intestinal lining becomes so tattered that it cannot absorb what tiny amounts of food are digested.

Millions of people throughout the world suffer from various degrees of *protein energy malnutrition (PEM).* The problem is especially acute in children in developing nations, both because of the high energy and protein demands of their growing bodies and because of cultural practices that often restrict their access to food. PEM is also common in people who are in poor health and have little appetite. PEM symptoms are divided into two categories, kwashiorkor and marasmus, depending on the severity of the kcalorie restriction.[17]

Kwashiorkor is a condition that results primarily from a lack of dietary protein. Kcalorie intake is usually marginal. The symptoms include lethargy, depigmentation (loss of color) of hair and skin, a characteristic flaky dermatitis, stunted growth, loss of muscle tissue, and edema. This last symptom accounts for the pot-bellied appearance of the children we often see in ads for world hunger relief programs. Malnourished children clearly are at greater risk of developing diseases and may die of infections like chicken pox that are usually harmless. (You will find a detailed description of the world hunger crisis in Looking to the Future.)

NUTRI QUIZ Explain how infection and dietary protein deficiency can produce diarrhea.

Marasmus results from near or total starvation. It is often seen in bottle-fed babies who are given overly diluted formula in poverty-stricken areas throughout the world. Marasmus is also observed in starving people of all ages, including persons with anorexia nervosa. Symptoms include loss of both muscle and fat, giving victims the appearance of a skeleton with skin. Growth is severely stunted in children, and there may be severe mental retardation, as the majority of brain growth occurs in the first 2 years of life. Once this critical time period is past, no amount of refeeding will reverse the intellectual damage.

Treatment of both kwashiorkor and marasmus begins with restoring fluid balance, then slowly introducing protein-containing fluids and finally solids.

Stress

Physiological stress leads to PEM in hospitalized patients recovering from trauma, surgery, cancer, and other debilitating illnesses. Apparently protein metabolism is altered by the hormonal changes that occur with prolonged stress (lack of food, need to repair tissue and fight disease, emotional upheaval). The long-term effects of emotional stress on health are not known with certainty, but such stress may affect longevity by decreasing the activity of the immune system.[24]

NUTRI NUGGET Scientists have confirmed what students have always known: Final exams cause emotional stress. Researchers have noted negative nitrogen balance in students during final exam time. The students' diets seemed to be more than adequate.

Protein Excess

What happens if I have too much protein in my diet?
Cells rapidly dismantle protein we consume in excess of the amount we need for growth or replacement. The nitrogen is excreted in the urine as **urea,** and the remaining carbons are used to produce energy. If the energy supply exceeds demand, the excess carbons are synthesized into fat and stored in the adipose tissue.

Excessive protein intake has been implicated in the development of both kidney and heart disease. Results of animal studies suggest that prolonged intake of high-protein diets leads to kidney disease because of the demands placed on these organs by nitrogen excretion. Although healthy humans do not show similar problems, people with preexisting kidney disease need to closely monitor their protein consumption.[4] A more convincing relationship has been established between diets high in animal-derived protein and the development of cardiovascular disease. This effect appears to result from the high levels of fat and cholesterol associated with animal proteins, not from the protein itself.[21] (This research is discussed in greater detail in Chapter 5, Lipids.)

Amino Acid Imbalances

What happens if I eat enough protein but too much of a particular amino acid?   Theoretically, you could create an amino acid **imbalance.** When amino acid imbalances have been intentionally created in the diets of experimental animals, severe metabolic disturbances have resulted. Although such imbalances have not yet been observed in humans, the possibility exists so long as amino acid supplements can be purchased without a prescription.[21-23]

Errors of Amino Acid Metabolism

Among the inherited errors of amino acid metabolism, the best known is **phenylketonuria,** or **PKU.**

Phenylketonuria (PKU)

People who are born with PKU are incapable of converting the essential amino acid phenylalanine to tyrosine. Consequently, phenylalanine accumulates in their body, causing many negative side effects, the most severe of which is mental retardation. If detected during the first few days of life, PKU can be successfully treated through diet, although not cured. (Most states require a PKU blood test for newborns.) A PKU diet provides the minimum amount of phenylalanine required to support protein synthesis. Phenylketonurics must stay on such a diet throughout their growth phase but often can eat a fairly normal diet as adults because their brain has formed and is no longer susceptible to damage by high levels of phenylalanine and aspartic acid.

In addition to restricting their intake of foods that contain phenylalanine, people with PKU must avoid using the sugar substitute NutraSweet™, a synthetic compound containing phenylalanine and aspartic acid.

Protein recap. Table 6-7 reviews the flow of protein from the foods you eat through your digestive tract and into your cells.

Why must people with PKU avoid NutraSweet™?
Hint: NutraSweet™ is composed of which two amino acids?

IN TODAY'S WORLD

Americans' heavy reliance on animal proteins has led to some unique ecological and food safety issues. Our animal-rearing practices include using highly nutritious grains and legumes to feed poultry and livestock and adding large amounts of antibiotics to animal feed to prevent the spread of infectious diseases in herds and flocks.[26] The use of nutritious food for animal feed is poor management of food resources. The use of antibiotics to control disease has had a more serious consequence—the evolution of new, more virulent strains of bacteria. The remainder of this chapter reviews how to select, handle, and prepare protein-rich foods while keeping an eye toward sound ecological and food safety practices.

anemia   lower than normal amounts of red blood cells or hemoglobin in the blood

edema   abnormal accumulation of fluid in the interstitial spaces of the body

protein energy malnutrition (PEM)   a condition that results when a person regularly consumes insufficient amounts of energy and protein; the deficiency eventually results in body wasting and an increased susceptibility to infection; also called PCM: protein calorie malnutrition

TABLE 6-7 Review of Protein Digestion, Absorption, and Utilization	
Structure	**Protein**
Mouth	Teeth crush
Stomach	HCl denatures protein; pepsin and renin hydrolyze protein
Small intestine	In the lumen, pancreatic enzymes (amylases, lipases, and proteases) digest dietary and endogenous protein to dipeptides and tripeptides; dipeptidases and tripeptidases on the intestinal cell surfaces digest these to amino acids
	Absorbed: **amino acids**—immature digestive tracts will absorb larger peptides, possibly contributing to the development of allergies
Circulatory system	Blood
Liver	Maintains plasma amino acid balance. Makes many essential proteins, including enzymes, lipoproteins, and albumin. Converts carbon skeletons of amino acid to glucose
Kidney	Synthesizes urea from surplus nitrogen and excretes it in urine
Cells	Make needed proteins; adipose cells store excess as fat (triglycerides)
Large intestine	Excretes undigested material

Ecology of the Nitrogen Cycle

As we saw at the beginning of the chapter, nitrogen is constantly passing from the environment, to plants, to animals including humans, and back into the environment.

In a balanced ecosystem, herbivores (plant-eating animals) keep the plant population in check. In turn carnivores (flesh-eating animals) control the herbivore population. However, modern agricultural efficiency, which has promoted and sustained the heavy consumption of animal products, has upset this delicate balance in two important ways. First, it has diverted nutrient-rich grains from the human food supply. Second, it has forced deforestation of vast acreage to provide grazing land.[12,26]

Meat Production

Plant matter that is marginally digestible by human beings is easily converted by herbivores into high-quality animal protein. Industrialized nations, however, feed beef animals high-quality grains and legumes to enhance both the rate of growth and the taste of the meat. Transformation of nutrients from these nutritious plant sources into animal tissue is very inefficient. It is estimated that 16 pounds of grain and soybeans are needed to produce 1 pound of usable beef. As shown in Fig. 6-5, 1 pound of beef will give four people one meal. This same 16 pounds of grain and soybeans could easily have fed 64 people!

NUTRI NUGGET Some people believe that meat is an ecologically unsound source of protein and that everyone should convert to vegetarianism. However, millions of acres that are not useful for cultivation can support grazing animals, which are useful for both labor and food (high-quality protein, as well as bioavailable iron and zinc). The trick is to use resources efficiently.

Land Use

Producing enough grain and legumes to meet both animal and human needs places an additional burden on the ecosystem. It takes 17 acres to produce 1 million kcalories of animal protein but only 1 well-developed acre to raise 1 million kcals of plant-based foods.[9] The demand for acreage on which to graze animals and grow their food has forced the clearing of enormous areas of forest that took millions of years to develop.

Many scientists believe this practice is doing irreparable harm to the ecology. It is destroying many species of plants and animals, and it is also turning once-green forests into deserts. Forest soil, which tends to be very shallow, is constantly replenished by decaying plant and animal matter. Once the forest is gone, so is the source of new soil and nutrients. After

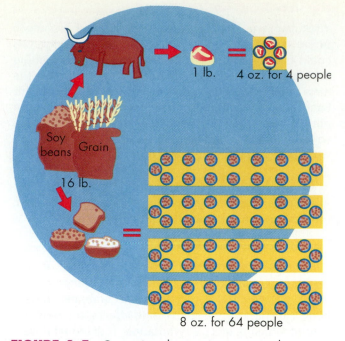

FIGURE 6-5 Converting plant nutrients to animal tissue: an efficient use of resources?

producing a few seasons of crops, the existing soil becomes unproductive; without plants to check erosion, the topsoil washes away, leaving a layer of hard clay that cannot be farmed. Forests also purify our air, ward off global warming, and maintain rainfall.[26]

What can we do?   Environmentalists and other concerned persons are urging us to decrease our reliance on animal products to help protect the ecosystem. We can all do our share by eating smaller portions of meat, observing one or more meat-free days per week, and whenever possible consuming range-fed rather than grain-fed animals.[9,26]

Processing

Processing of protein takes many forms: cooking, refining plant or animal foods, and producing purified amino acids.

Cooking

Cooking has little effect on the nutritional value of proteins, and most of the effect it has is beneficial. The heat used in cooking denatures protein, destroying potentially harmful microorganisms as well as enzymes that contribute to deterioration. Cooking is particularly important for plant proteins such as legumes and rice because it hydrates and softens their fibrous cell walls, facilitating release of the nutrients within. Cooking improves safety, palatability, chewability, and digestibility.

Refining (*re*-fine = *re*-move)

Purified proteins as well as individual amino acids can be refined from a variety of foods. As in any refining procedure, parts of the original material are taken away, resulting in the loss of valuable nutrients. What follows is a description of some of the proteins commonly refined from one food source for use in other products.

Gelatin. Gelatin is refined from animal collagen and is a poor-quality protein. Packets of purified gelatin can be purchased at the grocery store. Home cooks use it to give gelatin salads, pie fillings, and other desserts a firm texture. Gelatin is also added to many commercial products such as gelatin desserts, yogurt, reduced-fat sour cream, and ice milk.

Soy protein. One of the most widely used purified proteins is obtained from soybeans. It is used to make many products, including soy milk, tofu, soy grits, defatted soy flour, soy protein concentrate, soy protein isolate, and spun fibers, called **texturized plant protein (TPP),** which are used in vegetarian meat substitutes (Fig. 6-6). In many ways soy protein compares favorably with animal-derived protein. Its amino acid composition is close to that of meat. It has the added advantage of being lower in fat and cholesterol free.

A disadvantage of soy is that, unlike meat, it contains no vitamin B_{12}, and some of its valuable vitamins and minerals are removed during the refining process.

Soy flour is often added to baked goods to hold moisture and extend product shelf life. Unfortunately the properties that enable it to absorb water also allow soy to absorb fat. Extending meat with soy protein causes the dish to retain fat that cannot be drained off.

Dedicated label readers will find that refined milk (casein) and egg (albumin) proteins are also widely used by the food industry.

Aspartame. This sugar substitute, marketed under the brand names of Equal® and NutraSweet™, is a combination of two amino acids, phenylalanine and aspartic acid. (See Chapter 4, Carbohydrates, for details.)

Amino acid supplements. In general the human body needs high-quality protein, not individual amino acids, to stay in top form. Nonetheless, a wide variety of amino acid supplements are available in health food stores and fitness centers. They are touted as being able to enhance muscle strength, brain function, sleep, and overall health. In the best case, using amino acid supplements is simply a waste of money. In the worst case, they can produce serious physical harm.[21,23]

The best example of the dangers of self-administered amino acid supplementation is the toxic reaction suffered by some people who took supplements of the amino acid tryptophan as a natural sleep aid. The FDA in the late 1980s ordered vendors to remove tryptophan supplements from the market. The causes of these toxic reactions are still being investigated.[22]

Preserving

Salt, smoke, and nitrates have been used for centuries to cure and preserve meat. Luncheon meats, ham, bacon, hot dogs, and salami typically contain one or more of these preservatives. Recently these preservatives have come under scrutiny because of reports that they may be harmful to health. Excessive salt consumption has been associated with an increased incidence of high blood pressure (see Chapter 8, Minerals, for details). Eating too much meat that has been preserved with smoke or nitrates has been linked to stomach cancer. Chemicals formed on the surface of the meat during smoking, not the smoke itself, are believed to be the culprits in this instance.[3] The nitrates used to preserve meats are probably harmless. The human body makes a considerable amount of these chemicals, and many vegetables are naturally high in them. However, nitrates are converted in the stomach to cancer-causing chemicals known as nitrosamines.[21]

You can do two things to reduce your health risk: decrease the amount of cured meats you eat, and, when you do indulge, consume foods rich in vitamin C such as tomatoes and citrus. Vitamin C has no effect on salt or smoke-related compounds; however, it can prevent the conversion of nitrates to nitrosamines.

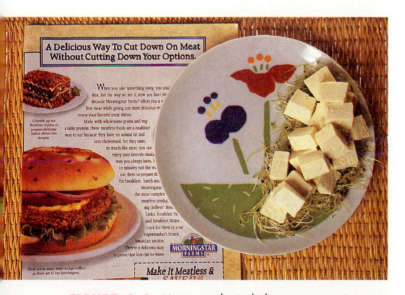

FIGURE 6-6 Many people, including nonvegetarians, enjoy the taste and texture of tofu and texturized plant protein.

IN MY DIET

How can I plan a diet that meets my protein needs?
Most people in industrialized nations obtain much of their dietary protein from meat, fish, poultry, and/or dairy products. There is also a sizable minority who practice vegetarianism. Whatever your eating style, many of the same considerations apply when you are selecting and cooking protein-rich foods.

At the Grocery Store

What protein-related concerns should I be on the lookout for at the grocery store?   The two major concerns for consumers are identifying specific sources of protein on food labels and handling animal products in a sanitary fashion.

Labels—Your License To Learn

Most of us eat too much rather than too little protein. Searching labels for protein content therefore is unnecessary unless you are allergic to a particular food protein; if so, you will need to scan the labels on any prepared food items.

Thanks to the 1990 Nutrition Labeling and Education Act, food labels must provide more specific information about standard food ingredients. Terms like "hydrolyzed plant protein," "animal protein," or simply "hydrolyzed protein" are no longer allowed. The precise source of this protein must be identified. Similarly, the labels on products that contain milk derivatives such as casein and whey must clearly state that they come from milk.[5,10,29]

Sanitation

The most important issue when shopping for proteins is *freshness*. Animal products deteriorate rapidly. It is essential to select fresh items that have been stored in well-maintained freezers or refrigerators.

Check the "pull dates" when shopping for animal products. Do not purchase items with an "off" odor or color.

Put meat, fish, and poultry into plastic bags to prevent dripping their juices, a potential source of bacteria, onto other groceries. Be sure to follow the handling procedures described on the package (Fig. 6-7).

Do not buy eggs with cracked shells or cheeses with mold spots (unless it is cheese like French Roquefort that is supposed to contain mold).

If you have many errands to run, the grocery store should be your last stop. Put refrigerated and frozen foods in the grocery cart last. Take the groceries directly home and store them promptly and properly.[16,19]

In the Kitchen

Are cooking and preparation techniques important? Because animal products are excellent breeding grounds for bacteria, it is important to practice good hygiene when preparing them. This includes (1) sanitary handling procedures to prevent spreading bacteria from contaminated foods around the kitchen and (2) cooking foods sufficiently to kill harmful bacteria and parasites.

Raw and undercooked animal tissue can carry a number of parasites. Pork was once notorious for harboring the parasite trichinosis, but veterinary technology has eradicated this parasite. Raw fish may carry worms and other parasites. In the last decade salmonella contamination of eggs and raw or undercooked poultry has become a significant health problem.[14,19]

The blood contained in animal tissue is another source of concern. Blood is rich in nutrients and as such is the perfect medium for bacterial growth. Because a bacteria-free environment is not possible under normal conditions, meats always have some bacteria on their surfaces. If meat remains at room temperature, these bacteria multiply, hastening spoilage and increasing the risk of food poisoning. Unfortunately, refrigeration or even freezing in the typical home appliance will not kill microbes. It simply puts them into a state of

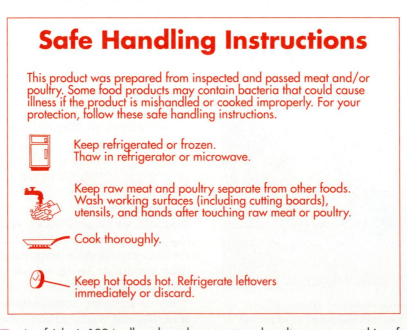

Safe Handling Instructions

This product was prepared from inspected and passed meat and/or poultry. Some food products may contain bacteria that could cause illness if the product is mishandled or cooked improperly. For your protection, follow these safe handling instructions.

Keep refrigerated or frozen.
Thaw in refrigerator or microwave.

Keep raw meat and poultry separate from other foods. Wash working surfaces (including cutting boards), utensils, and hands after touching raw meat or poultry.

Cook thoroughly.

Keep hot foods hot. Refrigerate leftovers immediately or discard.

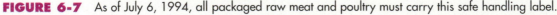

FIGURE 6-7   As of July 6, 1994, all packaged raw meat and poultry must carry this safe handling label.

suspended animation, stopping their multiplication. As soon as they warm up, however, their survivors multiply. To reduce bacterial growth, thaw meats only in the refrigerator, in a sink full of cold water, or in a microwave oven. Some of the bacteria on the surface of meats can be removed by rinsing in cool water. Bacteria are killed by high salt or acid concentrations. Rubbing salt inside and outside of poultry or pouring vinegar over meats and rinsing again will remove much of the bacteria.

NUTRI NUGGET In late 1992 food poisoning occurred at Jack-In-The-Box restaurants in several western states because of *E. coli*–infected hamburger meat. Although the source of this meat was found and is no longer being used, the USDA is considering tightening meat inspection regulations.[31]

To minimize opportunities for cross contamination, prepare fruits and vegetables before meats, ideally on a separate chopping board reserved for this purpose. Thoroughly clean counter tops, cutting boards, sink, hands, and any utensils used in meat preparation before fixing any other foods.[31]

After each use, wash any surface that comes in contact with meat with soap and hot water or a 1:10 dilution of chlorine bleach to water to kill all microbes.[14,16] The makers of Clorox bleach offer the following suggestions for thoroughly sanitizing kitchen work surfaces.

To sanitize a wooden cutting board: Wash with hot, sudsy water; rinse. Cover the surface with a solution made from 3 tablespoons of chlorine bleach per gallon of water. Reapply solution as needed to keep surface wet for at least 2 minutes. Rinse, let dry. For other items, soak in a solution of 1 tablespoon of bleach per gallon of water for 2 minutes; air dry.

Be sure to cook with enough heat to destroy bacteria (between 165° and 212° F). This is particularly important if you are using a slow cooking method such as a crockpot. Keep hot foods hot and cold foods cold until serving time. Temperatures *above* 140° F and *below* 40° F inhibit the growth of bacteria; unfortunately, within that range bacteria grow quite well. This is an important fact to keep in mind when serving buffet style or carrying foods to picnics. Store leftovers promptly, using shallow containers so that the food cools quickly. Reheat leftovers to at least 165° F. Boil sauces, gravies, stews, and soups for several minutes before serving a second time.

At the Barbecue

Humans have been grilling meat over open flames since we first discovered fire. Despite many advances in cooking techniques, grilling is still an extremely popular way to prepare meat. Scientists, however, charge

that, along with flavor, grilling adds potentially carcinogenic chemicals known as PAHs (polycyclic aromatic hyrocarbons). Fortunately for barbecue enthusiasts, there are some simple ways to reduce the amount of PAHs that form during grilling.[3]

PAHs form when fat drips onto a hot flame or cooking element. The resulting smoke distributes PAHs over the surface of the food. To minimize this problem:

- Grill mainly low-fat meats, like fish and poultry, instead of beef and pork
- Trim all visible fat from meats
- Use a drip pan to catch melting fat before it hits the coals
- Use only low-fat marinades and sauces.

At the Table

The biggest challenge for most people is limiting their meat and poultry intake to two 3-ounce servings (cooked weight) a day. Here's a way to stay on track: a standard audiotape cassette occupies the same amount of space as a 3-ounce serving of meat. Remember to fill up the rest of your plate with generous servings of grains and produce. Serving meat on top of starch or as part of a casserole is another way to help you cut down on your portions. Examples are meatballs with spaghetti, curried turkey and vegetables on a bed of rice, and clam sauce over pasta.

Eating Out

Serving size and food safety are often liabilities for restaurant diners. Many eating establishments have built their reputations as well as their revenue by serving extra-large portions of food. If you are eating in such a place, solve two problems at once by asking for a "doggie bag." You'll have your next meal already prepared, and you'll keep your kcalorie and fat intake in check.

Small portions are the norm in many trendy restaurants, but so are undercooked animal proteins. Despite the continuing craze for raw oysters and the Japanese seafood known as sushi, it is best to avoid raw animal tissue, including raw eggs. Undercooked animal proteins are just as much of a problem as raw ones. Many of the trendier restaurants serve game birds and lamb as well as beef on the rare side. Although trichinosis is not the problem it once was, other bacteria and parasites are as plentiful as ever. For your protection, request that your meat be well cooked.[16]

Also avoid any dish that contains raw eggs, such as freshly made mayonnaises and mousses.[14] Most restaurants have responded favorably to the campaign to discontinue the use of recipes that call for raw eggs. If you have any questions about how an item was prepared, ask your server.

When selecting food items from a salad bar, make sure they are well chilled and look fresh. Many eating establishments use containers suspended in a bed of ice. The contents of these containers heat up rapidly once the ice melts away and exposes the containers to the air. Avoid foods that appear to have warmed up or begun to deteriorate. If in doubt, choosing fruits and vegetables is safer than eating protein-containing salads, such as chicken, egg, seafood, and some pasta dishes. Use these tips to avoid potentially contaminated food at potlucks and picnics.[31] Just as at home, restrict the serving sizes of protein-rich foods you eat out—except for special occasions, of course!

Menu Matrix

Here are some suggestions for developing a meat-eater as well as a vegetarian menu matrix. Complete a week's worth of menus for the eating style you typically practice. To increase your familiarity with other food choices, complete 2 days' worth of menus you normally do not eat. For example, if you are a meat eater, plan 2 days' worth of vegetarian menus and vice versa.

Meat-Eaters Matrix

The Food Guide Pyramid suggests that 2 or 3 servings of dairy products plus 2 or 3 3-ounce servings (cooked weight) of meat or meat substitutes per day are sufficient to meet the typical person's protein requirements. It further stipulates that the majority of dairy and meat products consumed should be low-fat varieties. Because most Americans eat too much meat, the menu matrix will focus on limiting the number and size of servings of meat eaten each day. The easiest way to integrate these diet suggestions into your life is to plan meals on a weekly basis. This approach helps both to maintain variety and to achieve moderation. Using the above recommendations, you can have 14 to 21 servings per week of dairy products and 14 3-ounce servings of meat or meat substitutes. If you are like many Americans, you may need to make an effort to add milk products to your diet while cutting back on meat.

Where to begin? Work out your food selections from the milk group before turning your attention to the meat group. Although the Food Guide Pyramid suggests we consume no more than two 3-ounce servings of meat per day, you can split up your weekly intake any way you want. Just aim to keep it to a maximum of 42 ounces of meat or animal-based meat substitutes per week. This means you can have an 8-ounce steak for dinner occasionally, provided you make up for this indulgence somewhere else in your diet. If you find the 3-ounce serving size too skimpy for dinner, try having a smaller portion of meat at lunch. An ounce or two of thinly sliced lunch meat goes a long way. Also remember that eggs and cheese qualify as meat substitutes, so if you have eggs for breakfast or a cheese sandwich for lunch, you have already used up one of your meat choices for the week. To make your meat choices go further, leave the cheese out of sandwiches that al-

ready contain meat and restrict the number of cheeseburgers you eat. Think lean: try to select mainly low-fat meats or their equivalent (see Chapter 5).

After you have read the vegetarian menu matrix guidelines, develop 2 days' worth of vegetarian menus for your own use. Make a commitment to working at least 1 day's worth of vegetarian foods into future weekly menus.

Vegetarian Menu Matrix

Many people today choose to be vegetarians for ethical, environmental, or health reasons. This style of eating is probably as old as human civilization. Through trial and error, various ethnic groups around the globe learned to combine nuts, seeds, legumes, starchy vegetables, and grains in such a way that they provided amino acid patterns comparable to those found in animal products (see A Closer Look on p. 111). In some societies vegetarianism became part of the native religion and is still practiced today. People from these cultures are accustomed to vegetarian eating patterns that supply all of the necessary nutrients. On the other hand, people from meat-eating cultures who become vegetarians must learn how to plan nutritionally balanced meals.[2]

Whether you opt to become a vegetarian or simply choose to add a few vegetarian meals to your regular diet, you will find that a good vegetarian cookbook is an excellent investment. Not only do such books supply nutritious and tasty recipes, they also provide essential information for people trying to obtain their nutrients exclusively from plant products. (Appendix G lists some of the best cookbooks to try.)

There are two basic types of vegetarianism[2] with some variation within each group. Vegetarians are either **vegans** (those who eat *only* plant products) or **lacto-ovo-vegetarians** (those who eat dairy foods and eggs in addition to plant products). It is also possible to find fruitarians, lacto-vegetarians, and ovo-vegetarians. Not surprisingly, the more categories of foods you consume, the easier it is to meet your nutritional needs. Vegetarians who consume eggs and dairy products have a relatively easy time planning nutritious meals. Vegans, however, must make a concerted effort to con-

TABLE 6-8 Complementary Food Combinations		
Legumes	+	Cereals or grains
Legumes	+	Nuts and seeds
Seeds and nuts	+	Leafy vegetables and whole grains
Brewers' yeast	+	Peanuts, seeds, nuts, leafy vegetables, and whole grains

A CLOSER LOOK

Rediscovering Grains and Legumes

Throughout history, various combinations of grains and legumes have been the mainstay of people's diets. It is only in industrialized nations during the past 50 years that meat has become the centerpiece of the diet. In light of mounting evidence that the fat and cholesterol in meats may be linked to many of the illnesses common in industralized nations, health experts are encouraging people to rediscover grains and legumes.

Why grains and legumes?   In addition to being high-fiber, low-fat sources of energy and protein, **grains** and **legumes** complement each other's amino acid content. The grains featured in Chapter 4, Carbohydrates, in the section on Cooking Grains and Legumes, supply some of the iron, zinc, copper, and magnesium that legumes tend to be low in.

Many people's repertoire of grain and legume dishes begins and ends with rice, pasta, and pinto bean chili. Fortunately, just about all grains and beans work well as ingredients in soups and salads, so these dishes make good jumping-off points for your exploration of legume and grain combinations (see table). Traditional ethnic dishes also can provide inspiration for tasty pairings of grains and legumes. Curried lentils with rice, tofu and vegetable stir-fry served over rice, corn tortillas filled with beans and rice, and couscous topped with vegetarian stew are just a few examples of tasty and healthful combinations.

Learning about Legumes

Type	Color	Use
Black beans	Black	Baked, soups, stews, dips, casseroles, salads, vegetarian burgers
Black-eyed peas	White with a black spot	Casseroles
Garbanzo beans (chickpeas)	Golden brown	Dips, casseroles, salads, soups, stews, flour
Great northern beans	White	Baked, casseroles, chowder, soups, stews
Kidney beans	Red	Casseroles, chili, salads, soups
Lentils	Brown, green, or red	Casseroles, salads, soups, curries
Lima beans	White or green	Casseroles, soups
Navy beans	White	Baked, soups
Pinto beans	Pink	Baked, casseroles, soups
Red beans	Red	Casseroles, chili
Soybeans	Tan	Casseroles, salads
Split peas	Green or yellow	Soups

Adapted from Neiman DC, Butterworth DE, Neiman CN: *Nutrition*, Dubuque, Ia, 1990, William C Brown.

sume the appropriate amounts of grains and legumes to get a balanced amino acid pattern. Eating the complementary food combinations shown in Table 6-8 will provide a complete and balanced array of essential amino acids.

Lacto-ovo-vegetarians may use the Vegetarian Four Food Group Plan shown in Table 6-9. This plan emphasizes many of the features found in the Food Guide Pyramid. The major difference is that it replaces the meat group with grains, legumes, nuts, and seeds and recommends more servings from this category to meet nutrient needs. People who elect not to consume any animal products will need to modify this plan to compensate for the vitamins and minerals in which plant-derived foods are typically low. Fortified breakfast cereals and soy milk products can be used to provide vitamin D, vitamin B_{12}, and calcium. Eating extra servings of grains, nuts, and seeds will supply the necessary quantities of riboflavin, iron, and zinc.

TABLE 6-9   Vegetarian Four Food Group Plan

Food Group	Amount
Grains, legumes, nuts, seeds	6 servings
Vegetables	3 or more
Fruits	2 to 4
Milk	2 or more

lacto-   prefix meaning milk
ovo-   prefix meaning egg

Converting this food plan into meals would produce a menu that looks something like the one in Tables 6-10 and 6-11.

 Recent evidence has challenged the long-held belief that we need to consume a complete protein or its equivalent at every meal to sustain protein synthesis. It now appears that consuming an adequate balance of amino acids each day will support protein synthesis.

TABLE 6-10 Lacto-Ovo-Vegetarian Meal Plan

Breakfast	Whole wheat pancakes with ½ c. strawberries and maple syrup Milk 6 oz orange juice
Snack	Fruit and crackers
Lunch	Vegetable chili (beans, onions, green pepper, tomatoes) Cornbread Salad (lettuce, spinach, cucumbers, mushrooms, tomatoes) Beverage
Snack	Fat-free cheese, fruit and crackers, low-fat popcorn, tomato soup
Dinner	Vegetable moussaka (eggplant, potatoes, artichoke hearts, zucchini, low-fat cheese) Whole wheat couscous, bread sticks, whole wheat banana bread Beverage

TABLE 6-11 Vegan Meal Plan

Breakfast	Oatmeal with fortified soy milk Sliced fruit Whole wheat toast with fruit preserves Beverage
Snack	Fruit
Lunch	Peanut butter and jelly sandwich on whole-wheat bread Carrot, celery, and bell pepper sticks Calcium-enriched orange juice Fruit
Snack	Whole wheat apple Newtons and fortified soy milk
Dinner	Tofu, broccoli, red bell pepper, carrot, celery, and bean sprout stir-fry 2 servings of brown rice Dried fruit and nuts Beverage

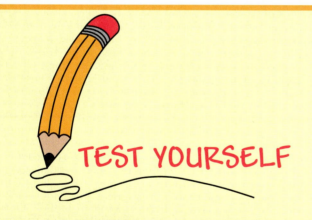

TEST YOURSELF

True or False. Put a **T** for true or an **F** for false in the space beside each question.

___ 1. Amino acids are the building blocks of protein.

___ 2. Protein is unique among the energy-providing nutrients because it contains nitrogen.

___ 3. Essential amino acids are made by your body from nonessential amino acids.

___ 4. Getting enough dietary protein is a problem for most Americans.

___ 5. Surplus protein is turned into fat.

___ 6. One of the main functions of protein in the body is the formation of body tissues, including bone.

___ 7. Soluble or globular proteins perform many regulatory functions in the body.

___ 8. Protein digestion begins in the stomach.

Short Answer

9. Explain the concept of using complementary proteins to create a healthy vegetarian diet. Give an example of a meal featuring complementary proteins.

10. List three ways to reduce the risk of food poisoning from contaminated animal protein.

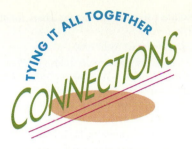

TYING IT ALL TOGETHER

CONNECTIONS

1. Identify the complementary protein categories to which the foods in each of the following combinations belong:

	Legume	Grain
Example:		
Peanut butter sandwich	peanut butter	bread
1. Red beans and rice	_____	_____
2. Macaroni and cheese with peas	_____	_____
3. Tofu, vegetable and rice stir-fry	_____	_____
4. Vegetarian chili and cornbread	_____	_____

2. Three childhood friends, Tom, Dick, and Harry, are college athletes. While home on vacation, they compare their training diets. (Assume they each weigh 180 pounds and each eat 3000 kcalories per day.)

- Tom eats anything he wants but uses amino acid supplements for muscle building, vitamin supplements for energy, and mineral supplements for strength.

- Dick is on a vegan diet. He uses no supplements at all. (See the Vegan Meal Plan in the Menu Matrix section.)

- Harry eats a diet based on the Food Guide Pyramid with some extra protein-rich food at each meal.

   a. List some possible sources of complete protein for each man.

   b. List some possible sources of complementary or supplementary protein for each man.

   c. Are they getting enough protein?

   d. Discuss the need or lack of need for amino acid and vitamin/mineral supplements for each man.

3. Which body tissues (water, bone, fat, or protein) are lost when dietary glucose is not available to the cells?

4. Which body tissue is increased when excessive dietary protein is available to the cells?

References

1. ADA Reports: Position of the American Dietetic Association: optimal weight as a health promotion strategy, *Journal of the American Dietetic Association* 89(12):1814, 1989.

2. ADA Reports: Position of the American Dietetic Association: vegetarian diets, *Journal of the American Dietetic Association* 93:1317-1320, 1993.

3. Ask the experts—is smoking meat harmful? *University of California Berkeley Wellness Letter* 9(3):8, 1991.

4. Blum M et al: Protein intake and kidney function in humans: effects of normal aging, *Archives of Internal Medicine* 149:211-216, 1989.

5. Browne MB: *Label facts for healthful eating*, American Dietetic Association and National Food Processors Association in cooperation with USDA, 1993.

6. Darby WJ, Jukes TH: *Founders of nutrition science*, vols 1 and 2, Rockville, Md, 1992, American Institute of Nutrition.

7. Dietary Guidelines for Americans, U.S. Department of Health and Human Services, Home and Garden Bulletin #232, 1990.

8. Epstein LH, Wing RR, Valoski A: Childhood obesity, *Pediatric Clinics of North America* 32(2):363-379, 1985.

9. FAO Agriculture Series #23, The state of food and agriculture 1990, Rome, 1991.

10. Focus of food labeling, FDA Special Report, *FDA Consumer*, 1993.

11. Food labeling update, *Food Safety Notebook* 3(12):110-115, 1992.

12. Gore A: *Earth in the balance: ecology and the human spirit*, Boston, 1992, Houghton Mifflin.

13. *Healthy vegetarian eating*, American Dietetic Association, Chicago, 1991, The Association.

14. How safe should you be with eggs today? *Sunset*, June 1991, pp 86-89.

15. Johnson S, Aguilur J: Essential amino acid patterns of quinoa, compared to wheat, soy, and FAO reference pattern for evaluating proteins in processing varieties of oilseed: report to Natural Fibers and Food Commission of Texas, 1979-1980.

16. Jones FT et al: A survey of salmonella contamination in modern broiler production, *Journal of Food Production* 54(7):502-507, 1993.

17. Latham MC: Protein-energy malnutrition. In Present knowledge in nutrition, ed 6, Washington, DC, 1990, International Life Sciences Institute, Nutrition Foundation.

18. Meredith CN et al: Dietary protein requirements and body protein metabolism in endurance trained men, *Journal of Applied Physiology* 66:2850-2858, 1989.

19. Missu B et al: Salmonella enteritidis gastroenteritis transmitted by intact chicken eggs, *Annals of Internal Medicine* 115(3):190-194, 1991.

20. National Research Council: *Recommended dietary allowances*, ed 10, Washington, DC, 1989, National Academy Press.

21. National Research Council: Diet and health: implications for reducing chronic disease risk, Washington, DC, 1989, National Academy Press.

22. Roufs JB: Review of L-tryptophan and eosinophilia-myalgia syndrome, *Journal of the American Dietetic Association* 92:844-850, 1992.

23. Safety of amino acids used as dietary supplements, Bethesda, Md, 1992, FASEB Life Science Research Office.

24. Sapolsky RM: *Why zebras don't get ulcers: a guide to stress, stress-related diseases, and coping*, New York, 1994, WH Freeman.

25. Senate Select Committee on Health: The dietary goals for the United States, ed 2, 1977.

26. *Smithsonian*, 20th Earth Day Issue, April 1990.

27. Steele RD, Harper AE: Proteins and amino acids. In *Present knowledge in nutrition*, ed 6, Washington, DC, 1990, International Life Sciences Institute, Nutrition Foundation.

28. The food guide pyramid, U.S. Department of Agriculture Home and Garden Bulletin #252, 1992.

29. The new food label, *FDA Backgrounder*, BG 92-4, 1992.

30. Waterlow JC et al: Protein turnover in mammalian tissues and in the whole body, New York, 1978, Elsevier North-Holland Biomedical Press.

31. Winter CK: Toxicologist, FoodSafe Program, UCD via Napa Solano, *Nutrition Council Newsletter* 2(1):1, 1993.

32. Zeman F, Ney D: Errors in amino acid metabolism. In Clinical nutrition and dietetics, Lexington, Mass, 1989, Callamore Press.

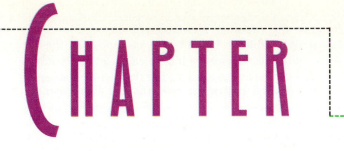

CHAPTER 7

VITAMINS
Separating Fact From Fiction

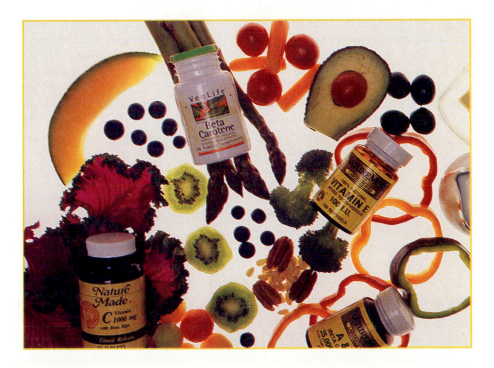

The cherry tomato is a
marvelous invention, producing
as it does a satisfactorily
explosive squish when bitten.

— Miss Manners (Judith Martin)

Upon hearing the word *nutrition*, many people immediately think of vitamins. Since their discovery in the early 1900s, the seemingly miraculous ability of vitamins to cure certain diseases has captured the popular imagination. When vitamins were discovered, little was known about the origin of contagious diseases or about the role of nutrients in preserving health. Consequently the history of the discovery of vitamins reads more like a combination of mystery tale and adventure story than like a technical work.

Like so many other scientific breakthroughs, the discovery of vitamins was accidental. In 1913 two teams of alert scientists found that rats fed a diet containing purified nutrients developed eye lesions and failed to grow.[6] Those fed the same diet with additional milk grew normally. The mysterious growth factor, which was isolated from the fat portion of the milk, was named *fat-soluble A*, or *vitamin A*. Not much later these researchers demonstrated that vitamin A could prevent the characteristic eye lesions seen in other animals and humans eating poor diets.

The discovery of vitamin A marked the beginning of an exciting era in nutrition science. Soon other diseases in animals were traced to dietary deficiencies. When the missing nutrient was replaced, the animal's health was restored. Buoyed by their success, scientists began to search for dietary causes of human disorders with symptoms mimicking those of animals that consumed nutritionally deficient diets. One breakthrough led to another. By 1940 all of the 13 currently recognized vitamins had been discovered, and thousands of people had been cured of debilitating and fatal diseases.

It is easy to see how the rapid succession of vitamin discoveries, each with seemingly magical curative factors, set the stage for today's multibillion-dollar nutritional supplement industry. Some manufacturers have tried to persuade the public that vitamins can cure all ills and that there is no such thing as too much of a vitamin. Vitamins do cure diseases, but only diseases related to the vitamins' metabolic functions. Moreover, the body is able to handle only certain quantities of these nutrients. Excessive intake can lead to disorders that are just as devastating as the deficiency diseases.

How did the individual vitamins get their names?

Initially scientists named vitamins with letters. The first one discovered they named vitamin A, the second one vitamin B, and so on. Later they found that vitamin B was not one but many vitamins, now collectively labeled the *B-complex* and distinguished from one another by numerical subscripts, as in vitamin B_1. Other vitamins received names rather than letters. Needless to say, confusion reigned. In the 1940s a committee of scientists established the present system of identification. It uses the letters A, B, C, D, E, and K (Danish for *koagulationsvitamin*) plus numerical subscripts where necessary.

What exactly are vitamins?

Vitamins are essential, organic, nonkcalorie molecules needed in very small amounts for cellular metabolism.

NUTRI NUGGET You may be wondering how an organic substance (a compound that contains the element carbon) can be nonkcaloric. The enzymes that liberate energy from protein, fat, and carbohydrate do not recognize the chemical structures of vitamins, so the kcalories contained in their carbon bonds are not accessible to the body.

IN THE DIET

Vitamins are divided into two broad categories based on whether they dissolve in water or fat (oil) (Fig. 7-1).

The water or fat solubility of a vitamin gives a clue as to:

- Which foods are likely to supply it
- How vulnerable it is to loss or destruction during cooking

TABLE 7–1 Review/Preview

| | Dietary Nutrient | |
	Water	Vitamins
Building block	H_2O	H_2O and fat-soluble molecules
Kcalorie content	0	0
Source	Fluid, foods	Unrefined, enriched foods
Nutrient intake standard	RDA, varies	RDA
Food intake standard	None	Dietary Guidelines, Food Guide Pyramid
In the body	Solvent, temperature regulation	Cofactors for enzymes, metabolic regulators, including release of energy from foods
Deficiency	Dehydration	Varies with vitamin
Excess	Electrolyte imbalances	Toxicity: Fat-soluble vitamins more often toxic than water soluble; symptoms vary with vitamin; dependence

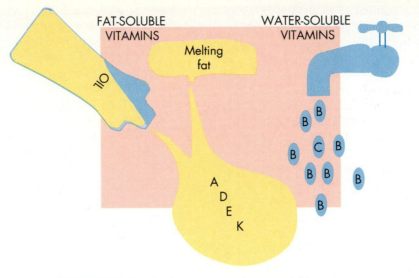

FAT-SOLUBLE
VITAMINS

WATER-SOLUBLE
VITAMINS

Melting
fat

OIL

A
D
E
K

B
B
C
B
B
B
B
B
B

FIGURE 7-1 The fat-soluble and water-soluble vitamins.

- How it will function in the body
- Whether the body stores significant quantities of it

Food Intake Standards

No one food is a good source of all vitamins. Every food group in the Food Guide Pyramid provides essential vitamins.[28] The vegetable and fruit groups are particularly rich sources of this nutrient class. To get the widest array of vitamins, select whole grain products and use the Food Guide Pyramid in conjunction with a produce selection guide such as the National 5-A-Day Program.[11]

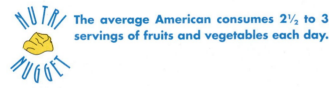 **The average American consumes 2½ to 3 servings of fruits and vegetables each day.**

The National 5-A-Day Program

The 5-A-Day Program encourages Americans to eat at least five servings of fruit and vegetables each day. The program specifies that we should eat at least one daily serving of vitamin C–rich fruit. We also should have one serving of cruciferous vegetables and one serving of beta carotene–rich leafy greens every other day.[11] Table 7-2 (on p. 118) is designed to help consumers make wise produce choices.

 Stress, either physical or emotional, increases the body's use of many vitamins as well as other nutrients. However, the vitamins supplied by a balanced and adequate diet are sufficient to meet the increased need.

Nutrient Intake Standards

How do I know how much of each vitamin I need?
The RDA provides information on desirable intake levels for 11 of the 13 vitamins currently recognized as being essential for human beings. The RDA also specifies safe and adequate intake levels for the remaining two vitamins, biotin and pantothenic acid, for which there is insufficient evidence to set an RDA.[16]

IN BETWEEN: DIGESTION AND ABSORPTION

Vitamins are released from food during the digestive process, but they themselves are not digested. The majority of water-soluble vitamins are freely absorbed across the intestinal membrane during water resorption. Two of the B-complex vitamins, folate and B_{12}, however, require special assistance.

 Don't take vitamin supplements on an empty stomach. Fat-soluble vitamins must be emulsified with bile to be absorbed because they do not mix well with the watery contents of the intestine. Because bile is released into the intestine only in the presence of dietary fat, vitamin supplements should be taken with a well-balanced meal.

IN THE BODY

Once inside the body, water-soluble vitamins can circulate freely in the water-based blood plasma and any ex-

TABLE 7-2 Fruits and Vegetables That Contain Vitamins A (Beta-Carotene) and C

FRUITS	Vitamin A	Vitamin C	Fiber
Apple			■
Apricots (3)	●		■
Banana			■
Figs (2)			●
Grapes (1 cup)			■
Grapefruit (½)		●	■
Kiwi fruit		●	■
Nectarine			■
Orange		●	■
Peach			■
Pear			●
Plums (2)			■
Prunes (4)			●

½ Cup Serving

	Vitamin A	Vitamin C	Fiber
Cantaloupe	●	●	■
Honeydew		■	
Papaya	■	●	
Pineapple			■
Raisins (¼ cup)			■
Raspberries		■	■
Strawberries		●	■
Watermelon (1 cup)		■	

JUICES ¾

	Vitamin A	Vitamin C	Fiber
Orange juice		●	
Grapefruit juice		●	
Tomato juice		●	

VEGETABLES ½ Cup Cooked	Vitamin A	Vitamin C	Fiber	Cruciferous
Asparagus		■	■	
Beans, green			■	
Bok choy	●	■	■	✔
Broccoli	■	●	■	✔
Brussels sprouts		●	■	✔
Cabbage		■	■	✔
Carrots	●		■	
Cauliflower		●	■	✔
Chile peppers (¼ cup)	●	●		
Corn			■	
Dried peas and beans			●	
Eggplant			■	
Green pepper		●		
Greens*	●	■	■	
Lettuce: (1 cup fresh)				
Spinach	●	■	■	
Romaine	■			
Red and green looseleaf	■			
Iceberg				
Okra			■	
Peas, green			■	
Potato (1 medium baked)		■	■	
Spinach	●			
Squash, winter	●		■	
Sweet potato	●		■	
Tomatoes (1)	■	■	■	
Zucchini			■	

■ These selections supply at least 25% of the U.S. RDA for vitamins A (as beta-carotene) or C or at least 1 to 3 grams of dietary fiber per serving.

● These selections supply at least 50% of the U.S. RDA for vitamins A (as beta-carotene) or C or at least 4 grams of dietary fiber per serving.

* Values are averages calculated using beet and mustard greens, swiss chard, dandelion, kale, and turnip greens. These foods are part of the cruciferous family.

Sources: USDA Handbook No. 8; Produce Marketing Association; and the Minnesota Nutrition Data System.

cess is easily excreted. Fat-soluble vitamins, on the other hand, must be transported through the blood by specialized carriers and tend to accumulate in the body's adipose tissue. Because fat-soluble vitamins are not transferred easily from the mother to the fetus, infants are born with minimal stores of these vitamins. These basic differences affect the body's ability to maintain balance and prevent toxicity.

Homeostasis—Maintaining Balance

How does the human body maintain a balance of water-soluble vitamins?   The body's main transport and purification system, blood plasma, is water based. Consequently, homeostasis of water-soluble nutrients is relatively easy to maintain. The water-soluble quality of the B-complex vitamins and vitamin C makes for easy absorption in the intestine, little accumulation in tissues, and efficient excretion in urine. The kidneys automatically excrete any water-soluble vitamin present in excess of the storage capacity. Typically, this is sufficient to rid the body of any surpluses. Toxicity symptoms, however, do occur in persons who take massive overdoses of some water-soluble vitamins such as vitamin B_6 and niacin. In such cases the amount of vitamin ingested overwhelms the kidney's ability to excrete it and the quantity remaining in circulation produces toxic side effects.

How does the human body regulate the levels of fat-soluble vitamins?   If you ever have seen a bottle of salad dressing separate into two layers, you know that water and oil (fat) don't mix. (See Fig. 5-6 in Chapter 5, Lipids.) This makes homeostasis of fat-soluble materials relatively complex. Fat-soluble vitamins A, D, E, and K require the presence of fat in the diet to stimulate the flow of bile. Bile aids in the digestion and absorption of fat and of these vitamins. Fat-soluble vitamins also require the help of protein to transport them in the blood plasma. For example, vitamin A attaches in the liver to a protein that ferries it safely through the watery bloodstream. Because no direct route exists for fat excretion, excesses of fat-soluble vitamins are stored in the liver and fatty tissues for use when dietary intake is inadequate. The small amounts of naturally occurring fat-soluble vitamins in foods, together with the restrictions on their absorption, keep storage levels from becoming excessive. Unless you have a liking for polar bear liver, which contains toxic levels of vitamins A and D, it is impossible to consume toxic levels of vitamins simply by eating whole, unprocessed foods. Eating too many fortified foods and/or taking *megadoses* of vitamin supplements, however, can produce symptoms of toxicity.

Deficiencies

What happens if I don't get enough vitamins?
Deficiency diseases and toxicity symptoms are presented in this chapter for each individual vitamin. As a rule, symptoms of vitamin deficiencies and excesses are noticed most readily in tissues that are easy to examine, such as skin, eyes, and blood.

Excesses

What happens if I consume too many vitamins?
Toxicity syndromes are presented for each vitamin. As a general rule, fat-soluble vitamins are more toxic than water-soluble ones because our bodies can't excrete fat.

Imbalances

Can vitamin supplements cause an imbalance?
An imbalance may occur when too much of a particular vitamin is added to an otherwise balanced and adequate diet, causing a relative deficiency of its helper nutrients. Some vitamins work alone; others, most notably the B-complex vitamins, function as part of a group. The success of their cooperative efforts depends on the body's maintaining a balanced quantity of B-complex vitamins. Excesses of individual B vitamins can throw off the body's biochemical balance, with profound metabolic consequences.[16]

The human body cannot distinguish between manmade and naturally produced vitamins. Natural vitamins, such as vitamin C extracted from rose hips, are *not* nutritionally superior to synthetic vitamins (manufactured in the laboratory).

Endogenous Sources of Vitamins

Does my body's ability to make certain vitamins increase my likelihood of developing a vitamin toxicity or imbalance? No. Given the appropriate **precursor** (starting material), the body can make some vitamins itself. These include niacin, from the amino acid **tryptophan;** vitamin D, synthesized from a cholesterol-like compound in skin exposed to sunlight; and vitamin A, from **carotene,** a yellow-orange plant pigment. The body stops producing the active forms of these vitamins when the dietary supply is adequate.

Vitamin K and the B-complex vitamins, biotin and pantothenic acid, also may be "produced locally." What sets these vitamins apart from niacin, vitamin D, and vitamin A is that the body itself does not synthesize them. They are manufactured by bacteria that reside in the colon (large intestine). Although your body can supply some of these vitamins, your diet should include food sources of each to ensure optimal health.[16]

Errors in Vitamin Utilization

Any disease or injury that affects digestion and/or absorption can alter the body's vitamin utilization. Genetic defects have been implicated in the utilization of two vitamins: B_{12} (related to pernicious anemia) and vitamin E (possibly related to asthma).

Functions

A vitamin's solubility determines in part how it will function in the body. Generally, fat-soluble vitamins regulate metabolic reactions, whereas water-soluble vitamins serve as *coenzymes.* Figure 7-2 on the following page shows how a coenzyme works.

The preceding discussion provides an overview of the general concepts that apply to all vitamins. Now it is time to turn our attention to the specific functions of each vitamin. To simplify learning, the vitamins in this book are divided into four categories according to the major function they perform in the body:

- Energy metabolism
- Tissue synthesis
- Red blood cell synthesis
- Antioxidant

Energy Metabolism

Which vitamins do I need to be full of energy?
Five of the B-complex vitamins—thiamin, niacin, ri-

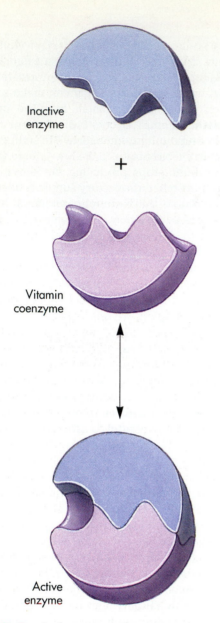

FIGURE 7-2 The functioning of a coenzyme.

boflavin, biotin, and pantothenic acid—play major roles in converting the kcalorie-containing nutrients (carbohydrate, lipid, and protein) into cellular energy.

Thiamin: B$_1$

Thiamin deficiency, **beriberi,** has been known for centuries, but not until this century were its cause and cure recognized. In the 1890s it was discovered that beriberi resulted from the consumption of hulled (white) rice, and that unhulled (brown) rice prevented or cured the disease. Later researchers found that thiamin in the hulls of whole grains prevents or cures the disease.

Functions. The major function of thiamin is to serve as a coenzyme in carbohydrate and energy metabolism. As part of its role in energy metabolism, it also assists in the breakdown of fatty acids.

Sources and recommendations. Small amounts are available in whole grains, brewer's yeast, organ meats, legumes, seeds, and nuts. The best natural source of thiamin is pork. Because of the small amounts available in most foods, people typically have had to make an effort to consume enough thiamin. In the United States enriched and fortified cereals, grains, and bakery products make a significant contribution to thiamin intake, eliminating thiamin deficiency as a health concern. The RDA for thiamin is linked to kcalorie intake because of its roles in carbohydrate and energy metabolism. Our need for thiamin increases as we consume more carbohydrate or expend more energy. The 1989 RDA recommend that men and women between ages 19 and 50 consume 1.5 and 1.1 mg of thiamin per day, respectively. This works out to 0.5 mg of thiamin per 1000 kcalories. Two servings of pork will provide the RDA for thiamin. For reasons of health, religion, or taste preference, however, most people get most of their thiamin from other sources.[16]

NUTRI QUIZ Why don't you need to take extra thiamin if you eat extra amounts of carbohydrate?

NUTRI NUGGET If you depended on a single food for your thiamin intake, you would need to eat 2 servings of pork, 4 to 8 servings of beef, lamb, poultry or legumes, or 15 to 20 servings of milk, eggs, fish, nuts, citrus fruits, starchy vegetables, or grains. Clearly the best approach is to consume a wide variety of whole foods daily.

Deficiency. Changes in the nervous and cardiovascular systems characterize beriberi, the disorder associated with thiamin deficiency. Initial symptoms include loss of appetite, muscle weakness, loss of reflexes, loss of sensation in the extremities, and mental confusion. Left untreated, symptoms progress to paralysis, an enlarged and irregularly beating heart, cardiac failure, and death.

Thiamin deficiency occurs most frequently in people who consume large amounts of unenriched white rice or white flour products. Thiamin is very vulnerable to destruction during cooking because it is easily destroyed by excessive heat. Additionally, it is easily lost from enriched grain products, like rice and pasta, if they are rinsed during the cooking process. In the United States, enrichment of refined flour has virtually eliminated thiamin deficiency. It is still common in alcoholics, however, because of decreased food intake and reduced intestinal absorption, coupled with the increased use of thiamin for alcohol metabolism.

Excess. There is no evidence that thiamin is toxic if taken orally, since the kidneys readily excrete any excess. However, there have been a few reports of toxic doses being administered intravenously. Adverse reactions include a rapid pulse rate, weakness, headache, and irritability.

Riboflavin: B₂

In 1897 a British chemist noticed a water-soluble, yellow-green fluorescent pigment in the whey of milk (the liquid that remains after cheese has been made from milk). It was not until 1932 that this compound was identified as vitamin B₂, or riboflavin.[6]

Function. Riboflavin, like thiamin, is an essential coenzyme for the conversion of food to fuel.

Sources and recommendations. Milk and milk products supply over half of the riboflavin consumed in the United States. Meat, fish, poultry, and organ meats are also good sources, as are broccoli, turnip greens, asparagus, and spinach. Grains are naturally low in this vitamin. However, enriched and fortified grain products, cereals, and baked goods all contribute significantly to Americans' dietary intake. For example, a cup of enriched wheat flour provides 25% of the DV for riboflavin compared with the 8% provided by an equal amount of whole wheat flour.

Your body's need for riboflavin depends on your total kcalorie intake, energy needs, body size, metabolic rate, and growth rate. The current RDA is 0.6 mg per 1000 kcalories. For healthy adults, this amounts to a daily intake of 1.3 mg for women and 1.7 mg for men. The requirement decreases slightly with age, reflecting decreasing energy intake. Pregnant women require an additional 0.3 mg of riboflavin per day to provide for the increased synthesis of both fetal and maternal tissues. Nursing mothers should consume 0.4 to 0.5 mg above the RDA to ensure adequate quantities in their milk.[16,23]

 How much of the % DV for riboflavin is supplied by the two to three servings of milk specified in the Food Guide Pyramid?

Deficiency. Riboflavin deficiency (ariboflavinosis) involves tissue inflammation and deterioration. Wounds fail to heal; cracks develop in the corners of the mouth and in the lips as well as in the skin folds around the nose; and the tongue becomes swollen and dark red. Extra blood vessels develop in the cornea of the eyes, followed by itching, burning, tearing, and sensitivity to light. Skin may develop a greasy, scaly condition, and in children, growth is impaired.

Excess. No documented cases of riboflavin toxicity have been reported, most likely because there is little intestinal absorption of this vitamin.[16]

Niacin: B₃

Niacin is available in foods as the active vitamin or as its precursor, the amino acid **tryptophan.** Vitamin B₆ is an essential cofactor for the conversion of tryptophan to niacin, once again demonstrating the interrelatedness of all nutrients.

Functions. Niacin occurs naturally in two forms, **nicotinic acid** and **nicotinamide.** Both of these compounds function as niacin in the body. Niacin serves as a coenzyme and partner to riboflavin in cellular reactions that promote conversion of glucose to energy.

Sources and recommendations. Both animal-derived and plant-derived proteins are good sources of niacin or its precursor, tryptophan. Meat is a major source of niacin and has the added advantage of being high in tryptophan. Peanuts, beans, peas, and enriched grains are also good sources of niacin. Unenriched white rice and corn are poor sources, as they lack both niacin and tryptophan.

The current recommendation is that healthy males and females consume 19 mg and 15 mg of niacin equivalents (NE) per day, respectively (1 NE = 1 mg niacin or 60 mg tryptophan). The RDA for niacin corresponds to kcalorie intake, in recognition of the role it plays in energy metabolism. During tissue growth, repair, and high physical activity, the body requires more.[16]

Deficiency. When whole wheat flour is refined to produce white flour, much of the niacin content is removed. Before the technology was developed to enrich white flour, the introduction of white flour caused some serious problems in parts of the world where corn was a staple. Corn has small amounts of the amino acid tryptophan (precursor to niacin), and unenriched white flour has very small amounts of niacin. The combination of these foods in the diet, plus low protein intake, contributed to the development of the niacin deficiency syndrome. As a result, the incidence of a disease called pellagra increased dramatically.

The hallmarks of pellagra, known as the "Three D's," are a flaky *dermatitis* that becomes black wherever skin is exposed to the sun; *diarrhea;* and inflammation of the mucous membranes. Severe cases progress to **dementia,** and eventually to a fourth "D," *death* (from fatal neurological damage).

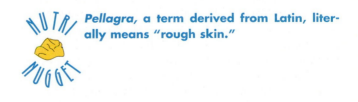 *Pellagra, a term derived from Latin, literally means "rough skin."*

dementia	loss of intellectual function

FIGURE 7-3 Food sources and RDA for 11 vitamins (µg, micrograms; *mg*, milligrams; 1 mg = 1000 µg).

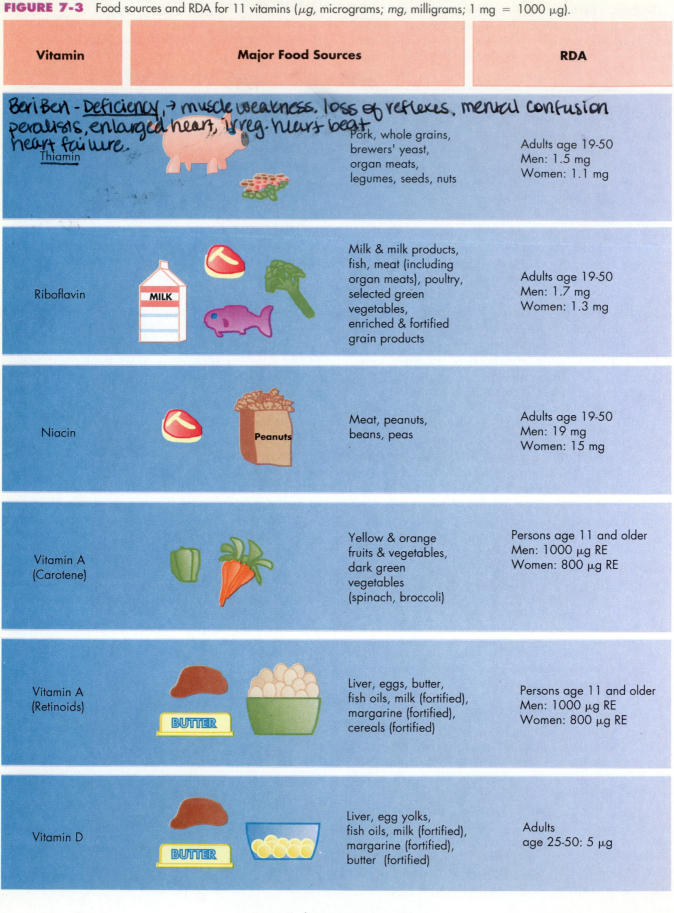

Vitamin	Major Food Sources	RDA
Thiamin	Pork, whole grains, brewers' yeast, organ meats, legumes, seeds, nuts	Adults age 19-50 Men: 1.5 mg Women: 1.1 mg
Riboflavin	Milk & milk products, fish, meat (including organ meats), poultry, selected green vegetables, enriched & fortified grain products	Adults age 19-50 Men: 1.7 mg Women: 1.3 mg
Niacin	Meat, peanuts, beans, peas	Adults age 19-50 Men: 19 mg Women: 15 mg
Vitamin A (Carotene)	Yellow & orange fruits & vegetables, dark green vegetables (spinach, broccoli)	Persons age 11 and older Men: 1000 µg RE Women: 800 µg RE
Vitamin A (Retinoids)	Liver, eggs, butter, fish oils, milk (fortified), margarine (fortified), cereals (fortified)	Persons age 11 and older Men: 1000 µg RE Women: 800 µg RE
Vitamin D	Liver, egg yolks, fish oils, milk (fortified), margarine (fortified), butter (fortified)	Adults age 25-50: 5 µg

(handwritten note across top of table:) BeriBeri - Deficiency, → muscle weakness, loss of reflexes, mental confusion, peralisis, enlarged heart, irreg. heart beat heart failure.

FIGURE 7-3, cont'd. Food sources and RDA for 11 vitamins.

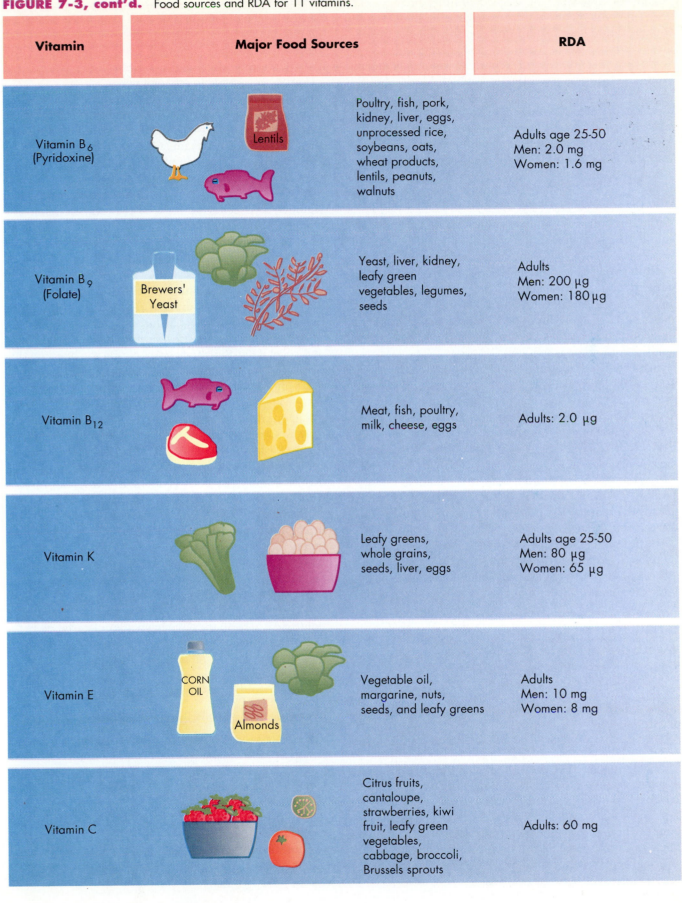

Vitamin	Major Food Sources	RDA
Vitamin B₆ (Pyridoxine)	Poultry, fish, pork, kidney, liver, eggs, unprocessed rice, soybeans, oats, wheat products, lentils, peanuts, walnuts	Adults age 25-50 Men: 2.0 mg Women: 1.6 mg
Vitamin B₉ (Folate)	Yeast, liver, kidney, leafy green vegetables, legumes, seeds	Adults Men: 200 µg Women: 180 µg
Vitamin B₁₂	Meat, fish, poultry, milk, cheese, eggs	Adults: 2.0 µg
Vitamin K	Leafy greens, whole grains, seeds, liver, eggs	Adults age 25-50 Men: 80 µg Women: 65 µg
Vitamin E	Vegetable oil, margarine, nuts, seeds, and leafy greens	Adults Men: 10 mg Women: 8 mg
Vitamin C	Citrus fruits, cantaloupe, strawberries, kiwi fruit, leafy green vegetables, cabbage, broccoli, Brussels sprouts	Adults: 60 mg

Excess. Ingestion of large quantities of nicotinic acid (but not nicotinamide) causes a number of adverse reaction: that can promote nerve damage, irregular heartbeat, facial flushing, and decreased blood lipids (fats and cholesterol). This last effect made nicotinic acid a popular treatment for high blood cholesterol levels during the late 1980s. Chronic megadoses of niacin aggravate peptic ulcers and cause liver damage. In a few cases liver damage has been severe enough to necessitate a transplant.[17] Once again this illustrates the dangers of self-administered supplementation.

Biotin

Biotin, a sulfur-containing vitamin needed in tiny amounts by humans and a few other species, gained notoriety in recent years as a "cure" for baldness.

Function. Biotin acts in carbon dioxide (CO_2) metabolism and as such participates in energy metabolism. Humans produce CO_2 as a by-product of burning food for fuel. Once produced, this carbon-containing molecule helps build some fatty acids as well as certain amino acids; some is exhaled.

Sources and recommendations. Bacteria that reside in the large intestine synthesize biotin. However, the amount produced and its bioavailability are unknown. The richest dietary sources of biotin are liver, yeast, egg yolks, soy flour, and cereal grains. No RDA has been established for this vitamin because there have been no definitive studies of human biotin requirements. An Estimated Safe and Adequate Daily Intake has been developed, however, and it recommends that adults of both sexes consume 30 to 100 micrograms of biotin per day.[16]

Deficiency. Naturally occurring biotin deficiency in humans is unknown. It has, however, been produced experimentally in both animals and humans by feeding large amounts of raw egg whites, which contain a protein that makes biotin unavailable for absorption.

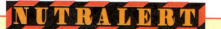

NUTRALERT

It is unlikely that anyone would eat enough raw eggs to cause a biotin deficiency. Contracting salmonella, food poisoning from raw egg whites, however, is a real possibility.

Biotin deficiency induced in the laboratory produces a wide variety of symptoms, including depression, anorexia, nausea, vomiting, dark-red swollen tongue, dry, scaly skin, and hair loss. This last symptom accounts for biotin's mistaken notoriety as a cure for baldness.

Excess. Biotin is not toxic, even when taken in doses up to 1000 times the RDA.

Pantothenic Acid

The presence of pantothenic acid in all living things accounts for its name, which is derived from the Greek *pantothen* meaning "from all sides." This usually forgotten vitamin does indeed occur everywhere, but never in abundance in any one place.

Functions. Pantothenic acid is in the "center ring" of metabolic activity. To obtain energy from the fuel-providing nutrients—carbohydrate, protein, and fat—their carbon skeletons must break apart. The resulting two-carbon particles combine with pantothenic acid (also known as coenzyme A) and become **acetyl CoA.** The word *acetyl* signifies two carbons; the term *CoA* signifies the coenzyme form of pantothenic acid. The acetyl CoA molecule then travels through the **tricarboxylic acid cycle,** producing cellular energy. Pantothenic acid also participates in the synthesis of sterols and steroid hormones.

Sources and recommendations. Pantothenic acid occurs in greatest abundance in protein-rich foods such as animal tissues, legumes, and whole grains. Smaller quantities are present in milk products, fruits, and vegetables. Scientists suspect that the bacteria that reside in the human intestine are capable of synthesizing pantothenic acid. As with biotin, however, the amount produced in this way as well as its availability are unknown. Instead of an RDA, the National Research Council has developed Estimated Safe and Adequate Intake levels of this vitamin, based on average dietary intake and excretion data. The suggested level for adults of both genders is 4 to 7 mg of pantothenic acid per day.[16]

Deficiency. There is no confirmed evidence of a naturally occurring pantothenic acid deficiency in humans. This is most likely because of its wide availability in foods and its possible synthesis by the intestinal bacteria. Symptoms of artificially induced deficiency in humans include listlessness and fatigue.

Excess. Pantothenic acid appears to be relatively nontoxic. Up to 10 mg have been administered daily for 6 weeks with no ill effects. At higher doses there is moderate evidence of toxicity. Researchers have reported that daily doses of 10 to 20 mg produce diarrhea or water retention in some subjects.

Tissue Synthesis

The role of vitamins is to support the growth and maintenance of the human body. Of the 13 vitamins required by humans, those most directly involved in tissue synthesis are fat-soluble vitamins A and D and water-soluble vitamins B_6 and C.

Vitamin A

Functions. Although it originally gained fame for its role in preserving vision, vitamin A is involved in a wide variety of other essential functions: growth and maintenance of body tissues, normal reproduction, and proper functioning of the immune system. These functions have been categorized into three major metabolic activities:[23]

1. *Synthesis of epithelial tissue.* Vitamin A is needed for **epithelialization,** the process by which our bodies form the cells that make up our skin and internal linings.
2. *Bone growth.* Bone grows through a process called **remodeling** that reshapes as well as enlarges the skeleton. Reshaping requires vitamin A to dismantle existing bone.
3. *Vision.* Vision is probably the best known function of vitamin A, which is why generations of parents have told their children: "Eat your carrots because they're good for your eyes." Vitamin A preserves vision by maintaining both the retina's sensitivity to light and the crystal-clear character of the cornea, the eye's outer covering.

Sources: carotenes (plants). Vitamin A exists in both precursor and active forms. The precursor forms of vitamin A, known as **carotenes,** are yellow-orange pigments produced by plants. Intestinal cells convert a small amount of carotene into active vitamin A (**retinoids**) and absorb the rest as is. The major carotene in plants is beta-carotene. Yellow and orange fruits and vegetables are excellent, easily recognizable sources of carotene. Equally good sources are dark green vegetables, such as spinach and broccoli. They are just not so obvious because the green pigment chlorophyll is masking the yellow-orange pigment in these plants.[16]

Sources: retinoids (animals). Only animal tissues and products are *natural* sources of vitamin A in its active form, retinoids. Liver, eggs, butter, and fish oils are all good, naturally occurring sources of retinoids. Fortified foods such as milk, milk products (retinoids), and margarine (carotene) also contain an ample supply of this nutrient. Some cereals and breakfast bars are fortified with vitamin A.

Recommendations. The RDA for vitamin A for males and females age 11 and older are, respectively, 1000 and 800 micrograms RE (retinol equivalents). One RE provides 1 microgram of retinol or 6 micrograms of beta carotene.

Deficiency. Vitamin A deficiency is a serious health problem worldwide. Deficiency may occur because of insufficient dietary intake or, more rarely, because of chronic (long-term) fat malabsorption. A solution is available: inexpensive supplements. Acute vitamin A deficiency causes dry, bumpy skin, poor immunity, and, in children, slowed growth. The most easily recognized symptoms of vitamin A deficiency are night blindness and, in extreme cases, xerophthalmia (dry eye), which can progress to total blindness. Vitamin A deficiency also can cause the skin and internal linings of the lungs, bladder, gastrointestinal tract, vagina, and the outer layer of the eye (cornea) to become dry and brittle. Dead cells accumulate and bacteria set up housekeeping, leading to infection. This phenomenon also may account for the increased incidence of skin, lung, and bladder cancers in people whose diets are deficient in vitamin A.

Excess. Some health experts believe there is a significant potential for vitamin A toxicity in the United States because of widespread use of supplements and vitamin-fortified foods. Symptoms of toxicity include headache, vomiting, double vision, hair loss, dryness of the mucous membranes, skin cell loss, bone abnormalities, and liver damage. On the other hand, single large doses (up to 300,000 RE) are used therapeutically in regions of the world where vitamin A deficiencies are common. Toxicity seems to be an issue mainly when large doses of vitamin A are consumed over a long period of time.

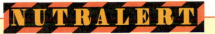

NUTRALERT

Acutane,™ a prescription drug that is very effectively used to treat cystic acne, and Retinaid,™ its nonprescription counterpart, are both *nonnutritive sources* of vitamin A that cause birth defects when used by pregnant women. Women who take either of these drugs must use a highly reliable form of contraception. So why not take vitamin A supplements for acne? Unfortunately, it will not cure or improve acne, and even if it could, it is toxic in excess.

Beta-carotene from natural food sources is not toxic because the body converts only as much carotene as it needs into vitamin A. Excesses of carotene, which can occur in people who drink too much carrot juice, for example, accumulate in body fat. Carotene stored in the subcutaneous fat gives the skin a harmless orange color, which disappears when intake levels return to normal.

Vitamin D

This vitamin is really a hormone in disguise. Given adequate exposure to either natural (sunshine) or artificial ultraviolet light, the body can manufacture its own supply of vitamin D by converting a form of cholesterol contained in the skin (Fig. 7-4). Fair-skinned people need about 30 minutes of daily exposure to sunlight to produce the RDA of vitamin D, but darker-skinned people can require as much as 3 hours. Clouds, smog, clothing, sunscreens, and window glass all filter out the ultraviolet light that produces vitamin D. This makes it necessary for certain people, such as invalids and some dark-skinned individuals, to rely on supplements.

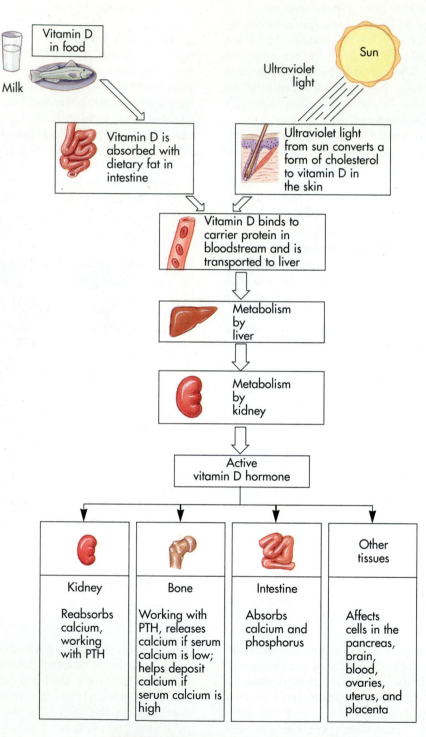

FIGURE 7-4 Vitamin D synthesis.

Functions. Vitamin D's primary function is to regulate the concentrations of calcium and phosphorus in plasma. In general, vitamin D raises plasma calcium levels. Acting as a hormone, it enhances calcium absorption by signaling intestinal cells to synthesize calcium-binding protein. It also increases plasma calcium levels by stimulating the release of calcium from bone stores as well as by limiting kidney excretion. Adequate plasma calcium is critical for the maintenance of normal heartbeat and muscle function and to promote calcification of bones.[16,23]

Sources and recommendations. Dietary sources of active vitamin D include liver, egg yolks, fish oil, butter, fortified milk, and fortified margarine. Many cereals and breakfast bars are also fortified with vitamin D. The RDA for vitamin D is 5 micrograms for healthy adult men and women ages 25 to 50. Twice that amount is recommended for younger adults and for pregnant or lactating women to promote bone mineralization.

Deficiency. In otherwise healthy people, vitamin D deficiency occurs because of a combination of inadequate dietary intake and insufficient exposure to sunlight. Worldwide, vitamin D deficiency is a major public health problem. It is especially prevalent in areas where people consume little animal protein and customarily dress in concealing clothing. Vitamin D deficiency contributes to poor mineralization or loss of calcium from bones and teeth. Severe deficiencies during childhood result in **rickets,** a skeletal deformity syndrome in which the breastbone protrudes (pigeon-chest) and the leg bones bow under the weight of the body. After fortification was introduced, there was little vitamin D deficiency in developed nations. Since the 1970s, however, there has been a resurgence of rickets, particularly among inner-city children of African descent and in children raised on a strict vegetarian diet. **Osteomalacia,** or soft bones, is a condition found in adults who lose calcium from their bones because they lack adequate vitamin D. Severe cases are associated with an increased incidence of bone fractures. In addition to skeletal abnormalities, a high incidence of **dental caries** occurs in people of all ages who have a chronic vitamin D deficiency.

Excess. Toxicity symptoms occur in people whose diet contains as little as five times the RDA, making vitamin D the most toxic of all vitamins. Acute toxicity symptoms include nausea, vomiting, and headaches. Chronic excesses result in fatal increases in calcium absorption and retention and decreased bone calcium stores. The extra calcium accumulates in body tissues, leading to a condition known as **soft tissue calcification** that eventually does irreversible damage to the kidneys and cardiovascular tissue. Typically the body is able to protect itself from excesses of vitamin D by restricting the quantity it activates, regardless of the amount of time one spends in the sun. Excess dietary vitamin D from supplements and vitamin-fortified food products, however, bypasses this built-in safety device and produces vitamin D toxicity.

Pyridoxine: B_6

During the late 1970s and early 1980s, vitamin B_6 gained popularity as a cure for PMS (premenstrual syndrome), carpal tunnel syndrome (a painful inflammation of the nerves in the wrist), and atherosclerosis. Many people with these ailments began to treat themselves with B_6 supplements. Few received the relief they sought; many developed signs of B_6 toxicity. Vitamin B_6 is not one but three related compounds, each of which converts to pyridoxal phosphate, the active coenzyme form, in the liver, red blood cells, and other tissues.

Functions. The primary function of vitamin B_6 is to serve as a coenzyme in more than 50 reactions that are essential for amino acid metabolism. B_6 is at work every time cells build or dismantle protein (amino acid reactions), change essential amino acids to nonessential ones, or make neurotransmitters from amino acids. It also serves as a coenzyme for fatty acid and carbohydrate metabolism.[23]

Sources and recommendations. The best sources of vitamin B_6 are protein-rich foods such as poultry, fish, pork, kidney, liver, and eggs. Other good sources are unprocessed rice, soybeans, oats, wheat products, lentils, peanuts, and walnuts. Vitamin B_6 is essential for amino acid metabolism. The RDA for B_6 for adults ages 19 to 50 is 1.6 mg per day for women and 2.0 mg per day for men.[16] These amounts are sufficient to provide for metabolism of twice the recommended daily protein intake. The B_6 requirement increases anytime tissue synthesis rises above maintenance levels, such as during recovery from surgery or injury and during pregnancy and lactation. The need for B_6 also increases when protein intake increases. Protein-rich foods tend to be naturally high in vitamin B_6; consequently people who obtain much of their protein from natural sources tend to have an ample supply of this vitamin.

NUTRI NUGGET **If a diet contained no vitamin B_6, all amino acids would become essential (see Chapter 6, Protein) because no cell could make a nonessential amino acid.**

Deficiency. A deficiency of vitamin B_6 rarely occurs alone because foods rich in B_6 are also good sources of many other B-complex vitamins. Isolated deficiencies have been observed, however, in people who consume purified diets. The most notable instance occurred in the 1950s. Some infants were fed a formula that had been inadvertently exposed to excessive heat, which destroyed the B_6 content. Symptoms included convulsions, intestinal distress, dermatitis, and anemia.

At least 40 different medications, including isoniazide and penacillamine, affect the bioavailability and/or metabolism of vitamin B_6. Currently it is unclear whether people who take these drugs have a greater than average risk of developing vitamin B_6 deficiency. However, people being treated for tuberculosis with the standard 6-month course of isoniazide receive B_6 supplements as a precaution. Numerous research projects focus on clarifying the role of drug interactions in deficiencies of this vitamin.[23]

How do the symptoms of vitamin B_6 deficiency reflect its functions in the body?

Excess. Vitamin B_6 seems to be the most toxic water-soluble vitamin, because megadoses produce permanent neurological damage in humans. People who took between 2 and 6 g per day (1000 to 3000 times the RDA) for extended periods of time have reported numbness in their extremities, sometimes progressing to the point where they could not walk. When B_6 supplements were discontinued, symptoms improved but never completely disappeared. Megadoses of this vitamin interfere with some medications, such as L-dopa, which is used to treat Parkinson's disease. Symptoms consistent with B_6 dependency (artificially induced deficiency) occur in some people who abruptly discontinue excessive use of this vitamin.

Red Blood Cell Synthesis

Which vitamins are needed to manufacture red blood cells? Production and maintenance of healthy red blood cells (RBCs) by the bone marrow depends on ample amounts of four vitamins: the water-soluble B-complex vitamins, folate and B_{12}, and the fat-soluble vitamins E and K. Blood cells are very metabolically active tissue. The typical RBC lives only 4 months, so maintaining an adequate blood supply demands a considerable amount of the body's resources. A deficiency of any of the vitamins mentioned above leads to anemia (see A Closer Look on p. 129). All anemias involve a deficiency of red blood cells. The type of anemia, however, depends on which vitamin is deficient. For instance, fragile normal-sized blood cells prone to rupturing characterize vitamin E–deficient anemia; folate and B_{12} deficiencies produce a small number of very enlarged cells. Loss of blood cells as a result of internal bleeding is indicative of vitamin K deficiency.

Folate: B_9 (also called folacin and folic acid)

In the 1930s folate was discovered to be an essential growth and antianemia factor for laboratory animals. Originally extracted from spinach, it was given the name *folic acid*, or *folate*, derived from the Latin word *folium* or leaf. The current name is *folate*.

Functions. Folate is required for the synthesis of amino acids, which are the building blocks of protein, as well as for synthesis of nucleic acids, which form the genetic material of the cell (DNA). Consequently, folate helps to make every type of cell in the body.

Sources and recommendations. Folate occurs in a wide variety of foods. The richest sources are yeast, liver, kidney, leafy green vegetables, legumes, and seeds. The RDA for folate for healthy adults is 200 micrograms for men and 180 micrograms for women.[16] But this standard is somewhat outdated.[1,15,18]

Deficiency. Folate deficiencies are often seen in poor people because of insufficient intake, in alcoholics as a result of decreased absorption, and in pregnant women because of their increased blood volume and demands for tissue synthesis. Deficiency can be related to diet, or it can be induced by the use of certain drugs. Several classes of medications are known to interfere with folate metabolism. These include aspirin, oral contraceptives, certain **chemotherapeutic** agents, and anticonvulsants used to treat epilepsy.

The effects of folate deficiency can readily be seen in cells that regenerate rapidly. A deficiency noticeably affects the formation of red blood cells because the average human body produces over 2 million RBCs per second. It also affects the gastrointestinal tract, where cells replace themselves every 2 to 3 days. The growth rate is lower in children who are deficient in folate. In adults the major symptoms of folate deficiency are **macrocytic** (large cell) **anemia** and abnormal gastrointestinal function, which in turn lead to a host of other symptoms, including irritability, exhaustion, and loss of appetite.

Studies have shown that women who were folate deficient during pregnancy had 10 times the normal incidence of producing children with **neural tube** defect (NTD), a group of brain and/or spinal cord defects of varying degrees of severity. A 1992 study showed a statistically significant decrease in the incidence of neural tube defects in infants of women who were given prenatal folate.

Neural tube damage often occurs before women realize they are pregnant. In 1992 the U.S. Public Health Service recommended that all women of reproductive age consume 400 micrograms of folate daily either in food or as a supplement to prevent them from bearing children with neural tube defects.[1] People are warned against taking more than 1000 micrograms a day, however, because it can cover up B_{12} deficiency.[8,15] The next edition of the RDA will reflect this new knowledge.

Excess. No toxic effects of folate supplementation occurred in healthy people consuming up to 100 times the RDA for folate daily for 4 months. Consequently, folate is thought to be safe. Nonetheless, megadoses of this vitamin are not advisable because they can mask the development of pernicious anemia.

Cyanocobalamin: B_{12}

Folate improves the appearance of red blood cells in people with **pernicious** anemia. It cannot, however,

What Is Anemia?

A CLOSER LOOK

Any disease or condition that alters the body's ability to manufacture or retain red blood cells (RBC) can produce anemia. For example, certain kinds of cancer and cancer treatments destroy the bone marrow's ability to make new blood cells. Similarly, dietary deficiencies of particular nutrients deprive the body of the starting materials needed to produce healthy blood cells. In other cases blood cell retention is a problem. Conditions such as bleeding ulcers, bleeding hemorrhoids, recurrent nosebleeds, and intestinal parasites, as well as the use of some anticoagulant drugs and overuse of aspirin, can cause sufficient blood loss to produce anemia.

There are also a few inherited forms of anemia. Two of these, thalassemia and sickle cell anemia, result from abnormal hemoglobin synthesis and are discussed in Chapter 8, Minerals. The third, pernicious anemia, is caused by an inherited inability to absorb dietary B_{12}.

cure the neurological degeneration associated with this disease.

In the 1940s researchers isolated a compound from liver that cured both the blood cell and neurological abnormalities associated with pernicious anemia. They named the new compound *vitamin B_{12}*. Because it contains the mineral cobalt, it also goes by the name *cyanocobalamin*.

Function. B_{12} is needed to convert folate into the form in which it can be used for production of red blood cells and nucleic acids for DNA synthesis.

Sources and recommendations. B_{12} occurs in foods of animal origin. Meat, fish, poultry, milk, cheese, and eggs are all good sources of this vitamin. The RDA for B_{12} is 2.0 microgram per day for healthy men and women. Pregnant women should consume an additional 0.2 microgram each day, and those who are lactating need an extra 0.6 microgram daily.[16]

Deficiency. Dietary deficiencies of B_{12} are rare because the vitamin is widely available in animal-derived foods. In addition, our bodies can store several years' worth of this vitamin, as compared to the 1- to 3-month supply typical of the other water-soluble vitamins.

Pernicious anemia has been documented, however, in vegetarians who eat no animal flesh or products, such as milk and eggs, for 5 years or more. It often goes undetected in the early stages because the vegetarian diet supplies sufficient folate to correct the blood abnormalities associated with B_{12} deficiency. Unfortunately, the neurological damage continues undetected and can result in permanent brain and nerve damage. Poor diet is only one cause of this condition. More than 95% of the cases of pernicious anemia result from a genetic defect in B_{12} absorption. Genetic pernicious anemia is distinguished from that induced by dietary deficiency because nutritional changes cannot alter the course of this disease. Instead treatment consists of periodic injections of B_{12}.

How does genetic B_{12} deficiency differ from the dietary form? B_{12} is an unusual water-soluble vitamin. Its absorption requires the presence of ***intrinsic factor (IF)***, a special transport protein synthesized by the stomach. Some persons have a genetic defect that causes them to stop producing IF, usually in midlife. Treatment consists of periodic injections of B_{12} to bypass the defective intestinal system.[23]

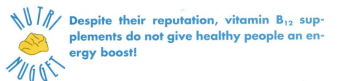 **Despite their reputation, vitamin B_{12} supplements do not give healthy people an energy boost!**

Excess. No toxic side effects of megadoses of B_{12} have been reported. In fact, it is so safe that it is sometimes used as a ***placebo*** because of its pretty red color and benign nature.

 NUTRI QUIZ

Why won't an increase in B_{12} intake cure pernicious anemia?

Extra for Eggheads
Why do people who have had a portion of their stomach surgically removed need to receive B_{12} injections?

chemotherapeutic   drugs used to fight disease, especially cancer
intrinsic factor   the protein-like compound produced in the stomach that enhances the absorption of vitamin B_{12}
neural tube   the column of tissue containing the spinal cord
pernicious   deadly; hidden danger
placebo   a substance containing no medication and given merely to humor a patient or used as a control in an experiment; from Latin: "I shall please"

Vitamin K

Discovered in Denmark in 1939, vitamin K was named *koagulationsvitamin* in recognition of its blood clotting properties. Vitamin K was later found to be several related compounds with similar functions in the body.

Functions. Vitamin K plays two important roles in the blood system. It is a cofactor for synthesis of proteins required for blood clotting and also for a protein that regulates the amount of calcium circulating in the blood.

Sources and recommendations. Intestinal bacteria synthesize almost half of the vitamin K used in the body. The other half comes from leafy greens, whole grains, seeds, liver, and eggs. The exact vitamin K content of many foods is unknown, so food consumption tables generally omit this information. Healthy adult men and women ages 25 to 50 need 80 micrograms and 65 micrograms of vitamin K per day, respectively. No additional vitamin K appears to be necessary during pregnancy or lactation.[16]

Deficiency. A deficiency of vitamin K is usually caused by diseases that reduce fat absorption or by the use of medications such as broad-spectrum antibiotics that kill the endogenous intestinal bacteria. Vitamin K deficiency manifests as hemorrhaging, often internally, which eventually leads to anemia. Newborns are vulnerable to vitamin K deficiency (and thus hemorrhaging) in part because they lack intestinal bacteria to synthesize the vitamin. As a preventive measure, U.S. hospitals routinely inject newborns with a water-soluble preparation of vitamin K.

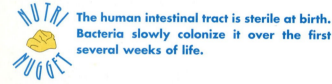

The human intestinal tract is sterile at birth. Bacteria slowly colonize it over the first several weeks of life.

Excess. Adverse effects of excessive vitamin K intake have not been reported in healthy adults. High doses, however, interfere with ***anticoagulant*** medications, such as those used to treat cardiovascular disease.

Antioxidants

Antioxidants became hot nutritional news makers in the late 1980s and early 1990s. Reports in the popular press suggest they are the cure-all for everything from cancer to heart disease to aging.

What are antioxidants? Essentially, antioxidants are chemical compounds that protect other substances from damage by free (singlet) oxygen. To date, five nutrients—beta carotene, vitamin C, vitamin E, and the minerals sulfur and selenium—have been identified as antioxidants.

If we need oxygen to live, why do we need protection from it? Usually oxygen travels in pairs. That is, the oxygen we breathe is actually composed of two individual oxygen atoms bound together. In this form it presents no hazard. But occasionally these oxygen pairs split up, yielding two individual or singlet oxygen atoms. It is this singlet oxygen that poses the health problems. Oxygen does not like being single and unattached, so it is constantly trying to find other chemical substances to join. Unfortunately, this turns out to be a kind of fatal attraction. Many substances that pair up with the singlet oxygen end up getting destroyed.

In addition to the damage singlet oxygen causes, it can combine with various chemicals to form even more damaging substances known as free radicals. Once a free radical forms, it starts a chain reaction that creates many more free radicals, so the potential for considerable cellular damage is high. Both singlet oxygen and free radicals have been linked to the development of cancer, arteriosclerosis, and cataracts, as well as the aging process.[5]

How do antioxidants help? The antioxidant nutrients can be thought of as cellular lifeguards. They protect membranes and other cellular components, such as DNA, from singlet oxidation and free radical damage by allowing themselves to be oxidized instead. Just as the President's bodyguards are trained to put themselves in the path of any weapons aimed at the Commander in Chief, antioxidant nutrients automatically intercept singlet oxygen and free radicals (Fig. 7-5).

In theory, dietary antioxidants can help combat cancer, arteriosclerosis, cataracts, and aging by preventing free radical damage to DNA molecules, the linings of the arteries, the membranes of the eye, and all other body tissues. Antioxidants have been proved to retard spoilage. In fact, they are used commercially to prolong the shelf life of many packaged food items. The real question in terms of human health is: can they retard the natural aging process by preventing damage to cellular components?

How effective is the protection antioxidants provide? Nobody knows for sure. What is clear is that people who eat large amounts of fruits and vegetables

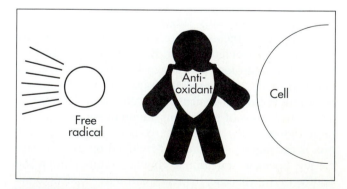

FIGURE 7-5 Antioxidants "take the hit" for cellular components by intercepting singlet oxygen and free radicals.

have lower incidences of diseases like lung cancer that are believed to be linked to oxidative damage. Because antioxidants perform a general function, it is difficult to design experiments that "prove" it is specifically antioxidants in the produce that cure or prevent any disease. It is clear, however, that protecting cellular integrity and function may go a long way toward promoting health!

Do I need antioxidant supplements, or can I get what I need in my diet? Even if you are one of the few Americans who consistently eat a nutritious diet, it is unlikely that you get all of the antioxidants that many health experts now believe are necessary. As a result several prestigious medical newsletters advocate selective supplementation.[12,20] But not all experts agree. Studies have shown that consuming high levels of antioxidant-rich foods reduces the risk of certain diseases, but this does not prove that the antioxidants in foods produce the benefits, nor has it been shown that supplements are helpful.[13,22]

Even the experts most opposed to supplementation were stunned by the results of a recently completed study evaluating the effects of beta-carotene and vitamin E supplementation on cancer and heart disease in 29,000 Finnish men who were long-term smokers. To everyone's surprise the men who took beta-carotene supplements had a greater incidence of cancer than those who did not, and the men who took vitamin E supplements had a higher incidence of stroke. The beta-carotene result is difficult to explain. It may be related to the combination of smoking and supplementation or some other factor(s). The vitamin E result may be due to the fact that people who have high blood pressure and clotting problems should not take vitamin E supplements.[2]

The take-home point is that the benefits of a well-balanced diet and healthy lifestyle outweigh those of selective supplementation. Rather than popping pills, evaluate your antioxidant state using the information in Box 7-1. With a little planning and practice, even fast food fanatics can improve their fare. Use the Food Guide Pyramid to help you establish a healthy foundation diet. Pay particular attention to reducing your fat intake and increasing your daily produce intake to a minimum of 5 servings (think "strive for 5"). Make a point of including several vitamin C– and beta-carotene–rich fruits and vegetables in each day's menu[20] (see Table 7-2 for sources).

Beta-Carotene

Beta-carotene, that appealing orange-yellow pigment found in plants, was encountered earlier in this chapter in the section on vitamin A. To date a total of 400 carotenes with differing levels of chemical activity have been identified in foods of plant origin. About 50 of these have been shown to have vitamin A–like capa-

---

BOX 7-1   Rate Your Antioxidant State

How many servings of fruits and vegetables do you eat daily? Give yourself 1 point for 0 to 2 servings, 2 points for 2 to 4 servings, and 3 points for 5 or more servings. _____

Using Table 7-2 determine how many of your fruit and vegetable selections are good sources of beta-carotene. Give yourself 1 point for zero servings, 2 points for 1 serving, and 3 points for 2 or more servings. _____

Do the same analysis for your vitamin C intake. _____

Now total your points. _____

INTERPRETATION

3 points: You are at high risk for poor vitamin, fiber, and mineral status. Use the Food Guide Pyramid and Table 7-2 as blueprints for developing a healthier diet.

6 points: You are probably meeting your RDA for vitamins A and C but you need to consume more beta-carotene and/or vitamin C–rich produce to reap their full antioxidant benefits.

9 points: Congratulations! You are well on your way to ensuring your dietary health. Consult the Food Guide Pyramid to determine how well you are doing with other aspects of your diet.

Why Didn't I Evaluate My Vitamin E Intake?

Vitamin E intake is hard to assess because many of its sources are hidden dietary fats. Most Americans meet their RDA for vitamin E because of the amount of fat they consume. As already noted, however, without supplements it is impossible to meet the level suggested for maximum antioxidant protection.

---

bilities. Carotene is enclosed in fibrous cell walls of plants. It is partially converted in the intestinal cell wall to vitamin A. The amount of conversion depends on vitamin A levels in the body.

Beta-carotene has captured the interest of scientists and public alike because of its reputed link with a reduced incidence of cancer and heart disease. For example, people with high levels of beta-carotene in their diets (6 to 15 mg daily) consistently have a lower risk of lung cancer.[3,20] However, it is becoming clearer with every report that beta-carotene is not universally protective against all cancers,[14] and some scientists question if it is carotene or some other component of fruits and vegetables that produces these healthful results.

---

anticoagulant   a drug that inhibits blood clot formation

Functions. Because of its chemical structure, beta carotene can neutralize hundreds of molecules of singlet oxygen (in the fat-soluble portions of cells) without being destroyed itself. This process may be the key to the vital protection carotene seems to supply to growing plant and animal cells.[5]

Sources and recommendations. Orange, deep yellow and dark green fruits and vegetables are the best sources of beta-carotene. No RDA has been set for beta-carotene; however, some scientists recommend about 15 mg per day (the amount in one baked sweet potato or one and a half medium-sized carrots) to help prevent cancer and heart disease.[20] See Table 7-2 for more information on beta carotene–rich produce choices.

Fool's Gold: Not all orange, yellow, and green fruits and vegetables are good sources of carotene. Corn, yams, and some lettuces, for instance, get their yellow color from pigments other than carotene.

Deficiency. A long-lasting but mild deficiency may increase the risk of initiation and development of certain forms of cancer (most notably lung, stomach, colon, prostate, and cervical cancer) and weaken the immune system. Research suggests that it is actually carotenes rather than active vitamin A that provide anticancer protection, so many health experts are urging us to consume plenty of carotene-rich foods.

Excess. Eating large amounts of carotene-rich produce seems to be harmless. High doses of carotene supplements, however, may be harmful.[2]

Vitamin C

Vitamin C may be the most famous of all nutrients. Scientists and quacks alike promote it as a cure for everything from the common cold to cancer, and advertisements constantly remind us to drink orange juice because it is rich in vitamin C.

Historical records dating from the time of Hippocrates (460 to 370 BC) indicate that epidemics of scurvy (a potentially fatal disease of the body's connective tissue) were common during famine, war, the Crusades, and long sea voyages. In 1747 a British naval physician found that citrus prevented and treated this malady.[6]

Sources and recommendations. The best sources of vitamin C are kiwi fruit, citrus fruits, cantaloupe, strawberries, leafy green vegetables, and vegetables of the cabbage family, like broccoli and Brussels sprouts.[16]

Other fruits and vegetables, like tomatoes, peppers, and potatoes, though not quite as rich in vitamin C, are nonetheless good sources of this vitamin. The RDA for adults of both genders is 60 mg. An additional daily 10 mg is recommended for pregnant women and 35 mg for lactating women.

Smokers need to consume nearly twice as much vitamin C as nonsmokers to compensate for increased losses of this important vitamin that result from alterations in metabolism induced by their tobacco habit. The extra vitamin C does not protect against the adverse effects of smoking; it simply replenishes the body's diminished supply.[16] Smokers also impair the vitamin C status of people around them. One study shows that people exposed to secondhand tobacco smoke need to increase their vitamin C intake by 50% to compensate for smoke's negative effect on their vitamin C status.[30]

It may be beneficial to consume more than the RDA level of vitamin C. Studies have shown that people whose diets contain 250 to 500 mg of vitamin C from fruits and vegetables have lower incidences of cancer and cardiovascular disease.[20-22] Eating this much vitamin C is easier than you might think. For instance, one kiwi fruit has 150 mg of vitamin C, and one medium orange about 70 mg.[20] Choose your own favorite sources of vitamin C using Table 7-2.

Most animals can manufacture their own vitamin C from blood glucose. However, humans, nonhuman primates, guinea pigs, fruit bats, and the red-vented bulbul bird lack the enzymes necessary for this conversion and thus require dietary vitamin C.

Functions. The eye, adrenal glands, and brain store high concentrations of vitamin C, reflecting this vitamin's role in the synthesis of compounds used in these tissues.[25] Vitamin C is a powerful antioxidant, active in amino acid metabolism and in the immune system. It increases mineral absorption and acts as a natural antihistamine.

1. **Antioxidant.** Vitamin C serves as an antioxidant in the water-soluble portions of cells. Oxygen destroys many nutrients and metabolites. Vitamin C protects them from this fate by being oxidized itself instead. In the digestive tract, vitamin C inhibits the formation of a cancer-causing compound formed from nitrates, which are used to preserve processed meats. These reactions may account for the fact that consumption of fruits and vegetables rich in vitamin C is associated with a decreased incidence of certain cancers and cardiovascular disease.[12,31] However, it is not clear whether it is the vitamin C or some other component of these foods that provides the protective effect.

2. **Absorption of minerals.** Vitamin C (ascorbic acid), along with other acids, increases absorp-

tion of nonheme iron and calcium in the digestive tract.

3. **Amino acid metabolism.** Vitamin C works in amino acid metabolism as an antioxidant, keeping iron and copper ions in their proper form. In this way it participates in the synthesis of **collagen,** a protein that forms the connective tissue of all body structures and scar tissue; and the breakdown of **thyroxin,** a hormone produced by the thyroid gland that regulates basal metabolic rate (BMR).
4. **Immune system.** Vitamin C aids the immune system's response, possibly through its antioxidant function with some hormones.
5. **Antihistamine.** Vitamin C acts as a natural **antihistamine** (it shrinks swollen tissues). It does not, however, cure the common cold, as some have claimed. If taking large doses of vitamin C when you have a cold makes you feel better, it is probably because of a placebo or antihistamine effect. Many health experts say most people can consume 1000 mg (or 1 g) a day for a few days without noticeable side effects. This may be a harmless way of helping people deal with a cold.

Deficiency. The maximum body storage of vitamin C is somewhere between 3000 and 4000 mg. Because about 35 mg are used every day, a maximum storage supply will last for about 100 days or 3 months. Vitamin C deficiency and its accompanying disease, **scurvy,** occur in any area of the world where famine, war, and/or poverty have diminished the food supply. In the United States scurvy occurs primarily in infants who are fed cow's milk exclusively and in elderly people who consume inadequate diets.

NUTRI NUGGET British sailors earned the nickname "Limey" because of their daily ration of lime juice, administered to help them combat scurvy caused by a lack of vitamin C.

TABLE 7-3 Vitamin Retrieval Chart

Nutrient	Major Source	Major Function	Deficiency	Toxicity
ENERGY METABOLISM				
Thiamin	Whole grains, MFP	Energy metabolism	Beriberi	
Niacin	Protein	Energy metabolism	Pellagra	Nerve, liver damage
Riboflavin	Milk, leafy greens, meats	Energy metabolism	Ariboflavinosis, cheilosis	
Biotin		Energy metabolism	Unlikely	Unlikely
Pantothenic acid		Energy metabolism	Unlikely	Unlikely
TISSUE SYNTHESIS				
A	Green and yellow vegetables, fruits, milk, and meats	Cellular reproduction and differentiation	Night blindness, xerophthalmia, increased cancer risk	Birth defects, liver damage
D	Sunshine, fortified milk products	Calcium absorption, plasma calcium levels	Rickets	Calcification of soft tissues, including kidneys
B₆	Protein	Amino acid metabolism		Nerve damage
RED BLOOD CELL SYNTHESIS				
K	Intestinal bacteria, leafy greens, whole grains	Blood clotting	Hemorrhage	Unlikely
Folate	Greens	RBC synthesis	Anemia, NTD	Megadoses mask pernicious anemia
B₁₂	Animal products	RBC synthesis	Pernicious anemia	None
ANTIOXIDANTS				
E	Oils, nuts, and seeds	Antioxidant RBC synthesis	Anemia	Diarrhea
Carotenoids	Orange and yellow fruits and vegetables, leafy green vegetables	Antioxidant	Increased risk of cancer	Yellow-orange skin tones
C	Citrus, berries, kiwi, melons, leafy greens	Antioxidant Tissue synthesis	Scurvy, increased risk of cancer	Diarrhea, death

Excess. People function on a wide range of vitamin C intake. Some can get by on as little as 10 mg per day (one sixth of the RDA); others can consume up to 1000 mg per day (16 times the RDA) with no observable ill effect. An excessive intake of vitamin C can irritate the stomach, cause diarrhea, give the urine a distinctive orange color, and interfere with anticoagulant drugs, diabetes tests, and colon cancer tests. In some cases reproductive failure also may occur. In rare instances megadoses of vitamin C contribute to iron toxicity.

Vitamin E

Vitamin E capsules and oil often are promoted as cures for sexual and reproductive dysfunctions and muscular dystrophy, and as age retardants. Vitamin E can improve fertility and muscular dystrophy in animals but not in humans. As for aging, vitamin E is often added to processed foods to extend their shelf life, but its ability to retard the human aging process is unproved.[3]

Functions. Vitamin E acts as an antioxidant in the fat-soluble portion of cells, just as vitamin C does in the water-soluble areas. It protects vitamin A and the polyunsaturated fatty acids (PUFA) in cell membranes from oxidative damage by being oxidized itself instead. Vitamin E's antioxidant properties are particularly important for maintaining the integrity of lung and red blood cell membranes, two tissues that are exposed to large amounts of oxygen. Studies also suggest that vitamin E may decrease the risk of oral and esophageal cancer[7] and cardiovascular disease.[24,32] Food manufacturers frequently take advantage of vitamin E's antioxidant property by using it as a preservative in cooking oils, margarines, salad dressings, and baked goods, where it prevents fats from becoming rancid.

Sources and recommendations. Wheat germ, nuts, seeds, leafy greens, vegetable oils, and products made from them, such as margarine and vegetable shortening, supply most of the vitamin E in the human diet. Vitamin E intake recommendations depend on body size because people have varying amounts of cell membranes. Accordingly, the RDA is 8 mg for women and 10 mg for men. The RDA for vitamin E covers normal variations in dietary intake of polyunsaturated fatty acids, but it may not be enough to provide the maximum antioxidant value. Several studies have shown that daily supplements of vitamin E ranging from 200 to 400 mg significantly reduced the incidence of heart attack.[3,4,24,32] Because it is not possible to consume this amount of vitamin E in food, many authorities began advising people age 30 and over to take daily supplements. Given the results of the Finnish study, however, no one should take vitamin E supplements unless advised to do so by a physician.[2]

Deficiency. Vitamin E deficiency is rare in healthy people because the vitamin is stored in the body's fatty tissue. It occurs occasionally in people with impaired fat absorption and in premature infants. Such infants may develop a form of anemia, as well as edema, rashes, blisters, and neurological damage.

Excess. In humans, large doses of vitamin E sometimes result in nausea, diarrhea, cramps, and bleeding. Megadoses of vitamin E also can interfere with blood-thinning (anticoagulant) medications.

PSEUDOVITAMINS

What about choline?   Health enthusiasts often tout choline, carnitine, inositol, lipoic acid, and taurine as essential dietary supplements. These vitamin-like substances are needed to maintain proper function of our bodies, but a healthy human body is able to make all of these substances it needs from starting materials like glucose and amino acids.[16] For more information about vitamin supplements, see A Closer Look on p. 135.

IN TODAY'S WORLD

Fruits, vegetables, and grains are major sources of dietary vitamins. Recent concern over chemicals used in farming may limit our intake of these valuable nutrient sources.

Chemical Issues

How do agricultural chemicals affect the wholesomeness of foods?   Ironically, at the same time nutritionists have been spotlighting the benefits of consuming fresh produce, the media has increased its coverage of the dangers of pesticide residues in food. In 1989 widespread concern developed over reports that Alar, a growth hormone commonly applied to apples, caused cancer.[25a] Of great concern with this *agrichemical* was the risk it posed to children, who are the biggest consumers of apples and apple products and whose immature detoxifying systems are less able to combat excessive intake of chemicals. The Alar scare caused many processors to stop using the chemical, and signs declaring that a product was "Alar free" or "pesticide free" became commonplace in produce departments. In 1993 the National Research Council reported that children are indeed at greater risk from pesticide residue in the food supply than are adults. This revelation did not create the public furor Alar did, but it did leave consumers wondering if eating five fruits and vegetables a day was going to destroy rather than improve their health.

The potential health benefits of a high-produce diet outweigh the pesticide risks, so by all means eat your 5-A-Day. With careful preparation, you can reduce your risk even further.

What steps can I take to reduce my personal risk quotient?   According to the American Dietetic As-

A CLOSER LOOK

Vitamin Supplements

Widespread and generally unfounded concerns about nutrient intake prompt many consumers to purchase vitamin supplements. Before investing in such items, ask: "Are these products really necessary?" "Are they beneficial?" "Can they be harmful?"

The consensus of health and nutrition experts is that supplements are no substitute for a balanced diet. The reasons are simple. First, food provides many dietary components that supplements do not; vitamins, minerals including trace elements, carbohydrate, protein, fat, and fiber are all "part of the package."[13] Second, new functions are continually being discovered for nutrients whose major metabolic function already has been identified. Until recently, for instance, generations of scientists thought that beta carotene was little more than a precursor (starting material) for vitamin A. Third, many nutrients work in concert. For example, vitamin C enhances iron uptake, vitamin D is needed to utilize calcium, and dietary fats increase absorption of fat-soluble vitamins. Fourth, the nutrients in supplements are not always as absorbable as those in food. Finally, chronic excesses of some nutrients can lead to health problems, including toxicity syndromes,[20,22] interference with medications and other nutrients, and dependence.[25]

Dependence is a special nutritional circumstance in which a person develops an artificially high requirement for a nutrient as a result of chronic overdoses. Dependence has been seen in people who take chronic megadoses of vitamins C or B_6. When their intake of these vitamins returned to normal they developed deficiency symptoms because their bodies had adapted to abnormally high levels.[25]

For this reason, experts recommend that only people with genetic abnormalities, chronic diseases, or special physiological conditions, such as pregnancy or lactation, should take supplements regularly—and then only under medical supervision.

If you believe you must take a supplement to ensure your health, use a product such as a multiple vitamin-mineral supplement that contains no more than 100% of the RDA of any given nutrient. Be sure to check the expiration date on the package before purchasing. Vitamins, like foods, have a limited shelf life. And *read the labels.*

Allegations have been made that many vitamin supplements pass through the stomach undigested. So save your receipt and, once you get your vitamin preparation home, try dissolving a single tablet in ½ cup of vinegar for 30 minutes, stirring every 5 minutes. If it is undissolved at the end of this time, return it for a refund and choose another brand.

---

sociation, you should take the following steps to decrease your pesticide exposure:

1. Buy undamaged produce; cuts, nicks, and bruises may allow pesticides to enter the food.
2. Wash all produce.
3. Peel produce whenever possible. Contrary to popular belief, peeling produce does not remove most of the nutrients. Other than reducing a food's fiber content, removing the peel has little impact on its nutrient content.
4. Eat a wide variety of produce to minimize your exposure to both natural and synthetic chemicals associated with a particular crop.
5. Raise much of your own fruit and vegetables.

What about buying organic produce? Organic produce is not guaranteed to be pesticide free. Organic farmers may use pesticides, typically chemicals found naturally in the environment such as copper and sulfur. The safety of these products has never been compared with that of synthetic pesticides.

What about buying produce that is certified "pesticide free"? This term is misleading. It conveys the impression that no pesticides are present, when what it means is that none of the pesticides *tested for* were present. Often a crop is tested for only one or two of the pesticides most commonly applied to that particular type of produce. There is some good news! Re-

searchers have developed agricultural techniques and plant strains that reduce the need for growers to use chemicals. Such new methods can be cost effective, and most of the people surveyed are willing to pay a slightly higher price to cover the expense of raising healthier produce.[25a]

Processing

Vitamins aren't processed per se; however, they are added to foods during processing, and their chemical stability can be affected by processing.

What do the terms enrichment and fortification mean? *Enrichment* usually means that nutrients that were lost during processing have been added back to the same level at which they were present in the unprocessed product. *Fortification* generally means that vitamins or minerals are added to a product that never contained them to begin with, or are added at a higher level than is found in the food naturally. These terms are sometimes used interchangeably.

---

agrichemical any chemical applied to agricultural plants, including fertilizers, pesticides, and spoil-retarding agents

A good example of the correct use of the terms *enrichment* and *fortification* is found in the federal Enrichment Act of 1941, which required that all refined white flour and white flour products crossing state lines be *enriched* with thiamin, niacin, riboflavin, and iron equal to that found naturally in whole wheat products. Subsequently the government mandated that milk be *fortified* with vitamins A and D to prevent the easily treatable deficiencies of these vitamins.[9,29]

Because folate deficiency represents a significant public health problem, the FDA is investigating the feasibility of adding folate to the list of vitamins added to enriched refined flour. Excesses of folate, however, could create another problem by masking vitamin B_{12} deficiency.[8] For this reason an enrichment program must be designed to prevent overdoses.

Some manufacturers try to make their products look nutritious by fortifying them with vitamins, minerals, and/or other nutrients like fiber. One example is cereals that contain 100% of the RDA for most vitamins and minerals even though they are little more than refined wheat, sugar, and salt. Another example is fruit-flavored beverages that are fortified with vitamin C but are composed mainly of water, sugar, and artificial color and flavorings.

In some instances vitamins are added to foods as preservatives. The antioxidant vitamins C and E are used in a variety of products to increase shelf life. For example, adding vitamin C to dehydrated mashed potatoes prevents the product from developing an unacceptable brown color. Adding vitamin E to vegetable oils prevents fats from becoming rancid.

How does food processing affect the vitamins in foods?   Refining decreases the vitamin as well as the mineral content of foods (nutrient density). As explained earlier, enrichment does not always replace all of the lost nutrients. You can see this clearly by comparing the vitamin content of whole wheat and enriched white flour. (See Fig. 4-10 in the Processing section of Chapter 4, Carbohydrates.)

Which vitamins are removed in refining wheat flour and not added back with enrichment?

IN MY DIET

At the Grocery Store

In this section we explain how to purchase, store, and prepare foods for maximum vitamin retention. The best sources of vitamins are fresh fruit, vegetables, meat, and unprocessed whole grains.

Pick of the Produce

When purchasing produce, avoid foods that show signs of aging (off color or odor, limpness) or damage (cuts and bruises). Buy frozen products if the quality of the "fresh" produce is questionable. Properly frozen produce contains just as many nutrients as the supposedly fresh produce, if not more.

To help retain the nutrients in frozen foods, make them the last items you pick out before leaving the store, then whisk them home to a freezer that will maintain the needed temperature.

Canned produce is the least desirable of the three choices. The processing required to can foods decreases their nutrient density, both because of the destruction of some nutrients (sterilization requires cooking at high temperatures for long periods of time) and because of the addition of others, such as salt and sugar. However, canned produce is preferable to no produce. The wise shopper can make healthier choices by selecting low-salt versions of canned products and by buying fruits canned in their own juice rather than those packed in heavy syrup.

Baked Bargains

Cereals and grains. When selecting baked goods, cereals, and grains, choose items made with whole wheat or unrefined grains (for example, brown rice) as often as possible to reap the maximum nutritional benefits. At the Grocery Store in Chapter 4, Carbohydrates, contains a detailed description of how to choose grain products wisely.

Dairy Decisions

Because riboflavin is extremely vulnerable to destruction by light, purchase only dairy products packaged in opaque containers.

Labels—Your License to Learn

Because of space limitations, not all of the vitamins contained in a food appear in the Nutrition Facts portion of the label. For instance, niacin, thiamin, and riboflavin content, once standard information on food labels, are required only if the food has been enriched. The reason is that deficiencies of these vitamins have virtually been eliminated by enriched flour.

The % DV for vitamins A and C must be indicated on all food labels. The % DV for other vitamins also must be shown on the label if the product has been enriched or fortified with vitamins or if a nutrition claim such as "rich in vitamin D" is being made. The % DV for other vitamins may appear if the manufacturer chooses.

Labeling law history was made in 1993 when the Nutrition Labeling and Education Act was expanded to include all dietary supplements. This means that only the descriptive terms and health claims approved for use on food labels can appear on supplement packages. Labeling of these products previously was unregulated.

To date no health claims for specific vitamins or classes of vitamins, such as "antioxidants prevent cancer," have been approved for use on food labels.[9,10,31]

How can I determine the vitamin content of fresh produce?   One of the best sources of vitamins is fresh produce, most of which is not individually labeled. However, in the produce section of your grocery store you should be able to find permanent placards or brochures stating the nutrient content of the 20 most popular fruits and the 20 most popular vegetables.

The vitamin and mineral content of produce is not the only information grocers must supply. You may be surprised to learn that your produce is often coated with waxes and resins. Under current labeling laws, produce retailers must declare the presence of such preservatives using one of the following phrases: "coated with food-grade animal-based wax to retain freshness" or "coated with food-grade vegetable-, petroleum-, beeswax-, and/or shellac-based wax or resin to retain freshness."[29]

How do waxes and resins promote freshness? Are they harmful?   Waxes and resins preserve freshness by preventing dehydration and oxidation. If you have ever grown your own vegetables only to be dismayed that the cucumbers fresh out of your garden deteriorated faster than those purchased at the grocery store, you have had a demonstration of the effectiveness of wax and resin preservatives. Although the federal government says these products are harmless, many health food advocates have raised questions about their safety. Of particular concern is the fact that antifungal agents and other kinds of chemical preservatives are often added to these coatings. Consumers have been largely ignorant of the presence of these coatings on produce, and the only effective way to remove them is by peeling.[26]

In anticipation of the consumer uproar that might greet the revelation that produce is coated with plastics and waxes, researchers announced in 1992 the development of a soy protein–based edible film that can be used to maintain the freshness of produce, meats, and packaged foods.[27]

Manufacturers of canned and frozen produce items must comply with the same labeling laws that apply to other packaged foods.

In the Kitchen

Vitamin's biggest enemies in the kitchen are cooking, water, and heat. Europeans and Americans tend to cook their vegetables in too much water for too long. Excessive cooking leaches out the water-soluble vitamins, and the prolonged exposure to heat destroys much of what remains. So don't pour the cooking water down the drain; save it and add it to soups!

Better yet, preserve the nutritional value of vegetables by adopting the Asian cooking techniques of stir frying and steaming. With both of these methods, vegetables are cooked until tender but still crisp. Of the two, stir frying is probably better. The high temperature seals in nutrients and the short cooking time reduces nutrient losses caused by heat exposure. Alternatively, steam vegetables in a very small amount of water until just tender. For example, 2 cups of broccoli flowerets can be cooked in 1 to 2 tablespoons of water in 3 minutes in a microwave on the high power setting. Although nutrients are not sealed in with this method, their losses are considerably reduced. Abandon the old practice of adding baking soda to green vegetables to help retain color. The alkali contained in the baking soda destroys many vitamins, and the sodium it adds is equally undesirable.

NUTRALERT

Store potatoes in a cool, dark place to prevent development of the green-tinged toxin solanine. This toxin is destroyed by heat, so cook all potatoes thoroughly, especially those with a green cast to their skin.

There are also some specific concerns regarding the effects of cooking on individual vitamins. For example, vitamin C is vulnerable to destruction by oxygen. Wrap or seal cut or cooked foods in airtight containers to preserve vitamin C. Take care when handling juices rich in vitamin C. Store them in well-sealed containers, and stir or shake them gently to prevent excessive mixing of oxygen with the juices.

At the Table

Vitamins appear in every food group in the Food Guide Pyramid. Ways to maximize the nutritional value of foods from the meat, milk, and grain groups are detailed elsewhere in the text, so in this chapter we will concentrate on making the most of your produce intake.

Fruits and vegetables add greatly to the visual appeal of a meal by making a colorful plate. They are also excellent sources of many vitamins. To make sure you get enough of these two important food groups, make produce at least one third of each meal. Fruit and vegetable garnishes count toward this goal. They add extra vitamins and minerals along with color.

Vegetables provide a variety of nutrients, especially

in combination. For instance, a tossed green salad composed mainly of lettuce contains too few nutrients to do much for your nutritional status. Adding bell peppers, tomatoes, carrots, broccoli, cabbage, or spinach can significantly increase the salad's nutritive value (think "salad bar").

Eating Out

Order a salad. If vegetables are not included in the meal, order one or more as side dishes. Simply prepared vegetables are preferable to those blanketed with high-fat sauces or butter. At the Table in Chapter 5, Lipids, contains suggestions for maximizing nutrient intake while minimizing fat consumption.

Menu Matrix—Weekly Servings

Until healthful eating becomes second nature, planning menus a week at a time helps you ensure that you include all essential nutrients. Make a list of all dietarily important vitamins before beginning the Menu Matrix for this class of nutrients.

By now you are aware of how many milk, meat, and grain products you should be eating, so the focus for this portion of the Menu Matrix will be the fruit and vegetable groups. Review Table 7-2 on p. 118. Remember that a healthful diet includes a daily source of vitamin C and a dark green leafy vegetable rich in folate and beta-carotene. Be sure to eat a cruciferous vegetable at least every other day.

Getting enough produce is easier than it seems. First, as with carbohydrates, the portion sizes are fairly small. Second, many foods you may not have considered can be used to meet your produce requirement. For example, did you think to count the tomato sauce that tops your spaghetti as a vitamin C–containing vegetable? Vegetable soup, fresh or frozen fruit toppings on yogurt, fruit added to cereal, and fruit and vegetable garnishes all count toward your daily total.

Vegans need to pay careful attention to their vitamin intake because vitamins present mainly in animal products will be missing from their diet. Vegans can prevent deficiencies of these vitamins by eating fortified cereals, using fortified soy milk, or taking a daily multivitamin supplement.

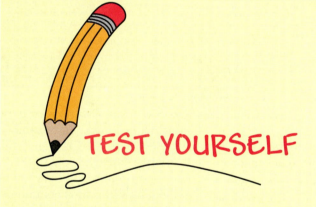

TEST YOURSELF

True or **False.** Put a **T** for true or an **F** for false in the space beside each question.

____ 1. In comparison to the energy-providing nutrients, vitamins are needed in very small quantities in your diet.

____ 2. Vitamins act as cofactors in many important metabolic reactions.

____ 3. Many of the B-complex vitamins are involved in the conversion of food to energy.

____ 4. Vitamins A, D, and B_{12} are present only in foods of animal origin.

____ 5. In general, fruits and vegetables are good sources of beta-carotene, vitamin C, and folate.

Short Answer

6. Identify two vitamins the human body can make if it has the appropriate precursors.

7. List two cooking techniques that can help preserve vitamins in your food.

8. Which food groups in the Food Guide Pyramid are sources of vitamins?

9. Why are we being encouraged to eat more fruit and vegetables?

10. List the appropriate vitamin next to each deficiency syndrome:

___ a. beriberi

___ b. rickets

___ c. scurvy

___ d. pellagra

___ e. pernicious anemia

___ f. night blindness

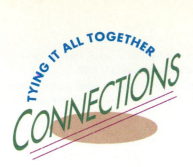
TYING IT ALL TOGETHER
CONNECTIONS

1. The waiter offers you a choice of mineral water with berry juice or raspberry-flavored mineral water. Which do you think is the healthier selection? Why?

2. Compare the label information from the mineral water bottles shown below. Now which beverage do you think is the better choice? Why?

Mineral Water with Raspberry Juice

per 6-oz. serving

| kcal | 60 | protein | 0 |
| carbohydrate | 15 | fat | 0 |

Contains less than 2% of the RDA for calcium, iron, vitamin A, vitamin C, riboflavin, niacin, and thiamin.

Raspberry-Flavored Mineral Water

per 6-oz. serving

| kcal | 0 | protein | 0 |
| carbohydrate | 0 | fat | 0 |

Contains less than 2% of the RDA for calcium, iron, vitamin A, vitamin C, riboflavin, niacin, and thiamin.

3. A 1-cup serving of fresh cranberries provides about $\frac{1}{4}$ of the RDA for vitamin C. An equal amount of apples supplies $\frac{1}{8}$ of the RDA for vitamin C. If you were choosing between applesauce and cranberry sauce to serve with your dinner, which would you select? Why?

4. Read the label information from the commercial applesauce and cranberry sauce cans shown below. Now which sauce would you select? Why?

Whole Berry Cranberry Sauce

per $\frac{1}{4}$ cup serving:

| kcal | 90 | protein | 0 |
| carbohydrate | 22 | fat | 0 |

Contains less than 2% of the RDA for calcium, iron, vitamin A, vitamin C, riboflavin, niacin, and thiamin.

Applesauce

per $\frac{1}{4}$ cup serving

| kcal | 28 | protein | 0 |
| carbohydrate | 7 | fat | 0 |

Contains less than 2% of the RDA for calcium, iron, vitamin A, vitamin C, riboflavin, niacin, and thiamin.

5. If you had to choose between a supplement containing beta-carotene and one containing preformed vitamin A, which would you choose? Why?

6. Why is food preferable to supplements as a source of vitamins?

7. Identify the two major functions of B vitamins in the body.

8. In which tissues of the human body are antioxidants most likely to help prevent destructive changes?

9. If a food label states that one serving of the product contains 25% DV of vitamin C, does the product supply 25% of your personal vitamin C requirement? Why or why not?

References

1. Adeprate P: Folic acid intake prevents neural tube birth defects, *Morbidity and Mortality Weekly Report* 40:513, 1991.

2. Alpha tocopherol, beta carotene cancer prevention study group: Effects of vitamin E and vitamin C on the incidence of lung cancer and other cancers in male smokers, *New England Journal of Medicine* 33(15):1029-1035, 1994.

3. Antioxidants and longevity, *Johns Hopkins Medical Letter*, Health after 50, p. 4, March 1992.

4. Antioxidants: Do they decrease the risk of cardiovascular disease? *Nutrition and the MD* 9:1, Aug 1993.

5. Antioxidants. In Vitamin Nutrition Information Service, FDA Backgrounder 1(5):1, 1991.

6. Darby WJ, Jukes TH: *Founders of nutrition science*, vols 1 and 2, 1992, Rockville, MD, American Institute of Nutrition.

7. E: the evidence grows, *University of California at Berkeley Wellness Letter* 9(5):2, 1993.

8. Focus on food labeling, FDA special report, *FDA Consumer*, 1993.

9. Folate enrichment of flour, *Federal Register*, Dec 27, 1993.

10. Food labeling update, *Food Safety Notebook* 3(12):110-115, 1992.

11. Healthy people 2000: National health promotion and disease prevention objectives, 1990, U.S. Department of Health and Human Services, Public Health Service Bulletin #91-50212.

12. Is vitamin C good for the heart? *Johns Hopkins Medical Letter*, Health After 50, p. 1, March 1992.

13. Kuller LH: Letters to the Editor: *American Journal of Epidemiology:* Antioxidants, fruits, and vegetables. Editor's reply, *American Journal of Epidemiology* 135(9):1068, May 1992.

14. Liebman B: *Nutrition Action Health Letter*, CSPI, pp 1 and 5, July/Aug 1992.

15. National Center for Nutrition and Dietetics, Finding out about folate, *Journal of the American Dietetic Association* 94:585, 1994.

16. National Research Council, *Recommended Dietary Allowances*, ed 10, Washington, DC, 1989, National Academy Press.

17. National Research Council report on diet and health: implications for reducing chronic disease risk, Washington, DC, 1989, National Academy Press.

18. New advice for 70 million American women, *University of California at Berkeley Wellness Letter* 9(2):1, 1992.

19. Omaye ST et al: Plasma ascorbic acid in adult males: effects of depletion and supplementation, *American Journal of Clinical Nutrition* 44:257-264, 1986.

20. Our vitamin prescription: the big four, *University of California at Berkeley Wellness Letter* Jan 1994.

21. Padah H: Vitamin C: newer insights into its biochemical functions, *Nutrition Reviews* 49(3):65-70, 1991.

22. Postscript on antioxidant pills, *Tufts University Diet & Nutrition Letter* 12:5-6, 1994.

23. *Present knowledge in nutrition*, ed 6, vitamin chapters, Washington, DC, 1990, International Life Sciences Institute, Nutrition Foundation.

24. Rim EB, et al: Vitamin E consumption and the risk of coronary diseases in men, *New England Journal of Medicine* 328(28):1450-1456, 1993.

25. Sauberlich HE: Ascorbic acid: a brief history of vitamin C. In *Present knowledge in nutrition*, ed 6, Washington, DC, 1990, International Life Sciences Institute, Nutrition Foundation.

25a. Sloan AE: Consumers, the environment, and the food industry, *Food Safety Journal* 47:72-75, 1993.

26. Soy-protein coating for freshness, *Food Safety Notebook* 4(3):32, 1993.

27. Stampfer MJ et al: Vitamin E consumption and the risk of coronary diseases in Women, *New England Journal of Medicine* 328(28):1440-1449, 1993.

28. The food guide pyramid, U.S. Department of Agriculture Home and Garden Bulletin #252, 1992.

29. The new food label, FDA Backgrounder, BG 92-4, 1992.

30. Tribble DL et al: Reduced plasma ascorbic acid concentration in nonsmokers regularly exposed to environmental tobacco smoke, *American Journal of Clinical Nutrition* 58:886-890, 1993.

31. Vitamin C: New roles, new requirements? *Nutrition Reviews* 51(12):450-451, 1993.

32. Vitamin E supplements and coronary heart disease, *Nutrition Reviews* 51(12):432-435, 1993.

C HAPTER

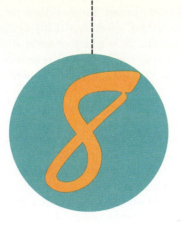

MINERALS
Gifts From the Earth

If this was adulthood, the only improvement she could detect in her situation was that now she could eat dessert without eating her vegetables.
— *Lisa Alther*, Kinflicks

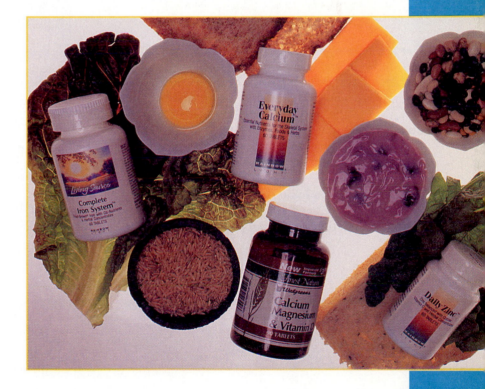

The familiar biblical phrase "for dust thou art, and unto dust shalt thou return" (Genesis 3:19) accurately describes what remains of a plant or animal body after death and decomposition. The dust referred to is minerals. After death, all the organic components of a plant or body decay and seem to disappear: water evaporates and the remaining minerals appear as a pile of ashes and dust. Burning plant material or animal bodies hastens this process, as we can see when we burn wood in our fireplace or charcoal in our barbecue.

Minerals are essential, inorganic, nonkcalorie nutrients (Table 8-1). Essential nutrients are those we must obtain in our diet because our bodies are unable to make them from other substances. *Inorganic* nutrients do not contain the element carbon and therefore contain no kcalories.

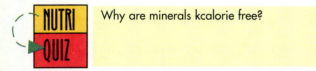

Why are minerals kcalorie free?

METALLIC MARVELS

Our bodies use various combinations of carbon, hydrogen, oxygen, and sometimes nitrogen to form water, carbohydrates, lipids, proteins, and vitamins. Minerals, the last class of nutrients we will cover, are not compounds like the other nutrients. Instead each mineral is itself a unique chemical element; most are from the group of elements known as metals. The minerals that are important to human nutrition are listed in Table 8-2.

Minerals are essential for the structure and function of human and animal bodies, as well as for the normal metabolic functioning of plants. We are all familiar with

the role of the mineral calcium in the formation of bones and teeth, and the importance of iron for healthy blood. Less well known are the many invisible functions of minerals that are equally important to our well-being. For example, a class of minerals known as electrolytes controls water balance; others are essential cofactors (assistants) in a variety of chemical reactions.

The Mineral Cycle

Where do minerals come from?   Minerals enter the food chain in water and plant-based foods. Water percolates through the Earth carrying with it minerals from the soil. Plants absorb these minerals along with water through their roots and incorporate them into their own tissues and fluids. Animals and people obtain minerals from the foods they eat and the water they drink (Fig. 8-1). Decaying plant and animal tissues return minerals to the soil.

TABLE 8-2 Minerals in Order of Quantities Generally Measured in the Human Body		
Major	**Trace**	**Ultra-trace**
*Calcium (Ca)	*Iron (Fe)	*Molybdenum(Mo)
*Phosphorus (P)	*Fluoride (F)	*Chromium (Cr)
Sulfur (S)	*Zinc (Zn)	Cobalt (Co)
*Potassium (K)	*Copper (Cu)	Arsenic (As)
*Chloride (Cl)	Silicon (Si)	Boron (B)
*Sodium (Na)	*Selenium (Se)	Nickel (Ni)
*Magnesium (Mg)	*Manganese (Mn)	Cadmium (Cd)
*Iodine (I)	Lead (Pb)	
Lithium (Li)		
Vanadium (Va)		

*The RDA provide guidelines for the intake of these minerals.

TABLE 8-1 Review/Preview			
Core Concepts	**Nutrient**		
	Water	**Vitamins**	**Minerals**
Building block	H₂O	Water- and fat-soluble molecules	Elements, ions
Kcal content	0 kcalorie/g	0 kcalorie/g	0 kcalorie/g
Source	Fluid, foods	Unrefined, enriched foods	Unrefined, enriched/fortified foods
Nutrient standard	RDA, varies	RDA	RDA
Food standard	None	Dietary Guidelines, Food Guide Pyramid	Dietary Guidelines, Food Guide Pyramid
In the body	Solvent, temperature regulation	Cofactors for enzymes, metabolic regulators	Structure (bones, teeth); cofactors (coenzymes)
Deficiency	Dehydration	Varies with vitamin	Varies with mineral
Excess	Electrolyte imbalances	Fat soluble and some water soluble are toxic; dependency	Varies with mineral

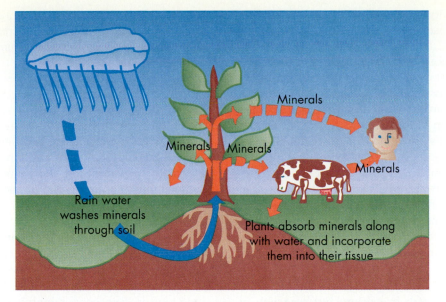

FIGURE 8-1 The mineral cycle: minerals cycle from soil to plants, to animals and humans, and back to the soil.

IN THE DIET

Traditionally, dietary minerals are divided into two broad categories, based on the amounts of them in our bodies. Those present in greater than 5 g quantities are referred to as **major minerals;** those present in less than 5 g quantities are called **micro,** or **trace, minerals.** Both major and trace minerals have identified roles in human metabolism. Additionally, there is a subgroup of trace minerals known as **ultra-trace minerals.** These minerals occur in minute amounts in the body, are widely dispersed in the diet, and are necessary for certain metabolic reactions in animals. Except for chromium, the functions of ultra-trace minerals in the human body are not yet well understood.

Nutrient Intake Standards— RDA and % DV

What standards are used to determine whether a diet contains enough minerals? Twenty-five minerals have been found in the human body, but dietary requirements have been determined for only 15 of them. The RDA is the most useful nutrient intake standard for minerals. It lists Recommended Dietary Allowances for seven minerals (calcium, phosphorus, magnesium, iron, zinc, iodine, and selenium); Estimates of Safe and Adequate Daily Intake for five others (copper, fluoride, manganese, chromium, and molybdenum), and Estimates of the Minimum Requirements for the three major electrolyte minerals (sodium, potassium, and chloride).[18]

Percent Daily Values (% DV) have been established for the minerals that appear in the RDA handbook. The % DV for sodium, calcium, and iron must appear on

food labels. Other minerals must be listed on the label only if the food is enriched or fortified with them.[3]

Food Intake Standards

As with vitamins, no single food is a good source of all minerals. Consuming a variety of unrefined foods is the best way to ensure adequate mineral intake because minerals are widely dispersed in plant and animal products. The Food Guide Pyramid emphasizes whole foods, particularly grains, fruits, and vegetables, to ensure adequate mineral, fiber, and vitamin intake. Further, small but nutritionally significant amounts of food from the milk and meat groups are required to meet our bodies' mineral needs.

IN BETWEEN: DIGESTION

Like vitamins, minerals are not digested; they simply need to be released from foods during digestion to be ready for absorption. The ease with which minerals are absorbed depends on a number of factors, including their potential toxicity and the overall nutrient composition of the diet. As a general rule, minerals with a low

TABLE 8-3 Intake Standards	
Foods	**Nutrients**
Dietary Guidelines **Food Guide Pyramid** 5-A-Day Program American Heart Association American Cancer Society	**RDA** % Daily Value (labels) Dietary Goals
People eat foods.	**Cells eat nutrients.**

potential for toxicity are readily absorbed and excreted, whereas those that are toxic in high doses are less absorbable.[18]

Phytates and **oxalates**, which are naturally occuring chemicals in dietary fiber and leafy greens, respectively, bind minerals and prevent their absorption. These binders can have a strong influence on the availability of minerals in foods. For example, the phytate found in whole grains binds most of the available zinc; and the oxalate present in leafy greens binds most of the calcium. Fortunately, the effect of both of these binders is restricted to the meal at which they are eaten and in some cases can be modified by the way the food is prepared.[28] For instance, fermentation with yeast breaks up the phytate molecule, allowing mineral absorption from yeast-raised breads to proceed unhindered.[17]

NUTRI NUGGET Spinach is rich in calcium but also rich in oxalate. The presence of oxalate means that calcium from spinach is poorly absorbed.

IN THE BODY

This chapter covers a number of individual minerals, each of which performs specific metabolic functions in our bodies. Despite their differences, minerals share certain properties, such as ionic charge, homeostatic mechanisms and dietary deficiencies, excesses, and imbalances.

Ionic Charge

The minerals in our bodies are in the form of **ions**—tiny electrically charged particles. The positively charged particles are known as **cations;** the negatively charged ones are **anions.** The ability of minerals to carry an electrical charge is the key to many of the functions they perform in the body. Maintenance of fluid balance, transmission of nerve impulses, and contraction of muscles require electrically charged particles.

Maintaining Mineral Homeostasis

How does the body maintain mineral homeostasis?
A series of metabolic checks and balances known as **homeostatic mechanisms** maintain mineral balance by regulating absorption, storage, and excretion. Most highly toxic minerals cannot be absorbed without the presence of a transport protein in the intestinal wall.

Maintaining mineral balance is also essential to preserve the body's pH, or acid-base, balance. The pH measures how much hydrogen (acid) a substance contains on a scale of 1 to 14. Except for our stomachs, which

produce hydrochloric acid to initiate food digestion, our bodies like to maintain a fairly neutral pH of 7.4. Maintaining mineral balance (especially electrolyte minerals) helps keep us neutral.

Deficiencies

Long-term consumption of a nutrient-poor diet reduces the body's ability to maintain mineral homeostasis, resulting in nutrient deficiencies. Deficiencies of certain minerals, chiefly calcium, zinc, iron, and magnesium, are relatively common in the United States because of the high intake of processed foods.

Excesses

In addition to promoting nutrient deficiencies, heavy reliance on processed foods, which as a group are notoriously high in salt and other sodium-containing compounds, can supply surpluses of the minerals sodium and chloride. Excessive mineral consumption also can result from overuse of supplements. In many cases, small to moderate excesses produce no discernible external symptoms. But when megadoses are consumed, toxic side effects are often easy to observe. For example, small excesses of zinc interfere with copper absorption and can result in copper deficiency and low HDL (good) cholesterol levels. Large excesses of zinc cause cramps, diarrhea and vomiting, and depressed immune function.[17,18]

Imbalances

Some nutrients work alone; others collaborate. Calcium and phosphorus work together to form strong bones and teeth. The electrolyte minerals (sodium, potassium, and chloride) have an interrelated effect on fluid balance. Such cooperative efforts depend on the body's ability to maintain a balanced quantity of these minerals; imbalances can have profound effects on metabolism. Imbalances occur when too much of a particular nutrient is added to an otherwise balanced and adequate diet, causing a relative deficiency of the other nutrients with which it works. Imbalances also have been observed in people who consume too much of a mineral whose size and chemical properties are similar to those of another mineral. For example, too much zinc creates a copper deficiency.

Errors in Mineral Metabolism

As with all nutrients, human requirements for minerals rarely differ significantly from the RDA. Unusual mineral requirements are seen in people with gastrointestinal tract disease, which alters nutrient absorption, and in people who take medications that alter mineral metabolism.

Genetics may account for the remainder of mineral requirements that differ from the norm. Some people require significantly more zinc or copper than the RDA to prevent deficiency symptoms. Many women of northern European descent tend to have poor bone mineralization, which can lead to osteoporosis. Hypersensitivities to particular nutrients also have been observed. For example, some people are very sensitive to dietary excesses of sodium or iron.

As in the vitamin chapter, we have categorized minerals in this chapter based on the major function they perform in the body: water balance, energy metabolism, tissue synthesis, red blood cell synthesis, and antioxidants.

Water Balance

Sodium, potassium, and chloride are a group of minerals known as *electrolytes.* Together they play a major role in maintaining both fluid balance and pH in the body. Individually they perform a variety of other important functions. Electrolytes are freely absorbed in the gastrointestinal tract. A normal, healthy person maintains homeostasis through the hormones aldosterone and antidiuretic hormone (ADH), which affect the kidneys' retention of these minerals. So long as fluid intake is adequate, hormones promote electrolyte retention by the kidneys during dietary deficiencies and excretion of excesses when a surplus occurs. Illness and certain drugs can interfere with these processes. For example, people with heart or kidney disease may have trouble disposing of excess sodium, which in turn leads to fluid retention. Conversely, diarrhea and vomiting or the use of drugs such as *diuretics, laxatives,* and *emetics* that increase fluid losses also promote electrolyte losses. Severe or prolonged losses cause dehydration and, if untreated, death.

> **NUTRI NUGGET** Many diuretics function by increasing excretion of sodium, which in turn pulls water from the body. Some diuretics, however, also remove other ions, such as potassium, iodine, and magnesium, which results in deficiencies of these minerals.

Sodium (Na)

The chemical element sodium is a gray metal. Dietary sodium actually is the ion sodium (Na^+), the majority of which enters the diet as table salt (sodium chloride). Sodium is also part of many food additives.

> **NUTRI NUGGET** Salt has been prized as a flavoring agent and preservative since ancient times. In fact, Roman soldiers were paid in salt because it was considered so valuable. A measure of social status in medieval Europe was the seating of a person "above the salt," which was a commodity of such value that it was used only by the host and honored guests.

Functions. Sodium is the major cation in the extracellular fluid, where its primary function is to regulate fluid balance. You already know that salt affects fluid balance. Sodium, along with chloride and other ions, helps the body maintain a neutral pH and allows molecules like glucose to enter the cells. Sodium also plays a role in transmitting electrochemical signals along nerves and muscle fibers.

Sources and recommendations. Meats, eggs, and dairy products are naturally high in sodium because of the vital role it plays in maintaining fluid balance in animal tissues. Whole, unprocessed produce, grains, and legumes also provide ample amounts of this nutrient. Consequently, it is possible to get all the sodium you need just by eating a balanced diet of natural foods. Processed foods typically contain large amounts of added salt as well as other sodium-containing compounds, which can result in excessive sodium intake if the diet is high in such products. Numerous health concerns have been generated by the widespread use of sodium in the American diet as a flavoring agent (sodium chloride, monosodium glutamate [MSG], sodium saccharin), dough conditioner (baking powder, baking soda), and preservative (sodium sulfite). A Closer Look on p. 146 discusses MSG in Chinese food.

The body can function on a wide range of sodium intake, so there is no RDA for sodium per se, but a safe minimum intake has been established.[18] According to the RDA, 500 mg of sodium (¼ teaspoon of salt) per day is sufficient for most people (Fig. 8-2). Because estimates of typical sodium intake range as high as 6000 mg (about 3 teaspoons),[23] the "safe minimum" quantity is far less than most Americans actually consume. Given the amount of processed food in the American diet as well as concerns about sodium-induced hypertension, the National Research Council determined that restricting sodium intake to 2400 mg (1¼ teaspoon of salt) per day is a desirable goal for the average healthy person, and that people with sodium-induced hypertension (high blood pressure) should use less.[19]

 NUTRI QUIZ Using your usual salt shaker, shake out salt on a piece of paper and measure it. How many shakes make ¼ teaspoon? How many shakes do you normally use in a day?

> **diuretics** substances that decrease fluid retention
> **electrolytes** the minerals involved in maintaining fluid balance in the body
> **emetics** medications that induce vomiting
> **laxatives** medications that promote bowel movements
> **phytates** compounds found in wheat bran that bind minerals

A CLOSER LOOK

MSG: Is It Safe or Sinister?

"No MSG," declare signs on the walls and menus of many Asian restaurants. If you dine in these establishments you may have found yourself wondering why you should be grateful for this omission. MSG (monosodium glutamate), a combination of sodium and glutamic acid, is one of the many amino acids found commonly in proteins. It was isolated from seaweed by a Japanese professor at the turn of the century. It soon became a popular ingredient in Asian foods and eventually found its way into many processed foods because of its ability to enhance flavor.

No one gave the safety of MSG a second thought until the 1970s, when an American researcher identified MSG as the cause of Chinese restaurant syndrome, a conglomeration of symptoms that include headache, flushing, palpitations, and numbness at the back of the neck and in both arms. According to the Chinese restaurant syndrome theory, eating MSG caused an excess of the amino acid glutamate, a neurotransmitter under normal conditions. This heightened level of glutamate altered brain and nerve cell function, producing the symptoms listed above.

Once the story appeared in the popular press, many people reported that they too had experienced these symptoms within 15 to 20 minutes of eating Asian foods and noted that they typically felt better within a couple of hours. Despite a growing body of evidence to the contrary, the concept of Chinese restaurant syndrome has remained firmly planted in many consumers' minds for the past generation.

The FDA acknowledges that some people may suffer something like Chinese restaurant syndrome if they consume large amounts of MSG, but the agency does not believe it is a public health problem. In fact, more recent research has shown that Chinese restaurant syndrome is a problem only for people who are deficient in vitamin B_6, which is needed for the proper metabolism of amino acids. Even in these people, excess glutamate has no ill effects on brain and nerve cells. The bottom line: Except for sodium-sensitive people, MSG is safe to use as a flavoring agent in foods.[5]

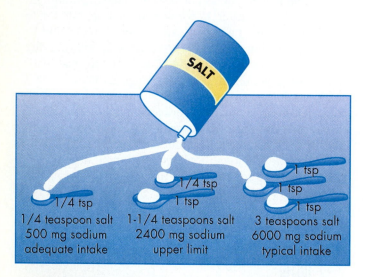

FIGURE 8-2 Minimum, maximum, and typical daily sodium intake.

Deficiency. Sodium deficiencies are rare because the kidneys are programmed by hormones to retain a minimum quantity of it. Dietary deficiencies have occurred, however, in people who restrict sodium intake too severely and use medications to treat cardiovascular or kidney disease. Sodium deficiency also occurs in people who suffer from prolonged gastrointestinal illness and in people who abuse diuretics, laxatives, and emetics.[18]

Excess. A surplus of sodium, in the form of salt or other compounds, is a common problem associated with consumption of highly processed foods. This presents no problem for healthy people provided they drink enough water because their kidneys can excrete any excess sodium. However, some genetically sensitive people as well as those with kidney or cardiovascular disease may experience problems when eating a high-sodium diet. (See the tables in the Grocery Store and Kitchen sections at the end of the chapter for a list of high-sodium foods and some low-sodium alternatives.)

The major symptom associated with excessive sodium consumption is chronic hypertension. Because research has shown that many people can consume large quantities of sodium without any ill effects, some health experts believe only a select group needs to restrict sodium intake. Most authorities believe, however, that everyone should monitor his or her sodium intake to prevent or reduce high blood pressure. The authors of a 1991 study estimated that decreasing sodium intake by 30% would decrease blood pressure by 5 points in healthy people and 7 points in people with hypertension. For Americans, this would mean reducing salt intake from 1½ to 1 teaspoon per day.

NUTRI QUIZ List three common food additives, besides salt, that contribute sodium to the diet. How much sodium does your favorite condiment contain? (HINT: check the label.)

A CLOSER LOOK

Hypertension: How High Is High?

Hypertension is the technical term for high blood pressure. When blood pressure is measured, two numbers are obtained: the systolic and the diastolic. Often a health care professional will say, "Your blood pressure is 110 over 75," which represents the systolic over the diastolic pressure readings. In the United States hypertension is defined as a systolic reading above 140 or a diastolic reading of 90 or greater.

How does hypertension relate to cardiovascular disease? Hypertension increases a person's chances of developing cardiovascular disease in two ways. As you learned earlier, high blood pressure worsens atherosclerosis by injuring and weakening the lining of the blood vessels, leading to further plaque formation. Chronic hypertension also can cause the walls of the blood vessels to weaken to such an extent that they balloon out, forming an **aneurysm.** Aneurysms eventually may bleed slowly or burst suddenly. The slow-bleeding type often causes pain because of the accumulation of blood outside the circulatory system, giving the affected person an important warning signal. People whose aneurysms burst suddenly are usually less fortunate. If their aneurysm is located in a major blood vessel, such as the aorta, it can cause fatal hemorrhaging; if it is located in a small vessel in the brain, it can produce a fatal stroke.

If my blood pressure is in the normal range, what is the value of reducing it by 5 points? Blood pressure can vary over a considerable range and still be considered normal. However, the lower the pressure, within acceptable limits, the less strain it puts on the cardiovascular system. The National Research Council's Food and Nutrition Board believes that because there is no advantage to eating extra salt, moderate use of salt and other sodium-containing compounds is advisable to reduce stress on the cardiovascular system and kidneys.

Are there any other dietary measures that help control blood pressure? For many people, maintaining a healthy body weight is an effective preventive measure. Losing excess weight is an equally effective treatment for others. A 1993 study that evaluated the effectiveness of different drug-diet combinations found that weight loss was the most effective method of controlling hypertension in moderately obese people with mild hypertension.[29] In addition to weight control, other factors that help control hypertension are moderate use of alcohol, adequate dietary calcium, decreasing lifestyle stress, and regular exercise (see A Closer Look on p. 147).

Potassium (K)

Functions. Potassium is nearly twice as prevalent as sodium in our bodies, reflecting the greater volume of intracellular than extracellular body water. It is also significantly more abundant in plants than in animal tissue. Potassium is the intracellular counterpart of sodium; its main function is to control fluid levels within cells. Intracellular potassium maintains intracellular fluid volume and acid-base balance. Although present in less than $\frac{1}{30}$ the concentration found inside the cells, potassium is also present outside the cells, where it plays an essential role in muscle contractions and neurological transmissions. Not surprisingly, given potassium's crucial jobs, the body carefully regulates extracellular potassium concentration to protect the functioning of the heart and other vital muscles.

Sources. Potassium is widely distributed in unprocessed plant foods. Legumes, whole grains, some fruits, leafy vegetables, and meats are all good sources of this mineral. Unprocessed foods are a better source than processed items because any procedure that damages cells causes loss of potassium. In addition, processing usually involves adding sodium-rich compounds, diluting the effective concentration of potassium in that food. There is no RDA for potassium; however, the minimum needed by healthy adults appears to be between 1.6 and 2 g per day.[18]

Deficiency. Dietary deficiency of potassium does not occur under normal conditions. Typically, potassium deficiency accompanies dehydration, such as occurs after prolonged gastrointestinal disease, use of diuretics, and abuse of emetics and laxatives. Deficiency symptoms include muscle weakness, mental confusion, irregular heartbeat, and eventual cardiac arrest. Potassium deficiency is particularly dangerous because the mental confusion that accompanies it can keep people from recognizing that they are becoming dehydrated or that their heart is beating irregularly.

Excess. If an excess of potassium is taken orally, it triggers a vomiting reflex to rid the body of the overload. If potassium overload occurs metabolically, such as with kidney failure, the heart quickly dilates to the point that it can no longer contract, leading to death by cardiac arrest. Potassium chloride–based salt substitutes have caused symptoms associated with potassium toxicity in many people, and they should be used only under medical advice. Several other flavoring agents are used as salt substitutes. (See In the Kitchen for a list.)

Chloride (Cl)

We do not consume chloride per se. Rather we obtain it from table salt (sodium chloride) and the salt substitute potassium chloride.

Functions. Chloride is the major anion in the intracellular and extracellular spaces. Like its cation counterparts, sodium and potassium, chloride participates in both fluid and acid-base balances. It is also an essential component of the hydrochloric acid produced by cells in the stomach lining. There is no RDA for chloride. Chloride intake should not exceed 2400 mg a day.[18]

Deficiency. A true case of *dietary* chloride deficiency has never been documented. Deficiencies of chloride (and of all electrolytes) can result from dehydration, gastrointestinal illness, or improper use of laxatives or emetics. A significant deficiency can cause the body chemistry to become relatively basic (a pH greater than 7.4). This condition can be fatal.

Excess. Extreme excesses of chloride are deadly. This poisonous property makes chlorine bleach a suitable disinfectant for swimming pools, spas, drinking water, countertops, and hospital laundries. Fortunately, the amount needed to kill bacteria is not high enough to be toxic to humans and is not encountered in foods. One study correlates chlorine in drinking water with an increased incidence of bladder cancer. The Centers for Disease Control and Prevention currently believes, however, that the benefits of chlorine outweigh any risks.[14] Moderate overloads of chloride may alter blood pressure. Some researchers believe that the chloride in table salt may be as important as sodium in the development of hypertension, if not more so.[19]

Energy Metabolism

Kcalories are provided by carbohydrates, lipids, and proteins. Both vitamins and minerals are needed to change these kcalories into usable energy. Phosphorus, magnesium, manganese, iodine, and chromium perform important functions in various aspects of energy metabolism. (Chapter 9, Energy, develops this topic further.)

Phosphorus (P)

The heads of matches are made of phosphorus; it is the phosphorus that sparks the match into flame when struck. As we will see, phosphorus plays a similar role in our bodies.

Functions. Phosphorus performs two major functions in the body: it lends strength to bones and teeth, and it participates in energy metabolism ("striking the match" to spark metabolism). It also performs a number of more specific functions. Eighty-five percent of the body's phosphorus is stored in bone and teeth. The remaining 15% is in every cell of the body, where it participates in energy reactions as part of adenosine tri-, di-, or monophosphates, more commonly known as ATP, ADP, and AMP. The ATP molecule is the power pack for almost every cellular activity. In addition to being part of the fuel molecule ATP, phosphorus:

- Activates nutrients such as glucose and thiamin (vitamin B₁)
- Is part of the lipoprotein transport mechanism for fats
- Is part of the genetic message carried in DNA and RNA
- Acts as a buffer system to maintain pH
- Is part of the phospholipid in cell membranes

NUTRI NUGGET — **ATP is to the cell what gasoline is to the automobile. Just as plant and animal fossils were compressed into crude oil that we humans later refined into gasoline, so the plant and animal foods we eat are transformed into two-carbon fragments that our cells further refine into ATP.**

Sources and recommendations. Protein-rich foods, including legumes and grains, are the major natural sources of dietary phosphorus. About half of the phosphorus consumed in the United States is from meat, fish, poultry, and milk products. Food additives supply an additional 10% of the phosphorus in a diet low in processed foods, and up to 20% to 30% of the phosphorus in diets that contain a high proportion of convenience foods. The remainder comes from grains, cereals, seeds, nuts, and legumes. Small amounts are also present in fruits and vegetables. We absorb 50% to 70% of the phosphorus we consume from a normal diet. The RDA for phosphorus for healthy adults is 800 mg.[18]

Deficiency. Because diets normally supply more than enough phosphorus, deficiencies are unlikely except during starvation. Deficiency symptoms occasionally appear in people who consume antacids that contain aluminum hydroxide, like Rolaids, for long periods of time. This is because aluminum competes with phosphorus for absorption.

Excess. The kidneys clear excesses of phosphorus, just as they do with sodium and potassium. Our bodies like to maintain approximately a one-to-one ratio of the plasma calcium and phosphorus concentration. Excessive dietary phosphorus decreases the calcium-to-phosphorus ratio. The body corrects this imbalance by pulling calcium from bone into the blood. In animals, such dietary excesses result in significant loss of bone calcium. Although not verified, a similar scenario has been proposed in people who routinely consume inadequate quantities of calcium and vitamin D in conjunction with excess phosphorus. This may occur when people replace the milk in their diet with carbonated soft drinks, which contain phosphoric acid.

Magnesium (Mg)

Magnesium, a silver-white metallic mineral, is an essential nutrient for plants and animals alike.

Functions. About 1% of the magnesium in our bodies is active in extracellular fluid. Close to 39% is in soft tissue, where it functions as cellular reserves. The remaining 60% of our magnesium stores are in bone, but only one third of this skeletal reserve is available to the rest of the body during dietary deficiencies. Many metabolic activities require magnesium. It is essential for mineralization of bones and teeth, protein synthesis, and neuromuscular activity. One of its most important functions is as a cofactor for both the synthesis and use of ATP. Magnesium therefore is needed whenever work (energy released from ATP) is being done within a cell, or whenever food energy is being packed away into the chemical bonds of ATP. Note that phosphorus and magnesium participate in these reactions.

Sources and recommendations. Nuts, seeds, whole grains, and the protein-rich cells of meat, fish, and poultry supply about two thirds of the dietary intake of magnesium. The other third is from green plants. Magnesium is an integral part of the green chlorophyll molecule, just as iron is part of hemoglobin, so one way to get magnesium in your diet is to eat green! The RDA for adult males is 350 mg, for females 280 mg.[18] The intestinal cells absorb 40% to 60% of dietary magnesium.

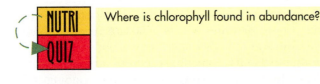

NUTRI QUIZ Where is chlorophyll found in abundance?

Deficiency. Alcoholism and gastrointestinal illness can lead to magnesium deficiency by depleting the body's cellular reserves of this nutrient. A naturally occurring dietary deficiency, however, is rare in healthy, nonalcoholic people because magnesium is widespread in food and the kidneys can conserve it by reducing excretion. Experimental magnesium deficiencies have been produced in humans fed purified diets. Symptoms include nausea, muscle weakness, irritability, mental derangement, and hallucinations. Magnesium deficiency may account for the hallucinations that accompany alcohol withdrawal. These symptoms are believed to result from a combination of insufficient dietary magnesium and an alcohol-induced increase in its excretion.

Excess. Dietary toxicities of magnesium are unknown, but large doses taken in the form of antacids or laxatives may cause diarrhea.

Manganese (Mn)

The metal manganese is a common trace element in the body, where it participates in numerous enzymatic reactions.

Functions. Energy metabolism, particularly carbohydrate metabolism, requires manganese. It also is needed for the activation of numerous enzyme systems and for the synthesis of tiny bones in the inner ear that are critical for balance.

Sources and recommendations. Manganese is most abundant in plant-derived foods. Whole grains and cereal products are excellent sources of manganese; fruits and vegetables rank a close second. There is no RDA for manganese, but 2 to 5 mg per day is considered to be a safe and adequate intake for healthy adults.

Deficiency. In animals, manganese deficiency is associated with poor reproductive rates, growth retardation, skeletal abnormalities, and lack of balance. Although only one case of possible manganese deficiency in a human has been recorded, the fact that this mineral is essential for all animal species studied strongly suggests that it is necessary for humans as well.

Excess. Excesses of manganese are not a dietary concern and occur only with exposure to industrial fumes and manganese dust. Nonethless, excessive dietary intake via supplements is not advisable because our body tissues readily concentrate this mineral. Toxicity results in nervous system disorders.

Iodine (I)

Before the days of iodized salt and modern milk processing techniques, iodine deficiency was common in some parts of the United States.

Functions. Iodine is part of the hormone thyroxin, which regulates basal metabolic rate. The thyroid gland, located in front of the windpipe, needs iodine to manufacture thyroxin. The thyroid gland releases thyroxin into the bloodstream. It travels to the various cells, where it sets the pace at which they work. If too little thyroxin is present, the cells work sluggishly. Too much, and they work feverishly.[13]

Sources and recommendations. Animals need iodide (the ionized form of iodine). Iodine is present in seawater and in any soil that was once covered by an ocean. Consequently, iodine is found in seafood as well as in plants grown on iodine-rich soils and the animals that feed on these plants. Conversely, foods grown in iodine-poor areas (usually mountainous or landlocked areas) contain little if any of this mineral. When people lived off the land, iodine deficiency was common in some areas. Today, however, iodine deficiency is rare in the United States because iodized salt is widely available, and various forms of iodine are used in food processing. The RDA for iodine is 150 micrograms for healthy adults; more is needed during pregnancy and lactation.[18]

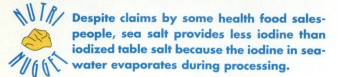

Despite claims by some health food salespeople, sea salt provides less iodine than iodized table salt because the iodine in seawater evaporates during processing.

The intestinal tract absorbs iodine freely, except in the presence of foods such as cabbage, peanuts, and soybeans, which contain a chemical that inhibits iodine absorption.

Deficiency. A dietary deficiency of iodine decreases the ability of the thyroid gland to make thyroxin. The body responds by enlarging the thyroid gland. As the deficiency continues, the gland grows bigger and bigger, eventually creating a noticeable bulge in the throat known as simple goiter (Fig. 8-3). Affected persons feel tired and cold, they gain weight, and their hair and nails become dry and brittle. Thyroxin deficiency during pregnancy is of particular concern because in some cases it results in a child with cretinism, which can cause severe physical and mental retardation.

Excess. People who use excessive amounts of iodized salt and eat a great deal of processed foods,

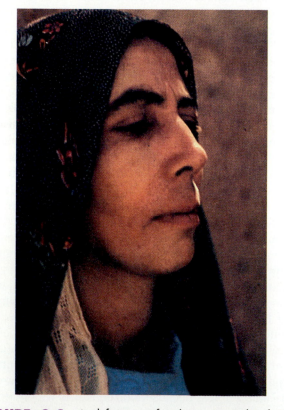

FIGURE 8-3 A deficiency of iodine causes the thyroid gland to enlarge, a condition known as simple goiter.

dairy products, and seafood may be at risk for developing iodine toxicity, which results in sluggish thyroid function. U.S. health experts encourage bakers and dairy farmers to restrict their use of iodine-containing compounds.

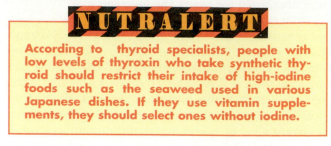

NUTRALERT

According to thyroid specialists, people with low levels of thyroxin who take synthetic thyroid should restrict their intake of high-iodine foods such as the seaweed used in various Japanese dishes. If they use vitamin supplements, they should select ones without iodine.

Chromium (Cr)

The metal chromium is the one ultra-trace mineral whose function scientists understand.

Function. Chromium is essential for optimal glucose metabolism because it serves as a cofactor for insulin production. Chromium is found in organ meats, whole grains, nuts, seeds, and beer. It is estimated that between 0.5% and 1% of the ingested chromium in a mixed diet is absorbed. Until more specific information is available, the best advice is to ensure adequate chromium intake by eating a wide variety of whole foods.

Sources and recommendations. There is no RDA for chromium, but 50 to 200 micrograms per day is safe and adequate for people age 7 and older.[18]

Deficiency. Chromium deficiency, which results in a diabetes-like syndrome characterized by poor glucose tolerance, has been observed in people who consume a poor diet and people who are receiving long-term intravenous feeding. Low body stores of chromium also have been linked with an increased incidence of coronary artery disease. In technologically advanced societies this may partially reflect a dietary chromium deficiency as a consequence of food processing and refining techniques that remove up to 80% of the chromium in some foods.[16]

Excess. Dietary excesses of chromium are unknown. Workers who are chronically exposed to *environmental* chromium, however, have an increased incidence of bronchial cancer.[6]

Tissue Synthesis

Normal growth, development, and tissue repair require an ample supply of all minerals. Calcium, phosphorus, and fluoride are particularly important for the structural integrity of bone; zinc is essential for formation of soft tissues like muscle, skin, and internal organs.

Calcium

Calcium is the fifth most abundant element in the body and the most abundant cation.

Functions. Calcium performs both structural and physiological functions in our bodies. One percent of the body's calcium is found in extracellular fluid, such as lymph and blood plasma. This extracellular calcium plays several vital roles, including the following:

- Conducting nerve signals
- Maintaining membrane permeability
- Stabilizing collagen strands by forming a "bridge" between them
- Acting as a cofactor in the synthesis of fibrin, a blood-clotting protein
- Serving as a cofactor in muscle contractions (one of calcium's most critical roles; either too much or too little free calcium results in cardiac arrest because the heart muscle is unable to contract and relax normally)

Bones and teeth contain 99% of the body's calcium and account for 1.5% to 2% of total body weight. Together they store approximately 10 years' worth of calcium in healthy, well-nourished people. Although hard like rock, these reserves are far from static. The calcium reserve is constantly being removed and replaced. Bones and teeth obtain their strength from a combination of calcium, phosphorus, and other minerals, such as zinc and magnesium.

NUTRI NUGGET What has happened to your baby bones? They were remodeled! The term bone remodeling describes the continuous breaking down and building up of bone tissue. Hormones, enzymes, and vitamins D and A all cooperate to dissolve the tiny bones and to deposit minerals on the growing ends of the bones.

Young people tend to put more calcium into bones than they remove. Sometime between the ages of 30 to 40, however, a metabolic shift occurs and adults start to remove more calcium than they replace, resulting in loss of bone tissue. Bone loss is exacerbated in women by the loss of estrogen that occurs with menopause. This heightened rate of bone loss lasts for about 5 to 10 years, then gradually returns to the same rate seen before menopause. Men, on the other hand, lose bone slowly and steadily from about age 30.[25]

NUTRI NUGGET Many people think bones are static like concrete. Actually they are quite lively. According to a noted bone specialist, the average person receives a new skeleton (but not new teeth) once every 8 years.[22]

Absorption. The phenomenon of adult bone loss may be caused in part by changes in calcium absorption. Children can absorb up to 75% of the calcium they ingest. The average adult, however, absorbs only 20% to 40% of dietary calcium to a maximum of 250 to 350 mg per day. New evidence suggests calcium absorption is further decreased in postmenopausal women.[25] How much calcium must an adult consume to absorb 250 to 350 mg? Table 8-4 presents the worst possible case (least total absorption and lowest rate of absorption) and the best possible case (most total absorption; highest rate).

Retention. Adequate dietary intake of phosphorus as well as calcium enhances calcium retention, as does weight-bearing physical activity, which puts stress on the bones (swimming doesn't do much!). Adequate fluoride intake also helps the body retain calcium by decreasing its resorption from bone.[5]

Sources and recommendations. In general, milk, stones, and bones are excellent sources of calcium! More than half of the calcium consumed in the United States is from milk and dairy products (Fig. 8-4).

This is because milk is one of the most concentrated sources of dietary calcium (Table 8-5). Other generous sources of calcium are the softened bones of canned fish like anchovies and sardines, tofu, broccoli, legumes, and calcium-enriched soy milk products. Stone-ground cornmeal and lime-processed tortillas (lime is calcium carbonate) provide some calcium, as do cream soups made with milk and tomato sauces in which bones have been cooked (the acid from tomatoes releases some bone calcium into solution).

At first glance, leafy green vegetables such as spinach (299 mg/cup) and kale (179 mg/cup) appear to

TABLE 8-4 Calcium Absorption

Absorption Rate	20%	40%
If maximum level of absorption = 250 mg	**Worst Case** 250 = 20% of how many mg? 250 = 0.2 times how many mg? 250/0.2 = 1250 mg intake needed	250 = 40% of how many mg? 250 = 0.4 times how many mg? 250/0.4 = 620 mg intake needed
If maximum level of absorption = 350 mg	**Best Case** 350 = 20% of how many mg? 350/0.2 = 1750 mg intake needed	350 = 40% of how many mg? 350/0.4 = 850 mg intake needed

TABLE 8–5 Milk and Milk Products as Sources of Calcium

Milk		Milk Products	
1 cup portion	**mg calcium**	**1 cup portion**	**mg calcium**
Human milk	79		
Nonfat milk	302	Nonfat yogurt	452
2% low-fat milk	297	2% low-fat yogurt	415
		2% low-fat yogurt with fruit	345
Whole milk	291	Whole yogurt	274
		Frozen yogurt (brands vary)	30 to 300

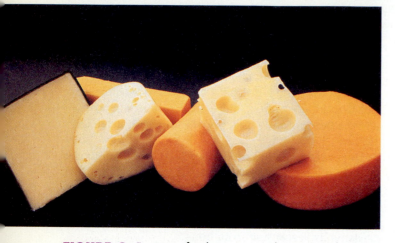

FIGURE 8-4 Dairy foods are a popular source of calcium in the United States.

be good sources of calcium. In actuality, the oxalate they contain keeps the calcium from being absorbed.[28] The recommended calcium intake is 1200 mg per day for people ages 11 through 24 and for pregnant and lactating women. The RDA for males and females over age 24 is 800 mg.[18]

What about people who can't drink milk? Researchers estimate that 70% of the world's adult population has some degree of difficulty digesting milk and milk products as a result of lactose intolerance. A small percentage of milk-sensitive people can handle lactose but are allergic to milk proteins. In some cultures an inability to consume milk presents few problems because of abundant use of other calcium-rich foods. But in the United States, western Europe, and Canada, where dairy products are the major source of dietary calcium, people who are unable to use milk must pay careful attention to their dietary calcium intake. See Chapter 4, Carbohydrates, for a complete discussion of lactose intolerance and alternative sources of dietary calcium.

Bone-building habits. Consuming sufficient calcium is only part of maintaining good calcium status. Equally crucial are developing habits, such as eating vitamin C–rich produce and exercising regularly, that promote calcium absorption and retention and avoiding behaviors, such as tobacco use and excessive al-

cohol intake, that reduce calcium absorption and retention.

Absorption is also hindered by low vitamin D levels, the hormonal changes of menopause that result in loss of estrogen, and excess phosphorus, phytate, and oxalate intake.

 Some calcium supplements are poorly absorbed because they do not dissolve in the stomach. To test for digestion, put one supplement pill in 6 ounces of cider vinegar. Stir every 5 minutes. It should dissolve within 30 minutes.

Deficiency. A deficiency of dietary calcium during the growth years results in reduced bone mineralization. The consequences are earlier and more severe symptoms of bone loss in later life. Many people consume enough calcium during their youth but neglect calcium intake during adulthood, reasoning that it is no longer needed because their bones are fully formed. This practice significantly increases their risk of developing osteoporosis in later life. (See A Closer Look on p. 153 for a more detailed description of this condition.) Low levels of calcium intake also have been linked with an increased risk of colon cancer and hypertension.

Excess. Surpluses (amounts greater than 2500 mg) of dietary calcium may create mineral imbalances by interfering with intestinal absorption of iron, zinc, and other essential minerals. Excesses of calcium also may contribute to constipation, urinary stones, and impaired kidney function.

 Why is osteoporosis more of a problem in long-lived populations? Why do heavier people usually have stronger bone structures than people who weigh less?

Fluoride (F)

Since the 1950s many American communities have chosen to fluoridate their water because of fluoride's proven effectiveness in reducing tooth decay in areas where ground water is naturally high in fluoride.

A CLOSER LOOK

Osteoporosis

Studies show that fair-skinned, postmenopausal white women of northern European descent with small bone structures are more susceptible to **osteoporosis** than are women of other races. The data suggest a genetic predisposition to bone loss. Thanks to widespread public health campaigns and advertising by food producers, the role of calcium in formation of healthy bones is firmly planted in the minds of most Americans.

What is less well known is that other nutrients, gender, race, age, and physical activity are equally important factors in determining bone strength. Low-calorie reducing diets and alcohol abuse affect bone health either through reduced food intake or decreased use of dairy products. Smoking also has been associated with a greater degree of osteoporosis because of alterations in hormone metabolism that ultimately affect bone strength. Long-term dietary calcium deficiency, in combination with the factors listed above, can lead to osteoporosis. This may result in height loss (Fig. 8-5) and pain from the pressure of collapsing vertebrae on nerves. Between 20 million and 25 million Americans are believed to have osteoporosis. This condition results in over 1 million bone fractures in elderly people each year. Bone fractures are not just a physical inconvenience. The cost in terms of human suffering and health care resources is high and in some cases even fatal: as many as 20% of elderly people who fracture their hips eventually die of fracture-related complications.

Osteoporosis is particularly prevalent in women because they lose estrogen at the time of menopause, which accelerates bone loss. Women also experience physiological conditions, such as pregnancy and lactation, that place large demands on bone calcium stores.[25] Women tend to live longer than men, so

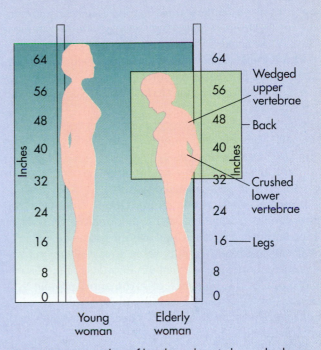

FIGURE 8-5 A loss of height and a misshapen body are common results of osteoporosis. Monitor yourself in adulthood to detect early signs of osteoporosis.

they have more time to lose bone mass, and they generally have smaller, less calcified frames than men.

Lifelong attention to dietary calcium intake, routine participation in weight-bearing exercise (lifting weights, even small ones, is ideal), using alcohol in moderation, avoiding smoking and, if you are female, receiving postmenopausal estrogen therapy are important steps that people can take to preserve their bone mass.

Functions. Fluoride is not considered an essential nutrient. Fluoride (and possibly iodine) does, however, increase retention of calcium in teeth and bones.[7]

Sources and recommendations. In addition to naturally and artificially fluoridated water, other dietary sources of fluoride are tea and seafood. People who live in areas without fluoridated water can obtain fluoride supplements. Such supplementation is particularly important for children because it strengthens their growing bones and teeth.

Deficiency. Although fluoride is not an essential nutrient for either plants or animals, low fluoride intake correlates with an increased incidence of tooth decay. No RDA has been set for fluoride, but 1.5 to 4 mg

is estimated to be safe and adequate for adults.[18] The upper limit for children is 2.5 mg daily.

Excess. Fluoride toxicity, more properly called *fluorosis*, has been observed in regions where the water contains natural excesses of fluoride (ranging from 2 to 8 ppm). Early symptoms include darkly stained, brittle teeth. Advanced cases result in bone disease and kidney damage.

osteoporosis a lack of calcium in the bone matrix; from Greek *osteon*, bone + *poros*, passage, hole

Zinc (Zn)

Zinc was first identified in 1939 as part of an *enzyme* required for carbon dioxide metabolism in rodents. Researchers have since established many links between zinc's biochemical mechanisms and specific deficiency symptoms, along the way providing valuable clues to the actions of other minerals.

Functions. Zinc is intimately involved in protein metabolism. It is essential for:

- Synthesis of the genetic material DNA during cell division
- Synthesis of the pigment needed for night vision
- Synthesis of the connective tissue collagen
- The immune response
- Insulin storage in the pancreas and as a cofactor in more than 200 enzyme systems

Sources and recommendations. Zinc is more bioavailable from meat, fish, and poultry than from plant sources. Legumes and whole grains (especially yeast-raised breads) supply some zinc. Galvanized water pipes contribute very small amounts. Zinc absorption requires the presence of a transport protein synthesized by intestinal cells. Milk, fiber, or phytates in a meal decrease zinc absorption. The RDA for males is 15 mg; for females, 12 mg.[17,18]

Deficiency. Zinc deficiency was shown to be responsible for dwarfism, anemia, and delayed sexual development in a group of Iranian males.[20] The kidney conserves zinc, although plasma levels drop within a day during dietary deficiencies. No available reserves exist in the body. Zinc deficiency symptoms have been closely linked to some of the specific biochemical functions already described.

Zinc's role in protein and DNA synthesis is especially evident in the deficiency symptoms associated with a lack of this mineral. Anorexia, diarrhea, slow tissue repair, mental lethargy, and night blindness are common symptoms of zinc deficiency in people of all ages. Some age-specific symptoms also have been noted. Maternal deficiencies of dietary zinc are associated with poor fetal development, including deformities and death of newborns. Slowed growth, dwarfism, and lack of sexual maturation are common in children who consume zinc-deficient diets; left untreated, this may lead to undeveloped sex organs and impotence in teenage males.

NUTRI NUGGET Because zinc plays a role in collagen synthesis and wound healing, physicians sometimes prescribe zinc for patients after surgery to promote good tissue repair.

Excess. Small excesses of zinc (a few milligrams above the RDA) interfere with copper absorption, alter cholesterol metabolism, and possibly weaken blood vessels. Moderate excesses cause vomiting, diarrhea, exhaustion, impaired coordination, kidney damage, and anemia. Greater excesses can be fatal. Toxicities have been observed in people who overdose on zinc supplements, consume acidic foods or beverages that have been cooked or stored in galvanized containers (zinc coated to prevent rust), and recently in children and pets that have accidentally swallowed pennies minted since 1988, when a new galvanization process was introduced.

NUTRALERT

Immediate medical attention must be sought for a child or animal who ingests a penny. The dose of zinc it contains can be lethal.

Red Blood Cell Synthesis

In addition to protein and vitamins, iron and copper also are essential for red blood cell (RBC) synthesis.

Iron (Fe)

Iron is a common material in tools and other everyday items. People tend to notice iron's presence after leaving items made of iron outside for several days or all winter—they rust! Scientists call this rusting phenomenon *oxidation* because it results from iron's interaction with oxygen. Iron within cells reacts just as easily with oxygen. Iron in the RBC protein hemoglobin binds with oxygen in the lungs and carries it to other cells in the body, where it is exchanged for carbon dioxide. Carbon dioxide then returns to the lungs for excretion. The oxygen thus delivered to the muscle cells then binds to the iron in the protein myoglobin. In muscle and other cells, oxygen "burns" or oxidizes the carbon-to-carbon bonds in carbohydrates, lipids, and proteins.

Thanks to widespread advertising by supplement manufacturers, the role of iron in red blood cell synthesis is one of the most readily recognized nutrient-health interactions. To some extent its reputation is well deserved. Our bodies produce approximately 2.5 million red blood cells per second, so a lack of any of the nutrients required for this process will really throw a wrench into this machine! Iron-deficiency anemia is the most prevalent worldwide nutritional problem.

Sources. Dietary iron comes in two forms: heme and nonheme. **Heme iron** is part of the protein hemoglobin from red blood cells and of the comparable muscle protein, myoglobin. Meat, fish, and poultry are the primary sources of heme iron in the modern diet (Fig. 8-6). The human body absorbs heme iron more easily than iron from other sources.

Nonheme iron is found in egg yolk, plants such as leafy greens (remember Popeye's spinach?), legumes,

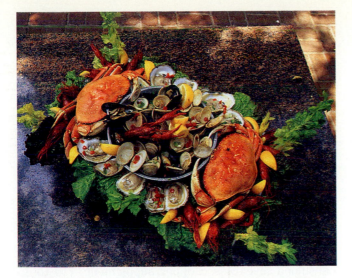

FIGURE 8-6 Animal proteins like meat, fish, and poultry are the best sources of heme iron and zinc.

TABLE 8-6 Dietary Factors That Affect Iron Absorption, Especially Nonheme Forms

Increase	Decrease
Vitamin C	Phytate (in fiber)
Acid in the stomach	Oxalate
Heme iron	Tannins (in tea)
High body demand for red blood cells (blood loss, high altitude, physical training, pregnancy)	Full body stores
	Great excess of other minerals (Zn, Mn, Ca)
Low body stores	Reduced stomach acid production
Meat protein (MFP)	Some antacids

whole and enriched grains, vegetables, nuts, and iron pots. (Anyone who uses rust-prone iron cookware consumes a tiny amount of the pot.)

 Is heme iron found in the animal kingdom or in the plant kingdom? Explain your answer.

Recommendations. The RDA for iron for adult men is 10 mg; for females of reproductive age, 15 mg, if the diet contains both some meat and vitamin C. Pregnant women need 30 mg per day. Vegetarians usually consume enough vitamin C in vegetables and fruits to aid in absorption of nonheme iron.

Why is heme iron more absorbable than nonheme iron? Absorption of heme iron is significantly greater than absorption of nonheme iron, averaging 25% to 40%. This is probably because the heme molecule is absorbed intact, which suggests that hemoglobin acts as an iron transport protein. In addition to supplying the body with more absorbable heme iron, meat, fish, and poultry contain a chemical known as the MFP (meat, fish, poultry) factor that enhances the bioavailability of nonheme iron. Vitamin C also increases the absorption of iron, so consider drinking a glass of orange juice when taking an iron supplement.

 How/why does vitamin C (ascorbic acid) increase iron absorption?

Absorption of nonheme iron is about 10%. Milk, cheese, tannins in tea, soy products, and unleavened whole-grain items decrease iron absorption. Phytates in bran and oxalic acid in vegetables can bind iron, preventing its absorption. Nonetheless, studies of vegetarians show no significant problems with iron stores.[19] Table 8-6 summarizes dietary factors that affect iron absorption.

Which minerals are more absorbable from animal-derived foods than from plant-derived ones? What dietary binding agent (other than phytate) have you encountered, and which mineral(s) does it affect?

Storage. Full-term, well-nourished infants have about a 2-month supply of iron and other minerals stored in their livers. However, milk is a poor source of iron, and it also blocks iron absorption. What is a baby to do? Currently, nutritionists recommend that babies be fed breast milk or iron-fortified infant formulas exclusively for at least the first 4 months of life.[10] Suggestions for feeding infants iron-rich foods are presented in Chapter 12, Life Cycle.

Deficiency. Iron is generally well conserved in the body because, unlike other minerals, it is not excreted in the urine. Iron is lost whenever blood is lost, and some is also lost when cells slough from epithelial tissue (cells covering the body or lining the digestive tract). Any condition that causes blood loss, whether natural like menstruation or pathological, such as a bleeding ulcer, also causes a loss of iron.

enzyme a protein produced by living cells that acts as a catalyst in chemical reactions in organic matter

What are the symptoms of iron deficiency?

Whatever the cause, the first sign of iron deficiency is a low plasma level. This is followed by a decrease in the number of red blood cells, and finally a full-blown anemia. Symptoms include lethargy, apathy, short attention span, irritability, and in children, decreased learning. The urge to chew ice cubes often signals iron-deficiency anemia, although no one knows why.

Who is likely to get iron-deficiency anemia?

Premature babies, growing children, women of reproductive age (because of menstrual losses), pregnant women (because of the expansion in blood volume and blood loss during childbirth), strict vegetarians, and people with hookworm, internal bleeding, or other blood loss are all susceptible to iron-deficiency anemia. Children who drink large amounts of milk, crowding out other foods, especially iron-rich ones, may develop "milk anemia."[10] Athlete's anemia is discussed in Chapter 10, Exercise.

Excess. Iron is the most toxic nutritive mineral. The body guards against toxicity by absorbing only small quantities of the iron in food. Iron overload, however, can occur in people who overdose on either iron or vitamin C supplements. **Hemochromatosis,** the official name for excessive iron storage, has occurred in males who ate a diet composed mainly of a tomato-rich stew cooked in iron pots or who drank beer made in iron containers. Some people develop hemochromatosis as the result of a genetic defect that enhances iron absorption. Eventually this condition leads to the failure of many body organs. It is estimated that about 4% of the U.S. population is affected, and an additional 7.5% may be carriers of this genetic trait.[19]

NUTRALERT

Keep all iron supplements out of the reach of children! About 2000 cases of accidental iron poisoning occur in American children every year.

Copper (Cu)

Jewelry made from the reddish-brown metal copper has been a popular folk remedy for arthritis for many years. Although there is no evidence that wearing copper improves joint disease, dietary copper appears to be essential for both plants and animals.

Functions. Copper and iron seem to work together. Copper appears to help iron absorption and assists in the synthesis of hemoglobin. Like calcium, it acts as a bridge or cross-link between strands of collagen. Copper also is important for regulation of blood lipid levels and the nervous system.

Sources and recommendations. Because copper is present in so many foods, it is impossible to plan a low-copper diet. Copper replaces iron in the blood protein of shellfish, so they are a good source for people who enjoy and can afford them. Other contributors to dietary copper intake are liver, whole grains, legumes, fruits, vegetables, chocolate (because it is cooked in copper pots), and copper water pipes. As with zinc, absorption of copper requires a specialized transport protein. The availability of this protein, as well as some other factors, limits copper absorption to about 25% to 40% of intake.[21] There is no RDA for copper; however, the safe and adequate intake for adults is 1.5 to 3 mg a day.[18]

Deficiency. Dietary deficiencies of copper are unknown under normal conditions; they do occur, however, in certain rare medical conditions and also have been observed in people who take megadoses of the mineral zinc.

Excess. Copper, like iron and zinc, is fairly toxic if consumed in excess. Copper supplements (10 to 15 mg) may cause vomiting and diarrhea. Larger amounts lead to rupturing of the blood cells and death.

Antioxidants

As you learned in Chapter 7, Vitamins, antioxidants protect cells and cellular activities from oxidation damage and participate in detoxification reactions. Two minerals, selenium and sulfur, are part of large antioxidant chemical complexes found in humans and animals. These minerals themselves, however, are not antioxidants.

Selenium (Se)

Selenium is a trace mineral that appears to work in concert with vitamin E as an antioxidant. Like iodine and fluoride, its prevalence in the diet varies by geographical region. Sources include plants grown in selenium-rich soil and the tissues of animals that eat these plants. The RDA for selenium is 70 micrograms for males and 55 micrograms for females.[18] The main symptom of selenium deficiency appears to be cardiac weakness. People who are maintained on intravenous feedings for prolonged periods of time as well as people who live in selenium-poor areas in central China, New Zealand, and Finland have exhibited such problems.

Excess. There is some concern that people who eat foods grown on or animals grazed on selenium-rich soils may be consuming an excess of this mineral. Because birth defects in animals low on the food chain have been attributed to selenium toxicity, measures have been taken to reduce the amount of selenium that leaches into the soil from manufacturing plants and agrichemicals.[29] The only confirmed cases of selenium toxicity in humans have involved industrial pollution, not dietary excesses. Nevertheless, selenium supplements, which some health enthusiasts advocate for cancer protection, are not recommended because the correct dose of this mineral is unknown and the toxic-

TABLE 8-7 Mineral Retrieval Chart

Nutrient	Major Source	Major Function	Deficiency	Toxicity
ELECTROLYTES				
Sodium	Table salt	Water balance	Unknown	Hypertension
Potassium	Plants	Water balance, muscle function	Cardiac arrest	Cardiac arrest
Chloride	Table salt	Water balance	Unlikely	Possible hypertension
ENERGY METABOLISM				
Magnesium	MFP, greens	Energy metabolism	Unlikely	Unlikely
Manganese	Plants	Energy metabolism	Unlikely	Unlikely
Iodine	Seafood, iodized salt	Energy metabolism (thyroxin)	Goiter	Unlikely
Chromium	Unrefined plants	Energy metabolism	Poor glucose tolerance	Unlikely
TISSUE SYNTHESIS				
Calcium	Milk/milk products	Tissue synthesis—skeletal	Osteoporosis	Unlikely
Phosphorus	MFP, milk	Energy metabolism	Unlikely	Unknown
Fluoride	Some water	Hardens bones and teeth	Tooth decay	Fluorosis
Zinc	MFP	Tissue synthesis, depressed immunity	Depressed growth	Copper deficiency
RED BLOOD CELL SYNTHESIS				
Iron	MFP (heme), nonheme	Red blood cell metabolism	Anemia	Death
Copper	Chocolate, shellfish	Red blood cell metabolism	Anemia, increased LDL	Death
ANTIOXIDANTS				
Sulfur	A few amino acids	Antioxidant	Unlikely	Unlikely
Selenium	Unrefined foods	Antioxidant	Unlikely	Unlikely

ity symptoms observed in animals, including neural damage, are relatively severe.

Sulfur (S)

Sulfur is found in a variety of enzymes where it works in conjunction with other nutrients as part of the body's drug detoxifying pathways, some of which include antioxidant reactions. Dietary sulfur is obtained from the sulfur-containing amino acids, methionine and cysteine. Sulfur also is part of the vitamins biotin and thiamin. No RDA has been established for this mineral. There are no known sulfur deficiency or toxicity symptoms, and a deficiency is unlikely if you are eating enough protein.[18]

Mineral recap. Table 8-7 is a retrieval chart that helps you collect and sort information about the minerals covered in this chapter. You may add to this chart, and you may use this format as a study aid by building your own retrieval charts.

IN TODAY'S WORLD

Variable distribution of sodium, calcium, iodine, fluoride, and selenium in the soil and underground water supply directly affects geographical differences in dietary intake. It is possible to identify areas that are either rich or poor in these minerals and to suggest the appropriate adjustments to the inhabitants' diets. The main environmental issue with respect to minerals concerns toxicity. Dietary deficiencies or excesses of the ultra-trace minerals aluminum, cadmium, nickel, tin, silicon, and vanadium are unknown, but toxicities of these minerals occur in people who are exposed to them through industrial pollution.[6] A better-documented public health concern is lead and mercury poisoning.

How can a person ingest lead or mercury? Nonnutritive minerals such as lead and mercury are highly toxic. They can enter the body through either ingestion or absorption through the skin. Lead toxicity has been traced to lead-soldered water pipes, cookware or dinnerware glazed with lead-containing paint, dust from lead-containing house paint, lead crystal glassware, and air polluted with automobile exhaust. We can avoid lead poisoning by replacing lead-soldered water pipes, minimizing our exposure to polluted air, and using domestically produced china and glassware, as the federal government carefully regulates the manufacturing of such items. Many people, however, inadvertently poison themselves by using imported pottery, which is not subject to the same controls.[11] Congres-

FIGURE 8-7 This is the lead warning that federal law requires be displayed on certain products.

sional hearings held in 1991 pointed out that lead toxicity is a more serious health problem than formerly believed (Fig. 8-7).

In response to this concern, public health messages about the dangers of lead poisoning have increased. Many local health departments hold lead testing fairs, pediatricians have stepped up screening of children for lead poisoning, and the FDA has proposed a ban on the lead foil used to cover the corks in wine bottles. Studies have shown that as the wine is poured it becomes contaminated by lead residue left on the rim of the bottle.[12] Symptoms of lead toxicity include nausea, hair and weight loss, and impaired reproductive function; and in children, depressed growth and mental retardation.

Mercury has crept into the water supply from industrial pollution, so some species of both freshwater and saltwater fish contain toxic amounts of this mineral. To protect yourself from mercury toxicity: (1) eat smaller (thus younger) fish, which have had less time to accumulate mercury than larger, older ones; (2) eat many different species of fish to reduce mercury exposure; and (3) consult your health department about mercury levels of fish caught in local waterways.[19]

NUTRI NUGGET All shipments of swordfish that enter the United States are tested for mercury content before being offered for sale. The reason is that this species was most strongly associated with an outbreak of mercury poisoning in Japan during the 1960s. In 1979 the FDA began to regulate levels of mercury in the U.S. food supply.

Processing

Most people in industrialized nations have more than enough food to eat. Excessive use of processed foods, however, can lead to deficiencies of calcium, iron, and zinc as well as to undesirable excesses of the most prevalent mineral, sodium. This is especially true in the United States where dining on fast food and highly processed items is a way of life.

Refining

What effect does refining have on the mineral content of foods?   The processing of whole wheat to white flour is a good example of how refining affects mineral content. Our love affair with white flour deprives us of more than just fiber and vitamins. Foods lose many valuable minerals during refining. Although iron is added back to the refined flour as mandated by the federal enrichment laws, other minerals, such as zinc and chromium, are not. Consequently, people who obtain most of their carbohydrate from refined products like white bread, refined cereal, and white rice can become deficient in these important minerals.

 NUTRI QUIZ List all the minerals removed from whole wheat flour during refining that are not fully replaced in white flour by the enrichment process.

HINT: Turn to Appendix A and compare whole wheat bread and white bread.

IN MY DIET

If you have completed a Menu Matrix at the end of each of the last five chapters, your diet should be in pretty good shape. But you may still have some "fine tuning" to do with respect to your mineral intake. Begin by reevaluating your diet. How would you describe the proportion of processed to unprocessed foods you are currently eating? If your consumption of processed foods remains high, you are undoubtedly getting too much sodium, fat, and sugar. Depending on what else you eat, your diet also may be low in calcium, iron, and zinc. Next consider whether you have any nutrient-robbing habits that you need to change. Is excessive intake of sodas and coffee keeping you from drinking more nutritious beverages? Do you smoke? Are you physically active, or are you a "couch potato"? Factor your answers to these questions into the food choices you enter in your Menu Matrix.

At the Grocery Store

Try to purchase whole foods, which are rich in calcium, iron, and zinc and low in sodium- and phosphorus-containing preservatives.

You can eliminate a certain amount of sodium from your diet just by reducing your consumption of foods that taste salty. But beware—sodium is tricky! Foods that contain salt, like many breakfast cereals, condiments, and baked goods, do not necessarily taste salty. Furthermore, sodium tastes salty only when it is part of the sodium chloride molecule. It often goes undetected in dough conditioners, saccharin, and preservatives.

TABLE 8-8 Examining Your Sodium Habits

Examine how the foods you eat and the way you prepare and serve them affect the amount of sodium in your diet.

How often do you:	Less Than Once per Week	1 or 2 Times per Week	3 to 5 Times per Week	Almost Daily
1. Eat cured or processed meats, such as ham, bacon, sausage, frankfurters, and other luncheon meats?	☐	☐	☐	☐
2. Choose canned or frozen vegetables with sauce?	☐	☐	☐	☐
3. Use commercially prepared meals, main dishes, or canned or dehydrated soups?	☐	☐	☐	☐
4. Eat cheese?	☐	☐	☐	☐
5. Eat salted nuts, popcorn, pretzels, corn chips, or potato chips?	☐	☐	☐	☐
6. Add salt to cooking water for vegetables, rice, or pasta?	☐	☐	☐	☐
7. Add salt, seasoning mixes, salad dressings, or condiments—such as soy sauce, steak sauce, catsup, and mustard—to foods during preparation or at the table?	☐	☐	☐	☐
8. Salt your food before tasting it?	☐	☐	☐	☐

The more checks you have in the last two columns, the higher your dietary sodium intake. However, not all items listed contribute the same amount of sodium. For example, many natural cheeses are relatively low in sodium. Most processed cheeses and cottage cheese are higher.

To cut back on sodium intake, you can start by eating some items less often, particularly those you checked as "3 to 5 times a week" or more. This does not mean eliminating foods from your diet. You can moderate your sodium intake by choosing lower-sodium foods from each food group more often and by balancing high-sodium foods with low-sodium ones. For example, if you serve ham for dinner, plan to serve it with fresh or plain frozen vegetables cooked without added salt, or use less salt when preparing other foods in the meal. Salt used in food preparation contributes greatly to sodium intake.

From *USDA Home and Garden Bulletin* No. 232-6, April 1986.

The self-test in Table 8-8 will help you examine how the foods you eat and the way you prepare and serve them affect the amount of sodium in your diet.

Labels—Your License to Learn

The biggest breakthrough in the labeling laws with respect to minerals is that nearly all packaged foods must supply information on their sodium, calcium, and iron content. These three minerals were chosen because of their impact on health. The remaining minerals are not required on food labels, unless added during processing, because of space limitations.

To improve your diet, learn to read the nutrient content panel on food containers. Don't get lazy and depend on general labeling terms like "low sodium" to help you choose low-salt foods. The legal definition of low sodium is less than 140 mg of sodium per serving.[3,8,27] Many health experts believe normal, healthy people should consume no more than 1 mg of sodium per kcalorie up to a maximum of 3000 mg per day. Note that this is slightly higher than the 2400 mg limit suggested by the National Research Council.[19]

Do you think all dairy products are automatically great sources of calcium? Let's check it out. As the label on this container of low-fat cottage cheese shows (Fig. 8-8), the product provides only 8% of the adult

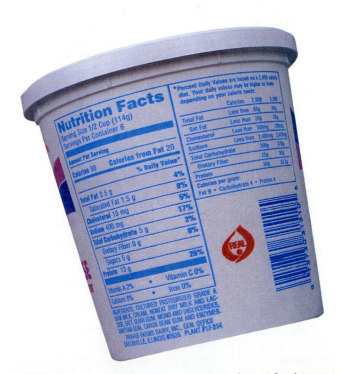

FIGURE 8-8 Check your assumptions about a food's nutrient content by being a careful label reader.

daily calcium requirement. And take a look at the sodium content: a whopping 400 mg per 90-kcalorie serving, or 4.4 mg of sodium per kcalorie.

You may decide to put this food back on the shelf; or, if the rest of your diet is fairly low in sodium, you may choose to buy this food. Remember that you need to consider your overall diet as well as the potential benefits and deficits of a particular food. In this case, a better choice would be plain, nonfat yogurt. The same serving size would yield 15% of the new RDA for calcium while supplying considerably less salt and fewer kcalories than the cottage cheese. The same labeling claims used for vitamins may be used in reference to minerals (Box 8-1).

Don't select a product on the basis of a single nutrient. Remember to look at the nutritional value of the food as a whole. Also consider how it fits into your diet. Is it one of your chief sources of nourishment, or is it a snack item you'll be eating in small quantities?

In the Kitchen

Unlike vitamins, minerals are not heat sensitive. Some cooking techniques, however, like boiling and stewing, leach minerals out of the foods and into the cooking water. Steaming and stir frying, the same techniques that help retain vitamin content, also will preserve minerals.[24]

The major challenges in food preparation where minerals are concerned are finding ways to increase the content of absorbable iron and calcium in your meals and to reduce your intake of sodium.

A simple measure like using cast-iron cookware can add iron to your diet. Adding powdered nonfat milk to casseroles, ground meats, and beverages provides an additional 50 mg of calcium per heaping tablespoon. (See the Resources section of Looking to the Future for how to obtain a calcium-enrichment brochure from Carnation Milk.)

Now for the biggest challenge: reducing your salt intake. Cut down on the amount of salt you use in a recipe. Don't use any additional salt if the recipe calls for canned tomato sauce or soy sauce (or use the low-sodium versions of these ingredients). Purchase seasoning blends designed to take the place of salt. Experiment with the salt substitutes in Table 8-9.

It will take about 6 weeks for your taste buds to adjust to a lower salt intake. Your patience will be rewarded! You eventually will begin to notice that you are more sensitive to the taste of salt. Foods you once seasoned with extra salt will seem sufficiently salty. To your surprise, you will find that many foods you once loved now taste too salty or send you running for a glass of water.

At the Table

Think variety. Are you eating virtually the same thing day after day, or do you vary your meals? Is your plate a mass of one color, or does it contain foods from several different groups?

BOX 8-1	Label Claims and Definitions
Label Claim	**Definition***
Good Source, Contains, Provides	10% to 19% of the Daily Value
High, Rich In, Excellent Source of	20% or more of the Daily Value
More, Fortified, Enriched, Added	Contains at least 10% more of the Daily Value, compared to the reference food

*Per Reference Amount (standard serving size). Some claims have higher nutrient levels for main dish products and meal products, such as frozen dinners and entrees.

TABLE 8-9 Salt Replacements	
Food	**Salt Substitute**
Eggs	Basil, dill, garlic, oregano, parsley, hot pepper
Beef	Basil, cumin, oregano, parsley, onions, garlic, hot pepper, red wine
Lamb	Rosemary, sage, mint, red wine vinegar, garlic
Pork	Orange juice, ginger, Italian seasoning, cumin
Fish	Basil, dill, fennel, parsley, sage, tarragon, thyme, hot pepper, onion, citrus juice, white wine
Poultry	Same as fish plus marjoram, rosemary, sage, poultry seasoning
Salads	Salad herbs, basil, parsley, tarragon, lemon juice, wine vinegar
Tomato sauce	Basil, bay leaf, marjoram, oregano, parsley, cinnamon, cloves, garlic, onion
Vegetables	Basil, garlic, oregano, parsley, thyme, rosemary, lemon juice
Barbecue blend	Cumin, garlic, hot pepper, oregano

Aim for food combinations that enhance mineral absorption. Be sure to include a source of vitamin C at each meal to increase iron and calcium absorption. Have calcium-rich foods several times a day to maximize absorption of this mineral. Get rid of your salt shaker to eliminate one source of sodium. If you can't bring yourself to do this, at least learn to taste your foods before salting them. You may find they don't need any flavor enhancement. If you have decided to eat less salt, give your palate a few weeks to adjust to the change in flavor.

Eating Out

The same steps that improve your mineral status at home apply when eating out. If eating out is routine for you, be sure to order dishes made with whole foods and include a source of vitamin C. If you are in the habit of going out for dessert, try ordering frozen low-fat or nonfat yogurt. Not only will this save you the fat, cholesterol, and kcalories found in many sweets, it also can contribute a good bit of calcium to your diet if you choose your brand carefully. A survey of national brands of frozen yogurt found that calcium content varies from a low of 15 mg per half cup to a high of 125 mg. Many manufacturers offer nutrition information, so read the label before you buy. By requesting a fruit topping, like berries, that is rich in vitamin C, you can turn dessert into a healthy treat!

Menu Matrix

The best course of action is to plan a diet that includes adequate sources of all minerals on a daily basis. If you plan a balanced diet and focus on obtaining less available zinc, iron, and calcium, you will automatically get enough of the easier-to-obtain minerals. The Menu Matrix for this chapter will focus on how to construct a diet that contains foods rich in these three minerals.

If you are not a vegetarian and you do not have a milk allergy, it is easy to meet your mineral requirements if you eat the right foods. If you are a vegetarian, it takes a bit more creativity to ensure adequate intake of certain minerals. Whatever your eating style, the best way to meet your calcium and iron requirements is to include a source of these minerals at each of your daily meals.

Don't ignore the value of snacks as you plan your diet. People are often admonished not to eat between meals, but a snack doesn't have to be synonymous with a junk food binge. A well-planned snack can be a valuable source of nutrients as well as energy.

Calcium

If you can consume dairy products, four servings of nonfat milk or yogurt can meet your daily calcium needs. However, it also supplies 400 kcalories and 40 g of protein (roughly the total protein requirement of the average adult female). If this is more kcalories and protein than you want to expend on dairy foods, consider consuming other calcium-rich foods.

For example, remember that you can satisfy part or all of your calcium requirement by eating canned fish with bones, tofu, selected green vegetables (broccoli and kale), or calcium-enriched orange juice. Because milk can limit iron absorption, you may prefer to have a dairy product for a snack rather than as a beverage at meals. An easy way to get all the calcium you need is to have two servings of milk or other dairy foods each day and to use a variety of other high-calcium foods. There is no need to overload on milk.

NUTRI NUGGET Tofu is isolated and purified soybean protein. Soy itself is not high in calcium, but the process of turning soybeans into protein adds valuable calcium.

Begin by entering two servings of dairy foods under calcium each day on your Menu Matrix (Appendix D). Now look at foods listed as rich sources of calcium. Select two or more servings of nondairy foods from this group daily. Vary your selections! For instance, on one day you may choose to have a canned salmon sandwich (cooked bones and all) and a glass of calcium-enriched orange juice for lunch and an Oriental vegetable stir fry with tofu for dinner. Another day you may elect to have calcium-enriched orange juice for part of a snack and a cup of steamed broccoli with dinner. By the end of the week you should have had 14 servings of dairy foods and at least 14 servings of other calcium-rich foods.

Fortunately, many of the foods that are rich in calcium are also good sources of iron and/or zinc. For instance, although milk is a poor source of iron, the amount recommended above will supply a little more than 10% of your daily zinc need. Broccoli and tofu are moderately good sources of both of these minerals. Meat eaters should be able to obtain adequate quantities of iron and zinc if they plan their diets well, since meat, fish, and poultry tend to be the richest and most absorbable sources of these minerals.

Now try planning several days' worth of calcium-rich meals without using any dairy products. Results of a study in mainland China[2] suggest it is possible for people to meet their calcium needs without eating any dairy products, but it takes careful planning. For generations Asians have consumed vegetarian diets, often without dairy products, with no ill effects. The secret of their success lies in both their food choices and their methods of preparation. Incorporating some of their practices with Western techniques can help produce a balanced diet. Vegetarians can consume legumes, cook in cast-iron pots, and eat the fruits and vegetables that are high in calcium, zinc, and iron (see Sources and

Recommendations for each of these minerals). Eating leavened (yeast-raised) whole-grain products will make mineral absorption easier because fermentation destroys mineral-grabbing phytates.[17] People who do not eat dairy products can use calcium-rich tofu or calcium-fortified soy milk and citrus juice.

How can I add iron and zinc to my diet?   Review the foods already entered on your Menu Matrix. Put an asterisk (*) beside any food that supplies zinc or iron as well as calcium. Add foods to the Matrix to cover your iron and zinc needs, indicating any that supply both zinc and iron with** so that you do not double up on servings. Animal proteins are good choices.

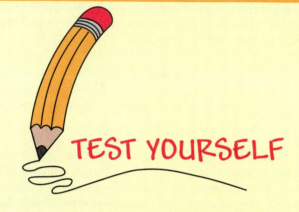

TEST YOURSELF

Because the mineral chapter is the last nutrient chapter in the text, this is a good time to discover connections between the various nutrients in your diet. To answer the questions for this chapter you must use your knowledge of the physiological functions of all six nutrient classes.

Short Answer

1. List three nutrients needed to form healthy bones.
2. Deficiencies of which nutrients lead to anemia?
3. Give two examples of how eating enough of certain vitamins helps your mineral status.
4. Which nutrients are involved in antioxidant reactions in the body?
5. What is the importance of antioxidant reactions?
6. Which vitamins and minerals are involved in converting food into fuel?

7. Night blindness may indicate a deficiency of which nutrients?
8. Which nutrients are involved in maintaining fluid balance in your body?
9. List three components of plant-based foods that can interfere with mineral absorption.
10. The nonnutritive minerals lead and mercury present a public health threat. Why?

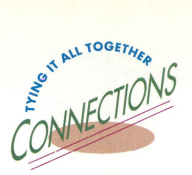

Read the recipe shown below.

Tamale Pie

Two 8-oz cans tomato sauce	1 tbsp sugar
One 12 oz can (1.5 cups) whole kernel corn, drained	1 tsp salt
1 lb ground beef	dash pepper
1 c chopped onion	3 tsp chili powder
1 c chopped green pepper	1 garlic clove, minced
6 oz sharp American cheese, shredded	$\frac{1}{2}$ c pitted ripe olives
$\frac{3}{4}$ c yellow cornmeal	1 tbsp margarine

Cook meat, onion, and green pepper until meat is lightly browned and vegetables are tender. Stir in all remaining ingredients except cheese, cornmeal, and margarine. Simmer 20 to 25 minutes or until thick. Add cheese; stir until melted. Place in a greased 9" × 9" × 2" baking dish. Make the cornmeal topper by stirring cornmeal and $\frac{1}{2}$ tsp salt into cold water. Cook and stir until thick. Spoon over meat mixture. Bake at 375° F for 40 minutes.

1. List all ingredients you think contain sodium.
2. Look up their sodium content in the Table of Food Composition in Appendix A.
3. List ways to reduce the sodium content of this recipe.
4. Reevaluate Connections questions 1 and 2 in Chapter 3, Water.
5. Which ingredients are good sources of iron, zinc, and calcium?
6. List food combinations in this recipe that either increase or decrease absorption of these minerals.
7. Which ingredients provide fat? How can the fat content of this dish be decreased?
8. How many sources of sodium can you identify on the following labels?

Chicken Bouillon
Salt, hydrolyzed vegetable protein, sugar, dehydrated chicken broth, monosodium glutamate (MSG), onion powder, turmeric, spices, disodium inosinate, disodium guanylate, natural and artificial flavor, BHA.

Matzo Ball Mix
Enriched wheat flour, sugar, salt, monosodium glutamate, onion, spices, vegetable shortening, garlic, monocalcium phosphate, baking soda, turmeric.

9. Why does kidney disease affect the skeletal system?
10. What effect does iodine deficiency have on nutrient metabolism?
11. What effect does zinc deficiency have on nutrient metabolism?
12. Yogurt is often recommended as a substitute for milk. Does it provide the same nutritional benefits? Are there any circumstances in which yogurt would be better than milk?

References

1. A new warning symbol for lead. *Food Safety Notebook* 4(3):33, 1993.

2. Campbell TC: A study of diet, nutrition, and disease in the People's Republic of China. Part 1. *Boletin-Asociacion Medica de Puerto Rico*, 82(3):132-134, 1990.

3. Browne MB: *Label facts for healthful eating.* American Dietetic Association, National Food Processors Association in cooperation with USDA, 1993.

4. Darby WJ, Jukes TH: *Founders of nutrition science*, vols 1 and 2, Rockville, Md, 1992, American Institute of Nutrition.

5. Fernstrom J: Dietary amino acids and brain function, *Journal of the American Dietetic Association* 94:71-77, 1994.

6. Fishbein L: Perspectives of analysis of carcinogenic and mutagenic metals in biological samples (As, Se, Cd, Cr, Ni), *International Journal of Environmental and Analytical Chemistry* 28(1 and 2):21-69, 1987.

7. Fluoride update, *Tufts University Diet and Nutrition Letter*, 11(8):2, 1993.

8. Focus on food labeling. FDA Special Report. *FDA Consumer*, 1993.

9. Food labeling update, *Food Safety Notebook* 3(12):110-115, 1992.

10. Fuchs G et al: Iron status and intake of older infants from formula vs cow milk with cereals, *American Journal of Clinical Nutrition* 58:343-348, 1993.

11. Greely A: Getting the lead out of just about everything. *FDA Consumer*, Reprint DHHS Pub # (FDA) 92-2249, 1991.

12. Health tips—Danger—Lead in wine bottle foils, *Johns Hopkins Medical Letter, Health After 50* 5(4):8, 1993.

13. Hetzel BS: Iodine deficiency: an international public health problem. In *Present knowledge in nutrition*, ed 6, Washington, DC, 1990, International Life Sciences Institute, Nutrition Foundation.

14. High tap water consumption may increase risk of bladder cancer, *Food Safety Notebook* 4(10):91-92, 1993.

15. Law MR et al: By how much does dietary salt reduction lower blood pressure? Analysis of observational data among populations, *British Medical Journal* 302:811-836, 1991.

16. Mertz W: Chromium in human nutrition: a review, *Journal of Nutrition* 123:623-633, 1993.

17. Moser-Veillen PB: Zinc: consumption patterns and dietary recommendations, *Journal of the American Dietetic Association* 90:1089-1093, 1990.

18. National Research Council: *Recommended dietary allowances*, ed 10, Washington, DC, 1989, National Academy Press.

19. National Research Council: *Diet and health, potential undesirable effects of dietary fiber: mineral bioavailability*, 1989.

20. Salt sensitivity and essential hypertension, *Nutrition and the MD*, 19:1, 1993.

21. O'Dell B: Copper. In *Present knowledge in nutrition*, ed 6, Washington, DC, 1990, International Life Sciences Institute, Nutrition Foundation.

22. *Outlook* magazine, Washington University School of Medicine, 30 (1):3, 1993.

23. Sanchez-Castillo et al: Estimates of sodium intake in a British population, *Clinical Science* 72:87, 1987.

24. Schroeder HA: Losses of vitamins and trace minerals resulting from processing and preservation of foods, *American Journal of Clinical Nutrition* 54:562-573, 1989.

25. Sowers MA et al: Calcium balance and osteoporosis in women, *Journal of the American Medical Association* 269:3130, 1993.

26. The Food Guide Pyramid. U.S. Department of Agriculture Home and Garden Bulletin #252, 1992.

27. The new food label. *FDA Backgrounder* BG 92-4, 1992.

28. Weaver CM et al: Human calcium absorption from whole-wheat products, *Journal of Nutrition* 121:1767-1774, 1991.

29. Wylie-Rosett E et al: Trial of antihypertensive intervention management: greater efficacy with weight reduction than with sodium-potassium intervention, *Journal of the American Dietetic Association* 93:408-415, 1993.

30. Yang GQ et al: Endemic selenium intoxication of humans in China, *American Journal of Clinical Nutrition* 37:872-881, 1983.

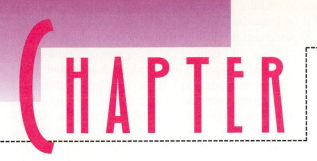

CHAPTER

9

ENERGY
Putting Nutrients to Work

Maybe counting calories is a science that is about as exact as handicapping horses.

— Calvin Trillin

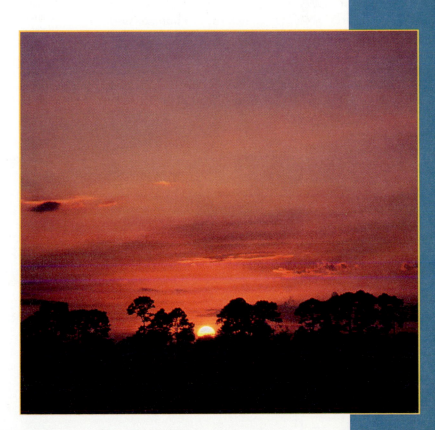

Energy is the ability to do work. It is measured in kcalories (kcal). A kcalorie is the amount of heat required to raise the temperature of 1 kilogram (about 1 quart) of water from 15° C to 16° C. Kcalories in the form of chemical energy are in the foods we eat and in our body tissues. For instance, 1 pound of body fat contains approximately 3500 kcalories. We expend kcalories in the forms of chemical and mechanical energy to maintain essential body functions and when we perform physical activities.

Energy cycles throughout the solar system. The energy found on Earth initially comes from the sun. This solar energy is captured by plants and transformed into chemical bonds between carbon atoms (Fig. 9-1). When humans and animals consume plant matter, their digestive enzymes break the carbon-to-carbon bonds, releasing the energy for their own use. Energy is neither created nor destroyed; it simply changes form. Some of the energy we obtain from food returns to the atmosphere as heat.

CARBON-TO-CARBON BONDS

What is the significance of carbon-to-carbon bonds?

All chemical bonds contain energy. It happens that the bonds between carbon atoms are the way in which energy is stored in organic matter. Because food is organic, carbon-to-carbon bonds are the major way in which the energy in food is transferred to humans and animals. Carbon-rich plant and animal foods are digested to their chemical building blocks (monosaccharides, amino acids, and fatty acids), which are then processed in cells to either three-carbon (C-C-C) or two-carbon (C-C) *intermediates.* These in turn are re-

fined in cellular "factories" to produce the energy-rich **ATP (adenosine triphosphate)** molecule.

In addition to ATP, our bodies manufacture two other forms of energy-rich adenosine molecules, known as **ADP (adenosine diphosphate)** and **AMP (adenosine monophosphate).** All three adenosine molecules store their power in high-energy phosphate bonds. Not surprisingly, the more phosphates the adenosine carries, the more energy it contains. Collectively these adenosine molecules serve as three different forms of cellular energy.

1. Where does the energy in high-energy phosphate bonds come from?
2. List three fuels we use in our homes, vehicles, schools, and businesses.

Why are there three different forms of adenosine?
The beauty of this system lies in adenosine's ability to carry a variable number of phosphates. As AMP it acts as an energy acceptor, picking up energy (phosphate) as it is released from the tricarboxylic acid cycle; as ATP it acts as an energy donor, releasing energy to power work; and as ADP it can perform in either capacity.

IN THE DIET

Why do some foods contain more energy than others?   Dietary carbohydrate, fat, protein, and alcohol all serve as sources of carbon-to-carbon bonds that can be burned to produce energy (ATP). Because fat and alcohol supply more carbon-to-carbon bonds

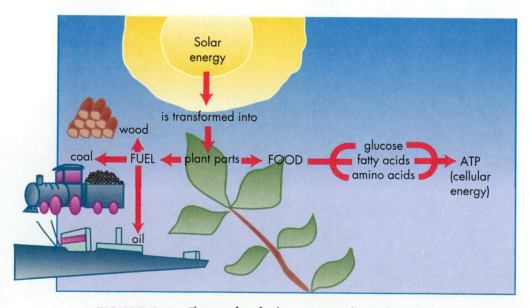

FIGURE 9-1   The transfer of solar energy to chemical energy.

than do equal quantities of protein or carbohydrate, they provide more kcalories per gram.

Sources

Which nutrients supply most of the energy in our diet?   For thousands of years, carbohydrates have been the major source of energy in most people's diets. This is true today in many developing nations where traditional foods are still consumed. In the United States and other industrialized nations, however, fat is becoming a major source of energy (Fig. 9-2)—often with serious health consequences.

Calorimetry

How do we know the kcalorie content of the various nutrients?   Scientists gradually realized that living things use energy and that foods supply it. To quantify the energy in foods, researchers developed **bomb calorimetry** (Fig. 9-3). With this technique they determined the kcalorie content of a given food or nutrient by burning a known amount of it in an insulated box (the bomb) in the presence of oxygen and then measuring the resulting temperature change in a known amount of water surrounding the box. The usable en-

ergy content of the major classes of organic nutrients[13] was found to be:

Protein	4 kcal per gram
Carbohydrate	4 kcal per gram
Fat	9 kcal per gram
(Alcohol	7 kcal per gram)

Now that the kcalorie values of the individual nutrients are known, it is no longer necessary to use this measuring technique to determine the energy content of a particular food. Instead we can determine the amount of each energy-supplying nutrient a food contains, convert this information into its kcalorie equivalents, and then sum the parts (Box 9-1).

Unless you have made something from scratch, you usually have no need to calculate the kcalorie content of your favorite foods. Detailed nutrient content information is provided on most food labels. There also are many books and computer programs that contain nutrient analysis data. If you want to get a rough idea of the number of kcalories you are eating each day, keep

intermediates   molecules that occur in the process of forming another molecule (such as glucose and acetyl CoA in energy metabolism within the cells)

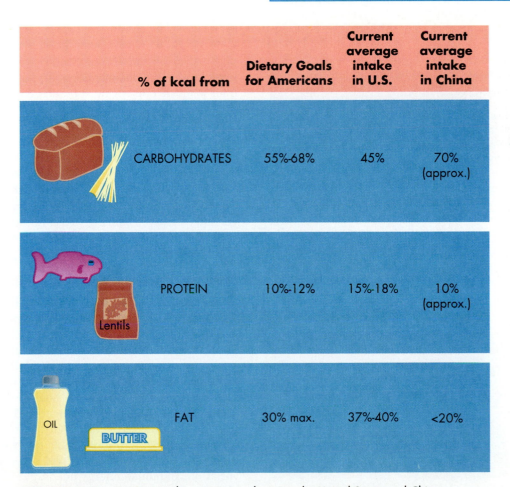

% of kcal from	Dietary Goals for Americans	Current average intake in U.S.	Current average intake in China
CARBOHYDRATES	55%-68%	45%	70% (approx.)
PROTEIN	10%-12%	15%-18%	10% (approx.)
FAT	30% max.	37%-40%	<20%

FIGURE 9-2   Nutrient intake comparison between the United States and China.

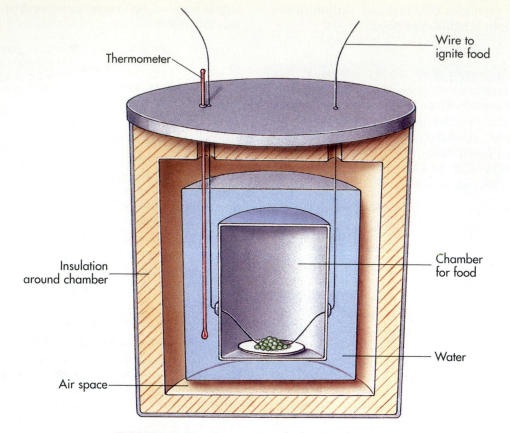

FIGURE 9-3 Cross section of a bomb calorimeter.

TABLE 9-1 **Kcal Content of Exchange Lists**

Exchange List	Serving Size	Kcals
Starch/bread	1 slice	80
Meat (lean)	1 ounce	55
Vegetable	½ cup	25
Fruit	varies	60
Milk (nonfat)	1 cup	90
Fat	1 teaspoon	45

track how much of what foods you eat and look up their kcalorie content in Appendix A.

Exchange Lists and Food Guide Pyramid

An even simpler though less accurate method is to estimate your kcalorie intake by using the exchange lists introduced in Chapter 4, Carbohydrates, or the Food Guide Pyramid food choices chart introduced in Chapter 2. Many people find these estimates more convenient than measuring serving sizes, calculating kcalorie content, or memorizing kcalorie counts. Complete exchange lists appear in Appendix C.

Energy Intake Standard—RDA

In contrast to the RDA for other nutrients, which are set to meet the upper level of requirements for the general population, the RDA for energy is set at the mean or middle-level requirement. An RDA for energy intake has been established for male and female adults in three age categories: 19 to 24, 25 to 50, and over 50. These RDA are for *groups* of healthy Americans who are of average height and weight and are performing light to moderate physical activity. The energy RDA are not designed to help individuals determine a kcalorie requirement because, as we will see, there are many variations in human energy needs.[16]

BOX 9-2   Method of Calculating Kcal Requirement

Body weight (in pounds) times **activity coefficient** (kcals/lb) minus **age factor** (kcals)

Activity coefficient

If you are **inactive**, multiply your weight in pounds by 9.

If you are **moderately active**, multiply your weight in pounds by 13.

If you are **very active**, multiply your weight in pounds by 20.

Age factor

Subtract 100 kcals from the answer for each decade of age over age 30, to adjust your kcal intake for the decrease in metabolic rate that accompanies aging.

Example: Joanne, a moderately active 50-year-old, weighs 150 lbs. Her kcalorie requirement = (150 lb. × 13 kcals/lb) − 200 kcals = 1750 kcals

Adapted from Anderson A: *Males with eating disorders*, New York, 1990, Brunner/Mazel.

How can I determine how many Kcalories I need each day?   Energy requirements vary considerably from person to person. You can make a rough estimate by using the formula in Box 9-2, which takes into account body weight, activity level (see p. 27 in Chapter 2 for definitions of activity level), and age.

IN THE DIGESTIVE TRACT

Digestion does not liberate energy from foods. Rather it refines the food (fuel) to the point where it can be used by individual cells in the body to produce energy. The end products of digestion for the energy-supplying nutrients are classified as potential sources of either glucose or fatty acids. Potential sources of glucose yield three-carbon units, whereas potential sources of fatty acids yield two-carbon units.

Why is this classification important?   This distinction is made because three-carbon units can be used to produce glucose, the only possible fuel for many tissues; whereas two-carbon units cannot be used to produce glucose but can be used to synthesize fat.

IN THE BODY

Why does my body need energy?   We use energy from various fuel sources in our homes, cars, and factories to keep us warm and to do work. The same is true within our bodies. For example, our bodies convert fuel-rich protein, fat, and carbohydrate into energy that is used to produce heat and perform physical and chemical work.

Energy Requirements

There are three major ways in which cells use energy:
1. basal metabolism
2. voluntary physical activity
3. dietary-induced *thermogenesis* (DIT)

A number of variables affect energy requirements: body size and composition, age, gender, genetics, kcalorie intake, and physiological state (pregnancy, lactation, recovery from injury, surgery, or disease).[13,17,20,24]

Basal Metabolism

Basal metabolism is the cellular activity required to maintain life. For all but the most active people, it is the body's largest energy expenditure. Asleep or awake, basal metabolic energy performs these vital functions:

- *Thermogenesis*—the heat our bodies generate to keep us warm
- *Movement*—involuntary muscle work (e.g., respiration and circulation)
- *Electrical work*—nerve signals
- *Chemical work*—purification, enzyme synthesis, and tissue repair

Basal metabolic rate (BMR) or resting energy expenditure (REE). The rate of cellular activity differs from one person to another. It is strongly influenced by age, genetics, gender, and by the percent of the body's mass that is composed of lean tissue. BMR decreases with increasing age. This effect is independent of gender. Our amount of lean body mass is influenced by gender and physical activity. In general, male gender and a high level of physical activity are associated with increased lean body mass and thus lead to a higher BMR.[20]

Measuring basal energy use. Just as kcalories can be measured, so can the amount of basal energy used in our bodies. The most accurate way of measuring basal energy expenditure is a technique known as **direct calorimetry.** A test subject is placed in a specially constructed room called a *calorimeter.* Thermostats built into the walls measure the heat given off by the subject's body. Because calorimeters are very costly, they are available at only a few research centers around the country, so scientists have developed a less costly but less accurate method of measuring basal energy expenditure known as **indirect calorimetry** or the **respiratory quotient (RQ).** This technique determines basal energy use by comparing the amount of

thermogenesis   heat production; from Greek *therme*, heat; *genesis*, birth, beginning

oxygen used by the test subject with the amount of carbon dioxide s/he produces.[20,24]

Activity

The second greatest energy cost for most people is that which we use to perform voluntary physical activities beyond rest, such as moving about, exercising, or doing any kind of physical labor. As with the basal metabolic rate, the larger the body, the more energy it uses to perform any kind of physical work. An easy way to understand this concept is to compare voluntary physical activity to moving a car. All other factors being equal, the larger the vehicle (body), the greater the cost of fuel (energy) to move it down the road. (See p. 189 in Chapter 10, Exercise, for a discussion of the value of sports and leisure activities in weight control.)

Dietary-Induced Thermogenesis (DIT)

The third major category of energy use is that we require to digest and absorb foods. Whoever created the popular clichés "There is no free lunch" and "You have to spend money to make money" could have been describing digestion and nutrient utilization. This scientific relationship was first noted about 100 years ago by a researcher who discovered that a person's metabolic rate is increased for as long as 4 hours after eating.[13] This increase represents the energy required to digest, absorb, transport, and metabolize nutrients. It is termed **dietary-induced thermogenesis.** This process, which is related to both the amount of food eaten and the composition of the meal, usually uses from 5% to 10% of the total energy we consume and represents the smallest of our bodies' energy expenditures.[13,17]

Energy Metabolism—Making and Using ATP

How are the Kcalories in food turned into usable cellular energy (ATP)?   The solar energy that was transformed into carbon-to-carbon bonds during photosynthesis is released and transformed into ATP, which fuels the work performed in our bodies' cells. First digestion transforms whole foods into individual nutrients. Carbohydrates, proteins, and fats are further digested into their individual building blocks, which are then absorbed across the intestinal lining into the bloodstream. Next cells extract these various nutrient building blocks from the blood and use them in **metabolism** either for building or replacing parts or for producing ATP.[12]

Metabolism—the work that goes on within cells—is the sum of two contrasting processes: catabolism and anabolism.

Catabolism

Catabolism (or *degradation* as it is sometimes called) is the process by which carbon-to-carbon bonds in food or in our bodies' energy reserves and protein tissues are broken down inside the cells. Sugars, glucose-producing (glucogenic) amino acids, or the glycerol backbone of fats are converted into a three-carbon fragment called **pyruvate.** Some ATP is formed during this process. Additional ATP is formed by breaking off one carbon from pyruvate. The remaining two carbons are used to produce additional energy in the same way as are the two-carbon fragments obtained from fatty acids, lipid-producing (lipogenic) amino acids, and alcohol. Two carbon units (acetyls) are joined to coenzyme A (CoA)—the coenzyme form of the B vitamin, pantothenic acid—to make acetyl CoA. The acetyl CoA is further oxidized (or burned) to carbon dioxide, water, and ATP through two consecutive chemical processes, known as the **tricarboxylic acid cycle (TCA)** and the **electron transport system.** These series of events complete the transformation of the sun's energy from carbon-to-carbon bonds found in foods into ATP, which fuels our bodies. In reality we are "solar powered": the warmth of our bodies comes initially from the warmth (energy) of the sun!

Anabolism

Anabolism, often referred to as *synthesis*, is the term used to describe the body's construction of a substance such as bone, muscle protein, or stored fat. Because anabolism is a process that requires energy, it uses some of the ATP formed during catabolism.

What happens to the rest of the ATP formed during catabolism?   It is used for basal metabolic activities (vital functions such as respiration and circulation), voluntary physical activity, and digestion and absorption of food.

Does my body turn ATP into fat?   Not exactly. It turns the acetyl CoA used to make ATP into fat. Here is how it works. When there is a surplus of energy, ATP begins to build up in the electron transport system and tricarboxylic acid cycle, preventing oxidation of additional acetyl CoA. Acetyl CoA molecules accumulate, signaling your body that it is time to synthesize fat. Through a complex series of events these molecules are then strung together, forming triglycerides for fat storage in specialized cells called adipose tissue.

BOX 9-3	**Uses of Metabolic Energy**	
METABOLISM =	**CATABOLISM +**	**ANABOLISM**
	Produces ATP	Uses ATP
	Breaks C-C bonds	Builds C-C bonds
	Uses molecules	Stores molecules
	Makes smaller pieces	Makes larger pieces

Energy Balance

What is energy balance?   **Balance** is the condition in which energy intake exactly equals energy expenditure for basal needs, voluntary physical activity, digestion, and absorption. An adult in energy balance has a fairly stable body weight and adequate but not excessive amounts of energy stored as fat in adipose tissue.

If the amount of energy consumed is less than the amount of energy spent, **negative energy balance** occurs. Protein will be used to produce glucose (gluconeogenesis), water will be lost, fat will be withdrawn from adipose tissue, and weight loss will follow. Conversely, if the amount of energy consumed exceeds the amount of energy spent, **positive energy balance** will ensue, fat will be deposited in adipose tissue, and weight gain will occur.[13]

Body Reserves

Our bodies' fuel reserves serve as protection from both short-term and long-term fasting. Our carbohydrate reserves (glycogen) are an important source of glucose between meals. During longer periods of fasting, protein is used to produce glucose. Both fat stores and protein tissues contribute kcalories during starvation. Plasma proteins are readily accessible to the liver. A significant decrease in plasma proteins accounts for the edema, anemia, and increased susceptibility of disease seen in the early stages of starvation. During prolonged food restriction, structural proteins are also depleted. This is a very dangerous situation. It weakens every muscle and organ in the body, often with fatal consequences.

How much potential fuel does a healthy person store?   Depending on hormonal signals, a healthy, trim, previously well-fed person has roughly the following tissue reserves:

Blood glucose	about 20 g (about 80 kcal)
Glycogen	about 400 g (about 1600 kcal)
Fat	15% of male body weight; 20% to 25% of female
Protein	15% of body weight

Body Fat and Health

Why is energy balance important?   Medical researchers, health practitioners, and insurance underwriters all have noted a strong correlation between body fat and health. Both low and high body fat content are associated with a variety of medical problems.

"Sudden death is more common in those who are naturally fat than in those who are lean."

— *Hippocrates, fourth century BC*

Excess body fat. *Overweight* does not necessarily mean *overfat*. For example, athletes with well-developed muscle mass can be overweight according to height-weight charts, but not overfat according to the body fat recommendation shown above. People who are truly overfat tend to have a greater incidence of high blood pressure (hypertension), diabetes, heart disease, certain forms of cancer, and pregnancy complications. Further, excessive body fat worsens many medical problems, such as arthritis, abdominal hernias, gallbladder disease, and respiratory problems.[3] In Chapter 11, Weight Control, we explore in more depth the physical, emotional, and social costs of *obesity.*

Inadequate body fat. It is difficult for many people in our weight-obsessed society to conceive of any problems associated with being too thin, yet this condition carries its own set of risks. People who consume too few kcalories to maintain an adequate body weight (such as elderly people in nursing homes and people with anorexia nervosa) are usually deficient in other nutrients as well. A severe and/or persistent lack of dietary energy results in loss of muscle as well as fat tissue, overall poor nutritional status, and depressed immune function. Children whose diets are low in kcalories are irritable, lethargic, have difficulty repairing and maintaining tissues, and show signs of retardation in growth as well as intellectual development. These symptoms of severe dietary energy deficiency are similar in adults, except that they have no effect on growth and no permanent effect on mental ability. Underweight people of all ages are generally the first to die in times of prolonged food shortages such as occur during a famine, war, or extreme poverty. They also have more difficulty recovering from diseases, injuries, and surgery. According to several studies, underweight people also are at greater risk for developing osteoporosis.[9] (See the section on stress fractures in Chapter 10.)

Energy Balance Classifications

The traditional way of assessing a person's energy balance has been to compare his or her weight and height with a standardized table of ideal weights for a range of heights. Using this table, some husky football players were rejected as being too fat to enlist in the armed services during World War II. In contrast, very petite women with low body weights but relatively high percentages of body fat were classified as underweight. Clearly something was wrong somewhere!

The problem was twofold. First, ideal weights for heights (Metropolitan Life Insurance Company Tables are on the inside back cover) were not determined scientifically. They were merely the average weight ranges for people of a given height who had applied for life insurance. Second, simply determining weight for height failed to take into account genetically determined dif-

obesity   body weight 20% or more above healthy weight for height

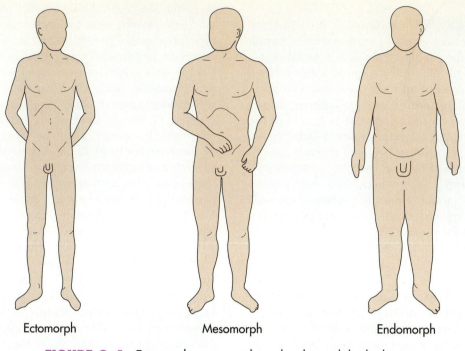

Ectomorph   Mesomorph   Endomorph

FIGURE 9-4   Ectomorph, mesomorph, and endomorph body shapes.

ferences in body build (muscle and bone size). Consequently, people with extremely light or heavy builds tended to be misclassified as underweight or overweight.

Body types. In the 1960s a researcher determined that human physiques could be grouped into three major categories: **ectomorph** (long and lean), **mesomorph** (solid and muscular), and **endomorph** (soft and rounded) (Fig. 9-4).[23]

Height/weight charts were adjusted to account for light, moderate, and heavy frame sizes, but it still is difficult to determine a person's build just by looking at him or her. Obesity can make a person with a slender frame appear to be endomorphic, whereas a very thin person with a moderate build may be misidentified as an ectomorph. The greatest value of the body type classifications is that they help us understand the extent to which we can reshape our physique. Regardless of diet or exercise regimen, our physical appearance is determined in part by the type of build we inherited. Endomorphs can be trim and firm, but they are never described as slender. Ectomorphs can "bulk up" their muscles considerably, but their frames will always be lean.

Determining frame size. A rough estimate of body

build can be obtained by measuring the width of a person's bones. One of the best bones to use for this purpose is the elbow bone, which, except in very obese people, is a good indication of skeletal structure. Extend your nondominant arm in front of you. Raise your forearm at a 90-degree angle to your upper arm. Keep your fingers pointing straight upwards. Turn your palm away from your body. Place the thumb and index finger of your other hand on opposite sides of the two prominent bones in your elbow. Measure the space between your fingers with a ruler. For greater accuracy, slip a tape measure under your fingers. Most accurate of all, measure your elbow width with a pair of calibrated **calipers.** Compare your measurement with those in Table 9-2.

How do you measure up?   Now that you know your frame size, weigh yourself at the same time of day at *weekly* intervals. The best time is first thing in the morning, after you urinate, and before you eat. Compare your weight to the height/weight chart shown on the inside back cover. Are you above, below, or in the range of your healthy weight?

Measuring percent body fat. Measuring your frame size is really an attempt to measure how much of your weight is lean tissue (bone and muscle) and how much is fat. Directly determining your percentage of body fat is a better way to measure energy balance because it more accurately reflects health risks than does body weight or body weight corrected for frame size. Several techniques are used to measure weight. **Underwater weighing** uses the tendency of fat to float in water. The difference between a person's body weight taken on dry land and that taken under water is used to

Compare the builds of Danny DeVito and Abraham Lincoln. Which body type is each of these men? How about Olympic figure skaters Nancy Kerrigan, Tonya Harding, and Kristi Yamaguchi? Which body type are you?

TABLE 9-2 Elbow Measurements for Medium Builds

The following measurements are the ranges obtained from men and women of varying heights with medium builds. Measurements greater than those shown for a given height indicate that the person in question has a large frame. Measurements smaller than those shown indicate a small frame.

Men		Women	
Height in 1″ heels	**Elbow Width**	**Height in 1″ heels**	**Elbow Width**
5′ 2″ to 5′ 3″	2 1/2″ to 2 7/8″	4′ 10″ to 4′ 11″	2 1/4″ to 2 1/2″
5′ 4″ to 5′ 7″	2 5/5″ to 2 7/8″	5′ 0″ to 5′ 3″	2 1/4″ to 2 1/2″
5′ 8″ to 5′ 11″	2 3/4″ to 3″	5′ 4″ to 5′ 7″	2 3/8″ to 2 5/8″
6′ 0″ to 6′ 3″	2 3/4″ to 3 1/8″	5′ 8″ to 5′ 11″	2 3/8″ to 2 5/8″
6′ 4″ and above	2 7/8″ to 3 1/4″	6′ and above	2 1/2″ to 2 3/4″

calculate the percentage of body fat. Underwater weighing is considered to be the "gold standard" for determining percent of body fat, but the equipment required makes it impractical for routine clinical use. Two drier, but less accurate, techniques are widely used. One method uses calibrated calipers to measure **skinfold thickness** at various sites on the body. These measurements are then compared with tables that interpret them in terms of percent of body fat (Table 9-3). Note: Women need more body fat than men for their reproductive systems to function normally. The other method, **bioelectrical impedance**, measures the amount of impedance (resistance) to the flow of a harmless low-voltage electrical current through the body and converts it to percent body fat. Because fat impedes the flow of electricity, the greater the fat stores, the greater the impedance of the electrical current.[3]

Hate to get wet but demand accuracy? Researchers have invented a new method of body composition analysis that is as accurate as underwater weighing but does not require dunking. The device is an airtight glass chamber with a built-in computer. The computer measures the air volume in the chamber when it is empty and again when the subject is seated inside. Using this information and the person's body weight, the computer calculates body fat content. Because fat weighs less than muscle, a person with high air volume but low body weight has a high percentage of fat.

NUTRI NUGGET

There is no such thing as cellulite. The dimpled appearance of fat on a woman's body occurs because women deposit more fat under the skin than do men; this fat is pulled on by the underlying connective tissue.

Healthy weights. Are you underfat, just right, slightly plump, or truly fat? In late 1990 the U.S. Department of Agriculture and the Department of Health and Human Services attempted to simplify the ideal-weight and body build controversy by issuing a more flexible standard known as the **Healthy Weight**

TABLE 9-3 Interpreting Skinfold Thickness

Gender	Ideal % Body Fat	Average	Triceps Skinfold Thickness
Female	20-25	22	1″
Male	13-18	18	1/2″

TABLE 9-4 Healthy Weights in Pounds

Height	19-34 years	35 years and up
5′ 0″	97-128	108-138
5′ 1″	101-132	111-143
5′ 2″	104-137	115-148
5′ 3″	107-141	119-152
5′ 4″	111-146	122-157
5′ 5″	114-150	126-162
5′ 6″	118-155	130-167
5′ 7″	121-160	134-172
5′ 8″	125-164	138-178
5′ 9″	129-169	142-183
5′ 10″	132-174	146-188
5′ 11″	136-179	151-194
6′ 0″	140-184	155-199
6′ 1″	144-189	159-205
6′ 2″	148-195	164-210

caliper a measuring device with two legs or jaws that is used to determine the distance between two surfaces

ectomorph a long, lean or slightly muscular human body

endomorph a human body with a predominance of abdomen and other soft body parts, short neck and fingers

mesomorph a human body characterized by powerful muscle or a predominantly bony framework

Table (Table 9-4). The separate height and weight tables for men and women have been replaced by a single table for both sexes. Additionally, size categories have been replaced with a much more lenient single-weight range of 30 pounds or more at each height. Finally, the table provides for a weight gain of up to 16 pounds at each height from age 35 on because some studies have shown that people who are a bit heavier in their later years have a longer life expectancy.

NUTRALERT

Body weight 100 pounds or more above average weight for height is classified as morbid obesity. This ominous-sounding term reflects the high rate of morbidity (illness) associated with such an extreme accumulation of fat.[3]

How do I interpret the data in this table?   In general, women and people with small frames should try to maintain their body weight at the lower end of the weight range for their height. In contrast, men and people with heavy bone structures should aim for the upper half of their weight range. A word of caution: be careful not to interpret the broad range of weights at your height to mean that you can safely weigh more than you currently do.

Body mass index. A highly reliable indicator of whether your body fat level presents any health risks is the **Body Mass Index** developed by obesity expert Dr. George Bray. You can calculate your own body mass index by dividing your weight in kilograms by your height in meters squared (or use Table 9-5). Health risks increase when the body mass index exceeds 25 (25 = low risk; 40 = very high risk).[3]

Fat distribution patterns. Researchers have noted that a person's fat distribution pattern is just as important as body weight or percent of body fat in terms of assessing health risks. Essentially, obese people can be classified as having either an *android* (also known as an apple or male) or *gynoid* (also known as a pear or female) pattern of fat distribution (Fig. 9-5).

Android obesity is the term used to describe the typical pattern of male fat distribution, which is characterized by a large abdominal fat deposit with small hips, buttocks, and thighs. This pot-bellied appearance is thought to be favored by male sex hormones and is associated with a greater incidence of heart disease, diabetes, hypertension, and in women breast cancer than is gynoid obesity.

By contrast, **gynoid obesity,** the typical female pattern, is characterized by large hips, buttocks, and thighs with a small abdomen. Deposition of fat in the lower rather than upper region of the body is favored

TABLE 9-5 Body Mass Index*

Height (in)	Body Mass Index (kg/m²)													
	19	20	21	22	23	24	25	26	27	28	29	30	35	40
	Body Weight (lb)													
58	91	96	100	105	110	115	119	124	129	134	138	143	167	191
59	94	99	104	109	114	119	124	128	133	138	143	148	173	198
60	97	102	107	112	118	123	128	133	138	143	148	153	179	204
61	100	106	111	116	122	127	132	137	143	148	153	158	185	211
62	104	109	115	120	126	131	136	142	147	153	158	164	191	218
63	107	113	118	124	130	135	141	146	152	158	163	169	197	225
64	110	116	122	128	134	140	145	151	157	163	169	174	204	232
65	114	120	126	132	138	144	150	156	162	168	174	180	210	240
66	118	124	130	136	142	148	155	161	167	173	179	186	216	247
67	121	127	134	140	146	153	159	166	172	178	185	191	223	255
68	125	131	138	144	151	158	164	171	177	184	190	197	230	262
69	128	135	142	149	155	162	169	176	182	189	196	203	236	270
70	132	139	146	153	160	167	174	181	188	195	202	207	243	278
71	136	143	150	157	165	172	179	186	193	200	208	215	250	286
72	140	147	154	162	169	177	184	191	199	206	213	221	258	294
73	144	151	159	166	174	182	189	197	204	212	219	227	265	302
74	148	155	163	171	179	186	194	202	210	218	225	233	272	311
75	152	160	168	176	184	192	200	208	216	224	232	240	279	319
76	156	164	172	180	189	197	205	213	221	230	238	246	287	328

Adapted from Bray GA: Obesity. In *Present knowledge in nutrition*, Washington, DC, 1990, International Life Sciences Institute—Nutrition Foundation.
*Each entry gives the body weight in pounds (lb) for a person of a given height and body mass index. Pounds have been rounded off. To use the table, find the appropriate height in the left-hand column. Move across the row to a given weight. The number at the top of the column is the body mass index for the height and weight.

TABLE 9-6 Comparison of Methods of Estimating Body Fat and Its Distribution

Method	Cost*	Ease of Use	Accuracy	Regional Fat
BMI	$	Easy	High	No
Height and weight	$	Easy	High	No
Skinfold measurements	$	Easy	Low	Yes
Density (immersion)	$$	Moderate	High	No
Impedance	$$	Easy	Moderate	No
Ultrasound	$$$	Moderate	Moderate	Yes

Adapted from Bray GA: Obesity. in *Present knowledge in nutrition,* Washington, DC, 1990, International Life Sciences Institute—Nutrition Foundation.

*$, Low cost; $$, moderate cost; $$$, high cost.

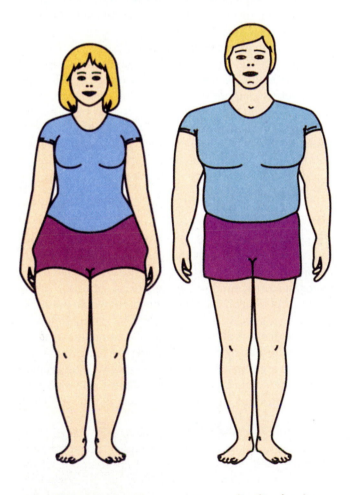

Lower body obesity (gynecoid obesity)   Upper body obesity (android obesity)

FIGURE 9-5 The gynoid and android patterns of body fat distribution.

by the female sex hormone progesterone. Although this fat distribution pattern is associated with a lower risk of heart disease, it seems to be more resistant than upper body fat to reducing diets and exercise.[3]

Am I an apple or a pear? *Apple* and *pear* are terms used to describe fat distribution patterns. People who store fat around their middle (most men) are apples; those who store fat around their hips (most women) are pears. If you're not sure which you are, measure the circumference of your waist (belly) and your hips (bottom). Divide your waist measurement by your hip measurement. You are an apple if you are a man and your belly to bottom ratio is greater than 0.9, or if you are a woman and your belly to bottom ratio is greater than 0.8. You are a pear if you are a woman and your belly to bottom ratio is less than 0.8.

 Our fat distribution pattern reflects our genetic makeup. Abdominal fat is mobilized more easily than fat at the extremities, so it tends to fill up the blood vessels around the heart with lipoproteins and cholesterol. This may account for the greater incidence of heart disease observed in apple-shaped as compared to pear-shaped people.[3]

Regulation of Energy Balance

How is energy balance regulated? The four major factors that contribute to energy balance are basal metabolic rate (BMR), dietary-induced thermogenesis (DIT), voluntary activity, and kcalorie intake. As yet, however, no one understands what regulates each of these factors; nor do we know how these factors affect each other or energy balance as a whole. Both nature (genetic inheritance) and nuture (environmental influences) have been cited as the primary regulator of energy balance. However, neither theory by itself provides a totally satisfactory explanation. The contemporary view is that a given person's energy balance results from a combination of nature and nuture.[6]

Nature—Genetics

Genetically determined obesity has been clearly demonstrated in certain strains of laboratory and domestic animals. The role of genetics in the determination of human energy balance, however, is not as well established. Genetics has been shown to influence familial body weight and fat distribution patterns, metabolic efficiency, and **body weight set point.** Each of these factors, however, also can be modified by environment.

Familial body weight patterns. Obesity or leanness tends to run in families. The high incidence of obesity in certain families, ethnic groups, and sets of identical twins has often been cited as evidence that genetics determines energy balance. More compelling evidence that "birth determines girth" are studies that show that the body weights of adopted children are typically more similar to the weights of their biological rather than adopted families.[6]

Metabolic efficiency. People vary greatly in the amount of energy they expend. Inborn differences in basal metabolic rate and activity levels can be detected in early childhood. During such investigations, some people's metabolisms have been found to be more efficient than others'. This means that if we examine two people of the same age, gender, height, weight, and general physical condition, the one with the "thrifty" metabolism (relatively low BMR and DIT) will require less energy to perform a given task than will the metabolic "spendthrift" (relatively high BMR and DIT).

Set point. People tend to maintain a stable body weight for years on end, regardless of changes in their kcalorie intake. Why, despite efforts to lose or gain weight, will a person's weight return to its original level once he or she ceases these efforts? Researchers theorize that the body somehow knows what weight it prefers and will fight to maintain that weight by altering eating behavior or metabolic rate. In other words, each of us has a personal set point at which our body weight tends to stabilize.[3,7]

Nurture—Environment

Experts now agree that genetics determines our body type, which in turn dictates our pattern of fat accumulation. But environmental factors, such as food intake and activity levels, alter what nature provided. For example, an ectomorph can overeat to the point of obesity or an endomorph can stay trim though solidly built with a healthful diet and consistent exercise program. Although physiques vary, widespread obesity does not occur in countries where food is scarce or hard physical labor is the norm. Further, a study of identical twins who were purposely overfed or underfed found that the combination of environmental and genetic factors had a greater effect on body weight than did either factor alone. In other words, body type (ectomorph, mesomorph, or endomorph) dictates our minimum amount of adipose tissue. The maximum amount, however, seems to be influenced heavily by eating behavior via environmental factors.[6,7]

Control of Food Intake

Food intake clearly has a major impact on energy balance. Scientists have been trying for decades to sort out what factors influence food intake and how these factors can be modified to control body weight. Eating is believed to be encouraged by two different mechanisms: inner drives, influenced by our individual physiological makeup; and external factors, influenced by our psychological makeup. Nutritionists separate these influences into two categories: **hunger,** or physiologi-cally motivated eating; and **appetite,** or externally motivated eating. Although there is some overlap between them, these designations are helpful when discussing eating behavior.[8]

Physiological—hunger. Hunger is defined as a physiological response to inner cues that trigger eating. Studies show that there are distinct areas in the brains of rats that regulate hunger. Stimulation of one site, known as the *feeding center*, will cause continuous eating. Stimulation of a nearby site, termed the *satiety center*, will cause the rat to starve itself to death in the presence of food.[8]

Psychological—appetite. Appetite is defined as the desire for a specific food or foods. It is thought to be caused by psychological or cultural responses to external cues. Common external eating cues are the time of day, physical location, presence of a favorite food, stress, and emotional stimulation, whether negative or positive. Many of our appetite cues appear to be learned, but we each seem to have an inborn preference for certain tastes and textures. From time to time, all of us eat in response to psychological cues. Such behavior is only a problem when a person eats primarily in response to appetite rather than hunger.

Some appetite-driven eaters can be helped simply by becoming aware of the situations that trigger them to eat. In others, appetite-driven eating behavior is so well entrenched that awareness of the problem has little impact on their habits. One explanation for this resistant behavior is that psychological factors may stem from or develop physiological responses, such as the production of various chemicals, that perpetuate eating behavior.[8]

Stress and Eating

In response to any physical or psychological threat, our bodies release hormones that prepare us for immediate action by increasing our metabolic rate, breaking down glycogen stores, and increasing glucose utilization. The need for fuel may be one reason some people eat in response to stress. Others may find that eating helps reduce the feeling of anxiety that accompanies stress. People who eat in response to stress tend to choose carbohydrate-rich foods. Interestingly, researchers have found that dietary carbohydrates stimulate the brain to produce opiate-like chemicals that induce a feeling of tranquility.[25]

If I only eat when I am hungry, will I stay trim?

No one really knows for sure. Although the factors that influence food intake have been identified, one of the most difficult questions for scientists to answer is whether people overeat because they feel hungry inappropriately or because their appetite has been stimulated. Some researchers, especially those who believe in the set point theory of obesity, think people become overfat because their body prefers being heavy so it signals them to eat (hunger). Others argue that people learn to overeat because they respond to appetite rather than hunger.

Errors of Energy Metabolism

A wide variety of illnesses can affect energy balance. Some, like cancer or gastrointestinal diseases, reduce food intake. Others, such as diabetes (discussed in Chapter 4, Carbohydrates) and thyroid dysfunction, affect the way the body uses energy. The thyroid gland produces the hormone thyroxin, which regulates the basal metabolic rate. Any change in its function therefore has a significant effect on energy metabolism. People who suffer from hyperthyroidism typically experience unexplained weight loss and hyperactivity and may constantly feel overheated. These people need a high-kcalorie diet that contains ample protein to prevent muscle wasting. Not surprisingly, the symptoms of hypothyroidism are just the opposite: unexplained weight gain, ongoing fatigue, and a sense of being cold all the time. In some cases a low-kcalorie diet is needed in addition to medication to achieve weight loss.

Psychological Disorders of Energy Balance

Eating disorders are conscious behaviors that produce alterations in energy balance, resulting in obesity or emaciation. Disorders range from eating too much to refusing to eat.

The four most common eating disorders are:

1. Obesity (body weight 20% or more above normal for height)
2. *Bulimia* (a binge/purge disorder)
3. *Anorexia nervosa* (self-imposed starvation)[8]
4. Baryophobia (purposeful underfeeding of a child by a parent who has a phobia about fat)

Many researchers who are familiar with these disorders believe they are a response to conflicting messages in our culture, which values thinness and at the same time encourages the consumption of rich foods. (A Closer Look on p. 178 traces some disturbing trends in the popular view of female beauty that may contribute to eating disorders.)

Obesity

Because obesity is such a widespread problem in industrialized nations, we devote a separate chapter (Chapter 12, Weight Control) to its possible causes and treatments.

Bulimia

Some people overindulge and suffer the consequences; others go on an eating binge, then purge their bodies of the excess food to prevent the undesirable outcome of obesity. According to the *Diagnostic and Statistical Manual of Mental Disorders*, people are bulimic if they participate in binge and purge behavior at least twice a week for several months. Using this standard, about 1 in 20 adolescent and young adult females can be classified as bulimic. However, the secretive nature of the disease and the fact that the diagnosis discounts people who binge and purge less frequently have led many health care practitioners to suggest that the number of bulimics is substantially greater.[7,9,18]

Most bulimics are single, well-educated, white women between 20 and 30 years of age and with body weight close to their ideal. Almost anyone, however, can be affected. Whether male or female, bulimic individuals are usually outgoing perfectionists who appear to have the world by the proverbial tail. In reality, their self-esteem is usually low and they feel disorganized and out of control. Food becomes a crutch to use in a crisis or when bored, lonely, depressed, or rejected. Bulimics are obsessed with food but repulsed by body fat. The combination of their strong desire to ease hurt feelings with food and their concern with meeting culturally approved standards of beauty leads to the characteristic binge/purge cycles.

 Excessive levels of the brain hormone vasopressin may be at the root of bulimic behavior, according to a National Institute of Mental Health Study.[9]

On a day-to-day basis, bulimics typically consume a very low-kcalorie diet to control their weight. But dietary control is only illusionary. In reality, they are obsessed by thoughts of food every waking moment. Eventually the deprivation of their low-kcalorie diet combined with some life crisis becomes too hard for them to tolerate, their resolve breaks down, and they secretly consume massive quantities of highly palatable foods (ice cream, pastries, candy) in a relatively short time. Later, feeling physically ill from overeating, shamed and disgusted by their lack of control, the bulimic induces vomiting and diarrhea.

At the very least, bulimia is a poor way to control weight. The bingeing and purging disturb the body's delicate physiological and biochemical balance. Ruptures may develop in the esophagus and stomach from repeating vomiting. The acidic vomit burns the lining of the mouth, esophagus, and pharynx, and destroys the enamel surface of the teeth. Repeated use of emetics (vomit-inducing drugs) is toxic to the liver and

anorexia   *an-*, without; *orexis*, a longing or a lack of appetite

bulimia   a cycle of binge eating and purging; from Greek *bous*, ox, cow; *limos*, hunger, famine

A CLOSER LOOK

The Changing Standards of Female Beauty

"Barbie's missing accessory: food," the title of an article in the *Tufts University Diet and Nutrition Letter,* perfectly sums up what's wrong with America's current ideal of female beauty. The article goes on to describe how when Finnish researchers transposed Barbie's measurements into those of a real woman, they found she would be amennorheic as a result of insufficient body fat, probably caused by anorexia. Other plastic beauties also need to gain weight. Since the 1960s, female department store mannequins have had only about 10% body fat, whereas mannequins manufactured between the 1920s and 1950s were proportioned more like real women. Even the Columbia Pictures woman, a long-time symbol of this motion picture corporation, has under gone a remake. Her rounded form was recently declared too matronly and discarded in favor of a leaner model.

Is it any wonder that this national obsession with unrealistic levels of female thinness has resulted in eating disorders and other poor health habits? A study conducted by the American Cancer Society found that despite well-publicized health risks, many young women smoke cigarettes to help control their body weight. This is not a case of wishful thinking. Researchers have found that changes in metabolism brought about by smoking can indeed keep off 10 to 15 pounds of body fat.

By contrast, cultural standards of the physically perfect male have changed little over the course of this century. The well-toned mesomorphic build still in vogue is realistically obtainable for the majority of men.

---

kidneys. Abuse of laxatives can damage the intestinal tract. Intense vomiting and diarrhea can result from overuse of emetics and laxatives, leading to fluid and electrolyte imbalances, which in turn cause the hands and feet to swell, induce abnormal heart rhythms, and damage the kidneys. In some cases these problems prove fatal. The emotional costs are just as high as the physical ones. The lack of self-esteem that underlies bulimia is reinforced by guilt over binge/purge behavior. The bulimic's inability to control disorder can lead to extreme feelings of despair and worthlessness and to suicidal depression.

Treatment consists of psychotherapy to help identify the roots of the bulimic's problem, in conjunction with nutrition education and behavior modification techniques to help extinguish the binge/purge behavior.

Anorexia Nervosa

Unlike bulimics, who recognize that their behavior is abnormal, some people, particularly adolescent females from affluent backgrounds, carry the quest for thinness to such extremes that they literally starve themselves to the point of emaciation, all the while insisting that they "feel fat." Interestingly, they apply this distorted judgment only to their own situation. It does not alter how they view others. When shown photographs, anorexics can correctly indicate whether other people are of normal weight for their height, yet insist that their own weight of 85 pounds is excessive for their 5'6" frame.

Though they deny hunger in the throes of their disease, recovered anorexics admit that they felt extremely hungry, were obsessed with thoughts of food, and would go to great lengths planning menus and preparing meals for others to consume but would never partake of the food themselves. When they do eat, anorexics restrict themselves to minuscule amounts of low-fat meats, nonfat dairy products, and low-kcalorie vegetables. They avoid starches and fats like the plague. Occasionally their resolve to starve deserts them and they binge. Like bulimics, anorexics feel very guilty about their loss of control, so they engage in purging behaviors, such as self-induced vomiting and the use of enemas, diuretics, and laxatives.

The compulsive perfectionism that fuels their drive to diet extends to other areas of anorexics' lives. They tend to exercise compulsively to burn off any of the kcalories they do manage to consume, usually choosing solitary activities such as jogging, swimming, or cycling that eliminate the need for social interaction. They become obsessed with obtaining perfection in their academic and leisure activities and with keeping their personal environment clean and well organized. As weight loss progresses, the anorexic begins to exhibit many of the clinical symptoms seen in famine victims[9]:

1. Loss of body fat and protein
2. Amenorrhea (failure to menstruate)
3. Alterations in sex hormones, growth hormone, insulin, and thyroid hormones. (Some researchers conjecture that alterations in these hormones may predate and thus predispose a person to anorexia. This theory does not explain, however, why the disease is only seen in developed countries or why it affects primarily affluent people.)
4. Lower body temperature, resulting from loss of insulating fat and decreased metabolic rate
5. Decreased muscle and bone mass, anemia, a low

white blood cell count, hair loss, and rough, dry, scaly skin (all resulting from poor nutrition)

6. Downy hair, called lanugo, appears all over the body to replace the insulation lost by the decrease in body fat

7. Constipation brought on by starvation and laxative abuse

8. Tooth decay and damage to the mouth and esophageal linings in anorexics who binge and purge frequently

The causes of anorexia are complex and not totally understood. In some cases the syndrome appears to be a reducing diet gone awry. The person may have started to diet when a friend or family member casually commented about the person's body weight. Alternatively, a new school, job, or social situation may have triggered the desire to diet to achieve a more socially acceptable weight. Because the majority of cases begin around the time of puberty, some researchers have suggested that anorexia is an attempt to stave off physical maturation. In this scenario the affected person reasons that if she can retain a childlike physique, she can avoid the pressures and responsibilities of adulthood.

Whatever the precipitating event, anorexics tend to share certain characteristics. In general, they are outgoing perfectionists from affluent backgrounds. They are proud of their dieting accomplishments and report that dieting gives them a sense of control. Their parents are often described as emotionally distant, controlling, demanding, and more concerned with external signs of achievement than with nurturing their child's self-esteem and independence. It has been theorized that anorexics diet to exert some control over their own lives and to overcome their fears that they cannot live up to their parents' unreasonably high expectations.

Currently about 1 out of every 200 teenage females in the United States is believed to be anorexic. According to one expert, this number will grow as more young women prepare to balance the roles of homemaker, wife, and career woman in a culture that values a woman's appearance over her intelligence and competence.[18]

Treatment requires nutritional support, psychoanalysis (Fig. 9-6), and in many cases family counseling. It is unclear whether anorexia is ever really cured or whether the anorexic is simply in a state of recovery. It is known, however, that the earlier the problem is diagnosed, the greater is the chance for a successful outcome. Helping an anorexic understand the basis for her behavior and educating family members about the role they may have played in the disorder are essential for successful therapy.

Bulimia-anorexia. Although bulimia and anorexia nervosa are usually two distinct disorders, they have certain similarities. Both are more prevalent in perfectionists from affluent, demanding families than in people from backgrounds with less lofty goals. There is a higher incidence of these disorders among people who are involved in body-conscious fields such as competitive athletics, professional dance, and modeling, than in people who engage in more academic pursuits. Finally, most—but not all—afflicted people are female.

Until recently both anorexia and bulimia were believed to occur rarely in males. Health care providers rationalized that this was because of the greater emphasis society puts on a woman's appearance as compared to a man's. Results of recent studies, however, are changing this stereotype. One group of researchers

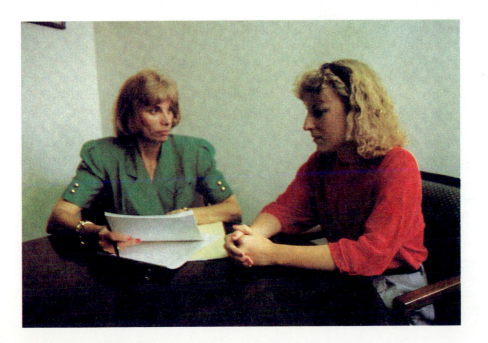

FIGURE 9-6 Personalized counseling sessions can help people with eating disorders discover the basis of their behavior.

TABLE 9-7	Comparison of Anorexia and Bulimia	
	Anorexia	**Bulimia**
Age of onset	Typically appears in teenagers	Usually seen in early adulthood
Dietary habits	Take pride in their ability to diet	Participate in self-imposed starvation, binge and purge
Concept of reality	Deny that their behavior is inappropriate; falsely believe themselves fat in comparison to others	Aware of abnormality of behavior; body image is more realistic

found that at least one third of all college athletes, male and female, suffered from eating disorders. Others have noted that many men in body-conscious fields indulge in eating disorder behaviors but that their illness often goes undiagnosed because of the perception that such syndromes are female disorders.[2,5]

What is the difference between bulimia and anorexia nervosa? Although there are several similarities between these disorders, there also are some important differences. Distinguishing characteristics are presented in Table 9-7. These symptoms occasionally overlap, resulting in a behavior pattern that is both bulimic and anorexic. Afflicted people subsist on a starvation diet, punctuated by binge/purge episodes. This disorder is extremely hard to treat, and the factors that contribute to its development are even less clear than those that result in anorexia or bulimia alone.

Baryophobia

Baryophobia is a relatively new disorder. The name, which means *fear of becoming heavy*, describes a set of symptoms identified in children who fail to grow in the absence of any underlying organic disease. In some instances the child has started a diet in an attempt to achieve a popular view of an ideal body. Most often, however, parents are the root of the problem. Many families with good intentions underfeed their children to "protect" them from carrying on a family history of obesity, heart disease, or diabetes. Unfortunately, the high-fiber, low-fat diet so beneficial for adult health provides too few kcalories for most growing children. In such cases parents and child alike need nutritional counseling to help them learn what makes up an appropriate diet and realistic body weight.[14]

NUTRALERT

Children and teens should go on a reducing diet only under medical supervision. Improper dieting in these age groups can permanently stunt growth and development.

IN TODAY'S WORLD

As we have seen, energy is closely connected to nutrition—so closely that we need to spend physical, chemical, and metabolic energy to obtain dietary energy. Energy is required to grow, harvest, process, and cook foods as well as to liberate the metabolic energy provided by foods.

Around the world, people are concerned that current agricultural practices will not be able to produce enough energy (kcalories) to meet the needs of the world's burgeoning population. (In the last chapter, Looking to the Future, we will explore the causes of the world food crisis and suggest some steps toward solutions.) In industrialized nations, environmentalists and energy policy experts observe that their countries use too much mechanical and fuel energy to produce highly processed convenience foods. In the United States, consumers worry about the safety of irradiation, a new form of energy, used in food processing. Calorie-conscious shoppers are dismayed to learn that the kcalorie content of a food that appears on the package label may be off by as much as 20%. On the home front, many people wonder if their microwave ovens really are a harmless energy source for cooking food.

IN MY DIET

One healthy choice each of us can make to improve our personal and global energy balance is to eat more whole, unprocessed foods and fewer processed items.

At the Grocery Store

Today most of us who live in industrialized countries have an amazingly wide variety of foods to choose from and places to find them, from huge supermarkets to rural roadside produce stands. The goods news—for our personal health and for our environment—is the growing popularity and availability of whole, unprocessed foods.

Processed Foods

What's wrong with processed foods? Consuming large quantities of processed foods is as bad for the Earth's energy balance as it is for our personal health.

Highly processed foods contribute very small amounts of nutrients to our diet but add an excessive amount of energy in the form of sugar and fat. On a global basis, the production of such foods consumes an excessive amount of the Earth's resources.

Consider for a moment the difference in personal and global energy costs between consuming a locally grown apple and a nationally distributed, individually packaged apple turnover. Solar energy, rain and irrigation water, human labor, and electrical and carbon fuels all have gone into producing an apple and getting it to your local market. If this apple ends up in a processing factory, becoming part of an apple turnover, instead of in your kitchen fruit bowl, its nutrient density will decrease considerably but its cost in terms of the Earth's energy resources will escalate dramatically. Fuel-burning vehicles will transport the apple to the factory, where it will be processed into a turnover, packaged by energy-gobbling machinery, and then transported to stores for sale. While in the factory, the apple will be combined with sugar, fats, flour, salt, spices, coloring, and preserving agents, each of which was produced in its own factory.

Eating "low on the food chain" by relying more on whole rather than processed foods is good for your health and the ecological stability of planet Earth.

Irradiation

Irradiation is the newest source of energy to be used in food processing. The word alone frightens many consumers who fear radioactive meals, yet government and food industry representatives claim irradiation is a safe and effective way to destroy a variety of bacteria and pests, thereby reducing the risk of foodborne illness and eliminating the need for potentially carcinogenic post-harvest pesticides. Irradiation also halts natural enzymatic processes within foods, extending product shelf life. The essential question is: Can you really zap pests away without introducing other undesirable health risks? First, it is important to establish the fact that irradiation does not make food radioactive. The process involves passing food through a chamber and bombarding it with a type of radioactive ray known as gamma radiation. Irradiation destroys bacteria, insects, and molds but leaves the food radiation free.[21]

Sounds great; what are irradiation's critics objecting to? Consumer groups are concerned about the safety of some of the chemical by-products of irradiation, loss of nutrients caused by the process, and environmental contamination at irradiation facilities. Irradiation disrupts cellular machinery, leaving behind fragments of DNA and RNA (pieces of genetic material that are similar to those found in untreated foods) as well as some atypical products called URP (unique ra-

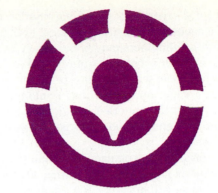

FIGURE 9-7 The federal government created this symbol, called the *radura,* for use on foods that have been irradiated.

diolytic products)—all of which most scientists claim are harmless. Some studies also have found that irradiation slightly diminishes the vitamin content of foods and chemically alters polyunsaturated fats.[10]

What is the status of irradiated foods today? In 1990 the FDA issued a ruling that irradiation is a safe and effective means to rid foods such as poultry and pork of dangerous microbes and worms, respectively.[11] This ruling was followed by the introduction of irradiated strawberries in early 1991. The FDA received so many written objections, however, that it has delayed use of irradiation until its safety has been further evaluated (Fig. 9-7).

NUTRI NUGGET Milk products change flavor when they are irradiated, so they must be sterilized by other means.

Labels—Your License To Learn

Is what I see on the label what I get in the food? By now you have developed some expertise in finding nutrition information on food labels. Food labels must carry nutrient content information as well as kcalorie counts.

One aspect of the food labeling laws we have not yet discussed is accuracy. How confident can you be that the information shown on the label reflects what you get when you eat the product? Consumers generally assume such information is accurate. Most would be surprised to learn that labeling laws require only that the product be within 20% of the specifications stated on the label.

This means that a food item whose label says it contains 500 kcalories per serving may actually contain anywhere from 400 (20% below) to 600 (20% above) kcalories. This is quite a difference for anyone who is trying to count kcalories! The 20% rule applies to all nutrients, not just energy. Labels on national brands tend to be more accurate than those on local brands.[1] Some flexibility in labeling accuracy is necessary because of variations from one batch to another. For example, even though processed foods are prepared according to an exact recipe, one batch may contain a little bit more sugar or fat than another. In addition, the vitamin and mineral content of foods vary with growing conditions and seasons.[4]

It is important to recognize that whatever standard is used today or adopted in the future, kcalorie information on labels will never be 100% accurate. This emphasizes the fact that counting kcalories is not the best way to control body weight. Rather than keeping track of specific kcalories, know the relative number of kcalories in a particular food group. For example, cereals, grains, and legumes provide roughly 100 kcalories per half-cup serving, whereas a similar serving of fruits and vegetables supplies about 50 kcalories.

In the Kitchen

Wise use of energy is needed not only in food manufacturing and transportation, but also in our personal daily routines.

Microwave Magic

Microwave ovens first became widely available for home use in the late 1960s and early 1970s: the same period during which the women's movement urged females to pursue careers other than housekeeping. The timing of these two events was coincidental. The speed and efficiency of microwave cooking, however, proved to be a good match for the quick-fix food needs of time-pressed working men and women. Today approximately 80% of American homes have a microwave oven. Despite their popularity, many owners are unsure of how they work and whether they are truly safe.

NUTRI NUGGET Microwaves are not allowed to leak more than 5 milliwatts of energy per square centimeter at a distance of 2"—a very safe level, according to FDA officials.

What is a microwave?   Microwaves are a form of energy wave related to sound and light waves, with which you are already familiar. They are able to penetrate foods, glass, paper, and certain plastics, but they cannot pass through metal.

How does a microwave oven cook?   Conventional ovens cook from the outside in; microwave ovens cook from the inside out. Microwaves penetrate partway into food, where they cause the water molecules in the food to vibrate, producing friction that in turn generates heat. Because it relies on water, microwave cooking is somewhat like steaming food from the inside.

The process itself is very safe, so safe that microwave cooking actually helps foods retain their nutritional value because it cooks them quickly, at a high temperature with little added water.[22]

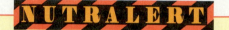

NUTRALERT

The FDA is analyzing data about the migration of chemicals from supposedly microwave-safe plastic wraps and containers into food. Until the results of these studies are in, it may be best to use only glass containers for microwave cooking.[15]

Food purists often refuse to cook in a microwave because of its meal-in-a-minute convenience food image. Julee Rosso and Sheila Lukins, of *Silver Palate Cookbook* and Catering Service fame, however, found the microwave to be a wonderful tool for producing menu miracles in minutes. Their book *The New Basics Cookbook* explains how to microwave preserves, dry beans, whole grains, meats, and vegetables—often with better results than are possible with conventional cooking techniques. If you love to cook but are on a tight time schedule, this may be the cookbook for you.

 NUTRI NUGGET A nutrition scientist has demonstrated that vegetables cooked in microwave ovens retain up to 100% of their vitamin content, whereas boiled vegetables retain only 40% to 60% of theirs. This benefit results from the short cooking time and small amount of water required for microwaving.

Microwave Safety Measures

- Use only glass containers or plastic and paper products that have been designated microwave safe.[15]
- Do not use metal containers or any items trimmed with metal.
- Do not cook eggs in their shells in the microwave. Steam will build up and cause the shell to explode.
- Before cooking thick-skinned vegetables such as potatoes and squash, puncture them to let steam escape.
- Use potholders when removing items from the microwave. Containers can get very hot.
- Never put food directly on the surface of the oven.
- Never attempt to deep fry items in a microwave. An oil-filled container is dangerous and awkward to handle, and the temperature of the oil cannot be controlled.
- Rotate and stir foods while cooking to eliminate cold spots, which can harbor harmful bacteria.
- When reheating, don't just warm food; get it steaming hot to ensure that dangerous microbes are killed.
- To minimize the risk of food poisoning, do not cook stuffed poultry in the microwave.

A generation ago home chefs had the choice of gas or electricity as their primary energy source for cooking. Improvements in technology have made it possible for the home cook to choose from a variety of energy sources in the kitchen. Most homes now have both conventional and microwave ovens; some well-designed kitchens include convection and infrared units as well. Table 9-8 summarizes the major forms of cooking energy and how they work.

TABLE 9-8 Common Sources of Cooking Energy

Appliance	Energy Source
Conventional ovens and ranges	Conduction, the transfer of heat from an energy source to food or to a cooking utensil (pot), then to the food
Convection ovens	Spreading of heat by the movement air; in convection ovens, fans speed the spread of heat
Microwave ovens	Radiation, the transfer of energy by waves from the energy source to the food
Infrared broilers	Radiation

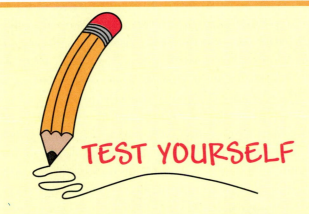

TEST YOURSELF

1. List the three basic categories of body builds.
2. What does the term *basal energy requirement* mean?
3. Give one reason why experts believe eating disorders like bulimia and anorexia are on the increase.
4. What do the terms android and gynoid obesity mean?
5. What is the Body Mass Index (BMI) used for?
6. How can you change the amount of energy you expend each day?
7. What is irradiation used for?
8. How does microwave cooking differ from cooking in conventional ovens?
9. How does bulimia differ from anorexia and baryophobia?
10. Is the nutrient content information on food labels 100% accurate? Explain.

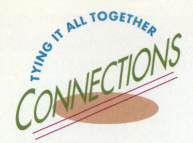

TYING IT ALL TOGETHER

CONNECTIONS

1. Growth can be thought of as *(circle one)* anabolism catabolism
2. List at least three kinds of work that cells do.
3. Work *(circle one)* produces energy uses energy
4. What kind/s of tissue is/are lost during periods of negative energy balance?
5. What kind/s of tissue is/are gained during periods of positive energy balance?
6. Why is oxygen required to release energy from food?
7. What effect if any would you expect respiratory disease to have on nutrient metabolism? (Hint: Oxygen is a prerequisite for, and CO_2 a byproduct of, cellular energy production.)

REFERENCES

1. Allison D et al: Accuracy of caloric labeling, *Journal of the American Medical Association* 270:1454-1460, 1993.
2. Anderson A: *Males with eating disorders*, New York, 1990, Brunner/Mazel.
3. Bray G: Obesity. *Present knowledge in nutrition*, ed 6, Washington, DC, 1990, International Life Sciences Institute Nutrition Foundation.
4. Browne MB: *Label facts for healthful eating: educator's resource guide*, National Food Processors Association, Dayton, OH, 1993, Mazer Corp.
5. Brownwell K et al: Eating disorders among athletes, *Physical Sportsmedicine* 18:116-121, 1990.
6. Buchard C, Pérusse C: Heredity and body fat. In *Annual Review of Nutrition* 8:259-277, 1988.
7. Carruth BR: Adolescence. In *Present knowledge in nutrition*, ed 6, Washington, DC, 1990, International Life Sciences Institute Nutrition Foundation.
8. Castanguay TW, Stern JS: Hunger and appetite. In *Present knowledge in nutrition*, ed 6, Washington, DC, 1990, International Life Sciences Institute Nutrition Foundation.
9. Comerci GD: Medical complications of anorexia nervosa and bulimia nervosa. *Medical Clinics of North America* 774:1293-1300, 1990.
10. Freidman M: *Nutritional and toxicological consequences of food irradiation*, New York, 1991, Plenum Press.
11. Irradiated food is coming to our stores. *Food Safety Notebook* 4(5):55, 1993.
12. Jones D et al: Coordinated multisite reguation of cellular energy metabolism. In *Annual Review of Nutrition* 8:327, 1988.
13. Kleiber M: *Fire of life: an introduction to animal energetics*, Huntington, NY, 1975, Krieger.
14. Lifshitz F: Children on adult diets: Is it harmful? Is it helpful? *Journal of the American College of Nutrition* 11:845-850, 1992.
15. Microwave wrap safety warning, *Federal Register* 54:373, 1989.
16. National Research Council: *Recommended dietary allowances*, Washington, DC, 1989, National Academy Press.
17. Nichols BL, Reed PJ: History of nutrition symposia: history and current status of research in human energy metabolism, *Journal of Nutrition* 121:1889-1890, 1991.
18. Patterson C et al: *Nutrition and eating disorders*, Van Nuys, Calif, 1989, PM Inc.
19. Rosenberg I, ed: National Institutes of Health Technology Assessment Conference Statement: Methods for voluntary weight loss and control, Mar 30-Apr 1, 1992, *Nutrition Reviews* 50(11):340-345, 1992.
20. Sawyer P: Assumptions used in the measurement of energy metabolism, *Journal of Nutrition* 121:1891-1896, 1991.
21. Shapiro J: Food irradiation: news and views, *Food Safety Notebook* 2(9):75-77, 1991.
22. Schiffmann RF: Understanding microwave reactions and interactions, *Food Product Design* 3(1):78-88, 1993.
23. Sheldon WH et al: *The varieties of human physique*, New York, 1963, Hafner.
24. Webb P: The measurement of energy expenditure, *Journal of Nutrition* 121:1897-1901, 1991.
25. Wurtman RJ, Wurtman JJ: Carbohydrates and depression, *Scientific American*, Jan 1989, 68-75.

CHAPTER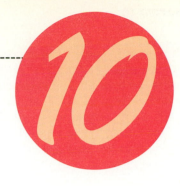

EXERCISE
Fueling Up for Fitness

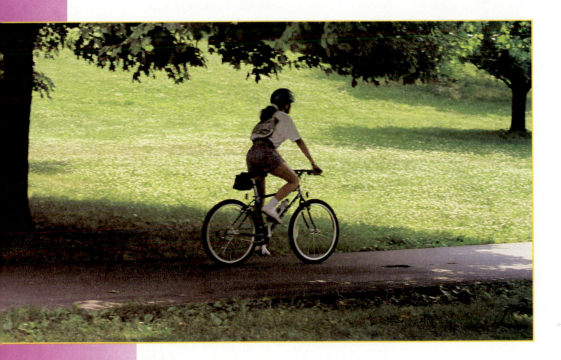

It was such a primitive
country we didn't even see
any joggers.

— *Hamilton cartoon captain*

Good nutrition is only one part of a healthy lifestyle. Other factors are equally important: regular exercise, adequate rest, good hygiene, and avoidance of self-destructive behaviors such as smoking and drug and alcohol abuse. Of all of these factors, exercise and nutrition are the most closely related—so closely that a regular exercise program maximizes the nutritional benefits of a good diet.

PHYSIOLOGICAL BENEFITS OF EXERCISE

The nutrition-related attributes of regular exercise affect all aspects of your body's condition and function. For many people the greatest benefit of exercise is weight control. Even more important, however, may be the impact of exercise on overall nutritional status through an improvement in general physiological functioning. A well-conditioned body enhances nutrient utilization and skeletal strength as well as decreasing the risk of cardiovascular disease and adult onset diabetes. Exercise also has been shown to promote emotional well-being. Although this effect is not directly related to nutrition, people who feel good about life in general and themselves in particular are more likely to pursue a healthy lifestyle, which includes a good diet.

NUTRALERT

Some 250,000 deaths per year can be attributed to lack of physical activity, according to the American College of Sports Medicine, the President's Council on Physical Fitness, and the Centers for Disease Control and Prevention.

How can exercise help me achieve these results? The metabolic changes that accompany exercise produce many of these benefits. Learning about exercise physiology will help you clarify these relationships.

Physiology of Fuel Utilization

Your body responds to the onset of exercise in much the same way it does to any form of stress. The heart and respiration rate speed up to ensure that an adequate supply of fuel and oxygen is delivered to the rapidly metabolizing tissues and the waste products are efficiently removed. The stress hormones, **epinephrine, norepinephrine,** and **cortisol,** begin to circulate in the bloodstream, signaling the liver, muscle, and fat cells to release their stored fuel. Initially the exercising muscle fuels itself with glucose obtained from its own glycogen stores and fatty acids from its stored triglycerides. As the muscles' own energy supplies dwindle, they switch over to glucose liberated into the bloodstream from liver glycogen stores and fatty acids released from your body's adipose tissue stores.

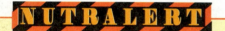 **Glucose or fat—which is the better source of fuel for exercise?** The answer depends in part on the athlete's oxygen supply. In general, fat is a better source of fuel for exercise, both because the body stores considerable amounts of it and because blood glucose levels cannot fall below a set limit without serious metabolic consequences.

The body's supply of glucose is quite small. A person in good shape and of a healthy weight can easily carry 20 to 30 pounds of spare body fat but only about 1 pound of glycogen. Because glycogen is an important source of glucose for many tissues, some of which are unable to use fat, your body tries to regulate glycogen utilization during exercise. At first the body's efforts in this regard seem rather ineffective. In fact, during the first 20 minutes of moderate exercise your body will use up about one fifth of its glycogen stores. Glycogen use gradually slows down as your body begins to conserve it by using more fat. Even with this economizing effort, glycogen stores can be depleted if the exercise is intense and/or prolonged. A high-carbohydrate diet together with a regular exercise program can help moderate the body's use of glycogen by enhancing body glycogen stores and increasing the body's ability to use fat for fuel. Together these changes in fuel utilization increase your endurance.[1]

Aerobic Metabolism

How does the oxygen supply affect my body's choice of fuel? The availability of stored fuel and the supply of oxygen determine whether your body uses glucose or fat for energy. When you are resting or performing light physical activity, ample oxygen is available and your body extracts energy from both fat and glucose by a process known as **aerobic** metabolism. During exercise, however, the availability of oxygen determines whether your muscles rely more heavily on glucose or on fatty acids as the source of fuel. Glucose can be partially burned to liberate energy in the absence of oxygen; fat cannot. When you perform light to moderate exercise, a healthy heart and lungs can supply all the oxygen your exercising muscles require. Both fat and glucose can be used as fuel. As the intensity of exercise increases, your heart and lungs work faster and faster, eventually reaching their maximum capacity.

Anaerobic Metabolism

When the need for oxygen exceeds the ability of the heart and lungs to supply it, your body can no longer burn fat for energy. Cells shift to **anaerobic** metabolism and rely mainly on glucose for energy. In the absence of oxygen, only a portion of each glucose molecule can be burned for energy. The remainder forms a by-product known as **lactic acid** that builds up in the muscle tissue, causing a painful, burning sensation. This quickly leads to muscle exhaustion, forcing you to slow down or stop completely to catch your breath. Once your activity level slows down, your oxygen intake catches up with demand and the lactic acid accumulating in muscle tissue is shunted to the liver where, in the presence of oxygen, it is converted back into glucose and aerobic metabolism is once again used to produce energy. The amount of oxygen required to clear the built-up lactic acid from your body is referred to as **oxygen debt.** Like all metabolic debts, it must be repaid for the body to function normally. Your elevated respiration rate after you stop exercising is evidence your body is doing just that.

Aerobic exercise. *How do the terms aerobic and anaerobic metabolism apply to exercise?* In aerobic exercise, your body is using oxygen to convert fuel into energy. Aerobic exercise routines use large muscle groups continually for 20 minutes or more. Most forms of exercise, such as walking, swimming, cycling, and jogging, are aerobic activities. Because oxygen is being used, fat is being burned. If aerobic exercise is performed too vigorously, however, your body shifts to an anaerobic state in which glucose is the predominant energy source. (See the In Today's World section of the chapter for details on designing an exercise program.)

Anaerobic exercise. Anaerobic activities are performed at a speed or intensity that exceeds the body's ability to supply oxygen. Some sports, notably weight-lifting and sprinting, fit the definition of anaerobic exercise because they require short bursts of intense effort. Anaerobic exercise does not help the body burn fat, so it is not useful for weight control but it does help increase muscle tissue.

Weight Control

Because aerobic activities can be performed for prolonged periods of time and rely heavily on fat for fuel, they are the best kinds of exercise for changing and maintaining body composition in the direction of less fat and more muscle. The weight-controlling effects of aerobic exercise extend far beyond a simple increase in fuel utilization. Food intake, fuel utilization, and the BMR all are altered by regular aerobic exercise.

Kcalorie Intake

Well-conditioned athletes typically increase their kcalorie intake to support their increased levels of physical activity. Many overfat people fear that initiating an exercise program will only increase their food intake. This does occur if the exercise triggers anaerobic metabolism, but fortunately this is not the case with aero-

bic exercise. Overfat people often eat no more kcalories when exercising than when they are not exercising. In some instances moderate exercise actually suppresses the appetite. In any case, exercise helps overfat people expend more energy than they take in, and fat loss ensues due to the resulting negative energy balance.

Kcalorie Output

Exercise helps your body burn kcalories two ways. There is an immediate increase in kcalorie usage to fuel the physical activity itself, and there is a long-term increase in the levels of fat-burning enzymes and BMR.

Metabolic rate increased. Because exercise requires fuel, clearly it burns kcalories. It is not just the fuel used during exercise, however, that contributes to weight loss. Your body continues to burn more kcalories than usual even after you stop exercising. This is partly because your metabolic rate stays elevated for several hours after an aerobic workout, expending more energy in the process. Some experts estimate that this residual increase in metabolic rate alone is enough to cause a 5- to 6-pound weight loss over the course of a year.[1]

Production of fat-burning enzymes stimulated. Even more long term are the effects of regular aerobic exercise on fat-burning enzyme activity and BMR. Regular aerobic exercise increases the amount of fat-burning enzymes in muscle tissue, which allows your body to use more fat for fuel both during exercise and at rest. Fuel utilization is further enhanced by an increase in the BMR.

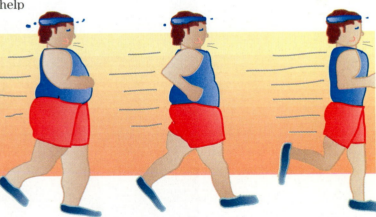

Jogging, a fat-burning aerobic activity, is a super way to shape up.

aerobic in the presence of oxygen
anaerobic in the absence of oxygen

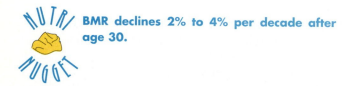

Regular exercise has been shown to increase both the number and size of the mitochondria (the energy-burning factory) in each muscle cell. It also increases the number of muscle fibers.

How does exercise increase the BMR?

In Chapter 9, Energy, you learned that your BMR is determined by heredity, age, gender, lean body mass, overall health, thyroid hormone level, and reproductive status (pregnancy and lactation both increase BMR). Of the factors affecting BMR, only lean body mass can be changed. Lean body mass is directly affected by your activity level. A consistent aerobic exercise program increases the amount of lean body tissue. Lean tissue (also known as muscle) is more metabolically active than fat. For this reason it requires more kcalories to sustain itself, even at rest, than does adipose tissue. As a result the more lean tissue you have, the greater your BMR. In contrast, inactivity, crash dieting (see Chapter 11), and the natural decline in muscle mass after age 30 all decrease lean body mass and BMR.

BMR declines 2% to 4% per decade after age 30.

How many kcalories can I burn while exercising?

The answer to this question depends on the frequency, duration, and intensity of your exercise, your size, your BMR, and how well trained you are in performing that activity. Not surprisingly, the more intense your exercise, the more kcalories you burn in a given time period. Similarly, as explained in Chapter 9, Energy, the bigger the athlete, the more energy s/he will need to perform a given activity.

Your BMR also helps determine how many kcalories you use while exercising. The higher your BMR, the more kcalories you will burn while exercising. For example, a person whose resting energy needs (BMR) are 60 kcalories per hour will burn about 300 kcalories during a brisk, hour-long walk, whereas a person who uses 80 kcalories per hour at rest will burn closer to 400 kcalories performing the same activity. Finally, the better conditioned you are to perform an activity, the more efficient you will be and the fewer kcalories you will expend. This does not mean that physically fit people obtain fewer weight control benefits from exercise than do people who are out of shape. The decrease in energy utilization during exercise by an efficient, conditioned body is more than offset by the exercise-induced increases in fat-burning enzymes and BMR. Because of these variables, it is impossible to give an absolute energy cost for the performance of a particular exercise, but we can make some generalizations. Box 10-1 gives approximate energy expenditures for a 154-pound person performing a given activity for 1 hour.

Being fit also can be fun.

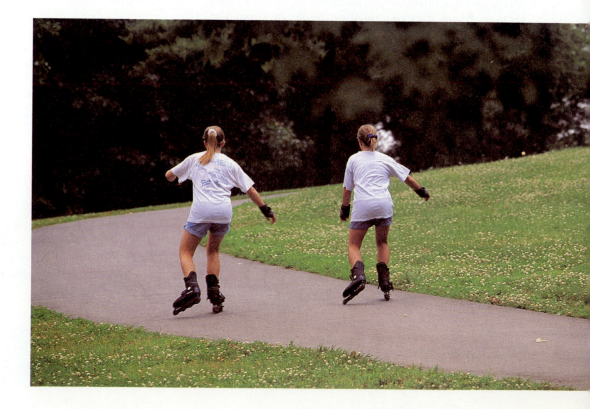

BOX 10-1 Kcalories per Activity Hour

Activity (1 hour)	Kcal
CYCLING	
Leisure, 5.5 miles per hour	264
Leisure, 9.4 miles per hour	420
DANCING	
Moderate tempo	216
Intense aerobics	708
JOGGING	
9 minutes per mile	816
7 minutes per mile	972
RUNNING	
11-minute mile, 5.5 miles per hour	640
5-minute mile	1212
STAIR CLIMBING	
Down, 1 step per second	204
Up, 1 step per second	864
WALKING	
Moderate, 3 miles per hour	264
Brisk, 4 miles per hour	396

NUTRI NUGGET You can actually consume more kcalories running in place than running distances because you never build up kcalorie-sparing momentum. As a result, you are constantly having to overcome inertia.

Overall Conditioning

The physiological benefits of exercise go beyond changes in fuel utilization. A regular aerobic exercise program benefits your entire body! Exercise strengthens the skeleton and connective tissue, the exercised muscle groups, and the cardiovascular and pulmonary systems; it also improves the function of muscle groups and body systems not directly involved in exercise—for example, the gastrointestinal, immune, and nervous systems—all while enhancing weight control.[1,18]

Bone Strength

Although adequate calcium and vitamin D consumption are vital to building a sturdy skeleton, one of the most effective ways to maintain strong bones throughout life is to stress them with weight-bearing exercise. The stress of exercising muscles pulling on the skeleton stimulates the bones to store more calcium, which in turn strengthens the skeletal structure.

What is weight-bearing exercise? Any exercise, including weight lifting, walking, or jogging, in which you are either moving an external weight or carrying the weight of your own body is weight-bearing exercise. Until recently it was believed that most aerobic exercises were good skeleton builders. This still appears to be true in children and young to early middle-aged adults. Research at the National Institutes of Health's Center for Aging, however, suggests that aerobics are great for weight control and cardiovascular conditioning but that strength-building exercises, such as weight lifting, are needed to maintain a healthy skeleton in later life.[11]

NUTRI QUIZ Is swimming a weight-bearing exercise? Why or why not?

General Muscle Strength and Function

Most people know that, within genetic limits, exercised muscles become larger and stronger. You can see proof of this at any athletic competition or body-building contest. What is less well known is that consistent exercise also strengthens the cardiovascular and pulmonary systems.

NUTRI NUGGET Growth of muscle tissue occurs during rest—not during the actual workout. Resting muscle fibers between workout sessions is mandatory for increasing muscle mass. Exercising at 70% of maximum strength will stimulate growth of muscle fibers.

Cardiovascular and pulmonary systems. The heart is a muscle and, like any muscle, it is strengthened by regular exercise. The demands of exercise cause the heart to grow larger and stronger, allowing it to pump more blood with less effort. This means that a well-conditioned heart beats less frequently than a poorly conditioned one, resulting in a decreased pulse rate and less wear and tear on this essential muscle. The muscles lining the walls of the arteries (the blood vessels that carry blood from the heart to the tissues) are similarly strengthened by exercise. They expand and contract more readily, resulting in a decrease in blood pressure. Likewise, the lungs (*pulmonary* system) become more efficient at their task. There is an increase in the volume of air inhaled and exhaled with each breath. The lung tissue itself becomes more efficient at extracting oxygen from the air. In response, there is an increase in blood volume to carry the additional oxygen. The combination of these physiological

pulmonary pertaining to the lungs

BOX 10-2   General Aerobic Exercise Recommendations

MAINTAIN FITNESS

Frequency:	3 times a week
Intensity:	70% of maximum heart rate (see p. 200 to calculate)
Time:	20 to 30 minutes

INCREASE FITNESS

Frequency:	4 to 5 times a week
Intensity:	71% to 90% of maximum heart rate (see p. 200 to calculate)
Time:	20 to 30 minutes

adaptations to exercise is known as **cardiovascular conditioning.** Unless there is a family history of heart disease, cardiovascular conditioning together with a healthy diet provide the best protection against cardiovascular disease. See Box 10-2 for exercise recommendations.

Exercise and Diabetes

Diabetes results in elevated blood glucose levels, either because the pancreas has lost the capacity to manufacture insulin (insulin-dependent diabetes) or because the cells have become less sensitive to the insulin that is produced (noninsulin-dependent diabetes). (A detailed description of diabetes is presented in Chapter 4, Carbohydrates.) Regular exercise reduces the risk of developing noninsulin-dependent diabetes and also improves control of both types of diabetes by increasing the cells' sensitivity to insulin.[14,18]

NUTRALERT

It is important for persons with diabetes to balance insulin, food intake, and exercise to prevent a precipitous drop in blood sugar. Persons with diabetes who exercise need to be alert for a drop in blood sugar during their activities, and take time out for a quick snack and some water. They should never exercise when their blood sugar is very low.

Other Body Systems

When you consider the body's response to exercise, it is easy to understand how physical activity enhances muscle as well as skeletal strength and cardiovascular conditioning. What is less apparent is how or why exercise improves the function of body systems that are not directly involved in the exercise process. Researchers are finding that exercise improves the physical condition of the entire body.

Gastrointestinal function. Although not directly involved in exercise, the muscles of the gastrointestinal tract are stimulated by the physiological changes that accompany exercise. As a result, people who exercise regularly report a lower incidence of constipation and constipation-related health problems, such as hemorrhoids and colon cancer, than do their sedentary counterparts.[18]

Immune function. Immune function is another example of how exercise improves the general physiological functioning of the body. Assuming you are otherwise healthy, your ability to perform a physical activity is not directly dependent on your immune system. Nonetheless, regular, moderately intense exercise appears to enhance immune function. Provided their workout is not too intense, physically active people suffer fewer infections than sedentary people and generally recover more quickly from illness. This disease-fighting advantage is lost, however, in people like marathon runners who exercise very intensely.[17] (See Exercise Addiction for more details.)

Neurological (nervous system) function. Using driving simulators, researchers have found that the reaction times of physically fit people of all ages are quicker than are those of age-matched inactive people. This benefit of exercise is particularly significant for older people, who typically experience an age-related decline in reaction time.[11]

PSYCHOLOGICAL BENEFITS OF EXERCISE

Exercise benefits both the intellectual and emotional components of our minds.

Mental Function

Your overall intellectual function clearly is enhanced by exercise. Studies have shown that both short-term and long-term memory are better in physically fit people than in sedentary ones. This finding is particularly important for senior citizens, because one of the better documented effects of aging is a decline in short-term memory.[11]

Self-Esteem

Your self-esteem significantly influences your emotional and mental outlook. Exercise enhances esteem by improving physical appearance, promoting a sense of accomplishment when a fitness goal is achieved, and providing opportunities for social interaction. Exercise has been found to reduce feelings of stress, to stimulate production by the brain of chemicals that induce a sense of well-being, and to promote sound sleep.[20]

Stress Reduction

Many studies have shown that exercise reduces stress and alleviates depression. Researchers have discovered a physiological basis for these seemingly psychological processes. As you learned earlier, your body responds to the onset of physical activity in much the same way it responds to stress. Because in earlier times most stresses were physical threats, the human body is primed to respond to stress with a burst of activity. In today's world most stress is psychological. No matter what the source of stress, however, the body's reaction to it is the same. We are able to suppress the outward manifestations of our natural stress response to flee or fight, but the internal responses—increased levels of stress hormones and circulating fuel—are not so easily turned off.

Some scientists believe exercise may reduce our perception of stress by burning up the excess fuel released as part of the stress response. Others believe that exercise metabolizes the stress hormones that accumulate in the bloodstream during stress or exercise. A few believe exercise is a successful antidote to stress because it both burns excess fuel and clears stress hormones from the bloodstream. However exercise reduces our perception of stress, the benefits seem to be very real. One study of people with high-pressure jobs reported a 14% decrease in their stress level after they exercised.[20]

Alleviating Depression

Chemicals released by the brain during exercise appear to explain why physical activity can help "chase away the blues." Exercise induces the brain to produce two substances, serotonin and endorphins. **Serotonin** is a hormone that promotes feelings of accomplishment and well-being. **Endorphins** are natural pain-killing hormones that are chemically related to opiates such as morphine and heroin. In addition to reducing the mind's perception of pain, they make people feel that everything is A-OK. The combined release of serotonin and endorphins appears to be sufficient to banish a garden-variety case of the blues.[11,20]

Sleep

No matter how well your life is going, sleep researchers have found that lack of rest causes irritability and a negative mental outlook. Regular exercise promotes sound sleep, so a physically fit person's positive, energetic personality may be partly related to a well-rested state.

NUTRI NUGGET Endorphins are believed to be responsible for the euphoric condition, known as runner's high, that is experienced by people who exercise vigorously.

NUTRITION AND PHYSICAL PERFORMANCE

Over the past 20 years, theories have changed drastically about the foods that promote peak athletic performance. The meat-and-potatoes diet, salt tablets, Gatorade, and "energy-boosting" candy bars generally have given way to high-carbohydrate diets and sports drinks made with dilute fruit juice. There is still, however, much controversy about performance-boosting dietary habits. Athletes and health care providers agree that top physical performance requires nutritional support. Less clear-cut is exactly what constitutes nutritional support. Many athletes tout the benefits of protein powders, amino acid supplements, pseudo vitamins (inositol, carnitine, lecithin), specially formulated vitamin/mineral concoctions, and sports drinks. Sports physicians, nutritionists, and researchers, on the other hand, contend that a well-balanced diet and adequate water supply all the nutrients required by most active people.[3,16,18]

Water

The most crucial nutrient for the athlete is water. During exercise, water is essential to cool and purify the body. Your body can tolerate only a very narrow range of internal temperature. Exercise raises internal body temperature far more quickly than does a hot environmental temperature. Your body typically maintains an appropriate internal temperature by dissipating heat into the environment. When this mechanism is no longer efficient, as occurs during vigorous exercise or with a high environmental temperature, the body cools itself by sweating. Sweat is formed by the movement of fluid (water and electrolytes) from the bloodstream to the surface of the skin via the sweat glands. Continuous sweating in the absence of fluid replacement leads to a disproportionate loss of blood volume in comparison to other body fluids. Loss of blood volume during exercise impairs the heart's ability to deliver an ample supply of oxygenated blood to the exercising muscles and to carry heat away from the muscles. At its most benign, **dehydration** (lack of water) impairs physical performance. As dehydration progresses, it forces the athlete to stop exercising altogether. In severe cases it can cause a loss of consciousness. Complicating this scenario is the fact that fluids are absorbed rather poorly during exercise because blood is shunted away from the stomach and intestine to the heart, organs, and the muscles directly involved in exercise.

How can athletes protect themselves from dehydration?   There are several precautions athletes can take to prevent dehydration. One of the most important is to gradually get themselves into good aerobic condition. The increase in blood volume that occurs in response to a regular aerobic exercise program provides some protection against fluid loss during exercise. Second, active people should carefully choose the environmental conditions in which they exercise. If they exercise outdoors in areas of extreme heat and/or humidity, they should work out during the coolest periods of the day. Third, exercise enthusiasts should avoid beverages containing either alcohol or caffeine before as well as immediately after exercise because both chemicals contribute to dehydration by increasing urine production. Fourth, if they will be exercising for more than 30 minutes, athletes should **hyper-hydrate** themselves by drinking 2 to 3 cups of fluid 2 hours before exercising and an additional 1½ cups 15 minutes before exercising. To maintain hydration during the event, athletes should consume about 1 cup of fluid every 15 minutes or so. Finally, after an event athletes should **rehydrate** themselves by consuming 1 pint of fluid for each pound of weight lost during exercise.[3,8,13,16]

NUTRI NUGGET Cool beverages are absorbed more readily than warm ones. The most absorbable fluid is cool water, which can be taken up through the stomach lining.

Which fluids are best for hydrating the body?

The answer depends on the duration and intensity of the exercise. A wide variety of sports beverages are available to today's athlete. Most contain water, some form of carbohydrate, and various kinds and quantities of electrolytes. Naturally, the manufacturers of these products would like to convince the public that everyone who exercises needs a special fluid-replacement beverage. In reality, only endurance athletes require these special drinks. For someone who exercises 1 hour or less, plain cool water is the beverage of choice to replace the volume of fluid that is lost as sweat. Nonendurance athletes do not need sports drinks because their regular diet will replace electrolytes lost in their sweat as well as the carbohydrate burned for fuel. As the duration of exercise increases, however, the addition of small amounts of electrolytes and carbohydrate is indicated. Table 10-1 provides guidelines for selecting a beverage appropriate to the exercise.

There is no need to buy costly sports drinks if all you need is a little sugar water. Athletes can make their own sports beverage by adding 2 tablespoons of sugar to 1 quart of water. Electrolyte replacement, however, is best left to the experts. A number of carefully formulated sports drinks manufactured by reputable firms are widely available. Athletes should select one geared to their level of physical exertion and sample it before a competitive event to make sure it agrees with their system.[3]

TABLE 10-1   Guide to Sports Beverage Selection

Duration	Beverage	Rationale
1 hour or less	Plain water	Prevent dehydration
2 hours	Water	Prevent dehydration
	Carbohydrate*	Enhance endurance
	Electrolytes (optional)	Enhance fluid balance, improve palatability
4 hours or more	Water	Prevent dehydration
	Carbohydrate*	Enhance endurance
	Electrolytes	Enhance fluid balance, improve palatability

*Carbohydrate concentrations should not exceed 10% of the beverage by weight. In many athletes, higher concentrations have been associated with cramps and other forms of gastrointestinal distress.

NUTRI NUGGET Salt tablets, once a staple supplement at many athletic events, should be avoided at all costs because they can contribute to dehydration by disrupting the delicate balance of fluid and electrolytes.

What about other nutrients?   Less clear-cut than an athlete's increased need for water are the requirements for protein, vitamins, and minerals. Conventional wisdom has maintained that athletes who eat a balanced and adequate diet are meeting all their nutritional needs. Newer findings, however, may change this advice.

Protein

Because the typical American diet exceeds the RDA for protein, sports physicians and nutritionists have long believed that this diet is adequate for the active person. Recent research indicates this is true for most fitness enthusiasts. Endurance athletes and marathon participants, however, may be consuming too little protein to adequately repair and build new muscle tissue. Scientists familiar with these findings have tentatively advised that the RDA for protein (0.8 g/kg of body weight) should be increased by 100% (1.6 g/kg) to 150% (2.0 g/kg) for endurance athletes. The American Dietetic Association supports these recommendations,[3] but not all members of the scientific community agree. As a result, the 1989 revision of the RDA did not change earlier recommendations that physically active people need no additional protein.[16]

While scientists debate the fine points of research, physically active people who read sports magazines, shop at health food stores, or work out at health clubs are bombarded with ads urging them to maximize their physical performance by taking protein supplements. Many athletes are left with the impression that no matter what their level of activity, their performance is suffering from lack of protein. Their question is not whether they need a protein supplement, but which of the numerous "performance building" protein powders and amino acid supplements they should be using. The answer is NONE!

Amino Acid Supplements and Protein Powders

Purified amino acid supplements are very costly, and few consumers know they typically supply only milligrams of amino acids (as opposed to the required grams). On the other hand, people who take excessive amounts of one or more purified amino acids run the risk of causing a metabolically disastrous amino acid imbalance. (See Chapter 6, Proteins, for more details.) Protein powders, although they lack the potential for creating an amino acid imbalance, are not a healthy choice either. They are often promoted as fat-free alternatives to natural foods. Unfortunately, the process that strips them of fat also divests them of their mineral and vitamin content so that in reality they are a low-nutrient density supplement. Routine substitution of these products for meat, fish, poultry, legumes, or milk can result in vitamin and mineral deficiencies. The best way to meet an increased protein requirement is with complete proteins obtained from natural foods. Either skim milk or cooked egg white (which avoids the fat and cholesterol associated with the yolk) can be used as protein supplements. Although these foods contain a balanced array of the essential amino acids, using either of them as the only sources of dietary protein can lead to vitamin and mineral deficiencies.[8,16]

NUTRI NUGGET Branched-chain amino acids are selectively metabolized by muscles as a carbohydrate-sparing mechanism, but supplementation with branched-chain amino acid supplements has no proven benefit for endurance athletes.

Vitamins and Minerals

As with protein, the need for increased amounts of vitamins and minerals by physically active people is a subject of considerable scientific debate. There are two schools of thought. One group believes sufficient amounts of vitamins and minerals can be obtained from an adequate, balanced, nutrient-dense diet. They add that increased food intake should help physically active people cover their increased vitamin and mineral needs. The other group contends that careful supplementation is advisable because several studies have shown that physically active people have a greater than average need for vitamins and minerals directly involved in energy use (most notably the B vitamins and the minerals magnesium and manganese). This group also argues that many competitive athletes restrict

their food intake to keep their body weight low, thereby placing themselves at risk for vitamin and mineral deficiencies. Both the American Medical Association (AMA) and the American Dietetic Association (ADA) recommend that physically active people who are interested in supplementation should choose products that contain no more than 100% of the RDA for any given vitamin or mineral, and should consume only one serving of the product per day.[3]

Many vitamins and minerals play important roles in fuel utilization, a fact that supplement manufacturers exploit to promote the use of their products. What they fail to mention is that excesses of these nutrients can cause an assortment of metabolic disturbances. (For details see Chapter 7, Vitamins, and Chapter 8, Minerals.)

 List as many vitamins and minerals as you can that are important to physical performance. Briefly state the function each performs.

Sports Supplements

Are great athletes born or made? Both, it seems. Athletic success requires a winning combination of inborn ability and state-of-the-art training. Because the margin of victory is often slim, athletes worldwide are always looking for "something extra" to guarantee them the competitive edge.

Serious athletes know that adequate carbohydrate and fluid intake both before and during an event are critical elements of success. To ensure a peak performance, many athletes turn to nutritional ergogenics. For the most part, the benefits claimed for these substances are more fantasy than fact. Studies intended to show the value of ergogenics often have been conducted in isolated cells grown in laboratories, in animals, or in people with serious illnesses. Not only are these items a waste of money, some have actually been shown to be harmful.[6,21] Table 10-2 summarizes the claimed versus actual benefits of some of the more popular nutritional ergogenics.

A variety of vitamin preparations formulated specifically for active people are widely available. Some of these so-called *ergogenic* preparations contain only manganese, magnesium, and the B vitamins because of the known involvement of these nutrients in energy metabolism.

Most of these products, however, provide hundreds to thousands of times the RDA for all the water-soluble

ergogenic energy producing

TABLE 10-2 Nutritional Ergogenics

Substance	Rationale	Actual Effect
Antioxidant vitamins	Increase aerobic endurance	No proven benefit
Alcohol	Decreases perception of pain and fatigue	Dehydration Decreases coordination
Bee pollen	Benefits linked to its high vitamin and mineral content	No proven benefit
Branched-chain amino acids	Spare glycogen	No proven benefit
Caffeine*	Enhances endurance Increases fat utilization Spares glycogen	Increases dehydration, anxiety, and stomach acid
Carnitine	Increases fat utilization and therefore endurance	No evidence of this effect
Coenzyme Q	Increases oxygen use and endurance in patients with cardiovascular disease	No proven benefit in healthy people
Vitamin/mineral supplements, including vitamin B_{15}	Enhance energy utilization	No proven benefit Potentially toxic

*Proven ergogenic effect at high levels. One to two cups of coffee are OK before competition, but higher levels are banned by the International Olympic Committee (IOC).

vitamins and fat-soluble vitamin E, as well as 100% of the RDA for the more toxic fat-soluble vitamins A and D. As we noted in Chapter 7, Vitamins, although the fat-soluble vitamins have a greater potential for causing serious toxic effects, excesses of water-soluble vitamins are not totally harmless. A variety of toxicity symptoms have been observed. At the very best, athletes who use these products are simply pouring money down the drain because they will urinate out most of the excess water-soluble vitamins. In more extreme cases they may be causing irreversible damage to their bodies, as has been observed in some people who ingested excessive quantities of vitamin B_6 and niacin.[6,16,18]

Many sports supplements contain large quantities of minerals as well as vitamins. In addition to promoting high intakes of manganese and magnesium for energy metabolism, supplement manufacturers often advocate increased zinc intake to sustain muscle protein synthesis. They also exaggerate the need for calcium and iron to prevent stress fractures and sports anemia, respectively. What goes unsaid is that minerals, particularly trace minerals, have a high potential for producing toxic side effects. Zinc is a good example. Studies have shown that the more protein the body synthesizes, the higher the body's zinc requirement. Megadoses of zinc, however, have never been proved to be beneficial and in fact are highly toxic. Most athletes can meet their zinc requirement by eating animal-derived foods, which are naturally high in this mineral. Vegetarian athletes, however, may benefit from taking small amounts of zinc supplements.[3]

Carbohydrate Loading

How does carbohydrate loading enhance physical performance? The principle behind carbohydrate loading is very simple. In essence it takes advantage of

the body's natural tendency to store excess dietary carbohydrate in the form of glycogen. Here is how it works. Ingested carbohydrate, whether sugar or starch, is rapidly broken down to monosaccharides in the intestine. These monosaccharides are then absorbed and transported to the liver, where they are converted into glucose. Glucose is released from the liver into the general circulation, where it is available to satisfy the immediate energy needs of muscle as well as other tissue. Excess glucose is stored in both muscle and liver in the form of glycogen.

When muscle glycogen stores are filled to their normal capacity, there is enough energy to fuel 90 to 120 minutes of vigorous exercise. Some additional glucose for muscle use also can be obtained from liver glycogen stores. Once glycogen stores are depleted, fatigue quickly sets in, curtailing the intensity and duration of physical activity. By consuming extra complex carbohydrate for several days before an event, athletes can increase their glycogen stores and thus prolong physical endurance.

 Note that carbohydrate loading is useful only for endurance events—activities lasting over an hour.

Used carelessly, carbohydrate loading can actually diminish endurance. Practiced properly, it is one of the safest and most effective dietary techniques for enhancing physical performance. The rapid changes in diet involved in the original carbohydrate loading method produced undesirable side effects. The modern approach advocates that athletes routinely consume the high-carbohydrate diet recommended for the general population to ensure adequate glycogen stores.

TABLE 10-3 Carbohydrate Loading Techniques

	Standard Method		Short Method	
Day	Exercise	Diet	Exercise	Diet
1	90 minutes	50% carbo		
2	40 minutes	50% carbo		
3	40 minutes	50% carbo		
4	20 minutes	70% carbo	Normal	70% carbo
5	20 minutes	70% carbo	Normal	70% carbo
6	Rest	70% carbo	Rest	70% carbo
7	4-6 hours before competition	70% carbo meal		
	During event	Carbohydrate-fortified beverages		

Eating extra carbohydrates for the 3 days before an event together with proper physical conditioning can increase muscle glycogen stores 20% to 40% above normal. This provides enough extra glucose to delay the onset of fatigue without any of the potential side effects associated with the original glycogen-loading method. Although everyone should strive to consume a high-carbohydrate diet for its numerous health benefits, carbohydrate loading is neither necessary nor beneficial for aerobic activities lasting 1 hour or less, or for single bouts of exercise that trigger anaerobic metabolism. Carbohydrate loading is useful, however, for marathon-like endurance events. Table 10-3 shows the two most popular carbohydrate loading techniques. The standard method produces slightly larger glycogen stores than does the short routine.[15] Pastas, whole-grain breads and cereals, and legumes are all excellent foods to use when carbohydrate loading.

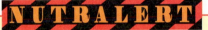

NUTRALERT

Because of alterations in carbohydrate metabolism, people with diabetes and hypoglycemia should not practice carbohydrate loading.

NUTRITION AND SPORTS-RELATED HEALTH PROBLEMS

The high incidence of stress fractures and anemia among endurance athletes has given nutrition supplement manufacturers plenty of ammunition to bolster sales of calcium and iron supplements. Both situations are good examples of how manufacturers can manipulate the truth to promote their products. You need to be aware that stringing together two or more true statements does not always make a conclusion valid.

Stress Fractures

Stress fractures are less the result of inadequate calcification of the bones than of repetitive, vigorous, weight-bearing exercise that exceeds the skeleton's

BOX 10-3   Validity of Rationale for Calcium Supplementation

RATIONALE

True: Calcium deficiency causes weak bones, which are prone to breaking.

True: Runners and aerobics instructors have a particularly high incidence of stress fractures in the bones of their feet and legs.

True: Females appear to be at greater risk than males for this kind of injury.

CONCLUSION

False: Stress fractures are caused by insufficient dietary calcium intake.

BOX 10-4   Validity of Rationale for Iron Supplementation

RATIONALE

True: Dietary iron deficiency results in anemia.

True: Compared with the general population, endurance athletes have lower concentrations of hemoglobin.

True: Typically, low hemoglobin levels are a sign of anemia.

CONCLUSION

False: All endurance athletes are prone to anemia.

ability to adapt. Typically exercise stimulates calcium deposition, thus increasing bone strength. In females, excessive exercise can cause body fat to decrease to such a low level that estrogen production and menstruation cease (*amenorrhea*) and false menopause follows. Just as in true menopause, osteoporosis develops, setting the stage for bone fractures. If a female athlete is suffering from osteoporosis secon-

amenorrhea   absence of menstruation

dary to false menopause, all the calcium supplements in the world will not improve skeletal strength. Rather she must be encouraged to gain enough weight for her body to resume normal reproductive functioning. Proper hormonal patterns together with adequate calcium intake can repair her weakened bone structure.[7]

Sports Anemia

A comparable situation exists with respect to sports anemia. Endurance athletes tend to have lower hemoglobin concentrations than the general population because expansion of blood volume is one of the first ways the body adapts to a consistent aerobic exercise program. This dilution phenomenon, known as **athlete's** or **sports anemia**, is a positive adaptation to exercise. It prevents loss of blood volume during exercise and causes blood to be thinner and easier to circulate so it can carry oxygen to exercising muscle tissue more efficiently.

Athletes also can develop genuine iron-deficiency anemia, which will impair their physical performance. Athletes with iron-deficiency anemia need advice about appropriate eating habits, with an emphasis on food combinations that enhance iron absorption. Iron supplements also may be needed on a temporary or ongoing basis.[21] Boxes 10-3 and 10-4 on p. 195 show supplement manufacturers' standard rationale and conclusions about the need for calcium and iron supplements together with comments about their validity.

Exercise Addiction

Yes, you can become addicted to exercise. In Chapter 9, Energy, you learned that bulimics and anorexics often exercise compulsively to burn off kcalories. In addition to such extreme cases, there are a significant number of people who get addicted to exercise because of the "high" they experience. Such people report feeling "down" if they do not exercise. As a result, they press themselves relentlessly, often sustaining overuse injuries in the process. Several studies have confirmed these reports. According to one clinical psychologist, when very physically active people are forced to discontinue their fitness program because of injury, they do indeed show symptoms of overall psychological distress and a tendency toward anger and depression.[5]

In addition to increasing an athlete's chance of physical injury, excessive exercise impairs immune function. As you learned earlier, your body responds to exercise as it would to any stress: by releasing a variety of stress hormones into the bloodstream. One of these hormones, cortisol, has been shown to suppress immunity. Earlier in the chapter you learned that the amount of stress associated with a moderate exercise program primes the body's defenses and enhances immune function. But when exercise is too intense, the body stays in a state of stress. Cortisol levels remain elevated for pro-

BOX 10-5   How To Avoid Negative Exercise Addiction

- Keep running sessions to 20-minute workouts, three or four times a week.
- If you want to increase mileage, do it gradually: no more than a 5% increase per month.
- Use the hard day/easy day method of training to ensure recovery.
- Build rest days into your weekly schedule.
- If you experience pain during or after a run, take some time off to allow your body to heal.

Adapted from Benyo R: *The exercise fix*, Berkeley, Calif, 1991, Leisure Press.

longed periods of time, and a significant decrease in immune function can be detected. One study found that runners who covered more than 60 miles a week were twice as likely to become ill as those who ran 20 or fewer miles per week.[17] In contrast, women who walked an average of 45 minutes per day 5 times a week were half as likely to become ill as their inactive neighbors.[12] Exercise addicts also may suffer from a syndrome known as **anorexia athletica,** which can worsen their already poor immune response.[3] Box 10-5 presents suggestions for preventing a negative addiction to running.

Steroids

For many athletes, particularly young men, the ultimate performance enhancer isn't a super sports drink or a megadose of vitamins—it's anabolic steroids. Purchased illegally, used carelessly and excessively, steroids have spelled the end, rather than the start, of many promising athletic careers. See A Closer Look on p. 197 for details about the frightening—and sometimes irreversible—consequences of self-dosing with anabolic steroids.

NUTRI NUGGET   There was no U.S. representation in a recent Mr. World contest because more sensitive tests are now used that detect steroid remnants over a longer period.

IN TODAY'S WORLD

By now you can see that exercise does more than just keep off excess body fat. You also know that a low body weight is not necessarily synonymous with a lean body or good physical conditioning. So, for all those people who want to know if they need to exercise even though their weight is OK, the answer is a definite YES! One of the toughest challenges for many people is find-

A CLOSER LOOK

"Roid Rage"

"I was playing football and looking for a scholarship. I figured steroids would give me a better chance. I gained so much strength and weight it was incredible—until my shoulder popped out." Mike Cestone, quoted in *USA Weekend Magazine*, May 15, 1992.

Canadian track star Ben Johnson forfeited his 1988 Olympic gold medals because of them. Former Los Angeles Raiders football star Lyle Alzado attributed his fatal brain cancer to them. Countless lesser-known athletes have suffered everything from violent mood swings to fatal diseases because of them. What causes these disasters? Anabolic-androgenic steroids, synthetic versions of the male sex hormone testosterone.

Why would people be willing to risk such harm? Because they work. When anabolic steroids are used in combination with a healthful diet and a weight training program, they cause rapid and dramatic increases in body weight as well as muscle size and strength. In a society that prizes fitness, glamour, and winning at all costs, steroids are the ultimate quick fix.

Who uses steroids? Steroids have many legitimate medical uses, including the treatment of certain blood and growth disorders. They first became popular among Soviet Olympic athletes in the 1950s. By 1983 their use was so widespread that 15 athletes from all over the world, including one from the United States, were disqualified from the Pan American Games for failing the steroid test. The publicity from this scandal alerted people to the dangers of steroids, but it also caused thousands of teens to search out these magic body-building bullets. Today steroids are used by male and some female athletes as performance enhancers as well as by some nonathletes purely for appearance's sake. Steroids' body-shaping ability has made them a popular confidence booster among male teens. A study by the National Institute on Drug Abuse estimates that 300,000 to 400,000 young people, some no more than age 12, have experimented with steroids.

The high levels of steroids used for body building have many dangerous side effects, including liver cancer, kidney and heart damage, severe acne, hair loss, shrunken testicles, impotence, sterility, permanent lowering of the voice, enlarged breasts, increased body hair, mood swings, and aggressive outbursts. Physicians who are familiar with steroid abuse say many users also suffer from a "reverse anorexia" syndrome. No matter how large they get, they still think they look small.[2] Knowing they will lose some muscle mass once they stop using steroids makes many people reluctant to stop no matter what the risks. In an interview published in the May 15, 1992, edition of *USA Weekend Magazine*, steroid expert Dr. Robert Goldman talked about a patient who had terrible acne all over his body, had developed female breast tissue, and was nearly impotent. When Goldman told the patient he must get off steroids, the 6' 5", 260-pound man replied, "Doc, I don't ever want to be small again."

Still tempted by steroids' quick-fix potential? Reread the side effects and ask yourself: Is a buff (well-muscled) body worth such risks?

---

ing ways to integrate a fitness program into their lifestyle or improve the one they already have.

Getting Going—Exercise!

Nature endowed us with bodies that require a good diet and regular exercise to achieve optimal health. Before the widespread mechanization of our modern times, people got all the exercise they needed finding and raising food, chopping firewood, and performing other tasks essential to life. We modern humans work just as hard as our ancestors, but much of the work we perform is mental as opposed to physical. To ensure good health, we need to incorporate physical activity into our daily schedules.

Can I just start exercising, or do I need a pre-exercise physical exam? The current advice is that healthy people age 35 and younger can undertake a regular exercise program without getting a physical exam first. People over 35 should consult their physician to be sure they have no underlying health problems that could be worsened by exercise.

Are you ever too old to start an exercise program? No. People of all ages benefit from physical activity. Aging modifies the recommendation for the intensity and duration of exercise, but not the need to be active.[11]

OK. I'm convinced I need to exercise, but which kind of exercise is best? The simplest answer is that the best exercise is the one you will do. No matter how good a particular kind of exercise is, it is worthless unless you perform it. Every year thousands of people begin an exercise program only to abandon it when it causes injury, fails to produce the desired results, or becomes too inconvenient. Do not underestimate the importance of personal preference when selecting an exercise program. Once you decide which

anorexia athletica depressed appetite caused by overexercise; reversible if exercise is cut back

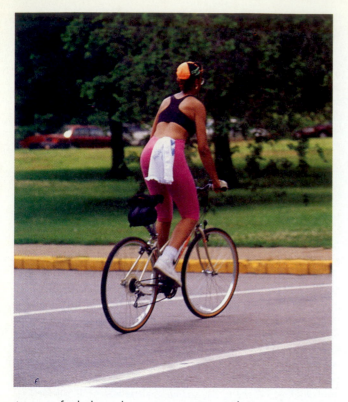

As part of a balanced exercise program, cycling is a great way to pursue fitness.

kinds of exercise fit best into your lifestyle, select the ones that appeal to you most. You are much more likely to stick with an exercise program you like than to endure one you consider pure drudgery.

Variety

When choosing an exercise program, you should consider several factors. Like a healthy diet, a good exercise routine requires variety. There are two reasons: to ensure a good overall workout and to allow muscles time to recuperate. There is no one perfect exercise. For example, joggers and cyclers often have well-developed lower limbs and poorly developed upper bodies. Swimmers usually develop all the muscle groups uniformly, but they may lack flexibility or strength. Weightlifters have strong, well-developed muscles, but unless they include an aerobic workout, they lack cardiovascular conditioning. A good fitness program includes exercises that promote flexibility (stretching), strength (calisthenics or weight work), and cardiovascular fitness (aerobic workouts) for all of the major muscle groups.[1,4]

As important as it is to develop muscles uniformly, it is just as important to protect exercised muscles from injury. Exercise causes a small but necessary amount of injury to muscle tissue and depletes muscles' fuel reserves. Muscles repair themselves and restore their fuel supplies within 24 to 36 hours of an exercise bout.

Over time this process of destruction and repair actually helps muscles grow stronger and use fuel more efficiently. Exercising the same muscle groups day after day, however, is a recipe for injury.

Alternating the muscle groups you exercise allows time for repair and refueling, thereby minimizing the chances of an exercise-curtailing injury. Some people choose to alternate different forms of aerobic exercise, such as brisk walking and cycling, as well as performing daily flexibility exercises and triweekly calisthenics or weight workouts. Others prefer to do flexibility exercises every day and alternate aerobic workouts with calisthenics/weight workouts.

Impact

Before settling on a particular form of exercise, consider the amount of impact involved. (Impact means the force with which the body hits the ground.) High-impact regimens, such as running and regular aerobic dance routines, are associated with a greater incidence of injury than are brisk walking, cycling, swimming, and low-impact aerobics. People with a history of joint injuries should avoid high-impact sports.

Convenience

Convenience for daily use is another important factor. If you choose an exercise program that does not fit easily into your lifestyle, you are not likely to stick to it. For example, if you decide to swim every day, but the nearest pool is an hour away, before long you will probably be an exercise dropout. Before deciding how to exercise, ask yourself if you would be more motivated to exercise if you joined a gym/health club or if you would be happier exercising on your own. If a health club is your choice, find one that has qualified instructors to familiarize you with the equipment. They can help you get the best workout with the least risk of injury. Considering buying a piece of home exercise equipment? Check out the equipment comparison chart in A Closer Look on p. 199.

Working out with a group provides motivation and encouragement.

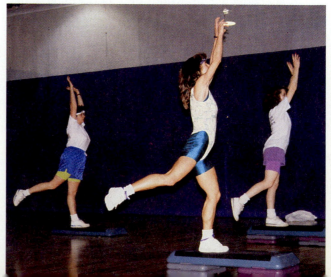

A CLOSER LOOK

Home Exercise Equipment

Which kind of home exercise equipment is the best buy?   Home exercise equipment has become one of the hottest trends in the fitness market. Selecting the right equipment, however, can be complicated. A wide variety of options make choosing difficult: rowing machines, cross-country ski simulators, stationary bikes, steppers, and treadmills with prices ranging from a few hundred to a couple of thousand dollars.

Cross-country ski simulators provide the best low-impact total-body workout. They exercise all the major muscle groups, especially the legs and arms. Learning to use one initially can be frustrating, and they are definitely not for people with balance problems, but if you stick with it you'll be rewarded by a leaner physique.

An investment of $429 will get you a Nordic Track Sequoia. It lacks some of the "bells and whistles" like the computerized distance and heart rate monitor found on the more expensive models, but the Sequoia does the job, folds up for easy storage, and comes with a free demonstration video to get you off to a safe start.

Ski simulators are available for less, but don't spend under $200. Simulators in this price range won't work well and may even cause injuries. Whichever brand you buy, choose one with independent foot action (this means the skis or foot platforms are not connected in any way).

Rowing machines, like ski simulators, exercise the whole body, but they tend to emphasize the arms and shoulders more than the legs (what does this mean in terms of kcalorie-burning potential?). They take up a lot of space (about 8 feet by 3 feet), make a roaring sound during operation, and are impossible to read on. It is easy to injure your back using one if you do not maintain proper form. They also tend to be expensive: $700 to $1000 is the typical price range. If you are not discouraged by the negatives, purchase a Concept II Rowing Ergometer. This model, which includes computerized feedback about your kcalorie expenditure and speed, has been used by generations of Olympic athletes with good results.

Treadmills are useful for everyone from distance walkers to marathon runners. The negatives: They exercise only the legs and buttocks, take up a lot of space (about 6 feet by 4 feet), and are costly. You need to spend at least $1300 to get a safe, reliable motorized model. Nonmotorized models can strain your hips and knees as you struggle to keep the belt moving.

When buying a treadmill, look for one with a safety lock so children can't injure themselves, and make sure the motor's top speed is high enough to meet your needs. A good choice is the Aerobics Pace Master, which sells for $1295.

Stationary bikes are great for everyone—especially overweight people who need to avoid extra stress on their knee and ankle joints. Bikes emphasize the leg, hip, and buttocks muscles. A few models even have moving handlebars for an upper body workout. Look for bikes with an easy-to-reach resistance setting and an adjustable seat. For $269 the Tunturi Executive Ergometer is a solid, reliable bike investment. Computerized models are available for between $500 and $1000, and the Cadillac of stationary bikes, the Lifecycle 5500R, goes for nearly $2000.

Steppers require relatively little space, 3 feet by 4 feet tops, and you can read while stepping. They are not a good choice, however, for people with balance or knee problems. Most models exercise only the legs and buttocks, but a few have optional ski pole attachments to give your arms a workout. Look for handrails for safety (not to rest on). Leaning on the rails will significantly reduce the kcalorie-burning value of your workout.

Dependent stair models (when you step down on one stair, the other comes up) are easier for beginners to use than independent models that require you to control both steps, but this feature is pricey. For instance, the Tunturi TriStepper 500, available for $249, comes with independent steps and wide foot supports, whereas a reliable dependent step model starts at $1695.

Where should I buy exercise equipment?   If possible, buy exercise equipment at a specialty store rather than at a department store or discount mart. Specialty stores have a wide range of equipment available for you to try out and employ well-trained clerks and technicians who can install the equipment in your home as well as make repairs.

Be sure to wear comfortable clothes while shopping and get advice from the sales staff about the benefits and drawbacks of the various pieces of equipment and how to use them. Select equipment that has any necessary safety features built in and that comes with a 1-year warranty on parts and labor.

Most manufacturers have toll-free phone numbers customers can call for brochures, information, and store locations. (Call 1-800-555-1212 for numbers of individual manufacturers.)

Adapted from Getting a leg up on home exercise equipment, *Tufts University Diet and Nutrition Letter* 12(1):3, 1994.

If you decide to go it alone, jogging, brisk walking, aerobic exercise videotapes, and a variety of exercise equipment geared to home use make getting in shape easier than ever. If you still need extra motivation, ask a friend to work out with you. Knowing that you are accountable to another person can help you keep going when you are feeling lazy.

NUTRI NUGGET No matter how committed you are to physical fitness, do not exercise when you are ill. Doing so can prolong your recovery time and in rare cases may cause an inflammation of the external lining of your heart.[1]

The Case for Aerobics

The most important thing to bear in mind is that the cornerstone of a good fitness program is one or more aerobic exercise routines, since only aerobic activities promote cardiovascular conditioning and weight control.

How can I tell if I am exercising aerobically? Aerobic exercise is any activity that raises the body's metabolic rate without exceeding its ability to supply sufficient oxygen with which to burn fat. A quick test of whether you are exercising too gently or too vigorously is to see if you can talk or sing. If you are getting a good aerobic workout, you should be able to speak normally, but you should not be able to sing. If you cannot talk, slow down! You have shifted to anaerobic metabolism. If you can sing, get moving! You are not exercising your heart!

Recent research has shown that prolonged aerobic exercise of moderate intensity promotes fat utilization. Vigorous brief aerobic activity burns less fat and more glycogen but provides a better cardiovascular workout.

What is the difference between moderate and intense aerobic exercise? Moderate aerobic activity is exercise that raises your heart rate to 55% to 70% of the maximum heart rate. Intense aerobic exercise increases the heart rate to between 71% and 90% of the maximum rate and increases cardiovascular conditioning.[1]

How do I know what my maximum heart rate is, and how can I measure it? Exercise stress tests provide a true measurement of maximum heart rate. Using the following equation, you can figure out your approximate maximum heart rate without the effort and expense of an exercise stress test:

> **220 beats per minute**
> **− your age in years**
> **= your maximum heart rate**

This equation is based on two assumptions:
- The average human heart has a maximum capacity of 220 beats per minute.
- Maximum heart rate decreases with age.

Next multiply the result of the preceding equation by your target heart rate for an intense aerobic workout. If you are 20 years old, your maximum heart rate is 200 beats per minute and your aerobic range is 71% to 90% of that, or 140 to 180 beats per minute. Alternatively, you can estimate your aerobic workout heart rate by doubling your resting heart rate. Once you know what range you are aiming for, measuring your heart rate is a simple matter of learning to take your pulse. Obtain a watch or clock with a second hand. Lie down or sit quietly for a few minutes before measuring your resting heart rate. Take your pulse immediately after finishing exercise to determine your workout heart rate. Take your pulse with your fingers, never your thumb (it has its own pulse), by pressing firmly but gently on a pulse point— on your neck directly below your jawbone on either side of your chin, over your heart, or on the inside of your wrist. Take your pulse for 10 seconds (count a beat that occurs on the tenth second as a half beat) and multiply by 6 to obtain beats per minute. Remember to update your exercise regimen as your physical condition improves to make sure you are still getting a good aerobic workout.

How much exercise do I need? Unfortunately, there is no "Recommended Exercise Allowance" or "Exercise Guide Pyramid" to help people plan an adequate and balanced workout. The good news is that you do not need to be in competition for an Olympic medal to reap the benefits of exercise. Most experts agree that 20 to 30 minutes of *moderate* aerobic exercise three times a week is the minimum amount needed to keep people in good shape. The latest research suggests that just 30 minutes a day of moderate exercise like walking, dancing, or cycling can reduce your risk of premature death nearly as much as can a vigorous exercise program. And the exercise need not be 30 consecutive minutes.[1,12]

DESIGNING A LIFESTYLE MATRIX

The Menu Matrix that we used in previous chapters to plan healthy meals now can be expanded to a lifestyle matrix by using the Exercise Matrix to help you plan a physical fitness program.

Because walking is one form of physical activity almost everyone can do, we will use the development of a fitness walking program as an example of how to use the lifestyle matrix. Our bodies are designed to walk considerable distances on a regular basis, so walking can be safely used as an aerobic workout day after day. It is important for sedentary people to begin an exercise program slowly. There is nothing to gain and much to lose (in the form of injured muscles) from attempting a crash fitness program. Using the Exercise Matrix in Appendix D as a model, you can develop a weekly exercise chart and use it to help you plan a safe exercise program. Read the advice below, then pencil in the appropriate routine one week at a time.

 Although some people believe that the harder you exercise, the greater the physical benefits, improvements in physical strength and biochemical indicators of fitness are seen with only moderate amounts of exercise. Unless you are in excellent physical condition, an all-out effort can actually do more harm than good.

If you are a beginner, start by walking 15 minutes a day every other day for 1 week. On alternate days, do

15 minutes of calisthenics or a light weight workout. End each exercise period with 5 minutes of stretching exercises: a cool-down routine. For years fitness experts have warned people to stretch before exercising to prevent injuries. Newer evidence suggests that stretching cold muscles may injure them. For this reason, you should stretch after an exercise period or after warming up with at least 5 minutes of walking or calisthenics.

During the second week, gradually extend your walking and strength workouts so that by the end of the week you are doing 30 minutes of exercise and 10 minutes of stretching. During the third week of the program, gradually extend the exercise period so that at the end of the week you are working out for 45 minutes a day with 15 minutes of stretching. Occasionally your schedule leaves no time to exercise on a particular day. Do not panic. It is all right to miss a day or two; just be sure to get in three aerobic workouts per week; to improve your conditioning, do four.

If you have been exercising and would like to improve your workouts, begin by alternating 30 minutes of aerobic exercise with 30 minutes of strength work and do 10 minutes of stretching each day for 1 week. Then follow the suggested routine for the third week.

Working With Weights

Like regular aerobic exercise, a consistent weight training regimen is an essential part of a balanced exercise program. In fact, research has demonstrated that weight training can prevent the decline in bone and muscle strength that typically occurs in later life.

NUTRALERT

Although some fitness experts advise people to use hand or ankle weights to increase their workout, many others caution against this practice because these kinds of weights increase stress on ankle, back, knee, and hip joints, increasing the potential for injury. A safer approach: wear a weight belt!

How can I develop a safe weight training program?

Weight training programs are not as easy to self-design as are aerobic exercise routines. Improper use of free weights (hand-held weights or barbells) can cause injury by pulling the body out of alignment or by causing you to drop a weight on part of your body. Working out on weight machines can prevent both of these kinds of injuries, but they are expensive and you need to know how to use them. The best way to get involved in weight training is to have a trained professional design a customized program for your needs and abilities.

Weight training experts can be found at health clubs and gyms. If this route seems too pricey, enroll in a beginning weight training course at the local community college, park and recreation department, or YMCA. Paying to have a weight training program custom designed is cheaper, ultimately, than sustaining an injury.

Won't weight training make me look like Arnold Schwarzenegger?

Not necessarily. The amount of muscle you develop depends on the type of build you have inherited, the amount of weight you use, and how often you work out. Some people can perform

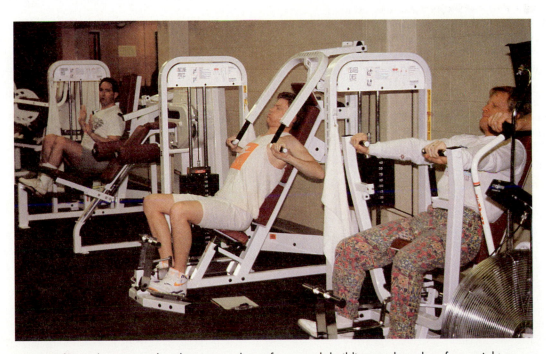

Weight machines provide a less intense but safer strength-building workout than free weights.

an intensive weight training routine for months or years and never achieve much bulk; other can bulk up quite readily. Muscle distribution and bulk are also a function of estrogen and testosterone levels. Women need not worry that they will bulk up significantly unless they use anabolic steroids. It is possible for men to tone and develop muscles without gaining a lot of bulk, even if they are prone to bulking up, by restricting the amount of weight they use as well as restricting the frequency and intensity of their workouts. For instance, to develop strength use light to moderate weights in conjunction with a circuit weight training approach: 30 seconds of lifting and 15 seconds of rest (rotate to next station) at 40% to 55% of maximum ability.

Persistence Pays

Exercise does not produce instantaneous results, but persistence pays. Fitness experts say it takes about 6 weeks for the benefits of a regular exercise routine to become apparent.[12] By that time a new exercise devotee should begin to look and feel better. Perhaps more important, your body will have become so adapted to exercise that it will crave activity. This craving can provide the motivation to make exercise a permanent part of your lifestyle. If you can stick with an exercise program for 6 weeks, you may find the key to ending the constant cycle of fitness starts and stops, and achieve the conditioning of your dreams.

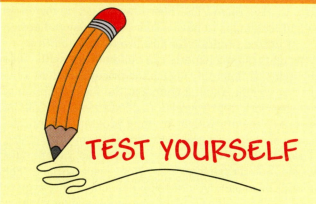

TEST YOURSELF

1. Which kind of exercise burns more fat: aerobic or anaerobic? Why?
2. Why is walking a good exercise?
3. What is the best diet for an endurance athlete?
4. Are ergogenic nutritional supplements necessary for peak athletic performance? Why or why not?
5. List three elements of a good exercise program.
6. At what age are you too old to begin exercising?
7. What is a quick test you can use to tell if you are exercising aerobically?
8. Why is adequate water intake necessary during exercise?
9. How long does it take for your body to adapt to a newly begun exercise program?
10. What factors should you consider when deciding which exercise program is best for you?

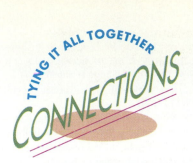

1. List three ways that a regular exercise program enhances nutrient metabolism.

2. List some ways that poor circulation may adversely affect nutrient utilization.

3. Approximately how many deaths per year could be prevented if all Americans exercised?

> **Case Study**
>
> Bill has an ectomorphic build. His friends always tease him about being a weakling, so he has decided to enroll in a weightlifting course at his college to help him "bulk up." He currently lifts weights for 1 hour 3 times a week. He does no other form of exercise because he does not want to burn up too many kcalories. He eats extra servings of high-fat foods and drinks a protein supplement.

4. What health traps do you see in Bill's current fitness program?

5. Is Bill's goal of "bulking up" realistic?

6. Suggest some ways Bill can improve his nutritional and physical fitness.

> **Case Study**
>
> Ms. Superbusy is a single mom. She supports two grammar school–aged children on the salary she earns as a long-distance operator for a major phone company. Her children take care of themselves after school. They spend the afternoons watching TV. Ms. Superbusy's life both at home and work is action packed and full of stress. The stress is so severe at times that even though exhausted she has trouble sleeping. She and her children have had a lot of colds this past year. To try to boost their immune systems she has put the entire family on a healthier diet: low in fat, high in carbohydrate, and rich in calcium and vitamins. Her doctor told her she and her kids should be more physically active but, given her current schedule, Ms. Superbusy just doesn't see any time for herself or her kids to exercise.

7. What would you tell Ms. Superbusy to convince her that exercise is vital to her health and the health of her children?

8. Suggest some ways Ms. Superbusy can work exercise into her family's everyday lives.

9. Do children need regular exercise to be healthy? Explain your answer.

10. Is exercise important for senior citizens? Why or why not?

REFERENCES

1. American College of Sports Medicine position stand: The recommended quantity and quality of exercise for developing and maintaining cardiorespiratory and muscular fitness in healthy adults, American College of Sports Medicine, 1991.

2. American College of Sports Medicine position stand: The use of anabolic androgenic steroids in sports, American College of Sports Medicine, 1984.

3. American Dietetic Association and Canadian Dietetic Association joint position: Nutrition for physical fitness and athletic performance for adults, *Journal of the American Dietetic Association* 93:691-693, 1993.

4. Allisen PE et al: Writing a weight control program. In *Fitness for life—an individualized approach*, ed 5, Dubuque, Ia, 1993, WC Brown.

5. Benyo R: *The exercise fix*, Berkeley, Calif, 1991, Leisure Press.

6. Body building supplements: false promises, *Nutrition and the MD* 18:7, 1992.

7. Brownwell K et al: Eating disorders among athletes, *Physician and Sportsmedicine* 18:116-121, 1990.

8. Clark N: Sports nutritionists practice what they preach. In For your information, *Journal of the American Dietetic Association* 92:419-420, 1992.

9. Does exercise prevent cancer? *University of California at Berkeley Wellness Letter* 9:6, 1992.

10. Edell D: Mental workout boosts strength, *Edell Health Letter* 4:2, 1992.

11. Evans W, Rosenberg I: *Biomarkers: the 10 determinants of aging you can control*, New York, 1991, Simon & Shuster.

12. Fries J (ed): Tips to help you stick with your exercise program, *Healthtrac Newsletter* 7(1):1, 1991.

13. Grandjean AC, Rudd JS: Fluid and electrolytes. In Mellion M, ed: *Sports medicine secrets*, Philadelphia, 1994, Hanley & Belfus.

14. Heimlich S et al: The use of exercise in the treatment and prevention of diabetes, *New England Journal of Medicine* 325:147-152, 1991.

15. Hoffman CJ: An eating plan and update on recommended dietary practices for the endurance athlete, *Journal of the American Dietetic Association* 91:325, 1991.

16. Institutes of Medicine's Food & Nutrition Board, Diet and physical performance, *Journal of the American Medical Association* 1994:271:98.

17. Neiman D: Exercise and immunity: are you running yourself into the ground? *Health Today*, Apr 1992, pp 131-135.

18. Nutrition and exercise: what your body really needs, *University of California at Berkeley Wellness Letter* 10:4-6, 1993.

19. Rock C, ed: Athletes and iron, *Nutrition and the MD* 20:3, 1994.

20. Sapolsky RM: *Why zebras don't get ulcers: a guide to stress, stress-related diseases and coping*, New York, 1994, WH Freeman.

21. Williams MH: Nutritional ergogenics: help or hype. In for your information, *Journal of the American Dietetic Association* 92:1213-1214, 1992.

CHAPTER 11

WEIGHT CONTROL
Finding a Healthy Balance

The two biggest sellers in any bookstore are the cookbooks and the diet books. The cookbooks tell you how to prepare the food, and the diet books tell you how not to eat it.

— Andy Rooney

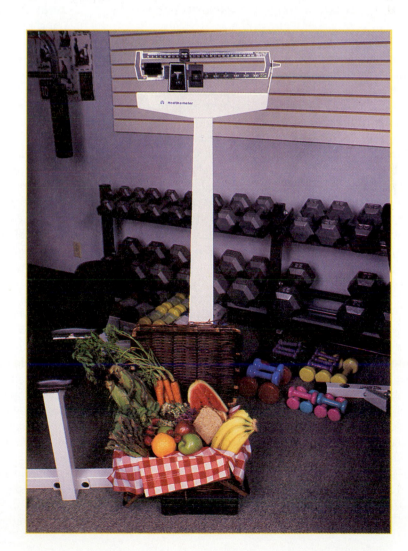

Americans are the most weight-conscious people on Earth. According to the National Institutes of Health, at any given time 20% to 24% of all men and 33% to 40% of all women report they are dieting. Fear of fat has even reached the grade schools. Many children report they have put themselves on a diet after deciding they were too fat.

 NUTRI NUGGET *Fat babies don't necessarily become fat adults. Obesity in late childhood and the teen years, however, may signal a lifelong weight problem. Forty percent of obese 7-year-olds and 70% of obese teens become overweight adults.*

Americans' fear of fat is well founded. The cost of obesity goes beyond the health risks identified in Chapter 9. For many people the social costs are just as great if not greater. Overfat people face discrimination at school, in the work force, when applying for health and life insurance, when seeking mates, and in a host of other social situations.[15]

Despite all this attention to our waistlines, Americans of all ages are getting fatter. Information from the National Center for Health Statistics indicates that between 1988 and 1991 the percentage of overweight Americans increased from 26% to 34%.[16] Health experts blame "an epidemic of inactivity" and improper dieting. Inactivity is a symptom of our highly mechanized society. Machines do much of the physical labor that still is done by people who live in less industrialized countries. Add to this the fact that Americans are watching more TV than ever (and the more TV they watch the fatter they get), and it is easy to see why inactivity is an epidemic.[11,17] The other part of the problem is the whole concept of controlling weight through dieting. Ninety percent of dieters regain all or most of the weight they lost within 2 to 5 years of ending their diet. An unfortunate few even end up fatter than before they dieted.[17]

Why don't diets work?   For one thing, diets are temporary. It is not surprising that people regain the weight they lost once they resume the lifestyle that caused them to gain the weight in the first place. Second, diets don't deal with the need to exercise.[1,17] Dieting without exercising is like taking only half the medicine you need to cure an illness. Third, diets tend to overlook the emotional factors that underlie the dieter's eating habits.[10] Often it is not so much *what* you eat but *why* you eat. Fourth, diet marketers and dieters alike develop unrealistic weight loss goals.[8] Genetic differences in build and body fat mean that no matter how hard some of us diet, we aren't going to look like swimsuit models. Finally, many diets are so low in kcalories that they actually make it harder to lose weight and keep it off.[18,19]

THE PROBLEM—DIETING

If low-kcalorie diets aren't the answer to weight control, why do people continue to use them?

Crash Dieting—A Nutritional Speed Trap!

When we explore the pitfalls of weight loss programs that focus only on a low-kcalorie diet, we can clearly see why the first dieter to reach the finish line is not the one who has won the weight-loss war. It can take months or even years to become significantly overfat, but most people expect to correct the situation in a matter of weeks. Considering the amount of time and effort it takes to lose 30 pounds gradually, using a program that includes diet, exercise, and behavior modification, we can easily see why so many people choose the "fast track" of a *quick weight-loss diet.*

NUTRI NUGGET *The search for a painless weight loss technique is endless. In the 1970s grapefruit was said to contain special enzymes that help the body dissolve fat. Today the mineral chromium is said to be a fat burner, and some researchers claim that rubbing a particular asthma medication on the thighs will dissolve fat.*

For all but people who are morbidly obese (more than 100 pounds over their healthy weight), health care experts agree that a safe weight reduction program should produce a weight loss of no more than 1½ to 2 pounds per week. Even at the maximum rate of 2 pounds per week, it would take about 15 weeks or 3½ months to lose 30 pounds with the safe, gradual approach. Someone who chooses instead to use a crash diet that promises a 5-pound-per-week weight loss might be able to shed all 30 pounds in 6 weeks, or 1½ months. Most crash dieters fail to realize (or care) that the 30 pounds they lose on a quick weight loss diet will be a combination of muscle and fat rather than the almost pure fat they could lose with a gradual approach based on both diet and exercise. Crash dieters are more likely to regain weight than are gradual dieters, and their future efforts to lose weight are made more difficult by undesirable metabolic changes that occur in response to the crash diet.[4,18]

Why do quick weight loss diets burn up muscle? Most experts agree that diets that lead to a weight loss of more than 2 pounds per week provide too few kcalories to meet the body's glucose requirement (to lose 1 pound of body fat you need to burn 3500 kcals). As a result, the body breaks down its own muscle tissue to obtain the amino acids that can be converted into glucose. In rare instances crash dieting causes enough loss of muscle tissue to damage the heart, sometimes fatally.[14]

A CLOSER LOOK

Surgical Solutions to Obesity

Most of us know that tummy tucks and liposuction are slenderizing surgeries. Both of these techniques remove a few pounds of unwanted fat. Their application, however, is more cosmetic than physiological, so they really can't be considered solutions to obesity. A separate category of surgical procedures has been developed to treat chronic morbid obesity.

The severe health problems associated with morbid obesity sometimes make drastic measures such as gastrointestinal surgery necessary. Such treatments have significant physical as well as psychological side effects, so they are undertaken only when all other therapeutic routes have been exhausted.

A variety of gastrointestinal surgeries have been tried.

Because of the severity of the side effects associated with procedures that cause food to bypass large sections of intestine, stomach stapling is now the most widely used technique. Stomach stapling irreversibly reduces the capacity of the stomach to about $1/4$ cup. Overeating becomes almost impossible because it causes intense pain and vomiting; however, a few patients who are psychologically unprepared to deal with weight loss have managed to maintain a surprising amount of weight by drinking very nutrient-dense beverages. The majority of patients who undergo the procedure lose 50% of their body weight within a year of surgery and are able to maintain their weight loss. Since stomach stapling is irreversible it necessitates permanent life-style changes and is usually accompanied by psychological counseling.

Whatever your weight loss goals, remember no surgical procedure should be undertaken lightly. All surgeries whether cosmetic or therapeutic carry a risk of complications, ranging from simple wound infections to death.

How does the loss of muscle tissue affect the dieter's metabolism? People on quick weight-loss diets do lose weight, some of which is fat. Because they also lose muscle tissue, however, their percent body fat may actually increase! The loss of metabolically active muscle tissue decreases the dieter's BMR, making it both harder to lose weight and more likely that the lost weight will be regained once the diet is over. Additionally, one study found that rapid weight loss stimulates overproduction of an enzyme that helps adipose tissue store fat. Some researchers believe increased production of this enzyme may explain why many crash dieters regain weight so quickly. Because the regained weight is primarily fat, crash dieters end up fatter than ever. Desperate to lose weight, they often try one "miracle" diet after another, establishing an unhealthful pattern of "yo-yo" dieting.[1]

 How does loss of muscle tissue from overly severe dieting affect a dieter's ability to lose weight and keep it off?

Yo-Yo Dieting

The term **yo-yo dieting** refers to the pattern of people who repeatedly lose and regain weight. With each diet they lose a little more muscle tissue, their BMR drops a little lower, and they regain a little more weight. This means each new diet has to be a little more drastic to produce weight loss. The desire to lose weight quickly can be so strong that some unsuccessful dieters are willing to contemplate fat-reduction surgeries (see A Closer Look above).

THE SOLUTION—A BALANCED LIFESTYLE

Can crash dieters and yo-yo dieters ever lose weight and keep it off? Yes, but only with a complete change in lifestyle. Not only must crash dieters learn to eat healthfully, they also must make physical activity part of their daily routine. A combination of aerobics and weight training will rebuild muscle tissue and increase BMR. If you completed the diet/exercise matrix, you have already developed a personalized nutrition and fitness plan. Your challenge now is developing the motivation to follow through with the changes you must make to achieve your health and fitness goals.

 If you have lowered your BMR through repeated crash diets, what can you do to revive your metabolism?

A Balanced Weight Control Program

For a few lucky people, losing excess body weight is simply a matter of making up their minds to eat less and/or exercise more. Unfortunately, for many people overeating has become an addictive behavior. As with any addiction, successful treatment typically involves more than simply acknowledging the destructive be-

> **quick weight-loss diet** any diet that causes a person to lose more than 2 pounds per week

havior and vowing to correct it. Proof of this fact is the failure of most reducing diet and exercise programs to provide sustained weight control. Weight control experts are now convinced that essential features of a successful weight control program are awareness of the underlying factors that trigger eating, behavior modification, and maintenance therapy. The best programs include a gradual reducing diet, based on a varied and balanced menu plan, a personalized exercise program, identification of environmental factors that trigger eating, behavior modification to help the dieter change when, where, why, and what is eaten, and a maintenance phase to ensure the successful transition from reducing-diet to free-choice eating in a manner consistent with long-term weight control.[2,9,18]

Several studies suggest that the greater a program's emphasis on behavior modification and maintenance support, the more successful the dieters.[17,18] This is probably because of the very nature of addictive overeating. Unlike other addictive behaviors, such as excessive use of alcohol, smoking, compulsive gambling, and drug abuse, overeating cannot be treated by abstinence. Compulsive overeaters must learn to overcome their addiction while participating in the addictive behavior. This underlies the need for intensive behavior modification and support.

Behavior Modification

Behavior modification has been a popular buzzword for the past decade. It has been used to sell a variety of self-help programs and to justify a wide range of treatment techniques, some of which have given a bad name to behavior modification therapy. In reality, behavior modification is a legitimate technique developed by mental health professionals to teach people how to substitute a beneficial behavior for a destructive one. It has been successfully used to treat physical and emotional disorders such as gambling, smoking, alcoholism, stress—and obesity.

Energy Intake—Awareness and Change

Behavior modification is based on the idea that most of our behavior is voluntary rather than instinctive. Once people are aware of the conditions that stimulate them to participate in an undesirable behavior, they can work at modifying their response. Treatment is a gradual process. The first step is to identify environmental factors that trigger the undesirable behavior.

Next the counselor and client set modest goals for behavioral change. After achieving a goal the client receives a predetermined reward, and new goals are developed to replace the ones the client has attained. Eventually the undesirable behaviors will have been completely replaced with beneficial ones. The example that follows shows how behavior modification therapy works in a weight control program.

Edward, nicknamed "Tubby Ted" by his classmates, has been battling his weight since high school. With 4 months to go until his 30th birthday, he has decided to beat his problem once and for all. He calls the American Dietetic Association Hotline and requests a referral to a dietitian in his area who treats obesity. Within minutes he has the information he needs and makes an appointment with a registered dietitian (RD) who specializes in weight management.

During the first visit the dietitian gathers information about Ted's personal and family health history and eating habits. Then the dietitian instructs Ted to keep a food and activity journal for the next week and bring it to the next appointment. At the second appointment Ted and the dietitian review the journal. They note that he gets virtually no exercise and rarely socializes. Most of his energy goes into his work. It is also clear that Ted eats when lonely and in response to negative stimuli, such as job stress or arguments. In further discussion Ted tells the dietitian that he keeps a journal. Together Ted and the dietitian decide that every time Ted feels like reducing stress or loneliness with food, he instead will write about his hurt or angry feelings in his journal, forcing him to look at the cause of his discontent rather than trying to lessen it with food. If Ted can successfully practice this new behavior for 2 weeks, he can treat himself to a recording by his favorite musical group.

Ted is understandably concerned about being able to stick to his new behavior for 2 weeks. The dietitian reminds Ted of one of the basic elements of behavior therapy: break your goal down into small, manageable pieces. Do not concentrate on maintaining your new behavior for 2 weeks; instead focus on maintaining it "just for today." Use this method each day.

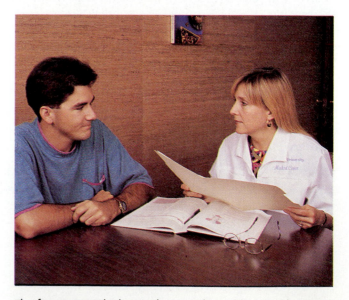

The first step in dealing with a weight problem is admitting it and asking for some help.

It takes Ted a few weeks of fits and starts to get comfortable with this new approach to stress management. To help him make the transition, the dietitian tells Ted that on days he is able to stick to his goal, he can reward himself with an activity he enjoys. When Ted has successfully avoided eating in response to loneliness and stress for 2 weeks, the dietitian suggests that it is time for Ted to start choosing healthier foods for meals and snacks. After reviewing Ted's current diet, he and the dietitian decide what specific changes Ted will try to make during the next 2 weeks and what the reward will be. Ted and the dietitian continue to examine aspects of Ted's eating and activity patterns, and alter them as needed to help Ted achieve his weight loss goal.

Strategies for Modifying Energy Intake

There is no single way to motivate people to reduce their reliance on food. Different tactics work for different people. Below we present behavior modification tips for reducing fat intake gathered from a variety of sources, including personal consulting experience. You may want to incorporate some of these activities into your new eating style, along with a formal weight reduction program.

Cultivating awareness. The first step in modifying eating behavior is to cultivate awareness of when, why, and how you eat.[2,3,9,25]

DO

- *Identify the factors that contribute to your overeating.* Do you nibble constantly, or do you fast all day only to gorge at night?
- *Keep a food intake diary for several days* to help make you aware of what, when, where, and why you eat. List every food you eat, the approximate amount, where you ate it, what you were doing while you were eating (for example, watching TV), and what you were feeling immediately before, during, and after eating (for example, were you angry over an argument with your boss, friend, etc., or were you celebrating a raise?)
- *Familiarize yourself with appropriate serving sizes* so that you can more accurately gauge your food intake. Overweight people tend to underestimate what they eat and overestimate how much energy they expend. You do not need to carry around a scale and measuring cups to accomplish this goal. The information below explains how you can learn to estimate serving sizes based on a knowledge of common household objects.
  - A 3-ounce serving of cooked meat, fish, or poultry takes up about as much space as a standard ¼-inch audiotape.
  - A 1/2-cup serving of rice or ice cream takes up about as much room as two golf balls sitting side by side.

- A 1-ounce serving of hard cheese or nuts takes up about as much space as two dice sitting side by side.
- *Learn to eat only when you are truly hungry.*
- *Learn to give your body a chance to feel full.* It takes about 20 minutes after consuming a meal for your brain to get the message that your body no longer needs fuel and to turn off the hunger signal. So hold off on the second helpings, and if you are still hungry have just a little bit more.
- *Chew your food thoroughly; put your fork down between bites.*

DON'T

- *Eat while standing up.* People consume many extra unnecessary kcalories while standing in front of an open refrigerator or kitchen cabinet.
- *Eat out of storage containers.* Serve yourself a given portion of food and sit down to eat it, thereby forcing yourself to confront what and how much you are eating.
- *Eat while doing other things* (like driving, working, watching TV). People who do this tend to lose track of how much food they consume. They also report that they feel less satisfied by the foods they eat under these circumstances than by foods they pay attention to consuming. This last point is particularly important if you are making an effort to reduce your food intake. Giving up favorite foods can make anyone feel deprived. Not enjoying the foods you do eat can make you abandon a diet.

Avoiding temptation. Although no single food is "bad," some foods are definitely better for you than others. Successful lifelong weight control requires that we learn to minimize our consumption of less nutritious foods. For people with a food addiction this may require giving up certain foods altogether until they feel confident they have gained control of their eating habits.

DON'T

- *Grocery shop while hungry.*
- *Indulge in food samples at the grocery store.*
- *Eat anything out of a package that is larger than your hand.*

DO

- *Make a list before going grocery shopping and stick to it!*
- *Keep the Food Guide Pyramid in mind when planning meals and shopping.*
- *Learn to shop on the edges of the grocery store. High-fat foods are generally in the center isles.*
- *Go through the cabinets in your house and get rid of the high-kcalorie, low-nutrient density foods*, like chips and cookies, in which you tend to overindulge.

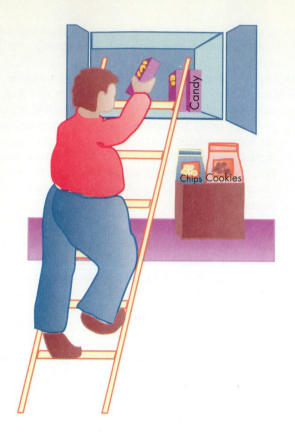

sticking with one. Sustaining motivation is one of the major challenges of weight loss. What follow are some ways to help you keep in mind why you are on the diet in the first place and to reward yourself for staying with the program.

DO

- *If you are just moderately overweight, it may help to tape an unflattering photo of yourself on your refrigerator or inside the cabinet where you keep favorite snack foods.* (Or you might use an attractive photo of yourself before you gained weight.) This can help strengthen your resolve when you are tempted to binge.
- *On the refrigerator or inside a cabinet, put a list of your favorite high-kcalorie snack foods and the amount of time you would have to exercise to burn off these kcalories.* For example, it takes 1 hour of moderately paced walking to burn off the average 257-kcalorie serving of cheesecake or a 260-kcalorie, 2-ounce Peter Paul Almond Joy candy bar.
- *Set realistic goals*, such as "I will stick to a balanced diet of 1500 kcalories per day and walk 3 miles 4 times per week."
- *Reward yourself* for sticking to your diet and exercise program with a favorite activity or nonfood item.
- *Look for other ways to measure improvement.* For example, decreasing body measurements and increased physical endurance are other important advantages of successful weight-control efforts.

DON'T

- *Replace meals with diet drinks or bars.* The way to take weight off and keep it off is to practice healthful eating habits at every meal.
- *Measure success only according to weight loss.* Scales do not tell the whole story. Your weight loss may slow down for a variety of reasons.
- *Get discouraged and give up.* Sticking with a realistic weight reduction plan eventually will yield the desired result.

- *If you live with people who cannot give up these foods, put them in a hard-to-reach area of the kitchen so you will have to make an effort to get them.* This gives you time to think about what you are doing. Better yet, replace traditional snack foods with more healthful low-fat versions. Everyone will benefit!
- *Try freezing candies and baked goods so that they will be less palatable.* If you do decide to eat one, you will have time while it is defrosting to consider the implications of what you are doing.
- *If you tend to graze mindlessly through the kitchen cabinets, put childproof locks on them.* The effort involved in opening the lock may help make you more conscious of what you are doing.
- *If possible, avoid walking through the kitchen as you move from one end of your house to the other.*

NUTRI NUGGET Even with lower-fat snack foods, be sure to pay attention to the size and number of servings you eat. Watch out for mini-versions of your favorite snacks; without thinking, you may be eating more pieces than you realize.

Sustaining dieting motivation. Getting started on a weight loss program is usually much easier than

NUTRALERT

Overweight people should go on a protein-sparing modified fast (liquid diet) only under medical supervision. Used improperly, such diets can lead to electrolyte imbalances and in some cases have even caused fatal heart attacks.

Developing new eating habits. Short-term dieting is not the solution to long-term weight control. The key to achieving lifetime weight control is to create healthful new eating patterns.[3,17,21]

DO

- *Learn to eat regular meals, especially breakfast.* All-day nibbling or the starve-all-day, gorge-all-night syndrome can add up to a hefty kcalorie intake.
- *Keep plenty of high-fiber, low-fat snacks readily available.* For example, keep a bowl of fresh fruit on the table so that you will have something to snack on. (For additional tips on reducing fat intake, see Chapter 5, Lipids.)
- *Serve a platter of raw vegetables with low-kcalorie dip or assorted fruits with meals to help take the edge off hunger.*
- *Carry an emergency snack,* such as low-kcalorie rice crackers or fruit, so that you will not end up heading for the candy machine if the urge to snack strikes when you are not at home.
- *Drink a glass of water or other low-kcalorie beverage just before eating.* It will help fill you up.
- *Drink plenty of water or other low-kcalorie fluids throughout the day.*
- *Plan ahead before you go out to eat.* If you are going to a restaurant, you can decide ahead of time that you are going to have fish or some other light dish. If the portion seems very large, ask for a "doggie bag" and divide the serving before you start to eat. This will help you reduce the temptation to overindulge.
- *If you will be eating at a friend's house, avoid high-fat hors d'oeuvre and stick politely but firmly to small portions.*
- *Eat a small, low-kcalorie snack before going out.* This will help you stick with your eating plan.
- *Avoid the temptation to binge by purchasing a single portion when it is time to treat yourself to a favorite food.*

Learning to enjoy. Foods that are low in kcalories do not have to be tasteless or monotonous.[3,19]

DO

- *Invest in one or two good "light" cuisine cookbooks* and follow the suggestions in Chapter 5, Lipids, for reducing the fat in favorite dishes you already cook.
- *Pay attention to aesthetics.* Foods served attractively are much more appealing to the senses than foods dished onto the plate with little thought given to color and form.
- *Consider buying small dinner dishes or serve food on salad plates.* Smaller portions look bigger when served on smaller plates.
- *Consider the impact of color on your eating habits.* Color is known to influence emotions and appetite. Red and orange tones stimulate the desire to eat, whereas blue and green tones suppress the appetite. If you are in the market for new dinnerware, you may want to consider these facts in selecting colors and patterns.

Principles of Energy Output

Obesity experts frequently remind us that heavy people are less active than lean ones. Additionally, overweight people tend to overestimate their level of activity while underestimating the amount of food they consume.[13] Inactivity sets up a vicious cycle that promotes additional weight gain. The less people move, the fewer kcalories they use and the more weight they gain. The heavier people get, the more quickly they tire while performing physical activities, so they tend to move less, which leads to further weight gain, and so on.

NUTRI NUGGET Exercise uses fat stored in adipose tissue throughout the entire body, not just around the "trouble spot." Spot reducing doesn't work. Want proof? "If spot reducing worked, people who chew gum would have skinny faces." (Covert Bailey, author of *The New Fit or Fat*.)

The combination of inactivity and excessive kcalorie intake can cause weight gain to escalate rapidly. Lifelong weight control depends in part on becoming more active. Exercise not only helps you take weight off, it keeps it off by increasing your body's ability to burn fat.[1,2,9,17]

Awareness of activity. Developing awareness of your activity patterns is just as important for changing energy output as recognizing your eating patterns is for controlling energy intake. Once again, the first step in cultivating awareness is to keep a diary. This time, instead of listing all foods eaten, the diary will focus on activity.

DO

- *Keep an activity diary for several days.*
- *List how much time you spend in various activities.*
- *Estimate how far you walk* from your car to class, your office, or the grocery store.
- *Keep track of any purposeful exercise routine.*

Strategies for Modifying Energy Output

Develop an understanding of how much activity it takes to burn off a given food item or a pound of fat. Many people sabotage their own weight loss efforts by deciding that if they exercise on a given day, they do not have to restrict their food intake that day. Unfortunately, our bodies are much more fuel efficient than some people realize. *After* reaching your target weight, however, you can use exercise to "purchase" treats for yourself without fear of weight gain.

ACTIVITY DIARY

March 10	Biked from dorm to school (1 mile) the big hill was tough, but I made it. After chem lab, walked to music building for chorus practice. In the p.m. it started to snow, so Greg gave me and my bike a ride home in his van.
March 11	No classes because of snow. Walked to golf course (1/2 mile), where several people were cross country skiing. Looked hard, but they were having fun. Walked to Frank's apartment (1/4 mile); he drove me home later.
March 12	Started working out to a video of "Sweatin' to the Oldies." Kept it up for 15 minutes-lots of sweat! Biked to and from school-18 minutes to get there, 24 minutes back (traffic).
March 13	23 minutes on the workout video. Took bus to school (running late because of workout); after class, walked the track with Karen: 8 times around, 30-35 minutes.

Keeping an activity diary is a good way to become aware of what you do and what you eat each day.

DO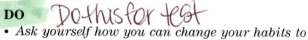

- *Ask yourself how you can change your habits to include more physical activity* once you determine your current activity level.
- *Establish a regular aerobic exercise program.* Aerobic activity burns kcalories and increases your body's fat-burning capacity.
- *Include weight training* in your fitness program to build fat-gobbling muscles as well as increase muscle and skeletal strength.
- *Stay active while sedentary.* You can increase your energy output by being more active while sitting still. While sitting at your desk you can flex your arm, leg, and back muscles. If your class schedule or job allows, you can take a brief walk once each hour. Some people take the term "relaxing" too literally. Watching TV does not have to mean being a couch potato. Doing calisthenics or using a rowing machine, stationary bike, or treadmill are just a few of the ways you can exercise while watching a favorite show.
- *Choose the road of most resistance.* Inactive people typically develop strategies to keep them

selves from using too much energy and/or effort. They usually choose the road of least resistance. You can change many parts of your daily routine into habits that use more energy (Box 11-1). Gradually they will become second nature and help you burn more kcalories.

Motivation to move. Sustaining motivation is an essential part of permanently incorporating exercise into your life.

DO

- *Select activities you enjoy and can fit easily into your lifestyle.*
- *Set realistic fitness goals.*
- *Reward yourself for reaching your goals with nonfood items or activities.*
- *Find an exercise buddy* to keep you honest when your determination weakens.
- *Start your exercise routine even if you feel tired.* If you are really too tired to exercise, you can always quit. Most likely, once you get moving you will feel revitalized and be able to complete your workout.

Support

Making permanent lifestyle changes is a major challenge. The more support dieters get, the better they tend to do. Ideally, family and friends should assist the dieter in any way they can. Sometimes, however, others have their own agendas that restrict the amount of support they can lend. For example, overweight friends and family members may be resentful of the dieter's attempt to deal with a weight problem and unconsciously will sabotage his or her efforts. Friends and loved ones may feel threatened by a change in the *status quo* and try to undermine, rather than bolster, the dieter's resolve. Often an organized weight loss program is a dieter's best support system. In an appropriately designed program a dieter can get encouragement from other participants, from staff members, and from successful graduates.

Over the long term. In addition to support during the weight loss process, many weight reduction experts now acknowledge that dieters need long-term support. Taking a lesson from Alcoholics Anonymous (that a person with an addictive behavior disorder is never really cured; s/he is simply in recovery), Weight Watchers always encourages members who have reached their goal weight and completed the maintenance program to attend monthly or even weekly meetings. The aim of this program is to provide lifelong support for people who face a weight control challenge and need support when the stress of everyday life tempts them to abandon their new lifestyle. This service is free of charge as long as the member remains within 2 pounds of his/her original personal weight loss goal.

When You Need More Personalized Help

If you have completed a reliable weight loss program only to regain weight for the umpteenth time, and you still are determined to be trim, you should find a therapist who specializes in weight control. The cause(s) of your overeating may be so deeply rooted in your emotional makeup that behavior modification alone will not be effective. For example, people who eat in response to stress may be able to gradually alter their behavior once they recognize it. On the other hand, people who suffer from deeply repressed anger, low self-esteem, or fear of their sexuality usually gain little benefit from behavior modification. To achieve long-term weight control, they need to deal with the true causes of their overeating.

CHOOSING A WEIGHT CONTROL PROGRAM

Deciding how to achieve lasting weight control depends both on how much weight you need to lose and on the factors that cause you to gain weight. If you have 5 to 10 pounds to lose, eat a generally healthy diet, and lead a sedentary lifestyle, all you may need is to start a regular exercise program. If you have more than 10 pounds to lose, you usually need to combine a reducing diet with an exercise program.

Self-Help Programs

Each year the marketplace is flooded with a seemingly endless supply of new diet books, articles, tapes, "miracle" pills, "weight-reducing" suits, passive exercise devices, and diet programs. Fortunately, you do not need to be a health expert to find out what works and what does not. You do need to be aware that successful weight control requires time, effort, and commitment. The most important thing is to proceed with caution. Be suspicious of any program, food, drug, or device that promises very rapid (more than 2 pounds per week) and/or effortless weight loss.

Comparing Commercial Programs

There are many commercial weight-loss programs. If you decide to go this route, you need to be a wise consumer. First of all, be wary of endorsements! People may have had initial success with a program, but how long did they keep the weight off? Celebrity endorsements are no guarantee of success. Celebrities are paid for their support. Do not let your opinion of their acting, writing, or athletic abilities influence your decision. A simple guideline is: If it sounds too good to be true, it probably is. Although most of us would love to find an easy way to stay in shape, the truth is that it takes work. Unfortunately, it is easier to sell people a miracle pill than to convince them that the only sure solution is a lifelong change in diet and exercise habits.

As the result of unethical practices during the 1980s, Congress in 1988 launched a 3-year investigation of the multibillion-dollar diet industry. In 1990 the Federal Trade Commission began its own investigation of advertising claims made by commercial weight-loss programs. Their findings led to revisions in the laws governing these programs' marketing techniques.[25]

If after evaluating all the available information you still believe a commercial or medically supervised diet program is the way for you to lose weight, proceed with caution. Before enrolling, visit several programs. After you leave each location, use the checklist on p. 214 to help you evaluate the program. An "ideal" program will have all "yes" answers; any "no" answers are cause for concern and perhaps further investigation.

Making the Commitment

A healthy body is yours if you want it. Yes, it takes time and commitment, but the rewards are often far beyond those you anticipate. Success with weight control frequently has a positive impact on other areas of a dieter's life. Not only do successful dieters/exercisers feel better about their physical appearance, they also tend to feel better about themselves in general. Conquering a weight problem teaches people that they have the ability to determine their own destiny. This often makes them more willing to take risks in job situations and interpersonal relationships. Think about this before you reach for that extra serving of food or tell yourself you'll begin an exercise program "tomorrow."

Too Thin To Be "In"

Thin is definitely "in," but there are some people who must fight to keep weight on. Unless there is a medical reason for their thinness, these people generally are active ectomorphs in their teens and twenties. They usually find it easier to keep weight on once their metabo-

status quo existing situation

To Gain weight - eat carbohydrates

BOX 11-2 Checklist for Evaluating Weight Loss Programs

CLIENT EVALUATION

YES   NO
- ☐ ☐ A preliminary health exam is given.
- ☐ ☐ It includes at least a complete physical and blood and urine tests.

CREDENTIALS OF STAFF

- ☐ ☐ The people who run the program are registered dietitians (RD) and/or medical doctors (MD).

DIET

- ☐ ☐ The diet provides a minimum of 1200 kcalories per day for women and 1800 kcalories for men.
- ☐ ☐ The diet is high in carbohydrate, moderate in protein content, and low in fat (30% or fewer kcalories from fat).
- ☐ ☐ The diet includes all food groups (avoid the carbohydrate-free diets that were popular during the 1970s).
- ☐ ☐ The diet has a varied and flexible menu plan so you can substitute foods you like for those you dislike. (Variety helps fight monotony and feelings of deprivation that can cause you to fall off the diet wagon.)

EXERCISE

- ☐ ☐ The program includes an exercise plan.

SUPPORT

- ☐ ☐ The program includes a substantial behavior modification component that teaches you how to keep weight off by changing how, when, and what you eat.
- ☐ ☐ The program is a balance of diet, exercise, and behavior modification.

YES   NO
- ☐ ☐ The program includes a maintenance phase to help you make the transition from a reducing diet to a maintenance diet. (Several studies have shown that the longer and more personalized the behavior modification and maintenance programs, the more likely dieters are to keep weight off.)

COST

- ☐ ☐ The total cost of the program is clearly specified.
- ☐ ☐ The cost includes the behavior modification program.
- ☐ ☐ The cost includes the maintenance program.

PAST RECORD

- ☐ ☐ A high percentage of people who enter the program complete it.
- ☐ ☐ A high percentage of people who complete the program achieve their weight loss goal.
- ☐ ☐ A high percentage of participants maintain their weight loss 1, 3, and 5 years after completion.
- ☐ ☐ A low percentage of people have adverse physical or psychological experiences.

GENERAL ISSUES

- ☐ ☐ The staff took time to answer any questions.
- ☐ ☐ The program puts more emphasis on weight loss than on selling prepackaged food items.
- ☐ ☐ The staff provided information about long-term success rates.

Adapted from *Consumer Reports* rates commercial weight loss programs, *Consumer Reports*, June 1993, pp 353-358.

---

lism starts to slow in their thirties. But what can they do in the meantime? If you are extra-lean, a balanced diet is a good start. Piling on the kcalories in the form of fat-laden fast food and desserts is just as unhealthful for a lean person as it is for someone who is overfat. To keep weight on, be sure you eat regular meals and sufficient snacks during the day to meet your energy requirements. You probably need to keep your fat intake at 30%, but most of it should come from heart-friendly unsaturated fat. Supplementing your exercise program with weight training can help provide more bulk in the form of muscle. A phone call to the American Dietetic Association Hotline can help an extra-lean person as much as it helped Ted lose weight.

IN TODAY'S WORLD

In our body image–obsessed society, weight watchers face a daily challenge to control the external factors that trigger overeating. Holidays and special events, however, can undermine even the most determined dieter's resolve. What follow are some practical tips for dealing with the food fests that are typical of holidays and celebrations.

NUTRI NUGGET According to the American Dietetic Association, the average American gains 5 to 7 pounds during the winter holiday season. For many, the overindulging begins with leftover Halloween candy and does not end until the last of the holiday debris is cleaned up on January 2.

Streamline for Less Stress

For people who do the planning and meal preparation, the hectic holiday pace often serves to escalate their stress levels. For someone who has a weight control problem, this added stress can trigger more overeating. If this description fits you, there are definite steps you can take to make sure you have a low-stress, healthful celebration.[13]

- Share responsibilities for holiday celebrations.
- Develop realistic expectations. Breathtaking decorations and gourmet foods don't make a holiday memorable. Sharing time and activities do.
- Don't let others set your agenda for you. Start your own holiday traditions!
- Have dinner catered. Many grocery store chains now offer this service.

Fat-Wise Gifts for Friends

- A basket of fruits, exotic vegetables, and/or herbs
- Assorted pastas with a jar or two of gourmet sauce
- Gourmet sauces for pasta, barbecue recipes, or dessert; exotic salsa (for example, cactus salsa)
- A dozen specialty bagels, gourmet English muffins, or a loaf of fancy bread
- A bottle of real maple syrup and a package of a gourmet pancake mix
- A gift certificate for a frozen yogurt shop
- Flavored gourmet coffee or tea

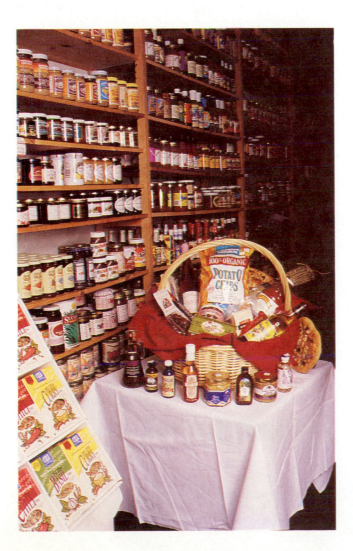

IN MY DIET

Learning to live lean at home is easier than you may think. It doesn't require major changes; you may already have incorporated some of these fat-trimming strategies while reading Chapter 5, Lipids. Here are some additional tips for planning healthful holidays at home.

Help on the Home Front

- Prepare some new low-fat, low-kcalorie dishes along with treasured family favorites.
- Be butter-wise! You can decrease fat by 25% to 33% in all of your cooking without affecting the quality of the finished product. If your recipe calls for 1 cup of butter, use ¾ to ⅔ cup instead.
- Use low-fat cheeses in all your sauces and casseroles.
- Use Neufchatel 25% reduced-fat cream cheese for baking. Lower-fat versions, like 50% reduced-fat cream cheese, do not cook well.
- Plan to have leftovers of healthy, low-fat foods only. Or, if you can't enjoy the food as much as you'd like on the holiday itself because of all the hubbub, allow yourself one meal's worth of leftovers to sit and savor.
- Give away or freeze all excess forbidden foods and treats.

Recipe Resources and Rewrites

There is an abundance of low-fat, low-kcalorie holiday dishes and recipes; some are listed below. Other good sources are the November and December issues of *Sunset*, *Eating Well*, and *Cooking Light* magazines from both the current and previous years.

Hors d'oeuvre. Even these tiny tidbits can quickly total up to big kcalories. For example, a miniature quiche contains about 150 kcalories and 15 grams of

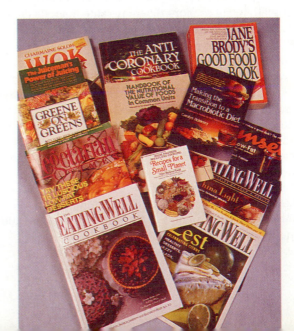

fat. One ounce of chips has about 100 kcalories and 9 grams of fat. Stuffed mushrooms can be anywhere from 75 to 125 kcalories, depending on size and filling. Here are some creative ways to take the edge off your appetite without paying such high kcalorie bills.

- Prepare a *vegetable tray* using unusual vegetables like steamed baby squash, snow peas or snap peas, sweet red and yellow peppers, or jicama.
- Make a *low-calorie dip* by reconstituting evaporated ranch dressing with nonfat milk and low-fat yogurt in place of the whole milk and mayonnaise called for on the packet. Chill for a couple of hours before serving. This version has 8 kcalories per tablespoon compared with 100 kcalories in the original recipe. For a festive touch, serve dip in hollowed-out red, yellow, orange, and/or green bell peppers.
- Save kcalories and fat wherever you can by serving *low-fat cheeses, crackers, chips, and dips.*
- *Other bottled skinny dips:* barbecue sauce and honey mustard have about 10 kcalories per dip (1½ to 2 teaspoons). Sweet and sour sauce is an additional 5 kcalories per dip.
- Your instructor may have lower-kcalorie recipes to share with you.

Dessert. When it comes to kcalories, dessert is a bottomless pit. Of the traditional holiday offerings, the most healthful is pumpkin pie at 200 kcalories for ⅛ of a pie, compared with pecan pie at 450 kcalories per serving. (But watch out for the whipped cream topping at 50 kcalories a tablespoon.)

If you are really on a strict kcalorie budget, nonfat frozen pumpkin yogurt, available at many local yogurt shops, runs only 90 to 100 kcalories per half-cup serving. For a more festive dessert, sprinkle it with a little crystallized ginger.

Dealing with Dining Out — *Know*

Eat a Snack Before you go

- Before the event, mentally review the temptations, plan what you'll allow yourself to eat, and stick to it.
- Offer to bring an hors d'oeuvre, side dish, or dessert that you can make to suit your diet restrictions.
- Don't arrive famished.
- Politely but firmly refuse well-meant pressure to overindulge.
- Eat small portions of everything. Remember: No second helpings of high-fat dishes!

Alcohol Alert

Whether eating out or at home, be extremely careful about drinking alcohol. It:

- Adds nonnutritive kcalories (7 kcalories per gram)
- Lowers your resistance to dietary temptations
- Interferes with medication, coordination, and judgment

Alcohol kcalories add up quickly. One beer averages 150 kcalories, a 3½-ounce glass of wine is about 75 kcalories, and 1 ounce of hard liquor is about 100 kcalories. Watch out for fruit-flavored wine coolers; they're usually high in sugar. So use alcohol sparingly, and consider alternatives like nonalcoholic brews and wines.

Holiday Weight Training

Plan! Plan! Plan!

Planning is the key to making it through the holidays healthy and happy. This includes planning for exercise and meals as well as for the traditional holiday events. You can plan to splurge on Thanksgiving, Christmas, Kwasanda, Hanukkah, and New Year's without paying for it later if you follow the guidelines below.

Save up for a splurge by:

- Paying close attention to your everyday diet. Try to limit fat to 25% of kcalories.
- Reduce your daily intake by 50 kcalories (for example, one small cookie, ½ ounce of chips). This adds up to 350 calories per week, which equals 1 piece of dessert per event.
- Make time for a daily exercise session, especially on the holiday itself (for example, mall walking, gentle aerobics, stationary cycling, dancing).
- Plan activities where eating is not the primary focus (for example, tree trimming, caroling, visiting hospitalized people, attending plays or movies).
- Focus on sharing with others who are less fortunate. In the San Francisco Bay Area, many weight-conscious people belong to a group known as Dieters Feed the Hungry. Rather than gorging on high-kcalorie treats, these people give food or the cash equivalent to the local food bank.
- Enlist a buddy to keep you honest. It can make the effort a lot more fun!

Give Yourself Permission to Eat

According to dietitian and eating specialist Ellyn Satter, MS, MSW, RD, trying not to eat can add to your stress. In fact, guilt about overeating and the attendant feelings of deprivation when you exercise self-control can actually spur you to eat more. Deactivate the guilt trap by giving yourself permission to eat and learning to savor those foods you choose to indulge in. Practice the focused eating exercise described below to enhance your enjoyment of food and curb "conveyor-belt" eating. Remember to repeat to yourself that you may eat as much food as you want.

Focused Eating Exercise[26]

1. Collect about five small crackers.
2. Allow yourself to examine their texture, color, and aroma.
3. Close your eyes and exhale.

4. Keeping your eyes closed, breathe in deeply, filling your entire chest. Simultaneously roll back and lift your shoulders to increase your lung capacity; continue to inhale.

5. Now slowly sample one cracker. Describe to yourself how it tastes and how the flavor and texture of this food affect your appetite.

6. Using a second cracker, move it around your mouth, considering how it feels to your tongue and how quickly it seems to be dissolving in your mouth.

7. Consider what your reactions would be like if the cracker were a chocolate chip cookie.

8. Learn to focus before you take your first bite.

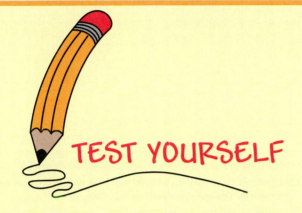

TEST YOURSELF

1. In terms of pounds per week, what is the safest rate of weight loss?
2. List three reasons why Americans tend to be overweight.
3. Why don't crash diets work?
4. Should children be put on reducing diets? Why or why not?
5. List three major pitfalls of most diets.
6. Why can crash dieting leave you fatter than before?
7. List three ways to cope with the temptation to overeat on holidays and during other celebrations.
8. What is behavior modification?
9. What can happen if you eat while watching TV or performing other tasks?
10. What might motivate family members and friends to sabotage your weight loss efforts?

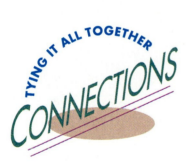

TYING IT ALL TOGETHER

CONNECTIONS

1. Assume your body weight is appropriate for your height. How can you apply some of the behavior modification techniques you have learned in this chapter to your fitness program? Give three examples.
2. How does a good exercise program improve the nutrient utilization of someone on a reducing diet?
3. Assume you eat a reasonably healthy diet. If you needed to lose 10 pounds and had to choose between changing your diet and changing your exercise habits, which would you change and why?
4. Argue (a) in favor of and (b) against the statement: "Some people are just born fat."
5. Assume you have decided to join a commercial weight loss clinic. List five features you should look for before you sign on the dotted line.
6. What eating habits are beneficial to both people who are trying to lose weight and people who are trying to gain weight?
7. Why do people who are trying to gain weight need to watch fat intake?

REFERENCES

1. Alfred B et al: Exercise is the key component of successful long-term weight control, *Journal of the American Medical Association* 2760:2547-2553, 1988.

2. Allisen PE et al: Writing a weight control program. In *Fitness for life—an individual approach*, ed 3, Dubuque, Ia, 1993, WC Brown.

3. American Dietetic Association Lean Toward Health, American Dietetic Association Foundation, Chicago, 1992.

4. American Dietetic Association position on very-low-calorie weight loss diets, *Journal of the American Dietetic Association* 90:722-724, 1990.

5. American Dietetic Association position on optimal weight as a health promotion strategy, *Journal of the American Dietetic Association* 89:1814-1817, 1989.

6. Bagley CE: Government should strengthen regulation of the weight loss industry, *Journal of the American Dietetic Association* 91:1255-1257, 1991.

7. Bray G: Obesity. In *Present knowledge in nutrition*, ed 6, Washington, DC, 1990, International Life Sciences Institute Nutrition Foundation, pp 23-38.

8. Buchard C, Perusse C: Heredity and body fat. In *Annual Review of Nutrition* 8:259-277, 1988.

9. Calloway W et al: A quartet of approaches to obesity, *Patient Care* 26(14):157,165, 1992.

10. Castanguay TW, Stern JS: Hunger and appetite. In *Present knowledge in nutrition*, ed 6, Washington, DC, 1990, International Life Sciences Institute Nutrition Foundation.

11. Dietz WH, Gortmaker SL: Do we fatten our children at the television set? Obesity and television viewing in children and adolescents, *Pediatrics* 75:805-810, 1985.

12. Fabulous feasts: how to pare Thanksgiving calories and still feast deliciously, *University of California at Berkeley Wellness Letter* 19(2):3, 1992.

13. Forbes GB: Diet and exercise in obese subjects: self-reported versus controlled measurements, *Nutrition Reviews* 51:296, 1993.

14. Forbes GB: Exercise and lean body weight: the influence of body weight, *Nutrition Reviews* 50:157-161, 1992.

15. Gortmaker SL et al: Social and economic consequences of obesity. *New England Journal of Medicine* 329:1008-1013, 1993.

16. Heavy news, *University of California at Berkeley Wellness Letter* 10(5):2, 1994.

17. Lavery MA, Loewy JW: Identifying predictive variables for long-term weight change after participation in a weight loss program, *Journal of the American Dietetic Association* 93:1017-1024, 1993.

18. NIH Task Force Report on the safety of very-low-calorie diets, *Journal of the American Medical Association* 270:967-972, 1993.

19. Pi-Sunyer FX: The role of very-low-calorie diets in obesity, *American Journal of Clinical Nutrition* 56:240S-245S, 1992.

20. Pi-Sunyer FX: Usefulness of low-calorie foods for weight control, *Nutrition Reviews* 48:94-98, 1990.

21. Rand C: Breakfast eating and weight loss success, *American Journal of Clinical Nutrition* 55:645, 1992.

22. Rand C, Kuidau J: Socioeconomic status (SES) and race influence both the prevalence and acceptance of obesity, *International Journal of Eating Disorders* 9:329-334, 1990.

23. Robinson I et al: Obesity, weight loss, and health, *Journal of the American Dietetic Association* 93:445-449, 1993.

24. Rodin J et al: Weight cycling and body fat distribution, *International Journal of Obesity* 14:303-307, 1990.

25. Rosenberg I (ed): National Institutes of Health Technology Assessment conference statement: Methods for voluntary weight loss and control, Mar 30-Apr 1, 1992, *Nutrition Reviews* 50(11):340-345, 1992.

26. Satter E: Symposia: the feeding relationship: implications for dietitians. Paper presented at the American Dietetic Association annual meeting, Washington, DC, Oct 1992.

CHAPTER

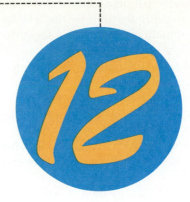

12

LIFE CYCLE

Nutrition From Infancy Through Adulthood

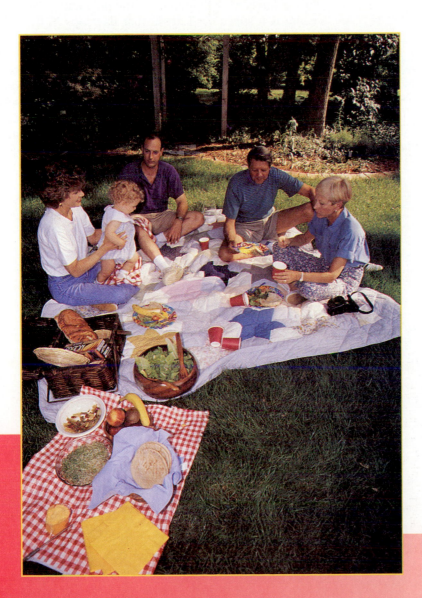

Food is our common ground, a universal experience.

— *James Beard*, Beard on Food

The impact of nutrition on our health begins before we are born and continues until we die. The basic nutrients we require remain essentially the same throughout our lives, but we need different quantities of nutrients to accommodate the metabolic and physiological changes that occur as we age.

Thus far we have concentrated on the nutrient requirements of healthy young to middle-aged adults. In this chapter we will explore how nutrient needs vary with age. From a nutritional standpoint, for purposes of this text we divide the human life cycle into seven categories:

1. The fetal period, which is represented by the expectant mother's nutrient needs
2. Infancy
3. Toddler years (1 to 4)
4. Childhood (5 to 12)
5. Teenage years
6. Young to middle-aged adult (20 to 50)
7. Older adult (age 51 and older)
   The RDA include eight additional age subdivisions.[19]

FETAL DEVELOPMENT

How does nutrition affect a person's health before s/he is conceived?   In an ideal world every child would be a planned child. Among other benefits, planning a pregnancy allows the prospective mother to be sure she is physically fit enough to have a healthy baby. A woman who is contemplating pregnancy should have a general physical checkup. She also should assess her weight, diet, fitness level, and overall health habits and should make any necessary changes at least a couple of months before trying to conceive.

Before Conception

A prospective mother's weight should be as close as possible to her healthy weight. Weight more than 10% below or 20% above normal is associated with a greater risk of complications for the pregnancy and birth. Body weight also can compromise fertility. Both very thin and very fat women often have trouble conceiving, let alone maintaining a healthy pregnancy.

Women with good diet and exercise habits tend to be at or near their healthy weight. But weight control is not the only reason to establish healthy eating patterns before conceiving. Nutrient-dependent developmental events occur even in the first few weeks of pregnancy, before most women know they are pregnant. Fig. 12-1 shows the stages of fetal development.

A woman's prepregnancy nutritional status influences her ability to grow a healthy **placenta,** which in turn influences the outcome of the pregnancy. The placenta is a specialized organ that develops in the first month of pregnancy. It carries nutrients, hormones, antibodies, and oxygen from the mother's bloodstream to the fetus. Because the fetus is growing in an enclosed environment and has no way to dispose of metabolic waste, the placenta also transports waste products from the fetus to the mother's bloodstream for detoxification and disposal. Additionally, the placenta manufactures more than 60 of its own enzymes and several

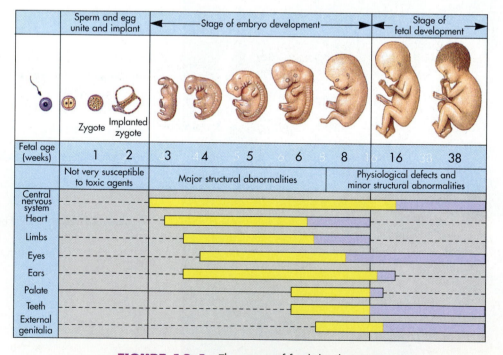

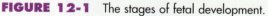

FIGURE 12-1 The stages of fetal development.

hormones needed to sustain the pregnancy.

Poor placental function leads to a poor pregnancy outcome—for example, a miscarriage or a low–birth weight baby. Once formed, a poorly functioning placenta cannot be repaired by good nutrition during the remainder of the pregnancy. (A pregnant woman with poor eating habits should make every effort to improve her diet, but she needs to realize that some harm already may have occurred.)[15] Poor maternal nutrition also can directly affect the developing fetus. Impaired development of a female fetus can permanently decrease her capacity to store nutrients, which in turn will jeopardize her own pregnancies.

Unlike poor diet, poor physical fitness does not directly affect the initial phases of pregnancy and can be improved with a carefully designed exercise program during the pregnancy. Because pregnancy can bring about many physiological changes, such as nausea and increased fatigue, staying in shape is easier for a woman with a well-established fitness program than for an exercise newcomer. Pregnancy and childbirth are less taxing for physically fit women than for those who are out of shape, so it is worth the effort to get in shape!

What about the father's role?   Alcoholism, drug abuse, and exposure to certain environmental chemicals are known to reduce male fertility and in some cases have been suspected as the cause of stillbirths and birth defects. Such problems usually were associated with the mother until the March of Dimes announced in 1993 that a higher percentage of fertility problems and birth defects than previously believed were the result of damaged sperm (about 40% of cases).[7] The new emphasis on the role of sperm in producing healthy children underscores the need for males who are contemplating fatherhood to practice sound health habits: eating a balanced diet, giving up tobacco, drinking in moderation or not at all, and taking precautions when working with environmental chemicals.[7]

During Pregnancy

Contrary to popular belief, pregnant women do not need to "eat for two." In fact, during the first 3 months a pregnant woman does not need any additional kcalories. A very modest additional 300 kcalories per day is all she requires from the beginning of the fourth month until delivery. Like the rest of the expectant mother's diet, these extra kcalories should be supplied by foods of high nutrient density and should provide:[19]

- An additional 10 g of protein and 3 mg of zinc per day to meet the needs of fetal tissue synthesis
- Extra thiamin, riboflavin, niacin, vitamin B_6, magnesium, and iodine to support the increase in energy metabolism
- Extra folate, B_{12}, and iron to support increased synthesis of red blood cells
- Extra calcium and phosphorus both to mineralize

the fetal bones and to lay down enough extra minerals in the mother's skeleton to support lactation See the RDA on the inside front cover for details on how much of each nutrient is required during pregnancy.

NUTRI NUGGET **Pregnant women often appear to be anemic because their red blood cell content is diluted by their greatly increased blood fluid volume. In reality, iron is conserved during pregnancy, because of both a lack of menstrual iron losses and physiological changes that enhance its retention.**

Do pregnant women need a vitamin/mineral supplement?   The 1989 RDA state that vitamin/mineral supplements are unnecessary during pregnancy, provided the woman is in good health and that her past diet was and present diet is nutritious.[19] In practice, most obstetricians advise their patients to take a vitamin/mineral supplement specifically formulated for pregnant women while trying to conceive and throughout their pregnancy. Not only does this ensure that the mother gets all the vitamins and minerals she needs, it also may prevent anemia and, if started before pregnancy, may prevent **spina bifida,** a birth defect in which part or all of the spine does not form properly. (See the discussion of folate in Chapter 7, Vitamins.)

Pregnant women need to consume more fluid as well as more food. Fluid needs increase very early in pregnancy because of a 25% increase in maternal blood volume as well as the formation of **amniotic fluid** (the fluid in which the developing baby floats). Pregnant women also need more fluid to aid in waste removal. As the fetus develops, the mother's body will be processing an increasing amount of fetal waste products. One of the best fluids for a pregnant woman to consume is water. She also should add to her daily diet an extra glass of milk to supply protein, phosphorus, and calcium.

NUTRI QUIZ How would a vegan or a woman with lactose intolerance get the extra calcium and protein needed for pregnancy?

Pregnant women have a tendency to retain fluid in their body tissues **(edema).** Earlier generations of physicians tried to combat this tendency by restricting their pregnant patients' sodium intake. It is now recognized that a certain amount of edema is normal during pregnancy. The increased fluid retention in body tissues, together with the increased blood volume and formation of amniotic fluid, actually *increase* a pregnant woman's sodium requirement. Because the American diet provides more than enough salt to meet the needs of both pregnant and nonpregnant women, however, there is no need to add any to the diet.

Weight Gain

Restricting maternal weight gain in the belief that it would result in a healthier pregnancy was popular during the 1940s and 1950s. Modern health care specialists, however, realize that adequate maternal weight gain is essential to produce a healthy newborn of appropriate size and weight. The National Academy of Science recommends that pregnant women gain from 25 to 30 pounds. If they are 10% or more above their ideal weight, they should restrict their gain to 16 to 24 pounds. Underweight women and teenagers should gain at least the amount of weight suggested and more, if possible. Box 12-1 shows how the 25 pounds typically gained during pregnancy are distributed.

The hormonal and emotional changes that accompany pregnancy affect many women's appetites. It is estimated that between 75% and 89% of all women suffer from morning sickness during the first 3 months of their pregnancy, and nearly every pregnant woman reports a variety of food aversions and cravings.

Morning Sickness

Morning sickness, that unmistakable sign of early pregnancy that has puzzled generations of scientists, is still not fully understood. Researchers appear, however, to be getting closer to a definitive answer. According to some experts, morning sickness is no accident; it is an adaptation to prevent women from eating foods that contain substances that can damage the fetus.[11,22] The nausea may be a reaction to a pregnant woman's intensified sense of smell. A highly acute *olfactory* sense may well be a way to prevent a pregnant woman from consuming toxins.[11] The top 10 offenders are: coffee, onion, garlic, herbs and spices, Brussels sprouts, barbecued foods, fried foods, fish, chili peppers, mustard, and canned meats and fish. Newly pregnant women show a definite preference for bland foods such as cottage cheese, toast, and roasted turkey or chicken breast.

NUTRI NUGGET Many studies have found that women who do *not* experience any morning sickness during a pregnancy are three times more likely to miscarry than those who do.

What about food cravings? Food cravings occur much later in pregnancy, after the fetus has developed. Cravings are much more individual than aversions and appear to having nothing to do with protecting the fetus. Experts believe food cravings are related more to hormonal changes or emotional needs than to nutritional necessity.[11] The exception is **pica**, the eating of nonnutritive substances, such as ice and clay, which often signals a deficiency of iron or other minerals.

Habits to Avoid

To ensure a smooth pregnancy and a healthy baby, pregnant women need to steer clear of substances that can harm the developing fetus.

Caffeine. Currently there is no general agreement among experts about caffeine intake during pregnancy. Consumption of more than 2 or 3 cups of caffeinated beverages per day,[4] particularly during the first 6 weeks of pregnancy, is associated with an increased risk of miscarriage and low–birth weight babies. If you are pregnant or are trying to become pregnant, restrict your caffeine intake and consult your physician for more advice.[6]

Alcohol. The best choice a pregnant woman can make is to abstain from alcohol during her pregnancy. Excessive consumption of alcohol during pregnancy results in a disorder known as **fetal alcohol syndrome** (FAS), which involves poor fetal and infant growth, physical deformities, and mental retardation. A milder form of this condition is known as fetal alcohol effect (FAE). Some experts believe pregnant women can tolerate small amounts of alcohol; others say even a sip can kill enough fetal brain cells to dull mental ability. To the American Academy of Pediatrics there are no two ways about it: the AAP's position is that pregnant women must abstain completely from alcohol because there is no amount that is known to be safe.

Smoking. In addition to abstaining from alcohol, pregnant women should strictly avoid smoking. Some studies even suggest that pregnant women should stay away from secondhand smoke. Mothers who smoke have long been known to produce low–birth weight babies, which decreases a child's chance for survival and impairs lung development. Some studies indicate that the children of women who smoke during pregnancy have an increased incidence of respiratory diseases.

BOX 12-1	Distribution of Weight Gain During Pregnancy	
Source	**Pounds**
Baby	7.5
Placenta	1.5
Amniotic fluid	2.0
Blood	3.5
Other fluid	3.0
Breast tissue	1.0
Uterus	2.5
Fat	4.0
Total	25.0

Drugs. Pregnant women also need to avoid all prescription and nonprescription drugs unless advised otherwise by their physician. The typical side effects of some drugs can be dangerous to a pregnant woman or her unborn baby.[15]

INFANCY

The first year of life is characterized by rapid growth and development, and by the change from a totally liquid diet to one that includes solid foods. Below is a brief summary of infant feeding recommendations.

Recommendations for Feeding Infants

- Breast milk for as much of the first year of life as possible

From 4 to 6 months and after, the diet also should include:

- Iron-fortified baby cereals (to prevent anemia)
- Strained, unsalted meats, fish, and poultry to supply readily absorbable iron
- Strained, unsalted, unsweetened fruits and vegetables to supply vitamin C
- Water, rather than other liquids, to quench thirst; juices only occasionally

Breast Milk

During most of this century food manufacturers and health experts alike pushed new mothers to abandon breast-feeding for bottle feeding.[2] By the 1950s nearly 70% of all infants were bottle fed. The tide turned dramatically during the 1980s. Nutritionists and the American Academy of Pediatrics now recommend that infants be fed breast milk for as much of the first year as possible.[3]

Why breast milk? Formula manufacturers try to "humanize" cow's milk by diluting its protein content and adding sugar and fat. Even the best commercial formulas, however, do not meet the infant's nutritional needs as effectively as breast milk. (Table 12-1 provides a nutritional comparison of cow-based infant formula with human breast milk.)

Benefits of breast-feeding for the infant. A breast-fed infant benefits in many ways. Among them are:

- Easily digested protein
- Correct cholesterol content
- Specialized mineral transport proteins
- Transfer of antibodies, which builds immunity
- Transfer of hormones, which aids in metabolism and in intestinal and nerve maturation
- Transfer of antibacterial, antiviral, and possibly antiparasitic factors
- The nutrient composition of breast milk changes as the baby grows. For example, protein content is highest during the first month of life when growth is fastest; it falls by about one third as growth slows.
- Prevention of obesity. Because a nursing mother cannot tell how much milk her infant is consuming, the baby learns to eat only until its appetite is satisfied. In contrast, mothers who bottle feed tend to urge their infants to consume all the formula they offer. This can result in a fatter baby as well as a child who ignores its internal cues for food intake.

olfactory pertaining to the sense of smell

TABLE 12-1 **Comparison of the Nutrient Content in 1 Liter of Breast Milk, Cow Milk, and Cow-Based Formula Milk**

	Human Milk	Cow Milk	Cow-Based Formula
Kcal	690	660	700
Protein (g)	9	35	15
Fat (g)	45	37	36
Carbohydrate (g)	68	49	72
Lactose (g)*	68	49	49*
Minerals			
Calcium (mg)	340	1170	445
Phosphorus (mg)	140	920	300
Sodium (mEq)	7	22	6

*The amount of lactose varies from brand to brand. Some manufacturers add lactose to increase their product's carbohydrate content; some use other sugars, like sucrose.

- Breast-fed babies have a lower rate of ear infections than bottle-fed ones.

Babies also benefit emotionally from breast-feeding because of the closeness that develops between them and their mother. The infant learns that humans can be relied on to provide love and care.

NUTRI NUGGET Infants who are breast-fed exclusively for the first 4 months of life have half as many ear infections as those who are bottle fed or have supplementary solid foods added to their diet.[3]

Maternal benefits of breast-feeding. Like her baby, a nursing mother derives both physical and psychological benefits from breast-feeding (Fig. 12-2).[3]

- Breast-feeding helps a new mother lose the fat her body stored during pregnancy.
- Nursing releases hormones that help the uterus recover from pregnancy and childbirth. Also, breast-feeding lets a new mom get some much-needed rest because she must sit quietly for several hours each day while she feeds her baby.

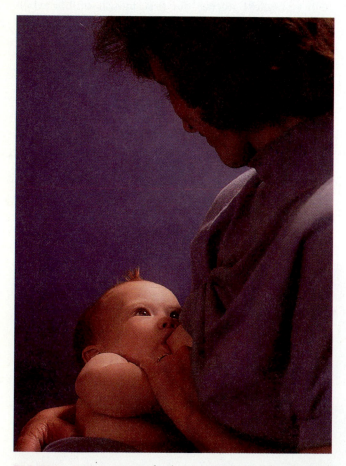

FIGURE 12-2 Breast-feeding provides benefits for both mother and baby.

- Breast-feeding fosters mother-child bonding. Similar bonding can be achieved by holding a baby during bottle feedings. Whether breast or bottle fed, all babies should be held while feeding.

NUTRI NUGGET About 20% of all babies, whether breast-fed or bottle fed, suffer from colic (crying and fussiness associated with gastrointestinal discomfort). A study showed that colic is often alleviated if cow milk is eliminated from the nursing mother's diet and/or from the formula of bottle-fed babies.

The Nursing Mother's Diet

Roughly 750 kcalories are needed each day to support **lactation** (production of milk for a nursing infant). About 500 of these kcalories should be supplied by the mother's diet and the remaining 250 from body fat stores. One of the best dietary sources of the extra 500 kcalories is milk to supply the required calcium. The nursing mother should continue to take pregnancy vitamin/mineral supplements to ensure that her stores of these nutrients are replenished.

Drugs can easily be passed to the infant through its mother's milk. Just as during pregnancy, a woman who is breast-feeding should not take any drug without her physician's approval. Caffeine and alcohol also pass easily through maternal milk to the infant. Women should not use either of these substances until the baby is fully weaned.

What if a woman cannot nurse her baby? After careful consideration, a new mother may decide not to nurse her baby, for either health or lifestyle reasons. She should *not* feel guilty. Commercial formulas, although not ideal, will promote normal growth and development.

Introduction of Solids

From 4 to 6 months of age and after, the infant's diet also should include iron-rich solid food to prevent anemia. Experts cite two reasons why solid foods should not be introduced until a baby is 4 to 6 months old. First, a newborn infant's gastrointestinal system is not equipped to digest and absorb solid foods. Second, early introduction of certain solids is associated with an increased incidence of food allergies in later life.[5,21]

Which solid foods should be fed first? Iron-fortified rice cereal, which is unlikely to produce an allergic reaction (**hypoallergenic**), should be the first solid food a baby is fed, followed by the gradual introduction of vegetables and meats. Many experts advise introducing fruits last to decrease the child's preference for sweet-tasting foods. For the same reason, baby foods should contain no added sources of sugar and salt. To control for allergies, only one new food should be introduced each week so that any adverse reaction can be easily detected. No mixed foods should be fed until each of the component foods has been tested.

 Reconstituting iron-fortified infant cereals using fruit juice enriched with vitamin C is an excellent way to improve a baby's iron status. Why?

Allergy Prevention

How can early introduction of solid foods predispose a baby to food allergies? During infancy, the lining of the gastrointestinal tract is unable to completely digest or to prevent absorption of large molecules, such as food proteins. Any food proteins (*antigens*) that make their way into the blood set off a chain of events similar to those used to fight disease. The body responds by producing *antibodies* to attack them. When foods containing these foreign proteins are fed at a later date the body senses the invader has returned and floods the system with antibodies, setting up an allergic reaction. Symptoms of food allergy include wheezing, a skin rash, itching, runny nose, vomiting, and/or diarrhea.

Up to 33% of Americans report they have a food allergy; the real rate, however, appears to be between 0.3% and 7.5%. The high incidence of reported food allergies reflects both the psychological reactions people have to food and food sensitivities (such as lactose intolerance) mistakenly identified as allergies. Remember: a food allergy involves the immune reaction, a food sensitivity does not.[5] For answers to specific allergy-related questions, call the AAAI Physicians' Referral & Information Line: 1-800-822-2762 (ASMA).

Food Safety

As babies reach 1 year of age, they begin to feed themselves. Self-feeding should be encouraged, despite the mess, because it is essential for development of manual dexterity, hand-eye coordination, and coordination of the tongue and jaw muscles. Certain precautions, however, are needed to ensure the child's safety.[21]

Choking prevention. Serve only tiny pieces of food to reduce the risk of choking. Offer foods that are easy to chew and to swallow, such as lifesaver-shaped cereal, bread, and bananas. Wait until your baby has at least eight teeth before allowing it to eat foods such as whole crackers on its own. No matter how many teeth a child has, however, the danger of choking is *always* present. Among the foods that are likely to choke young children are circular carrot slices, hot dogs, marshmallows, raisins, popcorn, nuts, and whole grapes. Stringy or fibrous foods, such as unpureed leafy vegetables, celery, and citrus fruits, also can be difficult

to chew and to swallow safely. Sticky foods like peanut butter and gum can lodge in a child's throat and promote choking. Any food, no matter what shape or texture, can block a baby's airway. Parents and other caregivers can learn emergency procedures for dealing with a choking victim from their local hospital or Red Cross.

Food poisoning. Children and elderly people are at greater risk from food poisoning than are young to middle-aged adults. This is because their bodies are less able to withstand the strain of dehydration that accompanies the vomiting and diarrhea induced by food poisoning. Also, what may be a relatively small dose of harmful bacteria for an adult can be an overwhelming dose for a small child. For instance, honey may contain botulism bacteria that can be fatal to infants. For this reason, honey or foods containing uncooked honey should never be given to children under 1 year of age. In Chapter 6, Proteins, we discussed procedures for hygienic food storage and preparation. Because infants cannot fight off even normal bacteria, their bottles and nipples must be sterilized for the first year of life.

Tooth Decay

Bottles should *not* be used as pacifiers! Putting a baby to bed with a bottle allows sugary liquid to pool around its teeth, eventually leading to severe tooth decay (bottle mouth). Almost as bad for a child's teeth as sucking on a bottle all night is drinking large quantities of fruit juice all day. The sugar in juice promotes a bacteria-friendly, tooth-decaying environment in the child's mouth.

Growth Rate and Energy Needs

The first year of life is when the most rapid growth occurs. In fact, a baby usually triples its birth weight by its first birthday. During their first year of life, babies have enormous appetites to meet the nutrient and energy demands of their rapid growth rate. Food intake decreases noticeably around the first birthday as growth slows, and varies widely during the remainder of childhood. At this stage wide swings in appetite are normal, but many parents worry that their children are not getting all the nutrients they need and encourage them to finish a set amount of food. This practice can lead to lifelong weight control problems by teaching the child to rely on external appetite cues, like the time of day or the presence of food. If a child is eating a nutritious diet, internal hunger cues can accurately determine how much food is needed.

> **antibodies** specialized proteins produced by the body that target and attack antigens
> **antigens** foreign substances that stimulate an immune response in the body

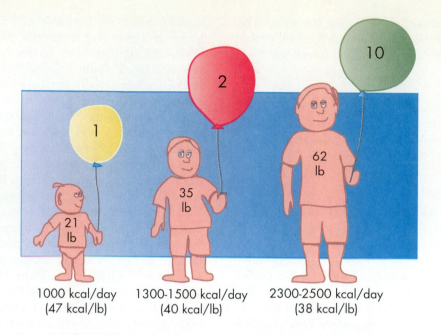

1000 kcal/day   1300-1500 kcal/day   2300-2500 kcal/day
(47 kcal/lb)   (40 kcal/lb)   (38 kcal/lb)

FIGURE 12-3 Kcalorie requirements for children at three ages.

NUTRI NUGGET The average birth weight is 7.5 pounds. By 1 year of age most babies weigh about 22.5 pounds. If this initial rate of growth were maintained, the baby would weigh about 67.5 pounds by its second birthday and a whopping 1822.5 pounds by its fifth birthday! (Real average weights at three ages are shown in Fig. 12-3, along with kcalorie requirements for each age.)

The Food Guide Pyramid and the dietary guidelines presented throughout the text can be used to develop a healthy meal plan for infants and children, with appropriate adjustments in serving sizes.

Parents need to be aware, however, that restricting a child's fat intake before age 2 is potentially dangerous. Both fat and cholesterol are needed for proper growth of brain tissue and formation of the protective sheath that surrounds nerves, as well as cell membrane formation. After age 2, a child's fat intake, like that of older family members, should be reduced to 30% of total kcalories or less. Low-fat or nonfat milk, reduced-fat cheeses, and other low-fat snack foods should be introduced gradually.

TODDLERS

The major goals in feeding a toddler are to make a happy transition from an all-milk diet to a solid diet and to establish a dietary pattern that will encourage normal growth and discourage unhealthful eating behaviors. The most effective way to achieve these goals is

for parents to set a good example by serving and eating nutritious foods.[21]

Feeding Recommendations for Toddlers

- Appetites vary. Generally a toddler's daily food intake should include:
    1 tablespoon each of fruits, vegetables, and meats per year of age per serving
    2 to 3 tablespoons of starches per year of age per serving
    2 to 3 cups of milk
- Serve water, rather than juice or soft drinks, to quench thirst (keep a small cup where the child can get some water for himself)
- Provide nutritious snacks such as fruits, vegetables, low-fat yogurt or cheese sticks, cooked beans, low-fat whole grain crackers (avoid fat-rich crackers)
- No more than 30% of total kcalories from fat
- No more than 10% of total kcalories or one third of fat intake from saturated fat
- Maintain regular meal patterns
- Be flexible. Eggs don't have to be served only at breakfast and sandwiches only at lunch. Children often respond well to inventive meals like pizza for breakfast or cereal for a snack.
- If the child rejects vegetables, offer mild-flavored ones like beans, corn, carrots, and peas; try giving vegetables cute names like trees for broccoli, grass for asparagus, and so on. Use low-fat dressings on both cold and hot vegetables to enhance flavor. Still no success? Give the child extra servings of nutrient-dense fruits like citrus, kiwi, and berries. This won't

replace all of the nutrients found in vegetables, but it will help. If all of these approaches fail, many pediatricians recommend giving children vitamin supplements.

- Strive for pleasant social interaction during meals

CHILDHOOD

Young children are quick to pick up nonverbal cues from the people around them. From the toddler years through childhood, many families find the dining table to be a battleground rather than a haven.

Food and Behavior

Parents and children often become involved in playing psychological games with food. When parents insist that a child eat a certain amount of a food, the child quickly learns to assert power by refusing to eat that food. Parents can cut conflict by calmly offering the food from time to time, without making an issue of the child's response.

Another unwinnable food game is the "clean plate club." Like bottle-fed babies, children should eat until their hunger is satisfied, not until they have eaten everything offered to them.

Parents also need to be wary of using food as a punishment, reward, or consolation. For example, withholding dessert because a child has not finished her dinner only makes the dessert seem more desirable than the foods in the main course. In the same way, bribing a child with food treats or using food to soothe hurt feelings teaches the child to use food for emotional comfort rather than to satisfy physical hunger and can lead to overeating problems in later life.

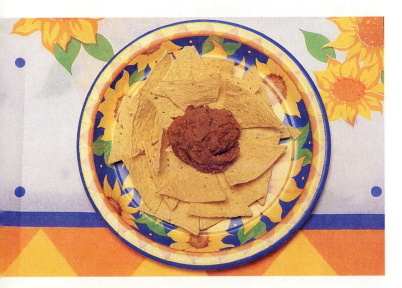

A healthy treat for kids is a "sunflower": a scoop of refried beans served on low-fat tortilla chips.

It is not just which food you feed your child that matters. *How* you feed it counts too. In addition to learning about good nutrition, childhood is the time when children form lifelong emotional reactions to food. Nutrition and feeding expert Ellyn Slatter has found that inappropriate feeding behaviors developed early in childhood are at the root of many of her adult clients' eating disorders. These observations emphasize the need for parents and childcare workers to be aware of the emotional cues they serve along with meals.[29] For more information on developing good mealtime interactions, read Slatter's *How To Get Your Kids To Eat But Not Too Much* (Bull Publishing, 1987).

Diet, Behavior, and Learning Potential

Parents, teachers, and childcare workers often say the foods children eat influence their behavior. To an extent they are right. Nutritional deficiencies such as a lack of iron, zinc, and/or B-complex vitamins can impair learning ability and lead to behavior problems.[13] The same is true of excessive intake of the metals lead and mercury (see Chapter 8, Minerals), exposure to environmental toxins,[17] or an irregular feeding schedule. Children's brains are nearly as large as those of adults, but their livers, which store the glucose essential for brain function, are only half the size of grownups'. To maintain an adequate level of blood glucose, children need to eat about every 4 hours. Lack of food leads to a decrease in blood glucose that in turn decreases the child's attention span and learning ability and contributes to behavior problems.[13]

One of the most widespread myths about childhood eating habits is that sugar and other food additives make children hyperactive. Carefully controlled studies, however, have shown there is no connection between hyperactivity and consumption of sugar, sugar substitutes, preservatives, or artificial colors and flavorings.[30]

TEENS

Not surprisingly, teenagers have the worst diet of any age group. Their eating habits are greatly influenced by peer pressure, acne control, weight control (especially among girls), and a quest for better athletic performance (usually in boys). There are two reasons to be concerned about poor diets in adolescence. During the teen years, nutrient needs are greater than at any time since infancy, so poor dietary habits can have serious health consequences. Further, health habits developed during the teen years often carry over into adulthood. Poor habits that are hard to break set the stage for many of the chronic illnesses seen in later life.[1,32]

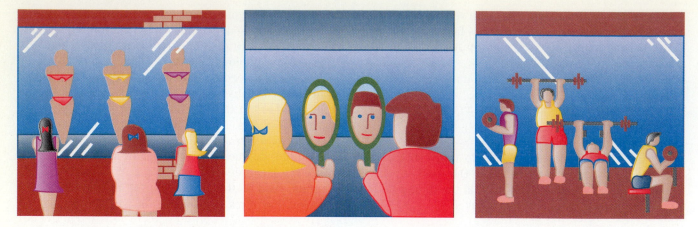

Teens want the perfect face and body—but they often go down the wrong diet path.

Gender-Related Differences in Nutrient Needs

Before puberty, gender-related differences in nutrient requirements are nonexistent. At puberty, females increase their percentage of body fat and begin to menstruate and males develop more bone and muscle mass. These natural physiological changes bring about alterations in nutrient requirements.

Males

By age 15 most females have finished growing, whereas males are just hitting their peak adolescent growth spurt. At this stage males need about twice as much food as do their female counterparts, but they tend to favor high-fat foods like burgers, fries, and milkshakes. Teenage boys can learn to make wise food choices if they are shown how healthful foods can bring about positive changes in other areas of their lives. Many young men, for instance, develop an interest in good health habits through their involvement in sports. Parents, physical education teachers, and coaches can encourage this interest by providing reliable nutrition information and psychological support. Chapter 9, Exercise, outlines the principles of good sports nutrition. Appendix G lists several reference books on the subject that are suitable for the home library.

Females

Young women are also more likely to make changes in their health habits if they believe it will improve their appearance. Many teenage girls, however, tend to be more interested in achieving a slender figure than in excelling at sports. As you have learned, this drive for thinness creates many health problems (see A Closer Look in Chapter 9). Both menstrual blood losses and inappropriate reducing diets place females at greater risk than their male peers for developing deficiencies of iron as well as other minerals and vitamins. The teen

years are a key time for females to build up the stores of iron and calcium they will need to see them through healthy pregnancies. To reduce their risk of mineral deficiencies, teenage girls should be encouraged to control their weight with a good exercise program rather than with a poorly thought out reducing diet.

 NUTRI QUIZ Why are women more likely than men to suffer from iron deficiency?

Diet and premenstrual syndrome (PMS). Many young women are concerned about the effect menstruation will have on their appetite and wonder if dietary changes can reduce symptoms of PMS. Research has shown that the kind of food a woman eats, but not the amount, is influenced by the phase of her menstrual cycle. Many women prefer carbohydrates, a good source of glucose, the week before menstruation.[8] Current thinking is that a stable blood glucose level may control some of the symptoms of PMS. To ensure a steady supply of glucose, women should divide their daily food intake among five to six small meals rather than three large ones, restrict their use of refined sugar products, consume naturally sugary foods like fruit with small amounts of fat and protein, and avoid caffeine-containing foods and drugs.[35]

Acne

The diet and acne myth is to teen nutrition what the hyperactivity myth is to childhood feeding practices. For many years physicians advised acne-prone teens to avoid fatty foods and chocolate. Repeated experiments, however, have failed to demonstrate a positive relationship between diet and pimples. Although a good diet is essential for healthy tissue and organs, no one food is responsible for poor skin. Acne sufferers can eat fried foods and chocolate in moderation without fear of triggering an outbreak of pimples. (The currently accepted theory is that acne is caused by an increase in oils and other secretions induced by the hormonal changes that occur at puberty.)

Drugs

A largely overlooked aspect of teenage nutrition is the impact of illegal drug use on nutritional status and health. Drug addiction often coincides with eating disorders. If a teen's eating habits change suddenly, parents should consider the possibility of drug use.

YOUNG ADULTHOOD

You have learned about typical adult nutrient requirements in earlier chapters, so we will focus here on the changes in dietary needs that accompany aging.

As people age, there is a natural slowing of their metabolism. Experts estimate that over age 30 the basal metabolic rate (BMR) slows by 2% to 4% each decade. For many years this change is too small to detect, but by the mid-50s it brings about noticeable differences in physical function that in turn alter nutritional needs.

OLDER ADULTHOOD

*"We do not stop playing because we grow too old;
We grow too old because we stop playing."*

— *Anonymous*

For researchers who are trying to develop nutrient intake standards for senior citizens, part of the challenge is that older people are more *unlike* their peers than are younger people. With the combined effects of illness, heredity, and health habits, some people are old and withered by their early 60s, whereas others are going strong well into their 70s and beyond (see A Closer Look on p. 230). In other words, chronological age is not necessarily an indication of biological age.[33] Nonetheless, everyone eventually experiences certain age-related changes in physical function related to nutrition. Below we review these changes and the effect they have on nutritional status and dietary habits.[27,31,34]

Energy Requirements

Aging leads to a natural decrease in basal metabolic rate, so kcalorie (energy) intake must decrease or physical activity must increase to prevent an increase in body fat content. The age-related decrease in the BMR also slows the rate at which body tissues, hormones, and enzymes are replaced. This in turn has far-reaching effects on many aspects of metabolism, ultimately altering the requirements for many nutrients and decreasing the requirement for energy.[36]

Protein Needs

The natural decrease in muscle mass that occurs with aging is largely a result of the diminished protein replacement that accompanies the decreased BMR. This loss of muscle tissue in turn diminishes an elderly person's protein requirement. Physical activity promotes retention of muscle tissue, preserving both physical strength and BMR, which in turn maintain protein requirements.

Vitamin and Mineral Needs

Vitamin and mineral needs can increase with advancing age as a result of decreased digestive function (see below). Gender-related differences in iron requirements disappear as women enter **menopause** (cessation of menstruation). The hormonal changes that accompany menopause, however, make women more vulnerable than men to calcium loss and thus to osteoporosis. Dietary calcium supplements alone appear to be of little use in reversing this trend. The most effective treatment to date seems to be a combination of oral calcium and estrogen replacement therapy together with a good weight-bearing exercise program. (For more details see the sections titled Bone Strength and Working With Weights in Chapter 10, Exercise.)

Diminished Digestive Function

Digestive function declines with increasing age. Practically speaking, this means the intestinal lining is not repaired as efficiently as it once was. This decreases digestion and nutrient absorption, which can result in gastrointestinal discomfort and constipation. In severe cases it can lead to malnutrition.

Decreased Mobility

Elderly people often decrease their physical activity because of failing health. Decreased mobility can cause several nutrition-related problems, including difficulty acquiring and preparing food, increased calcium loss from bone stores, decreased muscle mass, weight gain, and further suppression of digestive function.

Dental Problems

Loss of teeth, decaying teeth, ill-fitting dentures, and limited tongue and jaw motion can cause pain and difficulty when eating. If left unattended, such problems eventually contribute to malnutrition. Two ways to reduce the impact of poor dental health on an elderly person's diet are substituting soft, easy-to-chew, protein-rich foods like beans or peanut butter for meat, and chopping or mashing foods that are difficult to chew.

Decreased Sense of Taste, Smell, and Thirst

Aging is accompanied by a natural decline in the sharpness of all of the senses. With respect to nutrition, de-

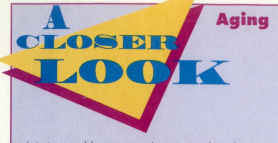

It is impossible to say with certainty how long a given person is likely to live. As you learned earlier in this chapter, the aging process is influenced by genetics, lifestyle, and environmental factors. Each of us has an aging timetable, depending on our own unique combination of these factors.

For scientists to develop methods to retard aging, they need to know what aging is and what causes it. Defining aging has proved easier than understanding it. Aging is a gradual decline in cellular function that ultimately results in death. Although most of us tend to think of aging as something that only happens to senior citizens, it actually affects each one of us from the moment of conception onward. In the first 20 to 30 years of life, aging is not detectable because it is masked by development and maturation of new tissue. A gradual decline in the efficiency of various body systems becomes apparent throughout the remainder of the adult years.

Theories about what causes aging include: slow cell renewal (so there are more old than new tissues), preprogrammed cellular death, an accumulation of toxic products, errors in copying of DNA, decreased immune efficiency, and increased autoimmune reactions.[31]

creased senses of taste, smell, and thirst are the most important sensory changes. Impairment of either taste or smell decreases a person's ability to enjoy food; in severe cases, it can even produce weight loss and malnutrition.[27,31,33]

Impairment of thirst is especially dangerous because dehydration can occur rapidly (see Chapter 3, Water). Some elderly people lose their sense of thirst, so they forget to consume enough beverages. They become dehydrated and mentally confused, which makes it even more unlikely they will remember to drink. Because kidney function also can decline with age, older adults may not be able to retain body fluids as well as younger ones so they produce relatively large amounts of urine even in the absence of adequate fluid intake, further increasing their chances of dehydration. Fluid requirements of the elderly are essentially the same as those for younger adults (about 8 cups per day) unless they are taking medications or have a medical condition that requires increased fluid intake.[12,19]

Loneliness

The longer a person lives, the more of his or her peers will have died or become physically incapacitated. Confronted with the loss of family, friends, and their own decreasing mobility, many older people feel lonely and isolated. Social isolation can have a profound effect on appetite. Some people respond by decreasing their food intake. Others gain comfort from overeating. The quality as well as the quantity of the food consumed is often affected. Too often the foods seniors do eat have low nutritional value or are not varied enough to create a balanced diet.

Meeting the Nutritional Challenges of Aging

How can older people compensate for their altered nutritional status and social situation? Unless

health problems indicate otherwise, the best diet for older people is the low-fat, low-cholesterol, moderate-protein, high-carbohydrate diet recommended throughout this text. Such a regimen should provide enough food to keep older people feeling satisfyingly full while at the same time keeping excess kcalories to a minimum.[27]

If decreased thirst is a problem, one way seniors can monitor their fluid intake is by purchasing pitchers they can fill with the amount of milk, juice, and water they should be drinking each day. When the pitchers are empty, they will know they have met their fluid needs.

Older people should make sure their diet contains plenty of fiber as well as fluid to help combat constipation. They also should discuss with their primary physician the value of a multivitamin/mineral supplement. Many health experts believe such preparations are useful to counteract the age-related decrease in digestive function as well as to prevent any nutrient deficiencies that can result from the decrease in food intake required to prevent obesity

Palatable and attractive food is just as important now as in earlier years. Many senior citizens find that the following suggestions can help counteract their decreased senses of taste and smell:[24]

- Use more seasonings (other than salt)
- Drink water to cleanse your palate as you eat
- Chew food thoroughly to release maximum amounts of flavor and aroma
- Alternate bites of one kind of food with bites of another
- Give up tobacco; in addition to its negative impact on health, it diminishes the senses of taste and smell
- Prepare a colorful meal for both nutritional and aesthetic value.

Even the tastiest and most attractive food can lose some of its appeal when eaten alone. If seniors find eat-

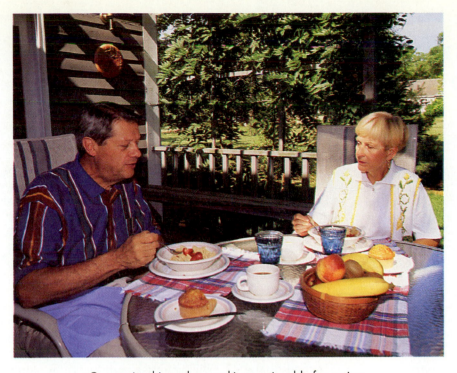

Companionship makes mealtimes enjoyable for seniors.

ing alone reduces the care they take in planning and preparing their meals, they should find others like themselves who would be willing to share food preparation and mealtimes; or they can investigate ***congregate meal*** programs available through senior citizen centers, religious organizations, and hospital community outreach programs.

Housebound patients can benefit from home-delivered meals through such programs as **Meals-on-Wheels.** Although lacking the social benefits of congregate meal programs, the Meals-on-Wheels system is a good way to ensure that at least some of an elderly person's daily nutritional needs will be met.

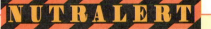

N U T R A L E R T

Congregate dining facilities and Meals-on-Wheels programs are not intended to provide all of an elderly person's dietary requirements. Such programs typically provide one meal a day on weekdays only. Seniors who rely on such a program as their sole source of food can quickly become malnourished.

It's Never Too Late

Scientists are finding that one of the biggest problems with the increased life span enjoyed by Americans is that, rather than increasing a person's useful years, longevity often means more time to suffer the ravages of disease. Starting life with sound nutritional status

and good exercise habits obviously carries certain health benefits, but it is never too late to reform! The National Institutes of Health's Center for the Aging has shown that even very elderly people can benefit from a sound diet and exercise program. They may not live longer, but they will live healthier.[34]

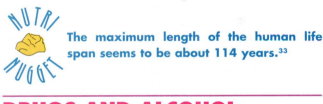

The maximum length of the human life span seems to be about 114 years.[33]

DRUGS AND ALCOHOL: CHALLENGES FOR ADULTS

Whether young or old, the nutritional status of adults as a group is significantly affected by their use of alcohol and caffeine, as well as by a variety of prescription and nonprescription medications. Despite the enjoyment they provide, alcohol and caffeine can have serious side effects. Many drugs affect appetite as well as the absorption or metabolism of specific nutrients.[25]

congregate meal a meal served to many people at a central location such as a senior center

A CLOSER LOOK

The French Paradox

In most countries, high levels of dietary fat and cholesterol are associated with high rates of heart disease. Researchers investigating low rates of heart disease in France, a country paradoxically known for rich cuisine, believe routine consumption of alcohol, particularly wine, may be the secret.[23] Subsequent studies have found that wine contains antioxidant substances that may protect against heart disease.[9]

Does this mean if you don't drink you should start? NO!

Alcohol consumption, particularly for women, is a double-edged sword. What the original study failed to point out is that although deaths from heart disease are down in France compared with the United States, deaths from liver disease and other alcohol-related maladies are up. In addition, American researchers have found an association between alcohol consumption and breast cancer in women. Further, no one has evaluated the protective effect of the heart-safe diet and exercise program emphasized throughout this text versus the protection conferred by wine drinking. So if you do not drink, there is no need to start to protect your health, and if you do drink, do so in moderation. Moderation is one drink per day for women, two per day for men, because of their larger size and greater alcohol metabolizing capabilities.

Alcohol

Providing little more than 7 kcalories per gram, alcohol is classified as a nonnutritive food and treated by the body much like dietary fat. Unlike most foods, which must be digested before being absorbed in the intestine, alcohol is absorbed in the stomach. This means it quickly enters the general circulation, from which it can reach the brain before being detoxified by the liver.

Although it provides little in the way of nutrients, alcohol can drain the body of several of them. Alcohol requires several of the B-complex vitamins to be metabolized and detoxified. It also alters the kidneys' ability to retain water, thereby depriving the body of necessary fluid. (See Chapter 3, Water, for a more detailed description of alcohol's effect on fluid balance.)

Does this mean people should never drink alcoholic beverages? No. As the Dietary Guidelines state, alcohol may be used in moderation. Small amounts (one to two glasses of wine or 1 to 2 ounces of hard liquor per day) can be useful as a tranquilizer and appetite stimulant. But excessive quantities quickly lead to malnutrition by replacing more nutritious whole foods, adding unnecessary empty kcalories to the diet, inhibiting nutrient absorption, and altering nutrient metabolism. Recent reports on the possible health benefits of moderate alcohol consumption have generated new discussion and controversy (see A Closer Look above).

Tobacco

Tobacco is a serious public health problem from the teen years on. As we saw in Chapter 9, Energy, many people, particularly women, smoke to maintain a low body weight. Body weight isn't the only thing that gets shortchanged by smoking. The nutritional value of

smokers' diets is often marginal both because tobacco takes the place of food and because people who are willing to risk their health by smoking are less likely to practice sound nutrition. As you learned in Chapter 7, Vitamins, smoking decreases the nutritional value of a diet by altering vitamin C metabolism and possibly interfering with the body's use of other nutrients as well.

Maintaining sound nutritional status is not the only reason to avoid tobacco. According to the American Cancer Society, using any form of tobacco presents significant health risks. Over 35% of all cancers are linked to cigarette smoke, and oral cancers are common in people who chew tobacco. Smoking or exposure to secondhand smoke also has been linked to an increased incidence of premature births, miscarriages, respiratory diseases, cardiovascular disease, and impotence in males.

If you don't smoke, don't start! If you do smoke, contact the local chapter of the American Cancer Society for advice on finding a smoking cessation program in your area. Eliminating tobacco from your life is easier if you give up caffeine at the same time, because tobacco users metabolize caffeine faster than nonusers, which can contribute to the nicotine-withdrawal jitters. Research conducted by the California Medical Association suggests women can further improve their chances of success if they give up tobacco during the first two weeks of their menstrual cycle.

Caffeine

Found naturally in coffee, tea, and cocoa beans, caffeine is one of the most widely consumed drugs in the world. Caffeine is often added to other foods and drugs, such as soft drinks, *analgesics* (for example,

Anacin), and stimulant preparations (for example, No Dōz). Moderate amounts of caffeine, such as the quantity contained in 2 to 4 cups of coffee or tea, appear to be safe for most people. A variety of undesirable side effects, however, have been reported in people who routinely consume larger amounts.[4,6]

In addition to interacting with water as you learned in Chapter 3, caffeine is a well-known metabolic stimulant that temporarily increases the metabolic rate by releasing stress hormones. This is why excesses of caffeine (more than 2 to 4 cups of coffee per day) can cause irritability and difficulty sleeping. Large amounts of caffeine have been tentatively linked to an increased incidence of cardiovascular disease and to benign fibrocystic breast disease in females.

NUTRALERT

Java junkies are in for an unwelcome jolt if they suddenly give up their caffeine-containing beverages, according to a study by a Johns Hopkins researcher. Even people who drink just 2 to 3 cups of coffee each day may feel depressed, anxious, sluggish, and headachy if they suddenly go cold turkey. If you want to cut down on your caffeine intake, do so gradually.[6]

Other Drug-Nutrient Interactions

Any drug can adversely affect nutritional status, just as a nutrient may affect the working of a drug. For example, some antibiotics become ineffective if they are consumed with calcium-rich foods. Certain diuretics, commonly known as water pills, increase the body's need for potassium. Other drugs, when combined with alcohol, either lose their effectiveness or produce harmful side effects. Aspirin or aspirin-like drugs may produce an increased need for iron because of increased intestinal blood loss.

BOX 12-2   Caffeine Content of Common Foods and Beverages

COFFEE

Brewed	100-150 mg per 5-oz. cup
Instant	40-110 mg
Decaf	1-5 mg

TEA

Brewed	10-50 mg per 5-oz cup
Instant	10-30 mg
Iced	20-40 mg

COLAS

	30-60 mg per 12-oz. can

CHOCOLATE

Milk or dark	1-35 mg per oz.
Hot cocoa	2-8 mg per 5-oz. cup

COFFEE ICE CREAM AND YOGURT

Ice cream	18-26 mg per ½ cup
Frozen yogurt	0-25 mg
Regular yogurt	0-22 mg

STIMULANTS

Vivarin	200 mg per tablet
No Doz	100 mg

PAIN RELIEVERS

Anacin caplets	35 mg per tablet
Excedrin Extra Strength	65 mg

PMS REMEDIES

Aqua Ban	100 mg per tablet
Maximum Strength Midol	60 mg

BOX 12-3   Preventing Food and Over-the-Counter (OTC) Drug Interactions

- To minimize stomach irritation, don't combine aspirin or other nonsteroid anti-inflammatory drugs (such as Nuprin, Advil, Motrin) with acidic beverages like coffee or fruit juice.
- To prevent oversedation and drowsiness, don't mix antihistamines (Con-Tac, Benadryl) with alcohol.
- To prevent increased blood pressure and heart rate and/or insomnia, don't mix caffeine-containing foods, beverages, and medications (coffee, colas, tea, chocolate, Anacin) with decongestants such as Con-Tac and Allerest.
- To reduce stomach upset, don't mix acid beverages such as fruit juice, coffee, and tea with antacid preparations like Mylanta or Tums.

Adapted from Allen AM: *Food-medication interactions*, ed 7, Tempe, Ariz, 1991, The author.

---

analgesic   a drug designed to provide pain relief

cancer   A group of diseases characterized by unchecked cellular growth

metastasize   to form a new site of disease in a distant part of the body

NUTRALERT

People over age 80, not toddlers, are the population most susceptible to accidental poisoning. This problem typically results from adverse reactions to certain combinations of medicines.[20]

To reduce your chances of experiencing an adverse drug-nutrient or drug-drug interaction, read the package inserts in your prescriptions and tell your physician or pharmacist about all medications you are taking, both prescription and over the counter (Box 12-3).

IN TODAY'S WORLD

Several studies have shown a connection between dietary habits and the development of liver, colon, breast, and stomach cancers. Scientists also suspect that diet may play a role in the development of prostate and lung cancers.

Nutrition and Cancer

Cancer, the second leading cause of death among adult Americans, is constantly in the headlines, yet most people have only a vague idea of what it involves. Cancer is not one disease but a group of diseases, each of which is characterized by unchecked cell growth. Cancer can affect any tissue in the body and is found in people of all ages; however, it is more common in adults than in children. Although no one knows the exact cause of cancer, a number of nutrients have been implicated in both its development and prevention.

How does cancer form?   Normally, the cells that make up body tissue reproduce in an orderly way. Old, worn-out cells are replaced by the correct number of new ones. The new cells stop growing in response to chemical signals produced by the body. In cancer, however, cell growth is unregulated. Rather than simply replacing aging cells, the new cells continue to multiply,

BOX 12-4   The Seven Warning Signs of Cancer

1. A change in bowel habits
2. A sore that fails to heal
3. Unusual bleeding or discharge
4. Thickening of a lump in the breast or elsewhere
5. Indigestion or difficulty swallowing
6. An obvious change in a wart or mole
7. A nagging cough or hoarseness

From The American Cancer Society.

eventually forming surplus tissue known as a **tumor.** Cancerous tumors grow in an irregular fashion, disrupting normal body functioning and robbing healthy tissues of their food and blood supply. Early detection (see Box 12-4, The Seven Warning Signs of Cancer) and treatment are the keys to cancer survival. Once a tumor penetrates the blood or lymph vessels, cancerous cells break free and are carried to other sites in the body, where they **metastasize,** reducing a patient's chances for survival.

What causes cell growth to go wrong?   Some types of cancer appear to be inherited; others seem to be caused by environmental factors. The National Research Council, however, suggests that most cancers arise from a combination of genetic and environmental influences. This is actually good news because it offers hope that we can reduce the incidence of cancer by controlling carcinogens in the environment.[18]

What are carcinogens?   **Carcinogens** are substances that cause cancer by altering DNA. Certain natural and manmade chemicals, **radiation,** and some viruses have been shown to be carcinogenic. Once the DNA in a cell has been altered, the cell no longer grows and functions normally. Sometimes the body reacts quickly enough to prevent any lasting damage. For example, some cells are sloughed off frequently (skin and intestinal cells); other cells contain substances that can repair damaged DNA. In addition, the body's immune system is often able to suppress reproduction of abnormal cells, effectively stopping the cancer before it gets started.[34]

Compounds that stimulate cell replication are also believed to have the potential to cause cancer either by reproducing new cells faster than the body can repair damaged DNA or by increasing the speed with which damaged cells are reproduced. Excesses of alcohol, kcalories, dietary fat, and estrogen all have been identified as stimulants of cell growth.[27,34]

How large a dose of a carcinogen is needed to produce cancer?   No one knows the precise answer to this question. Some carcinogens are thought to be dangerous after a single brief exposure; others are believed to take years of repeated exposure to have an effect. Individual variation in response to carcinogens is one of the factors that make it difficult for scientists to understand the dose-response effect. Another problem is the length of time between exposure to a carcinogen and development of cancer. Cancer typically takes years to develop, making it difficult to identify the factor that triggered it.

One thing that is known for sure is that carcinogens are often more harmful to children than adults because children's cells are actively dividing and growing, making them more vulnerable to any changes in DNA structure. Also, because of their smaller body size, children may receive a proportionately larger dose of a carcinogen than adults.

How can diet reduce the risk of cancer?

A number of individual nutrients have been identified as anticancer agents; however, no single nutrient appears to be the magic bullet. The best way to reduce cancer risk seems to be following an overall nutritious diet because different nutrients provide different mechanisms of defense. As you learned in Chapter 4, Carbohydrates, fiber appears to reduce the risk of colon cancer by restricting the amount of time that carcinogens present in feces are in contact with the surface of the colon. A calcium-rich diet also is believed to decrease the risk of colon cancer, but by different mechanisms. As you learned in Chapter 7, Vitamins, a diet rich in fruits and vegetables is believed to reduce the risk of many forms of cancer by preventing DNA damage.

Unhealthful eating habits, such as consuming high levels of dietary fat and excessive kcalories, are thought to promote the development of cancer by stimulating cell division. Diet is only one variable in the cancer equation. Other lifestyle factors, such as tobacco use, exposure to carcinogens, lack of physical activity, and obesity, all contribute to cancer risk.

How strong is the role of genetics in the development of cancer?

There is no simple answer to this question. Some cancers have a proven genetic component. Others seem to occur randomly. The majority of cancers appear to be caused by a combination of heredity and environment. The strength of the genetic component varies with the type of cancer.

The difficulty in separating genetic from environmental factors is illustrated by two of the more common forms of cancer: colon and breast. Japanese people have higher rates of stomach cancer but lower rates of colon and (in women) breast cancer than do Americans. Once they move to the United States and adopt a Western lifestyle, however, their rates of stomach cancer decrease whereas their rates of colon and female breast cancer increase. Both of these cancers have been linked to consumption of a high-fat, low-fiber diet, and both are known to have a genetic component.[14]

The typical American woman has about one chance in eight of developing breast cancer. Her chances double if she has a close female relative, such as a mother or sister, who has been diagnosed with breast cancer. The fact that breast cancer rates are higher in Japanese Americans than in Japanese who live in Japan suggests an environmental component to the disease. The fact that a family history of the disease increases a woman's risk illustrates a genetic component. It is important to note, however, that 75% of all breast cancer cases occur in women with no family history of the disease. An essential question for nutritionists and cancer researchers to answer is: How much can diet alter the risk of cancer in people with and without a genetic predisposition to the disease?

What is a cancer-wise diet?

A diet to reduce the risk of cancer is very similar to the heart-safe diet described earlier. The main difference is that a cancer-wise diet places more emphasis on fiber and vitamins (see American Cancer Society diet recommendations in Chapter 2, Consumer Concerns).

In the Grocery Store—Beating the Hype

Grocery stores sell more than just food—they also sell shelf space. With an average of 53 new food items being introduced each month (Food Marketing Association), shelf space in markets is at a premium. Grocers want to stock what sells. Because of the tremendous impact of advertising on consumer demand, what sells often translates into which foods have the most financial backing in the form of manufacturer promotions (advertising, coupons, rebates) and which producers can afford to pay the most money to obtain shelf space.

Grocers' profits depend on enticing shoppers to purchase products they neither need nor want. What can you do to avoid such traps? Make a shopping list and stick to it. Avoid the temptation to buy on impulse. Let the grocery store manager know which products you would like to see carried. Educate yourself and your family about nutrition. Carefully evaluate sales pitches. Ask yourself: Is a celebrity name being used to sell this product? Do the marketing claims seem too good to be true? Am I being influenced by a good-looking package? Is there a generic version that can offer the same performance for a fraction of the price?

NUTRI NUGGET It is only natural for children to want to try some of the foods they see advertised or watch their friends eating. Rather than forbidding all such items or purchasing foods that have more slick advertising than substance, help kids select healthy items for daily use. Then choose some "just-for-fun" food items to be eaten on weekends or special occasions. Remember to set a good example by doing the same with your own food choices.

radiation literally, energy emitted in all directions from a central source; examples include X rays, radioactive chemicals (such as those used to produce nuclear energy), and the ultraviolet light from the sun

In the Kitchen

In earlier chapters this section covered food safety issues and healthful cooking techniques. In this chapter we devote the section to maintaining personal safety in the kitchen.

The combination of sharp utensils, appliances that can deliver an electric shock, and heat make the kitchen one of the most dangerous rooms in the house. Following the guidelines below can help you reduce the risk.

- Store knives and other sharp utensils properly.
- Do not throw sharp utensils into a sink full of water where they can cut an unsuspecting cook's hand.
- Tie hair back to keep it out of flames and food.
- Do not wear flowing clothes in the kitchen; they can get caught on appliances or dangle into a flame.
- Be sure older family members are still capable of preparing healthful meals. Senior citizens whose senses and mobility may have been dulled by age or disease may require assistance in the kitchen.

The increase in dual-career families means that more kids than ever before are helping themselves in the kitchen. Food manufacturers, well aware of this trend, have developed many microwaveable items specifically aimed at the juvenile market. It is important to encourage children to learn how to use the kitchen. Doing so will help ensure their personal safety, provide a good opportunity to foster nutritious eating habits, and build children's feelings of competence.

- Put approved snack foods in a readily accessible area.
- Closely supervise children between the ages of 4 and 7. This means standing next to them as they cut foods and use the oven or microwave.
- A supervising adult should be in the same room with children between 7 and 12 years of age.
- Do not assume that because a child has mastered one cooking skill s/he can cook everything.

- Teach children how to safely handle sharp knives, can lids, and hot items. Insist on the use of potholders. Teach children to carefully remove the cover from cooked or cooking foods; escaping steam can cause painful burns. Instruct them to be especially careful with microwaveable foods that crisp because the packages can become extra hot. Using a damp dishcloth or sponge, demonstrate why children must dry their hands before removing food from the freezer.
- Emphasize that appliances are not toys. This means no swinging on doors, blowing flames on gas ranges, or playing with range or microwave switches.

Senior Cooking Skills

As people age, they may find that cooking seems to be more effort than it is worth. This attitude frequently leads to poor eating habits as well as poor health. Simple changes in food preparation techniques can help put the enjoyment and nutrition back into cooking for seniors.

- Learn to cook simpler, nutritionally dense foods such as brown rice, stews, and lentil or bean soups.
- Take advantage of community programs, friends, and family to help with shopping and food preparation.
- Find a neighbor or friend to share food preparation and mealtimes.
- Arrange your work space so you can prepare part of the meal while sitting down.
- Consider investing in labor-saving devices, such as a mini food processor.
- If you own a freezer, cook large amounts, then freeze individual servings.
- Shop for nutritious convenience foods. Look for products that are dense in nutrients but low in fat, sugar, and sodium. Several companies offer lines of health-oriented frozen meals.

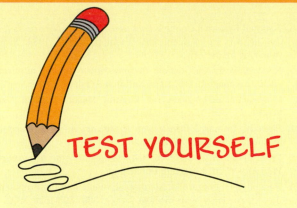

TEST YOURSELF

1. List three reasons why breast milk is better for a baby than a commercial infant formula.
2. Is there any truth to the statement that a pregnant woman must "eat for two"?
3. What is one possible explanation for the value of morning sickness?
4. What is a good technique for encouraging young men to eat a healthy diet?
5. What are some techniques seniors can use to deal with their decreased sense of taste and smell?

6. Why is it important to let babies feed themselves despite the mess?
7. List three nutritional challenges of aging.
8. Why is rice cereal a good choice for a baby's first solid food?
9. How old should a child be before you let him/her use the kitchen without supervision?
10. Does a high incidence of cancer in your family mean you are bound to get it too? Why or why not?

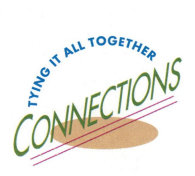

TYING IT ALL TOGETHER

CONNECTIONS

1. What steps should you take throughout your life to maintain a healthy skeleton?
2. List three dangers associated with excessive consumption of alcohol.
3. List three ways in which the diet you consume early in life can affect your health in later life.
4. Give three examples of how social interactions at mealtime influence your eating patterns throughout your life cycle.
5. What is the relationship between dietary sugar and behavior?
6. Why do young children need to eat at more frequent intervals than do older children and adults?

References

1. Anderson JB: The status of adolescent nutrition. *Nutrition Today* 26:7-10, 1991.

2. American Dietetic Association timely statement on marketing of infant formulas, *Journal of the American Dietetic Association* 89:268, 1989.

3. American Dietetic Association position on promotion and support of breastfeeding, *Journal of the American Dietetic Association* 93:467-469, 1993.

4. Caffeine: Grounds for concern? *University of California at Berkeley Wellness Letter* 10(6):4-5, 1994.

5. Dobler ML: *Food allergies*, Chicago, 1991, American Dietetic Association.

6. Facts after 50—caffeine withdrawal, *Johns Hopkins Medical Letter: Health After 50* 5(1):1, 1993.

7. Fathering healthy babies, *University of California at Berkeley Wellness Letter* 10(7):1, 1994.

8. Fong AKH, Kretsch M: Food intake and the menstrual cycle, *American Journal of Clinical Nutrition* 57:43-47, 1993.

9. Frankel EN et al: Inhibition of oxidation of human low-density lipoproteins by phenolic substances in red wine, *Lancet* 341:454-457, 1993.

10. Goldstein et al: Biologic theories of aging, *American Family Physician* 40(3):123,1989.

11. Hahn NI: Battling morning (noon and night) sickness: new approaches to treating an age-old problem, *Journal of the American Dietetic Association* 94:147-148, 1994.

12. Hallfrisch J: Fluid balance in the elderly, *Nutrition and the MD* 17:1, 1991.

13. Kanarek RB, Marks-Kaufman R: *Nutrition and behavior: new perspectives*, New York, 1991, Van Nostrand & Reinholt.

14. Kern SE, Pietenpol JA: Oncogenic forms of MNU inhibit growth regulated gene expression, *Science* 256(5058):827-830, 1992.

15. Little MT, Hahn P: Diet and metabolic development, *Federation of American Societies for Experimental Biology (FASEB) Journal* 4:2605-2611, 1990.

16. Moffatt J, Owens SG: Cessation from cigarette smoking: changes in body weight, body composition, resting metabolism, and energy consumption metabolism, *Clinical and Experimental Physiology* 40:165-170, 1991.

17. National Academy of Science: *Pesticides in the diets of infants and children*, Washington, DC, 1991, National Academy Press.

18. National Research Council: *Diet and heath: implications for reducing chronic disease risk*, Washington, DC, 1989, National Academy Press.

19. National Research Council: *Recommended dietary allowances*, ed 10, Washington, DC, 1989, National Academy Press.

20. Pharmaceutical Services at Virginia Mason Medical Center, Seattle.

21. Pipes PI, Trahms CM: *Nutrition in infancy and childhood*, ed 5, St Louis, 1993, Mosby-Year Book.

22. Profit M: *Morning sickness: why we get it, how to manage it*, Palo Alto, Calif, 1993, Bull Publishing.

23. Renaud S, de Lorgeril M: Alcohol, platelets, and the French paradox for coronary heart disease, *Lancet* 339:1523-1526, 1992.

24. Reviving your sense of taste, *Johns Hopkins Medical Letter, Health After 50* 4(8):6, 1992.

25. Roe D: *Diet and drug interactions*, New York, 1991, Van Nostrand Reinhold.

26. Rolls BJ, Phillips PA: Aging and disturbances of thirst and fluid balance, *Nutrition Reviews* 48(3):137-144, 1990.

27. Rosenberg IH (ed): Symposium on nutrition and aging, *Nutrition Reviews* 50(12):360, 1992.

28. U.S. Department of Agriculture: *School nutrition dietary assessment study*, 1993, USDA.

29. Satter E: Symposia: the feeding relationship: implications for dietitians. Paper presented at American Dietetic Association annual meeting, Washington, DC, Oct 1992.

30. Shaywitz BA et al: Aspartame, behavior, and cognitive function in children with attention deficit disorder, *Pediatrics* 93:70-75, 1991.

31. Smiciklas-Wright H: Aging. In *Present knowledge in nutrition*, ed 6, Washington, DC, 1990, International Life Sciences Institute Nutrition Foundation.

32. Story S et al: Adolescent nutrition, *Journal of the American Dietetic Association* 88:591, 1988.

33. Symposium on Aging, *Nutrition Reviews* 50(12), 1992.

34. Williams E, Rosenberg IH: *Biomarkers: the 10 determinants of aging you can control*, New York, 1991, Simon & Schuster.

35. Wurtman J, Wurtman R: A high-carbohydrate diet may lessen symptoms of premenstrual syndrome, *American Journal of Obstetrics and Gynecology* 161:1228-1233, 1989.

36. Young V: Energy requirements in the elderly, *Nutrition Reviews* 50:95-101, 1992.

LOOKING TO
THE FUTURE

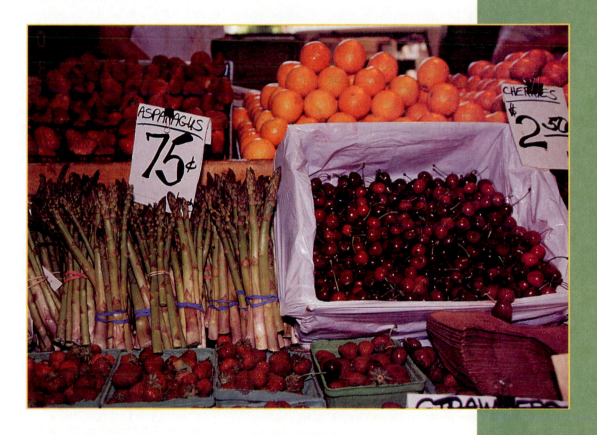

Most of the future lies ahead.

— *Denny Crum*, Louiseville Basketball Coach

FROM CURRENT KNOWLEDGE TO EMERGING TRENDS

Up to this point in the text we have focused on current knowledge in the field of human nutrition. In this final chapter we look toward the future of nutrition—in research, agricultural practices, and food marketing trends. In the section Preparing for Tomorrow's World we examine the world food crisis and explore the role of government and individuals in developing solutions. We give you the information you need to become a food package recycling expert, and we describe the food, fluids, and other items you should have on hand for emergencies.

NEWSMAKERS—IN THE NINETIES AND BEYOND

What will be the hot topics in human nutrition as we move into the 21st century? To predict the major trends that will emerge in nutrition, we need to know who we will be as well as what we may be able to achieve through advances in technology.

Demographic Changes

Four major demographic changes are emerging that will shape nutrition over the next generation. They are the "graying" (aging) of America, shifts in population trends, the restructuring of the American family, and changes in income distribution.[5,11,26]

The Graying of America

Statistics show that America is aging rapidly. By the year 2000 the majority of our population will be over age 50.[5] As people age and become more vulnerable to diet-related chronic diseases such as hypertension and heart disease, they typically become more willing to make diet and lifestyle changes. Food manufacturers are likely to find a growing market for special diet foods for older Americans.[15] For example, Kaiser Permanente, the West's largest health maintenance organization, through its pharmacy distributes low-sodium meals for people with hypertension. Through the Healthy Choice line, Dr. Dean Ornish is marketing low-fat, low-sodium foods for people who are undergoing cardiac rehabilitation. The makers of Centrum Silver vitamins for seniors now offer their preparation in a low-sodium version.

Shifts in Population Trends

America is not only graying but, to borrow a phrase from *Time* magazine, it is also browning.[26] According to U.S. Census projections, Caucasians are becoming the minority as nonwhite populations continue to grow. African-Americans will remain the largest nonwhite ethnic group, but Hispanic and Asian-American populations are expanding rapidly.[5,26] This shift in population trends will create greater demand for foods favored by these ethnic groups, including native produce. Over the past generation an increasing variety of ethnic foods and flavors have become part of the American mainstream. Depending on where you live, you can enjoy such multiethnic treats as Asian pasta or pizza, blueberry bagels, or Mexican burritos stuffed with Polish sausage.[7,13]

The Restructuring of the American Family

Dramatic changes have been taking place not only within population segments but also within the family itself.[5,11,15] The traditional picture of the American family—a breadwinning father, homemaker mother, and 2.4 children—has virtually disappeared and is being replaced by growing numbers of single-parent households, dual-career families, and single-person households. As a whole, these groups tend to have more money than time, so there will continue to be a high demand for convenience foods and foods in single-serving sizes. This trend promises to boost the profits of fast-food establishments, grocery store service delis, and producers of microwave meals.

A serious concern is the ongoing rise in illegitimate births among both white and nonwhite populations and the resulting creation of more and more single-parent families living at or below the poverty line. People in this situation often lack the money or the knowledge to buy nutritious foods and thus are vulnerable to a variety of problems caused by nutrient deficiencies.

Changes in Income Distribution: The Shrinking Middle Class

Changes in the work force and the shift from an industrial to a service economy are affecting Americans' economic status. There are now more women and older people in the work force than ever before. Workers in general have more years of education than in the past but often have not acquired the skills needed to perform competently in today's increasingly high-tech jobs.[5,11]

America's middle class is shrinking rapidly, whereas both the upper and working classes are growing. In the 1950s 60% of American households were classified as middle class, 10% as affluent, and 30% as working class (including 8% of households that were living at or below the poverty line). By the year 2000 only 30% of households will still be considered middle class. About 40% will be categorized as working class (half of whom will be at or below the poverty line), and 30% will be affluent.[5,11]

According to economists and marketing analysts, the decline of the middle class is expected to bring about the end of *mass marketing.* Instead of aiming products at a broad segment of the population, food manufacturers are beginning to exploit economic market segments with premium products aimed at affluent households and "no frills" and generic products for thrifty high-income people as well as people on tight budgets.

Health Care Challenges

As the population ages and as more children are born into poverty, more money than ever will be spent on health care. Americans in general receive the most advanced health care in the world—and also the most expensive. With health costs currently consuming 20% to 25% of the federal budget, public officials are increasingly receptive to messages from groups such as the American Dietetic Association (ADA). The ADA and other knowledgeable experts point out that preventive measures, like a healthy diet and regular exercise, could greatly reduce current health care costs. People involved in health care reform acknowledge the role of poor nutrition and tobacco, alcohol, and drug use in chronic disease, but there is no simple way to legislate more healthful behavior.[16]

What can government do to improve Americans' health-related behaviors? Government agencies can step up public health campaigns. Using finanical incentives like tax breaks or credits, they can encourage employers, educational institutions, food manufacturers, and restaurants to offer healthier food choices. A similar incentive system can be used to motivate schools and employers to offer excercise classes, routine health screenings, and wellness workshops. Businesses and schools in turn can develop incentives to encourage employees and students to participate in these programs.[16]

NUTRI NUGGET Some businesses already sponsor employee wellness programs. Such programs help reduce the cost of health insurance premiums, increase productivity, and reduce sick leave.

Regulatory and Technological Advances

Important nutrition-related changes also are taking place on the regulatory and scientific fronts. The American Dietetic Association states that future research projects will identify new metabolic roles for nutrients, clarify the role of brain chemistry in food choices, and uncover more information about how heredity affects nutrient-disease interactions.[12,15]

A 1993 survey of university professors and food company executives identified the "hot" food issues as the revised labeling laws (Nutrition Labeling and Education Act), biotechnology, irradiation, food safety,

natural or organic foods, and diet-health links.[8,12] Also cited was solid waste disposal/recycling.[8]

Consumers likewise rate environmental concerns as a top priority. Surveys show Americans have a strong interest in recycling, overpackaging, and solid waste disposal problems, but the desire for convenience and single-serving packages often outweighs environmental considerations at the time of purchase. Many people, however, are willing to recycle the packaging they purchase.[22]

Labeling Laws

It is hard to predict what effect the 1990 Nutrition Labeling and Education Act will have on food production and purchasing processes. Now that food manufacturers must disclose the truth about their products' sugar, fat, and sodium content, will they cut down on these ingredients to make their products more appealing to consumers? Marketing experts will observe how the expanded labeling information may influence consumer choices. Will more healthful foods win out over old favorites that are high in fat, salt, and sugar?

Food Safety

Over the past decade consumer confidence in the safety of the food supply has been weakened by an avalanche of news reports about the dangers of eating everything from chickens to eggs and by news of pesticide residues in food[19,27] and an outbreak of food poisoning at some fast-food outlets.[20] Given these events and the fact that many scientists have reversed their position on the benefits of nutritional "advances" such as partially hydrogenated margarine and vegetable shortening, consumers are understandably concerned about the safety of advances in food technology like irradiation (discussed in Chapter 9, Energy) and bioengineering.

NUTRI NUGGET Imported produce appears to be just as safe as that grown in the United States. A study conducted in 1990 by the FDA found pesticide residues in 64% of imported produce as compared to 61% of domestic produce. Further, the FDA and USDA have stepped up testing of imported produce to prevent banned chemicals from making their way into the U.S. food supply.[3]

mass marketing the practice of distributing a single product that meets the needs of the broadest segment of the population

Food Poisoning

The 1993 outbreak of food poisoning in Washington state caused by *E. coli* bacteria was traced to consumption of undercooked, contaminated ground beef used in burgers sold at fast-food outlets. This incident brought consumer, food industry, and government sectors together in a single force whose efforts resulted in new federal regulations for the labeling, handling, and commercial cooking of meat and poultry. The new rules allow the federal government and individual consumers to sue a food outlet that is linked to an outbreak of food poisoning. These new safe handling regulations are expected to be followed by changes in the U.S. Department of Agriculture's meat inspection system. Currently meat and poultry are accepted as safe if they pass visual examination by a USDA inspector, but manufacturers are developing test kits that can rapidly identify disease-causing agents such as bacteria.[20]

Growing Pesticide-Free Food

Only a decade ago there was great excitement about the success of American agriculture made possible by technological advancements. Little thought was given, however, to the toll on the environment being taken by "super-farming" techniques like extra-heavy use of chemical pesticides and fertilizers. More recently, farmers have begun to experience the downside of some of these super-farming methods. In many areas, loss of topsoil has left the ground as hard as cement, so rain pools on the surface rather than seeping into the soil. Pesticide-resistant strains of insects have begun to appear. Ground water once thought to be invulnerable has shown signs of contamination by **agrichemicals.**[9,23]

Long-term Research in Agricultural Systems (LTRAS) is a coalition of scientists committed to developing methods of producing food that are environmentally sensitive and result in long-term agricultural productivity.[29] As part of this program 300 acres of land have been dedicated to 100-year-long sets of studies of agricultural methods at several land-grant universities.

Overwhelmed by both the financial and environmental costs of super-farming techniques, many growers are looking to county agricultural programs and university agricultural extension services for guidance in converting to safer methods. One option is *organic farming.* Currently about 2% of American farmers use organic techniques.[23] These growers have replaced chemical fertilizers with natural ones like steer manure and plant matter. They use naturally occurring chemicals like nicotine and sulfur as pesticides, and they

plant cover crops in the fall to reduce the soil erosion that occurs in open fields. They remove weeds mechanically rather than with herbicides, and they rotate crops (a practice discouraged by government farm subsidy programs) on a 4- to 5-year cycle to allow the ground to recover and to prevent the multiplication of undesirable insects that target a particular plant species.[23] Some farmers even use beneficial insects to control the population of harmful ones.[1]

A large and increasing number of farmers use a method called **sustainable agriculture.** These farmers use many organic farming techniques, but they also use synthetic chemicals sparingly if the need arises. They also are restoring habitats around the perimeters of their fields for beneficial insects and animals. In addition to helping preserve the Earth's delicate ecological balance, these farming techniques save money. Some farmers say they have cut their operating costs up to 50% by using these methods.[19,23]

A new pesticide application technique known as electrostatic spraying can reduce pesticide use by 25% to 50%.

How can these positive changes in agricultural practices be encouraged? Progress already is being made in the area of research. The National Science Foundation has awarded a major university a grant of up to $10.4 million to establish a national biotechnology research center that will investigate the nature of plant diseases and develop ways to improve disease resistance in food crops.[29]

Some people believe natural pesticides are less harmful than synthetic ones, but this has not been proved for all chemicals currently in use. Further, genetic engineering techniques have produced strains of plants that manufacture high levels of endogenous pesticides. Many of these accumulate in plants at a higher level than would be permitted for exogenous pesticides. The ultimate health effects of these endogenous pesticides have not been thoroughly evaluated.[2]

In making decisions about pesticide use, we need to carefully consider both the potential risks and benefits. A Closer Look on p. 243 explains the concept of weighing the odds in analyzing a risk:benefit ratio.

Is anyone opposed to agricultural reform? The multibillion-dollar agrichemical industry is a powerful lobby in Congress. Between 1990 and 1992 the agrichemical industry sold $10 billion to $12 billion worth

A CLOSER LOOK

Risk:Benefit Ratio—Weighing the Odds

If researchers prove that very high levels of beta-carotene are good for me, should I begin taking supplements of this nutrient? Whether evaluating the nutritional merits of a food or supplement or deciding on the safety of a pesticide or medication, it is essential to consider the concept of risk:benefit ratio. In essence this means you need to determine whether the benefits provided by a particular process or product outweigh the risks associated with it. For example, the National Academy of Science has determined that eating large amounts of fruits and vegetables provides fiber, vitamins, and minerals as well as protection against cancer and other chronic diseases. These benefits greatly outweigh any theoretical risks associated with consumption of pesticide residues remaining on the produce.

The Aflatoxin story is a dramatic example of how the potential benefits of pesticide use outweigh the health risks associated with consuming the pest. Aflatoxin B_2 is one of the most potent human carcinogens known. This toxin is produced by Aspergillus fungi, which grow naturally on grains, peanuts, and unprocessed peanut butter. The pesticides that control Aflatoxin B_2 are also carcinogenic, but they are much less potent than Alfatoxin B_2.[2]

The dose of a chemical is often the key to determining its risk:benefit ratio. The fact that a toxic substance is present does not mean that it poses any danger. For example, alcohol, nutmeg, a variety of other foods, most medications, and even water are lethal if consumed in high enough doses—but harmless if used with care.

You can use the same kind of pro-and-con analysis in making decisions about whether to eat other items, such as chemically or biologically engineered low-fat foods. A high-fat diet carries the risk of cardiovascular disease, obesity, and several other chronic conditions, but it offers no real benefit except giving foods a rich, creamy texture. You may decide to ignore the health risks and eat as usual, use chemically modified foods to reduce your fat intake, or change your eating habits entirely. If you opt for chemically engineered foods, you must decide whether the taste justifies the caloric expenditure and whether you are willing to assume any health risks that may be associated with these ingredients.

---

of fertilizer and more than $4 billion worth of pesticides. These companies are not about to let their profits erode without a fight.[1,9,19]

Food Technology

Food technology involves intentional chemical or genetic manipulation of the food supply. Technological manipulation of the food supply is nothing new. Hydrogenation of vegetable oil to produce shortening and margarine has been common since the early 1900s, and farmers have been selectively breeding various plants and animals for food ever since purposeful agriculture began.

Chemically Engineered Foods

Chemical engineering has gone far beyond hydrogenation of vegetable oil. It has enabled food manufacturers to develop leaner versions of favorite edibles. Foods that contain chemically engineered sugar and fat substitutes have been greeted with enthusiasm by consumers, many of whom may believe that at last they can have their cake and eat it too. Other avenues of chemical engineering research include production of cholesterol-free or reduced-cholesterol versions of eggs, butter, and cream, as well as ways to reduce or convert the saturated fat in these products.

Bioengineered Foods

In general, **chemically engineered** foods (margarine and sugar substitutes) have been more readily accepted than those that are **bioengineered.** Some people hail the progress of science, but many others fear the long-term consequences of human alteration of animal and crop genetics. It is not yet clear how consumers ultimately will respond to bioengineered foods and what kind of labeling information will be required on such products. So far, however, there has been strong public resistance to the planned introduction of a bioengineered tomato[14] and to the sale of milk from cows treated with a bioengineered growth hormone.[4,18]

bioengineered foods plant or animal products that have been genetically altered by the addition of genes from another species to improve the food's shelf life, fat content, or in the case of plants, pest resistance

chemically engineered foods food items that have been chemically altered to improve shelf life, texture, or nutrient content; examples include margarine, artificial sweeteners, and fats

organic farming grown with fertilizers and mulch composed only of animal or vegetable matter, with no use of chemical fertilizers or pesticides

How Science Happens

The story of the discovery of **pellagra**, a nutrition-related disease, illustrates how good science happens.

Notice a change

In the early 1900s, in the southern and midwestern United States, Italy, and Spain, pellagra, a usually endemic disease (always a few cases around), became epidemic (massive outbreaks of disease). The first symptom was noticeable darkening of the nose and cheek skin, making the afflicted person's face look as if a butterfly had been painted on it. Other symptoms included flaky black dermatitis, diarrhea, and inflamed mucous membranes. Dementia and in many cases death soon followed. Neighbors and friends avoided victims for fear of contagion.

Ask questions

What caused pellagra: a germ or a toxin? People who ate large amounts of corn got pellagra, and people who lived in the same environment frequently developed it.

Considerable research failed to find a toxin in corn.

If at first you don't succeed, try, try again

By 1913 the pellagra epidemic in the United States had grown to 150,000 cases annually. Dr. Goldberger of the U.S. Public Health Service was assigned the task of finding the cause. He visited prisons and orphanages in the southern United States, where the incidence of the disease was particularly high.

Observe

Because Goldberger was a trained scientist, he made careful **observations.** He noted that pellagra was common among inmates and orphans, but nurses and attendants at the same institutions seemed to be immune. It therefore was clear to him that personal contact or an insect carrier did not spread the disease.

Pellagra was not contagious.

Develop an idea—Theorize

How were the people who got pellagra different from those who didn't? Goldberger knew that pellagra appeared most frequently in people who ate a poor diet

Old Foods and Nutrients—New Uses

Will new disease-preventing nutrients be added to the RDA? Most scientists believe all the nutrients required to sustain human health have been identified. A few additional ultra-trace minerals may prove to be essential for people who are sustained for many years on purified intravenous feedings. Because healthy people obtain these nutrients from the foods and beverages they consume, there is no concern about deficiencies in the general population. The real progress in the area of food and nutrient requirements is expected to be a greater understanding of the metabolic roles played by the already recognized nutrients. Researchers also may discover new disease-fighting uses for foods already in our diets.

Nutraceuticals: Foods Used as Drugs

The new term *nutraceuticals* refers to specific foods, individual nutrients, and nonnutritive chemicals isolated from foods that act like drugs.[10] There are many examples of disease-fighting foods and nutrients. High-fiber foods seem to reduce the risk of colon cancer. Vitamin C prevents and cures scurvy, and folate prevents the birth defect spina bifida. The use of nonnutritive components of food, known as phytochemicals, to fight disease, however, is a relatively new phenomenon.

All of the phytochemicals identified thus far come from plant-derived foods. Five common produce items (celery, grapefruit, broccoli, garlic, and soybeans), for instance, have been found to contain natural nonnutritive chemicals that inhibit the formation of cancer and in some cases cardiovascular disease. Scientists are investigating the effectiveness and safety of these and many other food-derived chemicals as ammunition against disease. A word of warning: Each of these "wonder foods" also contains hundreds of other chemicals of unknown function, so making any of these foods a major part of your diet is definitely *not* advised.

A CLOSER LOOK

How Science Happens—cont'd

that contained large amounts of corn, but not in people who ate corn as part of a good diet. Goldberger's guess (**theory** or **hypothesis**) was that pellagra was somehow related to the diet of greens, fatback, and cornbread fed to the inmates and orphans and consumed by the rural poor.

Test the idea—Experiment

How could this theory be tested? Goldberger instructed two orphanages to add fresh meat, milk, and eggs to the orphans' diet as an **experiment** to see if his theory was correct. The result was exhilarating! Goldberger published his findings after conducting another, better experiment in which some inmates ate the new diet while others, who served as **controls**, consumed the old diet. It was clear from the results that

A protein-rich diet either prevented or cured pellagra.

Read the work of others

What about other research? A researcher named Harris reported an experiment that demonstrated the transfer of pellagra from one monkey to another, thus showing it was a contagious disease.

Plan another test

How can it be proved that one human cannot "catch" pellagra from another? Goldberger found healthy volunteers who were exposed to pellagra through their work. Wipings from the mouths and throats of pellagra victims were applied to the mouths of the volunteers. The volunteers also were injected with blood from pellagra patients and fed pelleted scrapings of sores and feces from the pellagra victims.

None of the volunteers developed pellagra—clear proof that transmission of pellagra did not happen in humans!

Serendipity—Happy coincidence

Exactly what was it in the protein-rich food that cured or prevented pellagra? Researchers at the University of Washington broke a container of nicotinic acid that had been extracted from tobacco leaves. Their research animals, dogs with "black tongue," a disease similar to human pellagra, lapped up the powder. Their disease disappeared!

The researchers put two and two together correctly and realized that nicotinic acid (niacin) was responsible for curing pellagra. They knew that rice polishings contained this substance and rightly concluded that it must be part of others foods as well.

Patience

Then what did corn have to do with pellagra? Corn was the puzzle! In 1945 scientists at the University of Wisconsin solved the final part of the puzzle when they discovered that humans could synthesize niacin from the amino acid tryptophan. This finding explained why foods like milk that are low in niacin but rich in tryptophan prevent pellagra, whereas *diets high in corn, which is a poor source of both tryptophan and niacin, increase the risk of developing pellagra.*

Reflect

What did we learn? *Disease may be caused by a poor diet.* Science is being curious, asking questions, developing ideas, testing the ideas carefully, and sometimes discovering new things. As our understanding of science becomes more sophisticated, so do research techniques. There are a variety of ways to plan a study, to control variables, and to assess the validity of the data. There is always more to learn.

KEEPING CURRENT

Nutrition, like any modern scientific field, is an ever-changing discipline. Learning the facts as they are currently understood can help clarify today's nutrition dilemmas, but what about tomorrow's? Appendix G lists a variety of publications and services that can help you keep informed about developments in the field of nutrition. Wellness letters published by major universities are especially useful for consumers because the information they contain has been researched and approved by panels of experts.

Unless a government health agency issues a public warning, don't change your health habits based on evidence from a single study. One set of results does not conclusively prove an observation. See A Closer Look on pp. 244-245 to gain an understanding of the scientific process.

PREPARING FOR TOMORROW'S WORLD

In Chapters 1 through 12, the section titled In Today's World showed you how to apply what you learned in the chapter to your current lifestyle. In this final chapter, Looking to the Future, we have renamed this section Preparing for Tomorrow's World. We focus on three nutrition-related concerns that each of us can begin preparing for today so we will be ready to meet tomorrow's challenges.

As part of the global economy, the United States must participate in the development of solutions to the world hunger crisis. Here at home we need to learn to select foods and other items packaged in recyclable containers. On a personal level, each of us should store an emergency supply of food, water, and other essentials to tide us over in the event of a natural disaster or other emergency.

World Food Crisis

Widespread hunger and the resulting malnutrition have been with us since the beginning of time, and workable solutions do not appear close at hand. The problem is primarily a lack of energy (kcalories). When kcalories are scarce, your cells are forced to use dietary and body proteins for glucose production. The secondary effect, then, is protein deficiency, which in turn produces the common symptoms of starvation: anemia, edema, and diarrhea.

Causes

In earlier times, when most people grew and hunted their own food, hunger was often brought about by environmental conditions, such as drought or winter weather, that limited food availability.

Economics. In the industrialized era, however, poverty has replaced nature as the leading cause of hunger. Until 1990 the world's population was small enough that redistribution of resources coupled with a decreased reliance on animal-derived foods in theory could have provided adequate food for every person on the planet. By 1990 the Earth's population had reached an estimated 5 billion people. Experts conceded that even under ideal conditions the world hunger crisis could not easily be solved. Worldwide, 15 million to 30 million people are at risk of starving to death each year. Those segments of the population that have the lowest tissue reserves, such as children, pregnant and/or lactating women, elderly people, and the infirm, are at greatest risk. Alarmingly, it appears that in the near future the situation will worsen rather than improve. If the population analysts are correct, the Earth will be inhabited by 6 billion people by the year 2000, provided diseases such as AIDS (acquired immune deficiency syndrome) do not proceed unchecked.[3,24,28]

The problem is not just one for developing nations to solve. As the 20th century draws to a close, the industrial era is giving way to what many social scientists describe as the "information age." This new era is bringing dizzying technological advancements, creating a demand for well-trained workers and thus widening the gap between the "haves" and "have-nots," both within industrialized nations and between these nations and their less developed neighbors.

The situation in the United States is a microcosm of the problems experienced by other developed nations. In the past generation, a greater emphasis on women's rights has increased their numbers in the work force. At the same time the rising cost of living has outstripped wage increases, meaning a greater number of families need two incomes just to get by. Concurrently, changing moral standards have led to more divorces. Record numbers of households are now being headed by women. Because women traditionally have earned less than their male counterparts, many of these single-parent households are living in or on the brink of poverty. Thousands more families are just one paycheck away from financial devastation. Add to this the cuts in the federal government's domestic spending, including school breakfast and lunch programs, and we see emerging a whole new generation of poverty-stricken, malnourished Americans.[3]

Politics. Compounding the domestic crisis, many political and economic practices of developed nations have perpetuated and worsened the global hunger crisis. In earlier times, politically and economically dominant nations colonized less developed ones to exploit their resources. Although political colonization is now virtually nonexistent, economic colonization is alive and well. The ongoing struggle over control of the Middle Eastern oil fields is a well-publicized example of a widespread problem. The lifestyle that people in technologically advanced nations take for granted consumes more resources than these countries produce. To keep up with demands, these nations have invested in refineries, factories, and farms in less developed regions. On the surface this arrangement seems to benefit everyone involved. In-depth analysis reveals a different picture. Typically the developed nations obtain goods, such as lumber, rubber, and metals, at bargain-basement prices and often leave ecological devastation in their wake, thus depriving developing nations of the resources they need to improve their people's standard of living.[24,28]

Foreign demands for luxury products such as cocoa, coffee, tea, tobacco, and beef, coupled with the developing nations' enormous debt, encourages these nations to use their agricultural resources to grow cash crops for export rather than the food products they need to feed their own people.[24]

Results

Starvation and malnutrition are major problems worldwide. The term **marasmus** is used to differentiate kcalorie deficit from protein deficiency, which is called **kwashiokor** (see Chapter 6, Protein). The terms **protein energy malnutrition (PEM)** or **protein calorie malnutrition (PCM)** are more commonly used today. In either case the early symptoms may include anemia, edema, lethargy, and susceptibility to infection and disease. Later there is loss of body tissue, muscle and organ tissue, adipose tissue, and eventually death.

Recommendations

Agencies like the United Nations that have thoroughly studied the problem recommend solutions that involve widespread political and economic reforms in conjunction with improvements in health care, population control, education, and agricultural practices.[28]

Production. Developed nations can help by reducing their reliance on nonrenewable resources, rethinking their foreign aid and investment practices, assisting with the development of environmentally appropriate agricultural practices, and helping implement health care and family planning programs. Although the United States and Western Europe support only 10% of the world's population, they consume over 40% of the world's resources. By decreasing their reliance on animal-derived foods, increasing recycling efforts, and using energy-efficient transportation, lighting, heating, and building methods (the technologies for which are already available), the developed nations could greatly reduce the stress they place on the environment and their developing neighbors.

Simply sending food or trying to transplant western agricultural practices to nonindustrialized nations will not solve the hunger crisis. Developed nations previously have tried to improve third-world food production by introducing crops that require considerable amounts of chemical fertilizers, pesticides, and mechanical harvesting devices. These efforts have been largely unsuccessful because the developing nations have been unable to sustain these practices on their own. Instead developed nations should concentrate on helping their neighbors increase production of a variety of native crops using organic or semi-organic farming practices. (See the discussion of organic and sustainable farming on p. 242.)

Developed nations can better assist their developing neighbors by sending advisers along with the aid packages. Aid without education is a short-term solution to a long-term problem. Ideally industrialized nations would take inspiration from the Chinese adage: "Give a man a fish and he eats for a day; teach him to fish and he can feed himself for a lifetime." This approach would encourage investment in businesses that will lead to economic independence for the developing nation.

Demand. Although implementing the changes outlined above will help supply more food, it does not address the other half of the hunger equation: demand. Demand for food is at an all-time high and if forecasters are correct will only increase. An important aspect of ensuring adequate food supplies is to decrease the demand by restricting population growth. This can be accomplished only through a combination of health care to reduce the current death rate and family planning to decrease the current birth rate.

Decreasing the death rate may seem like a strange, even contradictory, way to decrease world population. It has been shown repeatedly, however, that the best way to decrease the birth rate is to have a better survival rate. Infant mortality rates in developing nations are two to three times higher than in developed countries. As if to compensate, the birth rate in developing nations tends to be many times higher, thus creating a vicious and unending cycle of suffering.

Most of the 40,000 children under age 5 who die daily succumb to a combination of infectious disease and malnutrition.[28] Many of these diseases, such as measles and diarrhea, can be treated relatively simply and inexpensively. Measles vaccines cost about 12 cents each, and the medication to treat diarrhea is just 10 cents per dose.[28] Family planning measures are similarly affordable. The success of any of these measures, however, depends on education. People must understand the need for medical care and inoculations. They also need to learn the role that good hygiene and breast-feeding play in reducing transmission of infections and the need for appropriate weaning foods to maintain a child's nutritional status (see Chapter 12, Life Cycle).

The sheer magnitude of the problem can make people in developed nations feel as helpless about finding a solution as the starving feel about finding a meal. Remember that one person can make a difference. Change comes about not just by governments making laws and funding programs, but by each of us doing our part to contribute to a healthier society.[28]

Recycling

From the grocery store to the kitchen to the restaurant, the ultimate goal of the ecologically conscious consumer is total recycling. The problem of solid waste disposal looms large for scientists, urban planners, and consumers alike. As of 1990 it was estimated that each person in the United States produced 3.5 pounds of trash per day, the majority of which ends up in landfills. But what happens when the landfills are filled, as is expected to happen by the year 2000 to half of those currently in operation? Approximately half of all trash is packaging, so we can truly reduce garbage production by not using items encased in excess packaging, opting for items in recyclable packaging, and making the commitment to recycle them.[6,22,23] To find out what kinds of recycling options are available in your community, look in the yellow pages of your phone book under "Recycling" or call your refuse company. If no recycling service is available, try to generate community interest in getting one started. Finally, always try to purchase products in recyclable containers because this sends a message to the manufacturer that you value recycling.

The 3 R's of recycling are:
- **Reduce**
- **Reuse**
- **Recycle**

Which product containers can be recycled? In reality almost anything can be recycled, but in some instances recycling is neither economically nor environmentally feasible. For example, the work involved in separating the wax from the cardboard on milk or frozen food containers and the time and chemicals involved in separating the numerous components of aseptic juice and milk boxes make it impractical to recycle these packages.

At the Grocery Store

How do I choose products with an eye toward recycling? A quick armchair tour through the grocery store brings the fine points of recycling into focus.[6,17]

Dairy Decisions

Choose milk in recyclable plastic jugs, eggs in pulp paper cartons, and soft-spread margarine in recyclable plastic tubs.

Meat Matters

There was a time when butchers waited on patrons and wrapped their selections in butcher paper. The self-serve era has done away with this tradition. Instead meat, fish, and poultry are presented on Styrofoam trays, wrapped in plastic film. Producing this packaging creates huge amounts of toxic waste; worse yet, most municipalities won't recycle Styrofoam. Consumers should encourage Styrofoam recycling efforts and patronize old-fashioned butcher shops.

Frosty Facts

Choose frozen foods with the smallest possible amount of packaging. Microwaveable frozen and shelf-stable items are some of the worst offenders when it comes to excess packing, so choose carefully.

Whenever possible, choose foods packed in plastic bags over those in waxed boxes because they are easier to recycle. If neither of these are recyclable in your area, choose the plastic bag: it will take up less room in the landfill. Purchase frozen concentrated juices. It is cheaper on the wallet as well as easier on the environment for you to add your own water at home.

 What environmental costs are involved in making, packaging, and marketing juices in plastic jugs?

Produce Pointers

Try to avoid packaging altogether. In particular, stay away from fresh produce in microwave-ready containers. Sometimes packaging is unavoidable, such as when you purchase a pound of green beans or 10 pounds of potatoes. Just be sure to reuse or recycle the plastic bags you do use.

Snack and Cereal Sense

Look for foods packaged in containers made from recycled paper. Many such products carry the recycle logo. You can confirm their recycle status by looking for gray on the inside of the packaging.

In the Kitchen

Minimize use of plastic wraps. Purchase reusable storage containers. Invest in microwave-safe cookware with matching lids.

Why are glass containers preferable to plastic ones for microwaving? Hint: See the In the Kitchen section of Chapter 9, Energy.

Use reusable containers to pack your lunch. Look for the new sip-and-serve-style reusable drink containers. If you must wrap your lunch in a one-time-use-only package, choose aluminum foil. After you eat, clean off the food remnants and recycle the foil.

Separate dry refuse from wet waste to cut down on the use of plastic garbage bags. Consider composting your fruit and vegetable trimmings as well as leftover grain and vegetable dishes. It saves room in landfills, cuts down on the use of plastic garbage bags, and returns valuable nutrients to the soil in the form of natural fertilizer.

Name an additional environmental benefit of using compost for fertilizer.

Eating Out

Ask to have leftovers wrapped in foil instead of packed in environmentally unfriendly Styrofoam. If you are eating in at a fast-food outlet, request that the Styrofoam packaging be omitted from your order.[17]

Disaster Preparedness

Since 1989 we Americans have experienced an unusual number of natural disasters, from devastating earthquakes in the San Francisco Bay area and Los Angeles to hurricanes that destroyed thousands of homes in South Carolina, Florida, and Louisiana. Severe flooding in the summer of 1993 left additional thousands of people homeless in riverside towns throughout the Midwest. People who live in disaster-prone areas should be prepared to get by on their own for at least 3 to 5 days. Putting the items listed in the Emergency Essentials box below in a readily accessible area will go a long way toward making it easier to live through a manmade or natural disaster.[21]

A Redipak Disaster Preparedness Kit is available from Redipak in Kensington, California, for about $95. Described as a no-nonsense survival pack for 2 adults for 3 days, it contains all the essentials in a waterproof container. A child's pack, which sells for $24, is also available. Similar kits are available from Earthquake Preparedness Supply in Oakland, California, 510-839-0617.[21]

WHERE DO WE GO FROM HERE?

As you have seen throughout this text, nutrition is an exciting and ever-changing field that affects every aspect of our lives. As you have moved through these chapters, we hope you have gained the knowledge you need to make good decisions about your diet, your exercise regimen, and your overall lifestyle. We also hope we have shown you how to think scientifically, critically, and constructively about the role of nutrition in our increasingly diverse American population and in the global village that our world is rapidly becoming.

EMERGENCY ESSENTIALS

FOOD BASICS

- 2 quarts to 1 gallon of water per person per day
- Canned food that can be eaten hot or cold (such as spaghetti and meatballs, chili, etc.)
- Shelf-stable cheese foods
- Peanut butter or prepackaged peanut butter or cheese-filled crackers
- Granola-style breakfast bars
- Freeze-dried or dehydrated foods (look for these at a camping supply store, and remember they will require water to reconstitute)
- Food for infants, pets, and anyone with special dietary requirements

COOKING SUPPLIES

- Manual can opener
- Camp stove or barbecue grill with appropriate fuel and lighter
- Sealable plastic bags
- Paper plates and plastic utensils or a camping mess kit
- Pots
- Utensils
- Paper towels and heavy-duty aluminum foil

MEDICAL SUPPLIES

- First aid kit
- Essential medications
- Extra eyeglasses
- Emergency survival blanket

SANITATION SUPPLIES

- Large plastic garbage bags
- Liquid detergent, shampoo, toothpaste
- Premoistened towelettes
- Toilet paper
- Powdered lime for sanitation
- Feminine hygiene supplies
- Baby diapers

TOOLS AND SAFETY SUPPLIES

- Battery-operated radio
- Flashlight
- Candles and matches
- Work gloves
- Fire extinguisher
- Tools, rope, and duct tape

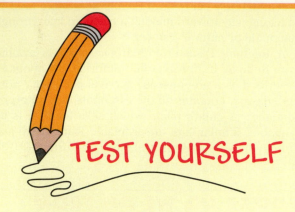

TEST YOURSELF

1. What are bioengineered foods?
2. What is the difference between organic farming and sustainable farming?
3. List three ways in which industrialized nations can help ease the world food crisis.
4. What is mass marketing? Why is it disappearing?
5. How many days' worth of food and water should you have on hand for emergencies?
6. Which age group is the fastest-growing segment of the population?
7. What are chemically engineered foods?
8. What are multiethnic foods? Give an example.
9. Why do food industry experts believe there will be a greater demand for convenience foods and takeout foods in the next decade?
10. What is a good way to keep abreast of new developments in the field of nutrition?

REFERENCES

1. ADA For your information: Working the bugs out: integrated pest management saves crops and the environment, *Journal of the American Dietetic Association* 92(8):931, 1992.
2. Chaisson P et al: *Pesticides in food,* Chicago, 1991, American Dietetic Association.
3. Campbell C: Food insecurity: a nutritional outcome or a predictor variable? *Journal of Nutrition* 121:408-415, 1991.
4. Consumers spill BST milk, *San Francisco Chronicle,* Feb 4, 1994, p. 1.
5. Current population survey, Washington, DC, 1990, U.S. Census Bureau.
6. *50 simple things you can do to save the planet,* Berkeley, Calif, 1991, Earth Works.
7. Food trends in the nineties, *San Francisco Chronicle* Food Section, Jan 12, 1994, p. 1.
8. "Hot" food issues, *Food Safety Notebook* 4(3)25:1993.
9. Gore A: *Earth in the balance: Ecology and the human spirit,* Boston, 1992, Houghton Mifflin.
10. Hunt JR: Nutritional products for specific health benefits: Foods, pharmaceuticals, or something in between, *Journal of the American Dietetic Association* 94:151-153, 1994.
11. Mandel TF: *American social trends in the 1990's,* Stanford, Calif, 1989, Stanford Research Institute, International Report #773.
12. Monsen ER: Forces for research, *Journal of the American Dietetic Association* 93:981-985, 1993.
13. Nathan J: The food of the future is ethnic and fast, *New York Times,* Mar 7, 1989.
14. "Flavr Saver" tomato ripe this month? *New York Times* section C3, Oct 26, 1993.
15. Owen AL: The impact of future foods on nutrition and health, *Journal of the American Dietetic Association* 90(9):1217-1222, 1990.
16. Opportunities in nutrition and food sciences: research challenges and the next generation of investigators, Washington, DC, 1993, Food and Nutrition Board, National Academy of Science.
17. Pack it right, *Nutrition Action Health Letter* 17(3):1, 1990.
18. Personal communication, FDA Press Office, Washington, DC, Feb 8, 1994.
19. Perspectives on pesticides and organic foods, *Food Safety Notebook* 2(5)37, 1991.
20. The USDA follow-up of an outbreak of food-borne illness, *Food Safety Notebook* 4(2):15, 1993.
21. Surviving the next BIG ONE, *San Francisco Chronicle* Home Section, Jan 19, 1994.
22. Sloan AE: Consumers, the environment, and the food industry, *Food Technology* 47:72-75, 1993.
23. *Smithsonian* magazine, 20th Earth Day Edition, Apr 1990.
24. Stout BA (ed): *Energy in world agriculture,* vol. 1, 1986, New York, Elsiver.
25. Thomas P, Earl R: Creating the future of nutrition and food sciences, *Journal of the American Dietetic Association* 94:257-259, 1994.
26. *Time* special issue: The new face of America: how immigrants are shaping the world's first multicultural society, Fall 1993, Time Inc.
27. Two years after alar: a survey of consumer attitudes toward food safety, Center for Produce Quality, Alexandria, VA, Mar 1991.
28. United Nations 9th Annual World Food Day Teleconference Study Packet, 1992.
29. University of California at Davis Agricultural & Environmental Science Outlook, Fall 1991.

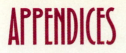

APPENDICES

A-1

A Food Composition Tables
B Dietary Advice for Canadians
C The Exchange System
D Dietary Intake Assessment
E Common Causes of Food Poisoning: Source, Symptoms, and Prevention
F Kitchen and Pantry Essentials
G Nutrition Information Resources

WT, weight; **KCAL,** kcalories; **PROT,** protein; **CARB,** carbohydrate; **FIBR,** fiber; **FAT,** fat; **SATF,** saturated fat;
MONO, monosaturated fat; **POLY,** polyunsaturated fat; **CHOL,** cholesterol; **SOD,** sodium; **POT,** potassium;

Food Name	Portion	WT (Gm)	KCAL	PROT (Gm)	CARB (Gm)	FIBR (Gm)	FAT (Gm)	SATF (Gm)	MONO (Gm)	POLY (Gm)
Baby Foods										
BABY FOOD-CEREAL-OATMEAL-MILK	OUNCE	28.4	33	1	4	0.7	1	0.4	0.8	0.9
BABY FOOD-CEREAL-RICE-MILK	OUNCE	28.4	33	1	5	0.3	1	t	t	t
BABY FOOD-DESSERT-BANANAS & TAPIOCA	OUNCE	28.4	16	t	4	0.7	0	0	0	0
BABY FOOD-DESSERT-CUSTARD CHOCOLATE-USDA	OUNCE	28.4	24	1	5	0.1	1	0.3	0.2	t
BABY FOOD-DESSERT-CUSTARD-VANILLA	OUNCE	28.4	24	t	5	0.1	1	0.3	0.2	t
BABY FOOD-DESSERT-MANGO/TAPIOCA	OUNCE	28.4	23	t	6	0	t	0	0	0
BABY FOOD-DESSERT-ORANGE PUDDING	OUNCE	28.4	23	t	5	0.1	t	0.2	0.1	t
BABY FOOD-DESSERT-PAPAYA/APPLE/TAPIOCA	OUNCE	28.4	20	t	5	0.1	0	0	0	0
BABY FOOD-DESSERT-PLUMS & TAPIOCA	OUNCE	28.4	20	0	6	0.3	0	0	0	0
BABY FOOD-DESSERT-PRUNES & TAPIOCA	OUNCE	28.4	20	t	5	0.7	0	0	0	0
BABY FOOD-EGG YOLKS	SERVING	28.4	58	3	t	0	5	1.5	1.8	0.5
BABY FOOD-FRUIT JUICE-APPLE	FL OZ	31	14	0	4	0.3	0	0	0	0
BABY FOOD-FRUIT JUICE-APPLE BLUEBERRY	OUNCE	28.4	17	t	5	0.1	t	0	0	0
BABY FOOD-FRUIT JUICE-APPLE PEACH-USDA	FL OZ	31	13	0	3	0.3	0	0	0	0
BABY FOOD-FRUIT JUICE-APPLE PRUNE-USDA	FL OZ	31	23	t	6	0.5	0	0	0	0
BABY FOOD-FRUIT JUICE-MIXED FRUIT-USDA	FL OZ	31	14	0	4	0.3	0	0	0	0
BABY FOOD-FRUIT JUICE-ORANGE	FL OZ	31	14	t	3	0.3	t	0	0	0
BABY FOOD-FRUIT-APPLESAUCE	OUNCE	28.4	12	t	3	0.7	0	0	0	0
BABY FOOD-FRUIT-PEACHES	OUNCE	28.4	20	t	5	0.7	0	0	0	0
BABY FOOD-FRUIT-PEARS	OUNCE	28.4	12	t	3	0.3	0	0	0	0
BABY FOOD-FRUIT-PEARS & PINEAPPLE	OUNCE	28.4	12	t	3	0.3	0	0	0	0
BABY FOOD-MEAT-BEEF	OUNCE	28.4	30	4	0	0	2	0.7	0.6	0.1
BABY FOOD-MEAT-BEEF & EGG NOODLES-STR	OUNCE	28.4	15	1	2	0.1	1	0.2	0.2	t
BABY FOOD-MEAT-BEEF STEW	OUNCE	28.4	14	1	2	0.3	t	0.2	0.1	t
BABY FOOD-MEAT-CHICKEN STEW-STR	OUNCE	28.4	22	2	2	0.2	1	0.3	0.5	0.2
BABY FOOD-MEAT-LAMB	OUNCE	28.4	29	4	0	0	1	0.7	0.5	0.1
BABY FOOD-MEAT-LIVER	OUNCE	28.4	29	4	t	0	1	0.4	0.2	t
BABY FOOD-MEAT-PORK	OUNCE	28.4	35	4	0	0	2	0.7	1	0.2
BABY FOOD-MEAT-VEAL	OUNCE	28.4	29	4	0	0	1	0.7	0.6	0.1
BABY FOOD-VEGETABLES-BEANS-GREEN	OUNCE	28.4	7	t	2	0.4	0	0	0	0
BABY FOOD-VEGETABLES-BEANS-GREEN/BU-STR	OUNCE	28.4	9	t	2	0.7	t	t	0	t
BABY FOOD-VEGETABLES-CARROTS-STR-USDA	OUNCE	28.4	8	t	2	0.7	0	0	0	0
BABY FOOD-VEGETABLES-GARDEN	OUNCE	28.4	11	1	2	0.7	t	0	0	0
BABY FOOD-VEGETABLES-PEAS	OUNCE	28.4	11	1	2	0.7	t	0	0	0
BABY FOOD-VEGETABLES-SQUASH	OUNCE	28.4	7	t	2	0.7	t	0	0	0
BABY FOOD-VEGETABLES-SWEET POTATOES	OUNCE	28.4	16	t	4	0.7	0	0	0	0
Beverages										
ALE-MILD-AMERICAN	CUP	230	98	1	8	0	0	0	0	0
BEER-BUDWEISER	FL OZ	30	13	t	1	0.2	0	0	0	0
BEER-LIGHT	FL OZ	29.5	8	t	t	0	0	0	0	0
BEER-MICHELOB	FL OZ	30	13	t	1	0.1	0	0	0	0
BEER-NATURAL LIGHT	FL OZ	30	8	t	1	0	0	0	0	0
BEER-REGULAR	FL OZ	29.7	12	t	1	0.1	0	0	0	0
BRANDY-CALIFORNIA	ITEM	30	73	*	*	0	0	0	0	0
BRANDY-COGNAC-PONY	ITEM	30	73	0	0	0	0	0	0	0
CARNATION INSTANT BREAKFAST-CHOCOLATE	ITEM	36	130	7	23	*	1	*	*	*
CARNATION INSTANT BREAKFAST-EGGNOG	ITEM	34	130	7	23	*	0	0	0	0
CARNATION INSTANT BREAKFAST-VANILLA	ITEM	35	130	7	24	*	0	0	0	0
CHAMPAGNE-DOMESTIC-GLASSFUL	ITEM	120	84	t	3	0	0	0	0	0
CHOCOLATE BEVERAGE POWDER-DRY MILK ADDED	OUNCE	28.4	100	5	20	0.5	1	0.5	0.3	0
CHOCOLATE BEVERAGE POWDER-NO DRY MILK	OUNCE	28.4	99	1	26	12	1	0.5	0.3	t
CIDER-FERMENTED	FL OZ	30	12	t	t	0	0	0	0	0

t = Trace of nutrient present   * = Not available

MAG, magnesium; IRON, iron; ZINC, zinc; VITA, vitamin A; VITC, vitamin C; THIA, thiamin; RIBO, riboflavin; NIAC, niacin; VB6, vitamin B-6;
FOL, folate; VB12, vitamin B-12; CALC, calcium; PHOS, phosphorus; SEL, selenium; VE-a, alpha tocopherol equivalents.

CHOL (mg)	SOD (mg)	POT (mg)	MAG (mg)	IRON (mg)	ZINC (mg)	VITA (RE)	VITC (mg)	THIA (mg)	RIBO (mg)	NIAC (mg)	VB6 (mg)	FOL (µg)	VB12 (µg)	CALC (mg)	PHOS (mg)	SEL (µg)	VE-a (mg)
0	13	58	10	3.4	0.3	6	t	0.14	0.16	1.7	0.02	3	0.09	62	45	1	0.2
0	13	54	13	3.5	0.2	6	t	0.13	0.14	1.5	0.03	2	0.09	68	50	1	0.2
0	3	25	3	0.1	t	1	5	t	0.01	0.1	0.03	2	0	1	2	0	0.2
0	7	24	3	0.1	0.1	1	t	t	0.03	t	t	1	t	17	14	0	0.1
0	8	19	2	0.1	0.1	2	t	t	0.02	t	0.01	2	t	16	13	0	0.1
0	1	17	1	t	t	19	35	0.01	0.01	0.1	0.03	1	0	1	2	0	0.2
0	6	24	2	t	t	3	3	0.01	0.02	t	0.01	2	0	9	8	0	0.1
0	1	22	1	0.1	t	2	32	t	0.01	t	0.01	1	0	2	2	0	0.2
0	2	24	1	0.1	t	3	t	t	0.01	0.1	0.01	t	0	2	2	0	0.2
0	1	50	3	0.1	t	13	t	0.01	0.02	0.1	0.02	t	0	4	4	0	0.2
223	11	22	2	0.8	0.5	107	t	0.02	0.08	t	0.05	26	0.44	22	81	5	0.5
0	1	28	1	0.2	t	1	18	t	0.01	t	0.01	0	0	1	2	0	0.2
0	0	20	1	0.1	t	1	8	0.01	0.01	t	0.01	1	0	1	2	0	0.2
0	t	30	1	0.2	t	2	18	t	t	0.1	0.01	t	0	1	1	0	0.2
0	2	46	2	0.3	t	1	21	t	t	0.1	0.01	0	0	3	5	0	0.2
0	1	31	2	0.1	t	1	20	0.01	t	t	0.01	2	0	2	2	0	0.2
0	0	57	3	0.1	t	2	19	0.01	0.01	0.1	0.02	8	0	4	3	0	0.2
0	1	20	1	0.1	t	0	11	t	0.01	t	0.01	1	0	1	2	0	0.2
0	2	46	2	0.1	t	5	9	t	0.01	0.2	t	1	0	2	3	0	0.2
0	1	37	2	0.1	t	1	7	t	0.01	0.1	t	1	0	2	3	0	0.2
0	1	33	2	0.1	t	1	8	0.01	0.01	0.1	0.01	1	0	3	2	0	0.2
4	23	62	5	0.4	0.7	16	1	t	0.04	0.8	0.04	2	0.4	2	24	3	0.1
2	8	13	2	0.1	0.1	31	t	0.01	0.01	0.2	0.01	1	0.03	3	8	3	0.1
4	98	40	3	0.2	0.2	95	1	t	0.02	0.4	0.02	2	0.15	3	12	3	0.1
8	114	26	3	0.2	0.1	50	1	0.01	0.02	0.3	0.01	t	0.04	10	14	3	0.1
0	18	58	4	0.4	0.8	7	t	0.01	0.06	0.8	0.04	1	0.62	2	27	4	0.1
52	21	64	4	1.5	0.8	3247	6	0.01	0.51	2.4	0.1	96	0.61	1	58	7	0.1
14	12	63	3	0.3	0.6	3	1	0.04	0.06	0.6	0.06	1	0.28	1	27	4	0.1
11	18	61	4	0.4	0.6	4	1	0.01	0.05	1	0.04	2	0.37	2	28	3	0.1
0	1	45	7	0.2	0.1	13	2	0.01	0.02	0.1	0.01	10	0	11	6	0	0.2
0	1	45	7	0.4	0.1	13	2	0.01	0.03	0.1	0.01	8	0	18	6	170	0.2
0	11	56	3	0.1	t	325	2	0.01	0.01	0.1	0.02	4	0	6	6	0	0.2
0	10	48	6	0.2	0.1	172	2	0.02	0.02	0.2	0.03	11	0	8	8	0	0.2
0	1	32	4	0.3	0.1	16	2	0.02	0.02	0.3	0.02	7	0	6	12	0	0.2
0	1	51	3	0.1	t	57	2	t	0.02	0.1	0.02	4	0	7	4	0	0.2
0	6	75	4	0.1	0.1	183	3	0.01	0.01	0.1	0.03	3	0	4	7	0	0.2
0	16	*	*	0.2	*	0	0	0	0.07	0.5	*	*	*	30	41	1	*
0	2	7	2	t	0	0	0	t	0.01	0.1	0.02	2	0.01	1	4	0	0
0	1	5	1	t	t	0	0	t	0.01	0.1	0.01	1	t	1	4	0	0
0	2	7	2	t	0	0	0	t	0.01	0.1	0.02	2	0.01	1	4	0	0
0	2	5	1	t	t	0	0	t	0.01	0.1	0.01	1	0	1	4	0	0
0	1	7	2	t	t	0	0	t	0.01	0.1	0.02	2	0.01	1	4	*	0
0	*	*	*	*	*	*	*	*	*	*	*	*	*	*	*	*	*
0	t	1	0	t	t	0	0	t	t	t	0	0	0	0	1	*	0
*	136	422	80	4.5	3	525	27	0.3	0.07	5	0.4	0	0.6	100	150	*	5
0	196	266	80	4.5	3	525	27	0.3	0.07	5	0.4	0	0.6	100	150	*	5
0	145	382	80	4.5	3	525	27	0.3	0.07	5	0.4	0	0.6	100	150	*	5
0	*	*	*	*	*	*	*	*	*	*	*	*	*	*	*	*	*
2	147	227	23	0.5	0.3	3	1	0.04	0.21	0.2	t	12	0.68	167	155	*	0.1
0	60	168	28	0.9	0.4	1	t	0.01	0.04	0.1	t	2	0	11	36	*	0.1
0	0	36	1	0.1	t	0	t	0.01	0.01	t	0.01	t	0	2	2	*	t

WT, weight; **KCAL**, kcalories; **PROT**, protein; **CARB**, carbohydrate; **FIBR**, fiber; **FAT**, fat; **SATF**, saturated fat;

MONO, monosaturated fat; **POLY**, polyunsaturated fat; **CHOR**, cholesterol; **SOD**, sodium; **POT**, potassium;

Food Name	Portion	WT (Gm)	KCAL	PROT (Gm)	CARB (Gm)	FIBR (Gm)	FAT (Gm)	SATF (Gm)	MONO (Gm)	POLY (Gm)
COCKTAIL-DAIQUIRI	ITEM	100	186	t	7	0	t	t	t	t
COCKTAIL-EGGNOG	ITEM	123	335	4	18	0	16	1.8	1.3	0.3
COCKTAIL-GIN RICKEY	ITEM	120	150	0	1	0	0	0	0	0
COCKTAIL-HIGHBALL	FL OZ	29	26	0	0	0	0	0	0	0
COCKTAIL-MANHATTAN	FL OZ	28.5	64	t	1	0	0	0	0	0
COCKTAIL-MARTINI	FL OZ	28.2	63	0	t	0	0	0	0	0
COCKTAIL-MINT JULEP	ITEM	300	212	0	3	0	0	0	0	0
COCKTAIL-OLD FASHIONED	ITEM	100	180	0	4	0	0	0	0	0
COCKTAIL-PINA COLADA-HOME RECIPE	FL OZ	31.4	58	t	9	0.1	1	0.3	0.1	0.1
COCKTAIL-PLANTERS PUNCH	ITEM	100	175	t	8	0	0	0	0	0
COCKTAIL-RUM SOUR	ITEM	100	165	0	0	0	0	0	0	0
COCKTAIL-TOM COLLINS	FL OZ	29.6	16	0	t	0	0	0	0	0
COFFEE SUBSTITUTE-PREPARED	FL OZ	30.3	2	t	t	0	0	0	0	0
COFFEE-BREWED	FL OZ	29.6	1	t	t	0	0	t	0	t
COFFEE-INSTANT-PREPARED	CUP	239	5	t	1	0	0	t	0	t
CORDIALS/LIQUEUR-54 PROOF	FL OZ	34	97	t	12	0	0	0	0	0
FRUIT PUNCH DRINK-CANNED	FL OZ	31	15	0	4	0	0	t	t	t
FRUIT PUNCH-POWDERED-PREPARED WITH WATER	CUP	262	97	0	25	*	t	t	t	t
GATORADE-THIRST QUENCHING DRINK	FL OZ	30.1	8	0	2	0	0	0	0	0
HOT COCOA-PREPARED WITH MILK-HOME RECIPE	CUP	250	218	9	26	3	9	5.6	2.7	0.3
LIQUEURS-ANISETTE	ITEM	20	74	0	7	0	0	0	0	0
LIQUEURS-APRICOT BRANDY	ITEM	20	64	t	6	0	0	0	0	0
LIQUEURS-BENEDICTINE	ITEM	20	69	*	7	0	0	0	0	0
LIQUEURS-CREME DE MENTHE	FL OZ	33.6	125	0	14	0	t	t	t	0.1
LIQUEURS-CURACAO	ITEM	20	54	*	6	0	0	0	0	0
OVALTINE-CHOCOLATE FLAVOR-PREPARED/MILK	CUP	265	227	10	29	0.2	9	5.5	2.6	0.4
OVALTINE-MALT FLAVOR-PREPARED WITH MILK	CUP	265	228	10	29	0.1	8	5.4	2.5	0.4
POSTUM-INSTANT GRAIN BEVERAGE-DRY MIX	OUNCE	28.4	103	2	24	0	t	0	0	0
SANKA-DECAFFEINATED COFFEE-PREPARED	FL OZ	29.8	t	0	t	0	0	0	0	0
SODA-CLUB-CARBONATED	FL OZ	29.6	0	0	0	0	0	0	0	0
SODA-COLA TYPE-CARBONATED	FL OZ	30.8	13	0	3	0	0	t	0	0
SODA-CREAM FLAVORED-CARBONATED	FL OZ	30.9	16	0	4	0	0	0	0	0
SODA-DIET COLA-NUTRASWEET-CARBONATED	FL OZ	29.6	t	t	t	0	0	0	0	0
SODA-DR. PEPPER TYPE COLA-CARBONATED	FL OZ	30.8	13	0	3	0	t	t	0	0
SODA-GINGER ALE-CARBONATED	FL OZ	30.5	10	0	3	0	0	0	0	0
SODA-GRAPE-CARBONATED	FL OZ	31	13	0	3	0	0	0	0	0
SODA-ROOT BEER-CARBONATED	FL OZ	30.8	13	0	3	0	0	0	0	0
SODA-TAB-LOW CALORIE COLA-CARBONATED	CUP	236	0	0	0	0	0	0	0	0
SODA-TONIC WATER/QUININE-CARBONATED	FL OZ	30.5	10	0	3	0	0	0	0	0
TANG-INSTANT BREAKFAST DRINK-ORANGE-DRY	OUNCE	28.4	104	0	26	*	0	0	0	0
TEA-BREWED	FL OZ	29.6	t	0	t	0	0	t	0	t
TEA-HERBAL-BREWED	FL OZ	29.6	t	0	t	0	0	t	0	t
TEA-INSTANT-PREPARED-SWEETENED	CUP	259	88	t	22	0	0	t	t	t
TEA-INSTANT-PREPARED-UNSWEETENED	CUP	237	2	0	t	0	0	0	0	0
WATER-MINERAL-PERRIER	CUP	237	0	0	0	0	0	0	0	0
WATER-MUNICIPAL TAP	CUP	237	0	0	0	0	0	0	0	0
WHISKEY/GIN/RUM/VODKA-100 PROOF	FL OZ	27.8	82	0	0	0	0	0	0	0
WHISKEY/GIN/RUM/VODKA-80 PROOF	FL OZ	27.8	64	0	0	0	0	0	0	0
WHISKEY/GIN/RUM/VODKA-86 PROOF	FL OZ	27.8	70	0	t	0	0	0	0	0
WHISKEY/GIN/RUM/VODKA-90 PROOF	FL OZ	27.7	73	0	0	0	0	0	0	0
WHISKEY/GIN/RUM/VODKA-94 PROOF	FL OZ	27.8	77	0	0	0	0	0	0	0
WINE COOLER-WHITE WINE AND 7UP	SERVING	102	55	t	6	0	0	0	0	0
WINE-CALIFORNIA/RED-GLASSFUL	ITEM	102	85	t	3	0	0	0	0	0
WINE-DESSERT	FL OZ	30	46	t	4	0	0	0	0	0
WINE-MADEIRA-GLASSFUL	ITEM	100	105	t	1	0	0	0	0	0
WINE-MUSCATEL/PORT-GLASSFUL	ITEM	100	158	t	14	0	0	0	0	0
WINE-RED-TABLE	FL OZ	29.5	21	t	1	0	0	0	0	0
WINE-ROSE-TABLE	FL OZ	29.5	21	t	t	0	0	0	0	0
WINE-SAUTERNE-GLASSFUL	ITEM	100	84	t	4	0	0	0	0	0
WINE-SHERRY-DRY-GLASSFUL	ITEM	60	84	t	5	0	0	0	0	0
WINE-VERMOUTH-DRY-GLASSFUL	ITEM	100	105	0	1	0	0	0	0	0
WINE-VERMOUTH-SWEET-GLASSFUL	ITEM	100	167	0	12	0	0	0	0	0
WINE-WHITE-TABLE	FL OZ	29.5	20	t	t	0	0	0	0	0

t = Trace of nutrient present   * = Not available

MAG, magnesium; **IRON**, iron; **ZINC**, zinc; **VITA**, vitamin A; **VITC**, vitamin C; **THIA**, thiamin; **RIBO**, riboflavin; **NIAC**, niacin; **VB6**, vitamin B-6; **FOL**, folate; **VB12**, vitamin B-12; **CALC**, calcium; **PHOS**, phosphorus; **SEL**, selenium; **VE-a**, alpha tocopherol equivalents.

CHOL (mg)	SOD (mg)	POT (mg)	MAG (mg)	IRON (mg)	ZINC (mg)	VITA (RE)	VITC (mg)	THIA (mg)	RIBO (mg)	NIAC (mg)	VB6 (mg)	FOL (µg)	VB12 (µg)	CALC (mg)	PHOS (mg)	SEL (µg)	VE-a (mg)
0	5	21	2	0.2	0.1	1	2	0.01	t	t	0.01	2	0	3	6	*	t
94	75	178	16	0.7	0.6	25	0	0.04	0.11	0	0.07	15	0.57	44	74	*	0.2
0	19	12	1	0	0.1	t	4	0.01	0	0	t	1	0	2	1	*	t
0	4	1	t	t	t	0	0	t	0	t	0	0	0	1	1	*	*
0	1	7	1	t	t	0	0	t	t	t	0	t	0	1	2	*	0
0	1	5	1	t	t	0	0	0	t	t	t	t	0	1	1	*	0
0	0	6	t	0.1	0.1	0	0	0.02	0.01	t	t	0	0	t	10	*	0
0	1	2	0	t	t	0	0	0.01	t	t	t	0	0	0	4	*	0
0	2	22	3	0.1	t	t	1	0.01	t	t	0.01	3	0	3	2	*	t
0	*	*	*	0.1	*	0	8	0.1	0	0	*	*	*	4	3	*	*
0	1	2	0	t	t	0	0	0.01	t	t	t	0	0	0	4	*	0
0	5	2	t	t	t	0	1	t	0	t	t	t	0	1	t	*	t
0	1	7	1	t	t	0	0	t	0	0.1	t	t	0	1	2	*	0
0	1	16	1	t	t	0	0	0	0	0.1	0	t	0	1	t	0	0
0	7	86	10	0.1	0.1	0	0	0	t	0.7	0	0	0	7	7	0	0
0	1	1	0	t	t	0	0	t	t	t	0	0	0	0	0	*	0
0	7	8	1	0.1	t	1	9	0.01	0.01	t	0	t	0	2	t	0	0
0	37	3	3	0.1	0.1	t	31	0	0.01	t	0	t	0	42	52	*	*
0	12	3	t	t	t	0	0	t	0	0	0	0	0	0	3	*	0
33	123	480	56	0.8	1.2	96	2	0.1	0.44	0.4	0.11	12	0.87	298	270	*	0.3
0	*	*	*	*	*	*	*	*	*	*	*	*	*	*	*	*	*
0	2	11	1	t	t	t	3	0.01	t	t	t	1	0	1	1	*	t
0	*	*	*	*	*	*	*	*	*	*	*	*	*	*	*	*	*
0	2	0	0	t	t	0	0	0	0	t	0	0	0	0	0	*	*
0	*	*	*	*	*	*	*	*	*	*	*	*	*	*	*	*	*
34	228	600	52	4.8	1.1	700	29	0.63	0.97	12.7	0.77	29	0.87	392	302	*	0.4
37	201	576	47	4.5	1.1	770	30	0.67	1.16	11.9	0.75	29	0.87	371	308	*	0.3
0	28	896	*	1.9	*	0	0	0.17	0.08	6.8	*	*	*	77	189	*	0
0	0	10	1	t	t	0	0	0	0	0	0	0	0	1	1	*	0
0	6	0	0	t	t	0	0	0	0	0	0	0	0	1	0	*	0
0	1	t	t	t	t	0	0	0	0	0	0	0	0	1	4	*	0
0	4	t	t	t	t	0	0	0	0	0	0	0	0	2	0	*	0
0	2	0	t	t	t	0	0	t	0.01	0	0	0	0	1	3	*	0
0	3	t	0	t	t	0	0	0	0	0	0	0	0	1	3	*	0
0	2	t	t	0.1	t	0	0	0	0	0	0	0	0	1	0	*	0
0	5	t	t	t	t	0	0	0	0	0	0	0	0	1	0	*	0
0	4	t	t	t	t	0	0	0	0	0	0	0	0	2	0	*	0
0	30	*	*	*	*	*	*	*	*	*	*	*	*	*	30	*	*
0	1	0	0	t	t	0	0	0	0	0	0	0	0	t	0	*	0
0	13	81	*	t	*	535	107	0	0	0	*	*	*	71	76	*	*
0	1	11	1	t	t	0	0	0	t	0	0	2	0	1	t	0	*
0	t	3	t	t	t	0	0	t	t	0	0	t	0	1	0	*	0
0	8	49	5	0.1	0.1	0	0	0	0.05	0.1	0.01	10	0	5	3	0	0
0	7	47	5	t	0.1	0	0	0	0.01	0.1	0.01	1	0	5	2	0	0
0	3	0	1	0	0	0	0	0	0	0	0	0	0	32	0	*	0
0	7	1	2	t	0.1	0	0	0	0	0	0	0	0	5	0	*	0
0	0	0	0	t	t	0	0	t	t	t	0	0	0	0	1	*	0
0	t	1	0	t	t	0	0	t	0	t	0	0	0	0	1	0	0
0	1	0	0	0	0	0	0	0	0	0	0	0	0	0	0	0	0
0	0	0	0	t	t	0	0	t	t	t	0	0	0	0	1	*	0
0	7	41	5	0.2	0.1	t	2	t	t	t	0.01	t	0	6	7	*	t
0	10	116	11	1	0.1	0	0	0.01	0.03	0.1	0.04	1	0.01	8	13	*	0
0	3	28	3	0.1	t	0	0	0.01	0.01	0.1	0	t	0	2	3	*	0
0	5	92	9	0.2	0.1	0	0	0.02	0.02	0.2	0	t	0	8	9	*	0
0	4	75	4	1.6	0.1	0	0	0.01	0.01	0.2	0.05	2	0	8	9	*	0
0	19	41	4	0.1	t	0	0	t	0.01	t	0.01	1	0	2	4	*	0
0	1	29	3	0.1	t	0	0	t	0.01	t	0.01	t	t	2	4	*	0
0	2	89	10	0.4	0.1	0	0	t	0.02	0.1	0.02	1	0.01	8	14	*	0
0	2	45	6	0.2	t	0	0	0.01	0.01	0.1	0.01	1	0.01	5	8	3	0
0	4	75	10	0.4	0.1	0	0	0.01	0.01	0.2	0.02	1	0.01	8	14	5	0
0	9	92	9	0.2	0.1	0	0	0.02	0.02	0.2	0	t	0	8	9	*	0
0	1	24	3	0.1	t	0	0	t	t	t	t	t	0	3	4	*	0

WT, weight; **KCAL**, kcalories; **PROT**, protein; **CARB**, carbohydrate; **FIBR**, fiber; **FAT**, fat; **SATF**, saturated fat;

MONO, monosaturated fat; **POLY**, polyunsaturated fat; **CHOR**, cholesterol; **SOD**, sodium; **POT**, potassium;

Food Name	Portion	WT (Gm)	KCAL	PROT (Gm)	CARB (Gm)	FIBR (Gm)	FAT (Gm)	SATF (Gm)	MONO (Gm)	POLY (Gm)
Breads										
BAGEL-EGG-3 INCH DIAMETER	ITEM	55	163	6	31	1.2	1	*	*	*
BAGEL-WATER-3 INCH DIAMETER	ITEM	55	163	6	31	1.2	1	0.2	0.4	0.6
BISCUITS-BAKING POWDER-FROM HOME RECIPE	ITEM	28.4	105	2	13	0.4	5	1.2	2	1.2
BISCUITS-BAKING POWDER-PREPARED FROM MIX	ITEM	28.4	104	2	13	0.5	5	3.3	1.3	0.2
BREAD STICKS-VIENNA TYPE	ITEM	35	106	3	20	1	1	*	*	*
BREAD-CRACKED WHEAT-ENRICHED	SLICE	25	66	2	13	1.3	1	0.1	0.2	0.2
BREAD-FRENCH-ENRICHED	SLICE	35	98	3	18	0.8	1	0.2	0.4	0.4
BREAD-ITALIAN-ENRICHED	SLICE	30	85	3	17	0.8	0	0	0	0
BREAD-MELBA TOAST-PLAIN	SLICE	4.67	16	1	3	0.3	0	0	0	0
BREAD-MELBA TOAST-WHEAT	SLICE	4.67	16	1	3	0.3	0	0	0	0
BREAD-MIXED GRAIN-UNTOASTED	SLICE	25	64	2	12	1.6	1	*	*	*
BREAD-PITA	ITEM	38	105	4	21	0.6	1	0.1	t	0.1
BREAD-PUMPERNICKEL	SLICE	32	82	3	15	1.9	1	*	*	*
BREAD-RAISIN-ENRICHED	SLICE	25	70	2	13	0.6	1	0.2	0.3	0.2
BREAD-RYE-AMERICAN-LIGHT	SLICE	25	66	2	12	1.6	1	*	*	*
BREAD-VIENNA-ENRICHED	SLICE	25	70	2	13	0.8	1	0.2	0.3	0.3
BREAD-WHEAT-FIRM	SLICE	21	59	2	11	2.4	1	0.1	0.2	0.3
BREAD-WHEAT-TOASTED	SLICE	22	68	2	12	2.5	2	0.2	0.3	0.8
BREAD-WHITE-FIRM	SLICE	23	61	2	11	0.4	1	0.2	0.3	0.3
BREAD-WHITE-FIRM-ENRICHED-TOASTED	SLICE	20	65	2	12	0.5	1	0.2	0.3	0.3
BREAD-WHITE-SOFT-ENRICHED-CRUMBS	CUP	45	120	4	22	1.2	2	0.3	0.5	0.5
BREAD-WHOLE WHEAT-FIRM	SLICE	25	61	2	11	2.8	1	0.1	0.2	0.3
BREAD-WHOLE WHEAT	SLICE	25	67	2	12	2.8	2	0.2	0.3	0.8
BREADCRUMBS-DRY-GRATED-ENRICHED	CUP	100	390	13	73	3.7	5	1	1.6	1.4
CORNBREAD-HOME RECIPE	SLICE	45	108	2	16	1.2	4	1.5	1.9	1.1
CRACKERS-ANIMAL	ITEM	1.9	9	t	1	t	t	0.1	0.1	t
CRACKERS-CHEDDAR SNACKS	ITEM	1.6	7	t	1	0.1	t	*	*	*
CRACKERS-CHEESE	ITEM	1	5	t	1	t	t	0.1	0.1	t
CRACKERS-CHEESE SNACKS	ITEM	1.13	6	t	1	t	t	0.1	0.1	t
CRACKERS-GRAHAM-PLAIN	ITEM	7	28	1	5	0.2	1	0.1	0.3	0.2
CRACKERS-GRAHAM-SUGAR-HONEY	ITEM	7	30	1	5	0.1	1	0.1	0.4	0.1
CRACKERS-OYSTER	ITEM	0.45	2	t	t	t	t	0	0	0
CRACKERS-RITZ	ITEM	3.33	18	t	2	0.1	1	*	*	*
CRACKERS-RY KRISP-NATURAL	ITEM	2.1	8	t	2	0.3	t	0	0	0
CRACKERS-RYE WAFERS	ITEM	6.5	23	1	5	1.1	0	0	0	0
CRACKERS-SALTINES	ITEM	2.75	13	t	2	0.1	t	0.1	0.1	0.1
CRACKERS-SESAME AND WHEAT-RALSTON	ITEM	1.9	9	t	1	0.2	t	*	*	*
CRACKERS-SNACKERS-RALSTON	ITEM	3.5	18	t	2	0.1	1	*	*	*
CRACKERS-TRISCUITS	ITEM	4.5	21	t	3	0.2	1	0.2	0.2	0.2
CRACKERS-WHEAT THINS	ITEM	1.8	9	t	1	0.1	t	*	*	*
FRENCH TOAST-FROM HOME RECIPE	SLICE	65	153	6	17	2	7	0.5	0.9	0.5
MUFFIN-BLUEBERRY-FROM HOME RECIPE	ITEM	40	110	3	17	0.9	4	1.1	1.4	0.7
MUFFIN-BRAN-FROM HOME RECIPE	ITEM	40	112	3	17	2.5	5	1.2	1.4	0.8
MUFFIN-CORN-FROM HOME RECIPE	ITEM	40	125	3	19	1	4	1.2	1.6	0.9
MUFFIN-ENGLISH-PLAIN-TOASTED	ITEM	53	154	5	30	1.5	1	0.3	0.4	0.4
MUFFIN-ENGLISH-PLAIN	ITEM	56	133	4	26	1.3	1	1.9	2.6	1.5
MUFFIN-PLAIN-FROM HOME RECIPE	ITEM	40	120	3	17	0.9	4	1	1.7	1
MUFFIN-SOY	ITEM	40	119	4	17	0.8	4	*	*	*
PANCAKES-BUCKWHEAT-FROM MIX	ITEM	27	55	2	6	0.6	2	0.8	0.9	0.4
PANCAKES-PLAIN-FROM HOME RECIPE	ITEM	27	60	2	9	0.5	2	0.5	0.8	0.5
PANCAKES-PLAIN-FROM MIX	ITEM	27	59	2	8	0.4	2	0.7	0.7	0.3
ROLL-BROWN & SERVE-ENRICHED	ITEM	26	85	2	14	1	2	0.4	0.7	0.5
ROLL-CINNAMON	ITEM	26	100	2	14	0.7	4	0.6	1.2	0.5
ROLL-CROISSANT-SARA LEE	ITEM	26	109	2	11	0.6	6	3.3	1.6	0.3
ROLL-HAMBURGER/HOTDOG-COMMERCIAL	ITEM	40	114	3	20	1	2	0.5	0.8	0.6
ROLL-HARD-COMMERCIAL-ENRICHED	ITEM	50	155	5	30	1.5	2	0.4	0.6	0.5
ROLL-SUBMARINE/HOAGIE-ENRICHED	ITEM	135	390	12	75	3.8	4	0.9	1.4	1.4
ROLL-WHOLE WHEAT-HOMEMADE	ITEM	35	90	4	18	1.8	1	0.4	0.6	1.4
WAFFLES-ENRICHED-FROM HOME RECIPE	ITEM	75	245	7	26	1.1	13	2.3	2.8	1.4
WAFFLES-FROZEN	ITEM	37	103	2	16	0.9	4	*	*	*
WAFFLES-OAT BRAN-NO CHOLESTEROL-EGGO	ITEM	39	110	3	16	2	4	0.7	1.1	2.1

t = Trace of nutrient present   * = Not available

MAG, magnesium; **IRON**, iron; **ZINC**, zinc; **VITA**, vitamin A; **VITC**, vitamin C; **THIA**, thiamin; **RIBO**, riboflavin; **NIAC**, niacin; **VB6**, vitamin B-6; **FOL**, folate; **VB12**, vitamin B-12; **CALC**, calcium; **PHOS**, phosphorus; **SEL**, selenium; **VE-a**, alpha tocopherol equivalents.

CHOL (mg)	SOD (mg)	POT (mg)	MAG (mg)	IRON (mg)	ZINC (mg)	VITA (RE)	VITC (mg)	THIA (mg)	RIBO (mg)	NIAC (mg)	VB6 (mg)	FOL (μg)	VB12 (μg)	CALC (mg)	PHOS (mg)	SEL (μg)	VE-a (mg)
8	198	41	11	1.5	0.3	24	0	0.21	0.16	1.9	0.02	13	0.05	23	37	*	*
0	198	41	11	1.5	0.3	0	0	0.21	0.16	1.9	0.02	13	0	23	37	18	*
0	175	33	6	0.4	*	0	0	0.08	0.08	0.7	*	*	*	34	49	5	1
1	221	33	3	0.6	0.1	37	0	0.1	0.07	1.8	0.01	2	0.04	34	99	5	1
0	548	33	*	0.3	*	0	0	0.02	0.03	0.3	*	*	*	16	31	*	*
0	108	33	9	0.7	*	0	0	0.1	0.1	0.8	0.02	*	0	16	32	11	t
0	193	30	7	1.1	0.2	0	0	0.16	0.12	1.4	0.02	13	0	39	28	10	t
0	152	22	*	0.7	*	0	0	0.12	0.07	1	0.02	11	0	5	23	8	t
0	30	11	2	0.1	0.1	0	0	0.01	0.01	0.1	t	1	0	5	10	*	t
0	30	11	3	0.1	0.1	0	0	0.01	0.01	0.1	0.01	1	0	5	10	*	t
0	103	55	12	0.8	0.3	0	0	0.1	0.1	1	0.03	16	0	26	53	11	t
0	215	45	8	0.9	0.3	0	0	0.17	0.08	1.4	0.04	22	0	31	38	*	t
0	173	139	22	0.9	0.4	0	0	0.11	0.17	1.1	0.05	*	0	23	70	14	0
0	94	60	6	0.8	0.2	0	0	0.08	0.16	1	0.01	9	0	26	23	*	*
0	174	51	6	0.7	0.3	0	0	0.1	0.08	0.8	0.02	10	0	20	36	9	*
0	138	22	5	0.8	0.2	0	0	0.12	0.09	1	0.01	9	0	28	20	7	t
0	153	42	23	0.8	0.4	0	0	0.07	0.05	0.9	0.05	13	0	17	63	11	t
0	91	87	24	0.7	0.6	t	0	0.06	0.04	0.8	0.05	13	0.03	20	64	11	t
0	118	26	5	0.7	0.1	0	0	0.11	0.07	0.9	0.01	8	0	29	25	6	t
0	117	28	5	0.6	0.1	0	0	0.07	0.06	0.8	0.01	8	0	22	23	6	t
0	231	50	9	1.3	0.3	0	0	0.21	0.14	1.7	0.02	16	0	57	49	13	0.1
0	159	44	23	0.9	0.4	0	0	0.09	0.05	1	0.05	14	0	18	65	11	t
0	89	85	23	0.7	0.6	11	0	0.07	0.04	0.8	0.05	12	0.03	20	63	11	t
0	736	152	32	3.6	*	0	0	0.35	0.35	4.8	*	*	*	122	141	20	*
0	126	42	8	0.7	0.2	7	0	0.08	0.08	0.7	0.03	5	0.08	49	44	5	0.6
0	8	2	t	0.1	t	0	0	0.01	0.01	0.1	0	t	t	t	1	0	t
*	14	2	t	0.1	t	t	0	0.01	0.01	0.1	t	t	0.01	1	2	1	t
t	12	2	t	t	t	t	0	t	t	0.1	t	t	0.01	1	2	0	t
t	10	2	t	0.1	t	t	0	0.01	0.01	t	t	t	0.04	1	1	1	t
0	33	28	4	0.3	0.1	0	0	0.01	0.04	0.3	0.01	1	0	3	11	1	t
0	33	12	2	0.2	0.1	0	0	0.02	0.02	0.2	0.01	1	0	3	8	1	t
0	5	1	t	t	t	0	0	t	t	t	0	t	0	t	t	0	t
0	32	3	*	0.1	*	*	*	0.01	0.01	0.1	*	*	*	5	8	*	t
0	19	10	3	0.1	0.1	*	0	0.01	0.01	t	0.01	1	*	1	7	1	t
0	57	39	*	0.3	*	0	0	0.02	0.02	0.1	*	*	*	4	25	1	t
1	37	3	1	0.1	t	0	0	0.13	0.01	0.1	t	t	0	1	3	4	t
0	17	4	1	0.1	t	0	0	0.01	0.01	0.1	t	t	0.01	1	3	1	t
0	24	4	t	0.1	t	t	0	0.01	0.02	0.2	t	t	t	1	3	1	t
0	24	6	3	0.2	0.1	0	0	0.02	0.01	0.2	0.01	1	0.04	1	9	1	t
0	*	*	*	*	*	*	0	*	*	*	*	*	*	*	*	0	t
t	257	86	12	1.3	0.6	22	0	0.12	0.16	1	0.04	18	0.29	72	85	*	0.4
21	252	46	10	0.6	*	18	0	0.09	0.1	0.7	*	*	*	34	53	*	*
21	168	99	35	1.3	1.1	40	2	0.1	0.11	1.3	0.11	17	0.09	54	111	*	*
21	192	54	18	0.7	*	25	0	0.1	0.1	0.7	*	*	*	42	68	*	*
0	414	364	12	1.8	0.5	0	0	0.24	0.21	2.4	0.03	21	0	105	73	15	0.1
0	358	314	11	1.6	0.4	0	0	0.26	0.18	2.1	0.02	18	0	91	63	15	0.9
21	176	50	11	0.6	*	8	0	0.09	0.12	0.9	*	*	*	42	60	*	*
0	*	*	52	0.9	*	40	0	0.08	0.1	0.5	*	*	*	35	56	*	*
20	160	66	5	0.4	0.2	12	0	0.04	0.05	0.2	0.06	3	0.36	59	91	2	*
20	160	33	5	0.4	0.2	6	0	0.06	0.07	0.5	0.06	3	0.36	27	38	2	*
20	160	43	5	0.3	0.2	8	0	0.04	0.06	0.5	0.06	3	0.36	36	71	3	*
0	144	25	5	0.8	0.2	0	0	0.1	0.06	0.9	0.02	10	*	20	23	8	0.2
0	96	36	5	0.5	0.1	4	t	0.07	0.07	0.4	0.02	6	t	8	22	5	0.3
29	140	40	7	1	0.2	8	0	0.28	0.1	1.2	0.02	9	0.05	12	32	*	0.1
0	241	37	8	1.2	0.2	0	0	0.2	0.13	1.6	0.01	15	*	54	33	12	t
0	312	49	12	1.2	0.3	0	0	0.2	0.12	1.7	0.02	30	0	24	46	15	t
0	761	122	*	3	*	0	0	0.54	0.32	4.5	0.05	*	*	58	115	41	0.1
0	197	102	40	0.8	0.6	0	0	0.12	0.05	1.1	0.08	16	0.05	34	98	16	t
45	445	129	17	1.5	0.7	28	0	0.18	0.24	1.5	0.05	14	0.37	154	135	11	*
0	256	78	8	1.8	0.3	95	0	0.17	0.2	1.9	0.1	1	*	30	141	*	*
0	220	194	39	1.8	0.7	100	0	0.15	0.17	0.8	0.2	16	0.6	20	135	*	0.6

WT, weight; **KCAL,** kcalories; **PROT,** protein; **CARB,** carbohydrate; **FIBR,** fiber; **FAT,** fat; **SATF,** saturated fat;

MONO, monosaturated fat; **POLY,** polyunsaturated fat; **CHOR,** cholesterol; **SOD,** sodium; **POT,** potassium;

Food Name	Portion	WT (Gm)	KCAL	PROT (Gm)	CARB (Gm)	FIBR (Gm)	FAT (Gm)	SATF (Gm)	MONO (Gm)	POLY (Gm)
Breakfast Cereals										
CEREAL-100% BRAN	CUP	66	178	8	48	19.5	3	0.6	0.6	1.9
CEREAL-100% NATURAL-PLAIN	CUP	104	489	12	65	3.8	22	15.1	4.3	2
CEREAL-40% BRAN FLAKES-KELLOGGS	CUP	39	127	5	31	5.5	1	0	0	0
CEREAL-40% BRAN FLAKES-POST	CUP	47	152	5	37	6.5	1	0	0	0
CEREAL-ALL BRAN	CUP	85.2	212	12	63	25.5	2	0.2	0.2	0.8
CEREAL-ALPHA BITS	CUP	28.4	111	2	25	0.3	1	0.1	0.2	0.3
CEREAL-APPLE JACKS	CUP	28.4	110	2	26	0.2	t	0	0	0
CEREAL-BRAN BUDS	CUP	85.2	220	12	65	23.6	2	0.3	0.3	1.1
CEREAL-BRAN CHEX	CUP	49	156	5	39	7.9	1	0.2	0.2	0.7
CEREAL-BRAN FLAKES-RALSTON	CUP	49	159	6	39	6	1	0	0	0
CEREAL-C.W. POST-PLAIN	CUP	97	432	9	69	2.2	15	11.3	1.7	1.4
CEREAL-C.W. POST-WITH RAISINS	CUP	103	446	9	74	2	15	11	1.7	1.4
CEREAL-CAP'N CRUNCH	CUP	37	156	2	30	0.4	3	2.2	0.4	0.5
CEREAL-CAP'N CRUNCH-CRUNCHBERRIES	CUP	35	146	2	29	0.4	3	1.9	0.4	0.5
CEREAL-CHEERIOS	CUP	22.7	89	3	16	0.9	1	0.3	0.5	0.6
CEREAL-COCOA KRISPIES	CUP	36	139	2	32	0.2	1	0	0	0
CEREAL-COCOA PEBBLES	CUP	32.5	133	2	28	0.2	2	1	0.6	0.1
CEREAL-CORN BRAN	CUP	36	125	2	30	6.8	1	*	*	*
CEREAL-CORN CHEX	CUP	28.4	111	2	25	0.5	t	0	0	0
CEREAL-CORN FLAKES-KELLOGGS	CUP	22.7	88	2	20	0.5	t	0	0	0
CEREAL-CORN FLAKES-LOW SODIUM	CUP	25	100	2	22	0.3	t	0	0	0
CEREAL-CORN FLAKES-RALSTON	CUP	25	98	2	22	0.5	t	0	0	0
CEREAL-CORN GRITS-REGULAR-ENRICHED-HOT	CUP	242	145	3	32	0.6	t	0.1	0.1	0.2
CEREAL-CORN GRITS-REGULAR-UNENRICHED-HOT	CUP	242	145	3	32	0.6	t	0.1	0.1	0.2
CEREAL-CORN-SHREDDED-ADDED SUGAR	CUP	25	95	2	22	1.5	0	0	0	0
CEREAL-CRACKLIN BRAN	CUP	60	229	6	41	9.1	9	5.6	0.8	1.5
CEREAL-CRACKLIN OAT BRAN-KELLOGGS	SERVING	28.4	110	3	20	2	4	1	3	0
CEREAL-CREAM OF RICE-COOKED	CUP	244	127	2	28	0.4	t	0	0	0
CEREAL-CREAM OF WHEAT-INSTANT	CUP	241	153	4	32	2.2	1	0	0	0
CEREAL-CREAM OF WHEAT-PACKET SIZE	ITEM	150	132	3	29	2	t	0	0	0
CEREAL-CREAM OF WHEAT-REGULAR-HOT	CUP	251	133	4	28	1.9	1	0	0	0
CEREAL-CRISP RICE-LOW SODIUM	CUP	26	105	1	24	0.4	t	0	0	0
CEREAL-CRISPY RICE	CUP	28.4	112	2	25	1	t	0	0	0
CEREAL-CRISPY WHEATS AND RAISINS	CUP	43	150	3	35	2	1	0	0	0
CEREAL-FARINA-COOKED-ENRICHED-HOT	CUP	233	117	3	25	3.3	t	t	t	0.1
CEREAL-FORTIFIED OAT FLAKES	CUP	48	177	9	35	1.2	1	0	0	0
CEREAL-FROOT LOOPS-GENERAL MILLS	CUP	28.4	111	2	25	0.3	1	0	0	0
CEREAL-FROSTED FLAKES-KELLOGGS	CUP	35	133	2	32	0.8	t	0	0	0
CEREAL-FROSTED FLAKES-RALSTON	CUP	38	149	2	34	0.8	1	0	0	0
CEREAL-FROSTED MINI WHEATS-KELLOGGS	ITEM	7.1	26	1	6	0.5	t	0	0	0
CEREAL-FROSTED RICE KRISPIES-KELLOGGS	CUP	28.4	109	1	26	0.1	t	0	0	0
CEREAL-GRANOLA-HOMEMADE	CUP	122	594	15	67	12.8	33	5.8	9.4	17.2
CEREAL-GRANOLA-NATURE VALLEY	CUP	113	503	12	76	4.2	20	13	2.9	2.8
CEREAL-GRAPE NUTS FLAKES-POST	CUP	32.5	116	3	27	2.1	t	0	0	0
CEREAL-GRAPE NUTS-POST	CUP	114	407	13	94	5.5	t	0	0	0
CEREAL-HEARTLAND NATURAL-PLAIN	CUP	115	499	12	79	5.4	18	9.5	3.5	3.7
CEREAL-HONEY BRAN	CUP	35	119	3	29	3.9	1	0	0	0
CEREAL-HONEY NUT CHEERIOS-GENERAL MILLS	CUP	33	125	4	27	1.3	1	0.1	0.3	0.3
CEREAL-HONEYCOMB-POST	CUP	22	86	1	20	0.3	t	t	0.1	0.2
CEREAL-KING VITAMAN	CUP	21	85	1	18	0.3	1	0.7	0.2	0.2
CEREAL-KIX	CUP	18.9	74	2	16	0.3	t	0.1	0.1	0.2
CEREAL-LIFE-PLAIN/CINNAMON	CUP	44	162	8	32	1.4	1	0	0	0
CEREAL-LUCKY CHARMS	CUP	32	125	3	26	0.6	1	0.2	0.4	0.5
CEREAL-MALT O MEAL-COOKED	CUP	240	122	4	26	0.6	t	0	0	0
CEREAL-MAYPO-COOKED-HOT	CUP	240	170	6	32	1.2	2	*	*	*
CEREAL-NUTRI GRAIN-BARLEY	CUP	41	153	5	34	2.4	t	0	0	0
CEREAL-NUTRI GRAIN-CORN	CUP	42	160	3	36	2.6	1	0.1	0.2	0.5
CEREAL-NUTRI GRAIN-RYE	CUP	40	144	4	34	2.6	t	0	0	0
CEREAL-NUTRI GRAIN-WHEAT	CUP	44	158	4	37	2.8	1	0	0	0
CEREAL-OAT BRAN-COOKED	CUP	219	88	7	25	1.8	2	0.4	0.6	0.7
CEREAL-OAT BRAN-KELLOGGS	SERVING	28.4	100	4	22	1.5	1	*	*	*
CEREAL-OAT BRAN-QUAKER	CUP	85	270	18	51	12.3	6	0.8	1.7	2.1

t = Trace of nutrient present   * = Not available

MAG, magnesium; **IRON**, iron; **ZINC**, zinc; **VITA**, vitamin A; **VITC**, vitamin C; **THIA**, thiamin; **RIBO**, riboflavin; **NIAC**, niacin; **VB6**, vitamin B-6; **FOL**, folate; **VB12**, vitamin B-12; **CALC**, calcium; **PHOS**, phosphorus; **SEL**, selenium; **VE-a**, alpha tocopherol equivalents.

CHOL (mg)	SOD (mg)	POT (mg)	MAG (mg)	IRON (mg)	ZINC (mg)	VITA (RE)	VITC (mg)	THIA (mg)	RIBO (mg)	NIAC (mg)	VB6 (mg)	FOL (µg)	VB12 (µg)	CALC (mg)	PHOS (mg)	SEL (µg)	VE-a (mg)
0	457	824	312	8.1	5.7	0	63	1.6	1.8	20.9	2.1	47	6.3	46	801	20	1.5
0	45	514	125	3.1	2.4	6	0	0.31	0.56	2.4	0.19	31	0.13	181	383	*	0.7
0	363	248	71	11.2	5.1	516	0	0.5	0.6	6.9	0.7	138	2.1	19	192	4	0.2
0	431	251	102	7.5	2.5	622	0	0.6	0.7	8.3	0.8	166	2.5	21	296	5	0.2
0	961	1051	318	13.5	11.2	1125	45	1.11	1.28	15	1.53	301	0	69	794	25	1.3
0	219	110	17	1.8	1.5	375	0	0.4	0.4	5	0.5	100	1.5	8	51	10	t
0	125	23	6	4.5	3.7	375	15	0.4	0.4	5	0.5	100	0	3	30	18	0.1
0	523	1425	271	13.5	11.2	1125	45	1.11	1.28	15	1.53	301	0	57	740	25	0.9
0	455	394	126	7.8	2.1	11	26	0.6	0.26	8.6	0.9	173	2.6	29	327	10	0.6
0	456	191	118	7.8	2	649	26	0.6	0.7	8.6	0.9	173	2.6	27	273	*	1
0	167	198	67	15.4	1.6	1284	0	1.3	1.5	17.1	1.7	342	5.1	47	224	*	0.7
0	160	260	74	16.4	1.6	1364	0	1.3	1.5	18.1	1.9	364	5.5	51	232	*	0.7
0	278	48	15	9.8	4	5	0	0.66	0.71	8.6	1	238	2.34	6	47	*	0.2
0	243	49	14	9	3.6	5	0	0.59	0.67	8.1	0.93	128	2.51	11	47	*	0.2
0	246	81	31	3.6	0.6	300	12	0.3	0.34	4	0.41	5	1.2	39	107	10	0.2
0	275	53	12	2.3	1.9	477	19	0.5	0.5	6.3	0.6	127	0.02	6	47	*	t
0	155	54	13	2.1	1.7	430	0	0.42	0.49	5.7	0.59	115	1.72	6	25	*	t
0	310	70	18	12.2	4	8	0	0.37	0.7	10.9	0.86	232	1.39	41	52	2	*
0	271	23	4	1.8	0.1	14	15	0.4	0.07	5	0.6	100	1.5	3	11	2	0.1
0	281	21	3	1.4	0.1	300	12	0.3	0.34	4	0.41	80	0	1	14	1	t
0	3	18	3	0.6	0.1	10	0	t	0.05	0.1	0.02	2	0	11	12	1	t
0	239	22	3	0.6	0.1	10	13	0.1	0	1.1	0.02	2	0	2	10	1	0.1
0	0	53	10	1.6	0.2	*	*	0.24	0.15	2	0.06	2	0	0	29	24	t
0	0	53	10	1.6	0.2	*	*	0.24	0.15	2	0.06	2	0	0	29	24	t
0	247	*	4	0.6	0.1	0	13	0.33	0.05	4.4	0.45	88	1.33	1	10	2	0.1
0	487	355	116	3.8	3.2	794	32	0.8	0.9	10.6	1.1	212	0	40	241	10	0.7
0	140	160	60	1.8	1.5	180	15	0.38	0.43	5	0.5	100	1.5	20	150	*	1.2
0	2	49	7	0.5	0.4	0	0	0	0	1	0.07	7	0	7	42	*	*
0	6	48	14	12	0.4	0	0	0.2	0.1	1.8	0.03	11	0	59	43	*	t
0	241	55	9	8.1	0.2	1250	0	0.4	0.2	5	0.5	100	0	40	20	*	0.7
0	2	43	10	10.3	0.3	0	0	0.25	0	1.5	0.04	10	0	50	42	*	t
0	3	20	10	0.8	0.4	0	0	0	0.05	0.4	0.04	3	0	17	27	4	t
0	208	27	12	0.7	0.5	0	1	0.11	0.03	2	0.04	3	0.08	5	31	4	t
0	204	174	35	6.8	0.5	569	0	0.6	0.6	7.6	0.8	15	2.3	71	117	6	11.4
0	0	30	5	1.2	0.2	*	*	0.19	0.12	1.3	0.02	5	0	5	28	*	2
0	429	343	58	13.7	1.5	636	0	0.6	0.7	8.4	0.9	169	2.5	68	176	10	0.3
0	145	26	7	4.5	3.7	375	15	0.4	0.4	5	0.5	100	0	3	24	18	0.1
0	284	22	3	2.2	0.1	463	19	0.5	0.5	6.2	0.6	124	0	1	26	*	*
0	247	24	3	1	0.8	503	20	0.5	0.6	6.7	0.7	3	2	4	9	*	*
0	2	24	56	0.4	0.4	94	4	0.09	0.11	1.3	0.13	25	0	2	19	*	t
0	240	21	5	1.8	0.3	375	15	0.4	0.4	5	0.5	100	0	1	27	4	t
0	12	612	141	4.8	4.5	10	1	0.73	0.31	2.1	0.43	99	0	76	494	3	5.7
0	232	389	116	3.8	2.2	8	0	0.39	0.19	0.8	0.09	85	0	71	354	37	3.4
0	250	113	36	5.2	0.7	430	0	0.42	0.49	5.7	0.59	115	1.72	13	97	10	0.1
0	792	381	76	5	2.5	1500	0	1.48	1.71	20.1	2.05	402	6.04	43	286	34	0.3
0	294	385	147		3	7	1	0.36	0.16	1.6	0.19	64	0	75	416	*	0.8
0	202	151	46	5.6	0.9	463	19	0.5	0.5	6.2	0.6	23	1.9	16	132	*	0.8
0	299	115	39	5.2	0.9	437	17	0.4	0.5	5.8	0.6	22	1.7	23	122	*	0.2
0	166	70	8	1.4	1.2	291	0	0.3	0.3	3.9	0.4	78	1.2	4	22	*	0.1
0	161	26	7	12.7	0.2	717	33	0.92	1.06	12.9	1.18	286	4.13	2	27	*	6.7
0	226	30	8	5.4	0.2	250	10	0.25	0.28	3.3	0.34	67	1	24	26	*	t
0	229	197	14	11.6	1.5	3	1	0.95	1	11.6	0.08	37	0	154	238	*	0.3
0	227	66	27	5.1	0.6	424	17	0.4	0.5	5.6	0.6	6	1.7	36	88	*	0.2
0	2	31	5	9.5	0.2	0	0	0.4	0.3	5.9	0.02	6	0	5	23	*	0.3
0	9	211	51	8.4	1.5	702	28	0.7	0.8	9.4	0.9	9	2.8	125	248	*	*
0	277	108	32	1.5	5.4	543	22	0.5	0.6	7.2	0.7	145	2.2	11	126	27	10.8
0	276	98	27	0.9	5.5	556	22	0.5	0.6	7.4	0.8	148	2.2	1	120	3	t
0	272	72	31	1.1	5.3	530	21	0.5	0.6	7	0.7	141	2.1	8	104	*	t
0	299	120	34	1.2	5.8	583	23	0.6	0.7	7.7	0.8	155	2.3	12	164	7	t
0	2	201	88	1.9	1.2	0	0	0.35	0.07	0.3	0.06	13	0	22	261	*	0.4
0	270	115	40	4.5	3.8	180	*	0.38	0.43	5	0.5	*	1.5	*	150	*	*
0	15	540	180	5.4	3.6	1028	0	0.9	0.31	15	1.49	48	5.18	60	600	*	2

WT, weight; **KCAL**, kcalories; **PROT**, protein; **CARB**, carbohydrate; **FIBR**, fiber; **FAT**, fat; **SATF**, saturated fat;
MONO, monosaturated fat; **POLY**, polyunsaturated fat; **CHOR**, cholesterol; **SOD**, sodium; **POT**, potassium;

Food Name	Portion	WT (Gm)	KCAL	PROT (Gm)	CARB (Gm)	FIBR (Gm)	FAT (Gm)	SATF (Gm)	MONO (Gm)	POLY (Gm)
CEREAL-OAT BRAN-RAISIN/SPICE-HOT	OUNCE	28.4	100	3	19	3.8	1	*	*	*
CEREAL-OATMEAL-COOKED	CUP	234	145	6	25	2.1	2	0.4	0.8	0.9
CEREAL-OATMEAL-RAW	CUP	81	311	13	54	4.6	5	0.9	1.8	2.1
CEREAL-OATS-APPLE/CINNAMON-QUAKER-PACKET	ITEM	149	135	4	26	1.4	2	0.3	0.6	0.7
CEREAL-OATS-BRAN/RAISIN-QUAKER-PACKET	ITEM	195	158	5	30	1.8	2	0.3	0.7	0.8
CEREAL-OATS-CINNAMON/SPICE-QUAKER-PACKET	ITEM	161	177	5	35	1.5	2	0.3	0.7	0.8
CEREAL-OATS-MAPLE/SUGAR-QUAKER-PACKET	ITEM	155	163	5	32	1.4	2	0.3	0.7	0.8
CEREAL-OATS-PLAIN-QUAKER-INSTANT-PACKET	ITEM	177	104	4	18	1.6	2	0.3	0.6	0.7
CEREAL-OATS-PUFFED-ADDED SUGAR	CUP	25	100	3	19	2.7	1	0.2	0.1	0.5
CEREAL-PRODUCT 19-KELLOGGS	CUP	33	126	3	27	0.4	t	0	0	0
CEREAL-RAISIN BRAN-KELLOGGS	CUP	49.2	154	5	37	5.3	1	0.1	0.1	0.5
CEREAL-RAISIN BRAN-POST	CUP	56.8	174	5	43	6	1	0.2	0.2	0.5
CEREAL-RAISIN BRAN-RALSTON	CUP	56	178	4	47	7.1	t	0	0	0
CEREAL-RALSTON-COOKED-HOT	CUP	253	134	6	28	4.2	1	0	0	0
CEREAL-RICE CHEX	CUP	25.2	100	1	23	0.2	t	0	0	0
CEREAL-RICE KRISPIES-KELLOGGS	CUP	28.4	112	2	25	0.1	t	0	0	0
CEREAL-RICE-PUFFED-ADDED SUGAR	CUP	28.4	115	1	26	0.2	0	0	0	0
CEREAL-RICE-PUFFED-PLAIN	CUP	14	56	1	13	0.1	t	0	0	0
CEREAL-ROMAN MEAL-COOKED	CUP	241	147	7	33	2.3	1	*	*	*
CEREAL-SPECIAL K-KELLOGGS	CUP	21.3	83	4	16	0.2	t	0	0	0
CEREAL-SUGAR CORN POPS-KELLOGGS	CUP	28.4	108	1	26	0.2	t	0	0	0
CEREAL-SUGAR SMACKS-KELLOGGS	CUP	37.9	141	3	33	0.5	1	0	0	0
CEREAL-SUPER SUGAR CRISP-POST	CUP	33	123	2	30	0.5	t	0	0	0
CEREAL-TASTEEOS	CUP	24	94	3	19	0.8	1	0	0	0
CEREAL-TEAM	CUP	42	164	3	36	0.4	1	0	0	0
CEREAL-TOASTIES-POST	CUP	22.7	88	2	20	0.4	t	0	0	0
CEREAL-TOTAL-GENERAL MILLS	CUP	33	116	3	26	2.4	1	0.1	0.1	0.3
CEREAL-TRIX-GENERAL MILLS	CUP	28.4	109	2	25	0.3	t	0	0	0
CEREAL-WHEAT CHEX	CUP	46	169	5	38	3.4	1	0.5	0.1	0.3
CEREAL-WHEAT FLAKES-ADDED SUGAR	CUP	30	105	3	24	2.7	0	0	0	0
CEREAL-WHEAT GERM-BROWN SUGAR AND HONEY	CUP	113	426	25	69	5.7	9	1.6	1.3	5.5
CEREAL-WHEAT GERM-TOASTED	CUP	113	432	33	56	14.6	12	2.1	1.7	7.5
CEREAL-WHEAT-PUFFED-ADDED SUGAR	SERVING	38	138	6	30	2.1	t	*	0.1	0.1
CEREAL-WHEAT-PUFFED-PLAIN	CUP	12	44	2	10	0.4	t	0	0	0
CEREAL-WHEAT-ROLLED-COOKED-HOT	CUP	240	180	5	41	2.9	1	0.2	0.1	0.5
CEREAL-WHEAT-SHREDDED-BISCUIT	ITEM	23.6	83	3	19	2.2	t	0	0	0
CEREAL-WHEAT-WHOLE MEAL-COOKED-HOT	CUP	245	110	4	23	1.6	1	0.2	0.1	0.5
CEREAL-WHEATENA-COOKED	CUP	243	136	5	29	2.6	1	*	*	*
CEREAL-WHEATIES	CUP	29	101	3	23	2	1	0.1	0.1	0.2
CEREAL-WHOLE WHEAT NATURAL	CUP	242	150	5	33	2.7	1	0.2	0.2	0.4
OATS-ROLLED OR OATMEAL-DRY	CUP	81	311	13	54	3.8	5	0.9	1.6	1.9

Combination Foods

Food Name	Portion	WT (Gm)	KCAL	PROT (Gm)	CARB (Gm)	FIBR (Gm)	FAT (Gm)	SATF (Gm)	MONO (Gm)	POLY (Gm)
BEEF POTPIE-HOME RECIPE-1/3 OF 9" PIE	SLICE	210	515	21	39	3.9	30	7.9	12.9	7.4
BEEF STEW-WITH VEGETABLES	CUP	245	220	16	15	3.2	11	4.9	4.5	0.5
BEEF-RAVIOLIOS-CANNED WITH MEAT SAUCE	OUNCE	28.4	28	1	4	0.2	1	0.1	0.2	0.3
BURRITO-BEANS AND CHEESE	ITEM	93	189	8	28	8.3	6	3.4	1.2	0.9
CHEESE SOUFFLE-HOME RECIPE	CUP	95	207	9	6	0.1	16	6.6	5.8	2.5
CHICKEN A LA KING-COOKED-HOME RECIPE	CUP	245	470	27	12	1.2	34	12.9	13.4	6.2
CHICKEN AND NOODLES-COOKED-HOME RECIPE	CUP	240	365	22	26	1.3	18	5.9	7.1	3.5
CHICKEN CHOW MEIN-CANNED	CUP	250	95	7	18	0.9	0	0	0	0
CHICKEN CHOW MEIN-HOME RECIPE	CUP	250	255	31	10	0.5	10	2.4	3.4	3.1
CHICKEN POTPIE-BAKED-HOME RECIPE	SLICE	232	545	23	42	4.2	31	11	13.5	5.5
CHILI CON CARNE-WITH BEANS-CANNED	CUP	255	340	19	31	5	16	7.5	7.2	1
CHILI WITH BEANS-CANNED	CUP	255	286	15	30	6.9	14	6	6	0.9
CHIMICHANGA-BEEF	ITEM	174	425	20	43	4.3	20	8.5	8.1	1.1
CHOP SUEY-WITH BEEF AND PORK-HOME RECIPE	CUP	250	300	26	13	*	17	8.5	6.2	0.7
CORN DOG-PLAIN	ITEM	175	460	17	56	2.8	19	5.2	9.1	3.5
ENCHILADA-CHEESE	ITEM	163	320	10	29	3.2	19	10.6	6.3	0.8
ENCHIRITO-CHEESE/BEEF/BEAN	ITEM	193	344	18	34	3.4	16	8	6.5	0.3
HAMBURGER-BACON AND CHEESE-GENERIC	ITEM	150	464	25	29	1.8	27	*	*	*
HOT DOG-PLAIN WITH BUN-GENERIC	ITEM	98	242	10	18	0.9	15	5.1	6.9	1.7
MACARONI & CHEESE-BAKED-HOME RECIPE	CUP	200	430	17	40	*	22	11.9	7.3	1

t = Trace of nutrient present   * = Not available

MAG, magnesium; IRON, iron; ZINC, zinc; VITA, vitamin A; VITC, vitamin C; THIA, thiamin; RIBO, riboflavin; NIAC, niacin; VB6, vitamin B-6; FOL, folate; VB12, vitamin B-12; CALC, calcium; PHOS, phosphorus; SEL, selenium; VE-a, alpha tocopherol equivalents.

CHOL (mg)	SOD (mg)	POT (mg)	MAG (mg)	IRON (mg)	ZINC (mg)	VITA (RE)	VITC (mg)	THIA (mg)	RIBO (mg)	NIAC (mg)	VB6 (mg)	FOL (µg)	VB12 (µg)	CALC (mg)	PHOS (mg)	SEL (µg)	VE-a (mg)
0	10	100	43	0.7	0.8	0	t	0.06	0.05	1.2	0.08	24	0	16	148	*	0
0	1	132	56	1.6	1.2	7	*	0.26	0.05	0.3	0.05	9	0	20	178	20	3.5
0	3	284	120	3.4	2.5	10	0	0.59	0.11	0.6	0.1	26	0	42	384	22	0.2
0	222	107	34	6.1	0.7	435	0	0.48	0.28	5.1	0.7	137	0	158	117	13	0.9
0	247	236	57	7.6	1.4	479	0	0.56	0.63	8.1	0.76	155	0	173	206	17	1.2
0	280	104	51	6.7	1	475	0	0.56	0.34	5.7	0.77	153	0	172	146	14	1
0	280	102	42	6.4	0.9	451	0	0.53	0.32	5.4	0.74	145	0	162	143	13	0.9
0	286	100	43	6.3	0.9	455	0	0.53	0.29	5.5	0.74	150	0	163	133	15	1.1
0	294	*	28	4	0.7	275	13	0.33	0.38	4.4	0.45	6	1.33	44	102	6	0.2
0	378	51	12	21	0.5	1748	70	1.7	2	23.3	2.3	466	7	4	47	*	34.9
0	359	256	64	6	5	500	0	0.49	0.59	6.7	0.69	133	2.02	17	183	5	1.1
0	370	350	97	9	3	750	0	0.74	0.85	10	1.02	201	3.01	27	238	6	1.3
0	486	287	84	6.7	1.7	556	2	0.6	0.6	7.4	0.7	148	2.2	27	247	6	*
0	4	153	59	1.6	1.4	0	0	0.2	0.18	2.1	0.11	18	0.11	14	148	*	2
0	211	29	6	1.6	0.3	2	13	0.33	0.01	4.4	0.45	89	1.34	4	25	4	t
0	340	30	10	1.8	0.5	375	15	0.4	0.4	5	0.5	100	0	4	34	4	t
0	21	43	8	0	1.5	300	15	0	0	0	0.5	99	1.48	3	14	2	0.2
0	t	16	4	0.1	0.1	0	0	0.02	0.01	0.4	0.01	3	0	1	14	1	0.1
0	3	302	109	2.1	1.8	0	0	0.24	0.12	3.1	0.11	24	0	30	215	*	*
0	199	37	12	3.4	2.8	280	11	0.28	0.32	3.8	0.38	75	0.01	6	41	13	0.1
0	103	17	2	1.8	1.5	375	15	0.4	0.4	5	0.5	100	0	1	28	*	t
0	100	56	18	2.4	0.4	500	20	0.49	0.57	6.7	0.68	134	0	4	41	*	*
0	29	123	20	2.1	1.7	437	0	0.4	0.5	5.8	0.6	116	1.7	7	60	26	0.1
0	183	71	26	3.8	0.7	318	13	0.31	0.36	4.2	0.43	9	1.27	11	96	10	0.2
0	259	71	19	2.6	0.6	556	22	0.5	0.6	7.4	0.8	7	2.2	6	65	7	0.1
0	238	26	3	0.6	0.1	300	0	0.3	0.34	4	0.41	80	1.2	1	10	*	0.1
0	409	123	37	21	0.8	1748	70	1.7	2	23.3	2.3	466	7	56	137	*	34.9
0	181	27	6	4.5	0.1	371	15	0.37	0.43	5	0.51	3	1.51	6	19	*	0.1
0	308	174	58	7.3	1.2	0	24	0.6	0.17	8.1	0.8	162	2.4	18	182	*	0.2
0	368	81	33	4.8	0.7	330	16	0.4	0.45	5.3	0.54	9	1.59	12	83	3	0.1
0	3	803	272	7.7	14.1	0	0	1.41	0.7	4.7	0.83	298	0	38	971	*	20.5
0	5	1070	362	10.3	18.8	50	7	1.89	0.93	6.3	1.11	398	0	51	1295	*	15.9
0	2	132	55	1.8	0.9	0	0	0.08	0.09	4.1	0.07	12	0	11	135	*	*
0	t	42	17	0.6	0.3	0	0	0.02	0.03	1.3	0.02	4	0	3	43	*	0.1
0	535	202	53	1.7	1.2	0	0	0.17	0.07	2.2	*	26	*	19	182	*	2.5
0	t	77	40	0.7	0.6	0	0	0.07	0.06	1.1	0.06	12	0	10	86	*	0.1
0	535	118	54	1.2	1.2	0	0	0.15	0.05	1.5	*	27	*	17	127	*	2.6
0	5	187	49	1.4	1.7	0	0	0.02	0.05	1.3	0.05	17	0	10	146	58	*
0	363	108	32	4.6	0.7	384	15	0.4	0.4	5.1	0.5	9	1.5	44	100	3	0.1
0	1	171	54	1.5	1.2	0	0	0.17	0.12	2.2	0.18	27	0	17	167	58	2.6
0	3	284	120	3.4	2.5	20	0	0.59	0.11	0.6	0.1	26	0	42	384	43	1.2
44	596	334	*	3.8	*	344	6	0.3	0.3	5.5	*	*	*	29	149	*	1.2
72	1006	613	*	2.9	*	480	17	0.15	0.17	4.7	*	*	t	29	184	*	0.5
*	131	46	*	0.3	*	50	t	0.03	0.02	0.4	*	*	*	5	*	*	t
14	583	248	40	1.1	0.8	118	1	0.11	0.36	1.8	0.13	41	0.45	107	90	*	0.9
137	346	115	14	1	1	152	0	0.05	0.23	0.2	0.06	14	0.35	191	185	*	1.4
186	759	404	*	2.5	*	226	12	0.1	0.42	5.4	*	*	*	127	358	*	0.9
96	600	149	*	2.2	*	80	0	0.05	0.17	4.3	*	*	*	26	247	*	0.2
98	722	418	*	1.3	*	30	13	0.05	0.1	1	*	*	*	45	85	*	0
98	717	473	*	2.5	*	56	10	0.08	0.23	4.3	*	*	*	58	293	*	0
72	593	343	*	3	*	618	5	0.34	0.31	5.5	*	*	*	70	232	32	0.9
38	1354	594	*	4.3	*	30	*	0.08	0.18	3.3	0.26	*	*	82	321	*	*
43	1330	932	115	8.8	5.1	86	4	0.12	0.27	0.9	0.34	58	0.03	119	393	*	1.4
9	910	587	62	4.6	5	15	5	0.48	0.64	5.8	0.27	31	1.52	63	123	*	4.5
64	1052	425	*	4.8	*	120	33	0.28	0.38	5	*	*	*	60	248	*	0
79	972	262	17	6.2	1.3	36	0	0.29	0.71	4.2	0.1	60	0.44	101	166	*	1.3
44	784	240	50	1.3	2.5	186	1	0.09	0.42	1.9	0.39	34	0.74	324	133	*	1.7
49	1251	560	71	2.4	2.8	134	5	0.18	0.69	3	0.21	254	1.63	217	224	*	*
68	660	339	35	3.7	5.3	75	2	0.15	0.27	4.9	0.24	26	1.8	116	302	23	0.1
44	671	143	13	2.3	2	0	t	0.24	0.27	3.7	0.05	30	0.51	24	97	*	*
68	1086	240	36	1.6	1.8	258	1	0.15	0.31	1.5	0.15	17	0.46	362	322	*	1

WT, weight; **KCAL,** kcalories; **PROT,** protein; **CARB,** carbohydrate; **FIBR,** fiber; **FAT,** fat; **SATF,** saturated fat; **MONO,** monosaturated fat; **POLY,** polyunsaturated fat; **CHOR,** cholesterol; **SOD,** sodium; **POT,** potassium;

Food Name	Portion	WT (Gm)	KCAL	PROT (Gm)	CARB (Gm)	FIBR (Gm)	FAT (Gm)	SATF (Gm)	MONO (Gm)	POLY (Gm)
MACARONI & CHEESE-ENRICHED-CANNED	CUP	240	230	9	26	1.4	10	4.2	3.1	1.4
MACARONI & CHEESE-ENRICHED-HOME RECIPE	CUP	200	430	17	40	1.2	22	8.9	8.8	2.9
MEAT LOAF-WITH CELERY AND ONIONS	SERVING	87.6	213	16	5	0.1	14	5.3	5.9	0.6
MIXED FRUIT-CANNED-HEAVY SYRUP PACK	CUP	255	184	1	48	2.9	t	t	t	0.1
MIXED FRUIT-FROZEN-SWEETENED	CUP	250	245	4	61	3	t	0.1	0.1	0.2
NACHOS-CHEESE	SERVING	113	345	9	36	2.2	19	7.8	8	2.2
PEAS & CARROTS-CANNED-DIETARY-LOW SODIUM	CUP	255	96	6	22	7.1	1	0.1	0.1	0.3
PEAS AND CARROTS-CANNED	CUP	255	97	6	22	8.6	1	0.1	0.1	0.3
PEAS AND CARROTS-FROZEN-BOILED	CUP	160	77	5	16	7.1	1	0.1	0.1	0.3
PEAS AND ONIONS-CANNED	CUP	120	61	4	10	4.3	t	0.1	t	0.2
PEAS AND ONIONS-FROZEN-BOILED	CUP	180	81	5	16	4.7	t	0.1	t	0.2
PIZZA-CHEESE-BAKED	SLICE	63	140	8	21	1.6	3	1.5	1	0.5
PIZZA-CHEESE/MEAT/VEGETABLE	SLICE	79	184	13	21	1.8	5	1.5	2.5	0.9
PIZZA-PEPPERONI-BAKED	SLICE	71	181	10	20	1.5	7	2.2	3.1	1.2
PORK AND BEANS WITH FRANKFURTERS-CANNED	CUP	257	365	17	40	12.8	17	6.1	7.3	2.2
PORK AND BEANS WITH SWEET SAUCE-CANNED	CUP	253	281	13	53	14	4	1.4	1.6	0.5
PORK AND BEANS WITH TOMATO SAUCE-CANNED	CUP	253	248	13	49	13.8	3	1	1.1	0.3
RICE-FRIED (NASI GORENG)	OUNCE	28.3	55	1	7	t	2	0.3	0.5	1.1
SALAD-CARROT RAISIN-HOME RECIPE	CUP	268	306	4	56	16.7	12	6.8	12.8	23.4
SALAD-CHEF-WITH HAM AND CHEESE	SERVING	200	196	13	7	2.4	13	7	4.1	0.7
SALAD-CHICKEN	CUP	205	502	26	17	2.2	36	4.3	7.2	10.1
SALAD-COLESLAW	TBSP	8	6	t	1	0.3	t	t	0.1	0.1
SALAD-CRAB	SERVING	100	145	12	5	0.3	9	1	1.7	3.5
SALAD-FRUIT-CANNED-JUICE PACK	CUP	249	125	1	33	1.6	t	t	t	t
SALAD-FRUIT-CANNED-WATER PACK	CUP	245	74	1	19	4.5	t	t	t	0.1
SALAD-GREEN SALAD-TOSSED	SERVING	207	32	3	7	2.1	t	t	t	0.1
SALAD-MACARONI	SERVING	28.4	51	1	5	0.3	3	0.2	0.4	0.7
SALAD-MANDARIN ORANGE GELATIN	SERVING	28.4	23	t	6	0.6	0	0	0	0
SALAD-POTATO	CUP	250	358	7	28	5.3	21	3.6	6.2	9.3
SALAD-TACO	SERVING	198	279	13	24	2.8	15	6.8	5.2	1.8
SALAD-THREE BEAN-ALEX	SERVING	28.4	33	1	7	2.1	t	*	*	*
SALAD-THREE BEAN-CANNED-DEL MONTE	OUNCE	28.4	22	1	5	1.5	t	0	0	0
SALAD-WALDORF GELATIN	SERVING	28.4	27	2	5	0.3	t	0	0	0
SANDWICH-BLT-WITH MAYONNAISE	ITEM	148	282	7	29	2.9	16	6.8	5.5	4.9
SANDWICH-CHICKEN/SALAD/MAYONNAISE	OUNCE	28.3	81	6	3	0.4	5	0.6	1	1.4
SANDWICH-CLUB	ITEM	315	590	36	42	4.2	21	14.5	11.6	10.5
SANDWICH-HAM AND CHEESE	ITEM	146	353	21	33	3.3	16	6.4	6.7	1.4
SANDWICH-ROAST BEEF-PLAIN	ITEM	139	346	22	34	3.4	14	3.6	6.8	1.7
SANDWICH-ROAST BEEF-WITH CHEESE	ITEM	176	402	32	27	2.7	18	9	3.7	3.5
SANDWICH-STEAK	ITEM	204	459	30	52	5.2	14	3.8	5.4	3.4
SANDWICH-SUBMARINE-ROAST BEEF	ITEM	216	411	29	44	4.4	13	7.1	1.8	2.6
SANDWICH-SUBMARINE-WITH COLDCUTS	ITEM	228	456	22	51	5.1	19	6.8	8.2	2.3
SANDWICH-TUNA/SALAD/MAYONNAISE	OUNCE	28.3	64	5	5	0.3	3	0.4	0.7	1.1
SPAGHETTI IN SAUCE/CHEESE-FRANCO	OUNCE	28.4	11	1	5	*	t	*	*	*
SPAGHETTI/TOMATO/CHEESE-CANNED	CUP	250	190	6	39	2.5	2	0.5	0.3	0.4
SPAGHETTI/TOMATO/CHEESE-FROM HOME RECIPE	CUP	250	260	9	37	2.5	9	2	5.4	0.7
SPAGHETTI/TOMATO/MEAT-CANNED	CUP	250	260	12	29	2.8	10	2.2	3.3	3.9
SPAGHETTI/TOMATO/MEAT-FROM HOME RECIPE	CUP	248	330	19	39	2.7	12	3.3	6.3	0.9
SPINACH SOUFFLE	CUP	136	219	11	3	0.8	18	7.2	6.8	3.1
TACO	ITEM	171	370	21	27	2.7	21	11.4	6.6	1
TUNA-SALAD-CELERY/MAYONNAISE/PICKLE/EGG	CUP	205	350	30	7	1	22	4.3	6.3	6.7
VEGETABLES-MIXED-CANNED-DRAINED	CUP	163	77	4	15	8.1	t	0.1	t	0.2
VEGETABLES-MIXED-FROZEN-BOILED	CUP	182	107	5	24	6.9	t	0.1	t	0.1

Dairy Products

Food Name	Portion	WT (Gm)	KCAL	PROT (Gm)	CARB (Gm)	FIBR (Gm)	FAT (Gm)	SATF (Gm)	MONO (Gm)	POLY (Gm)
CHEESE FOOD-AMERICAN-PASTEURIZED PROCESS	OUNCE	28.4	93	6	2	0	7	4.4	2	0.2
CHEESE SPREAD-AMERICAN-PROCESSED	OUNCE	28.4	82	5	2	0	6	3.8	1.8	0.2
CHEESE-AMERICAN-PASTEURIZED PROCESS	OUNCE	28.4	106	6	t	0	9	5.6	2.5	0.3
CHEESE-BLUE	OUNCE	28.4	100	6	1	0	8	5.3	2.2	0.2
CHEESE-BLUE-CRUMBLED-UNPACKED	CUP	135	477	29	3	0	39	25.2	10.5	1.1
CHEESE-BRICK	OUNCE	28.4	105	7	1	0	8	5.3	2.4	0.2
CHEESE-BRIE	OUNCE	28.4	95	6	t	0	8	4.9	2.3	0.2
CHEESE-CAMEMBERT-WEDGE	ITEM	38	114	8	t	0	9	5.8	2.7	0.3
CHEESE-CARAWAY	OUNCE	28.4	107	7	1	0	8	5.3	2.4	0.2

*t = Trace of nutrient present   * = Not available*

MAG, magnesium; IRON, iron; ZINC, zinc; VITA, vitamin A; VITC, vitamin C; THIA, thiamin; RIBO, riboflavin; NIAC, niacin; VB6, vitamin B-6; FOL, folate; VB12, vitamin B-12; CALC, calcium; PHOS, phosphorus; SEL, selenium; VE-a, alpha tocopherol equivalents.

CHOL (mg)	SOD (mg)	POT (mg)	MAG (mg)	IRON (mg)	ZINC (mg)	VITA (RE)	VITC (mg)	THIA (mg)	RIBO (mg)	NIAC (mg)	VB6 (mg)	FOL (µg)	VB12 (µg)	CALC (mg)	PHOS (mg)	SEL (µg)	VE-a (mg)
42	729	139	*	1	*	52	0	0.12	0.24	1	*	*	*	199	182	*	0.4
42	1086	240	52	1.8	*	172	0	0.2	0.4	1.8	*	*	*	362	322	28	0.3
107	103	182	14	1.9	3.1	12	1	0.05	0.15	3.2	0.16	11	1.52	23	112	1	0.1
0	10	214	13	0.9	0.2	49	176	0.04	0.1	1.5	0.09	8	0	3	26	1	0.7
0	8	327	14	0.7	0.1	81	188	0.04	0.09	1	0.06	19	0	18	30	1	*
18	816	172	55	1.3	1.8	92	1	0.19	0.37	1.5	0.2	10	0.82	272	276	*	3
0	10	256	37	1.9	1.5	1471	17	0.19	0.14	1.5	0.22	47	0	58	116	3	0.1
0	663	255	36	1.9	1.5	1471	17	0.19	0.14	1.5	0.22	47	0	59	117	*	0.1
0	109	253	26	1.5	0.7	1242	13	0.36	0.1	1.9	0.14	42	0	37	78	*	0.2
0	530	115	19	1	0.7	19	4	0.12	0.08	1.5	0.23	32	0	20	61	*	t
0	67	211	23	1.6	0.5	63	12	0.27	0.12	1.9	0.16	36	0	25	61	*	0.2
9	336	110	16	0.6	0.8	74	1	0.18	0.16	2.5	0.04	59	0.33	116	113	*	*
21	382	178	18	1.5	1.1	101	2	0.21	0.17	2	0.09	27	0.36	101	131	*	0.8
14	267	153	8	0.9	0.5	54	2	0.14	0.23	3.1	0.05	53	0.19	65	75	*	*
15	1105	604	72	4.5	4.8	39	6	0.15	0.14	2.3	0.12	77	0	123	267	*	0.6
18	850	673	86	4.2	3.8	28	8	0.12	0.15	0.9	0.22	95	0	154	266	*	0.6
17	1113	759	88	8.3	14.8	62	8	0.13	0.12	1.3	0.18	57	0	141	297	*	0.6
7	126	41	4	2.2	0.1	70	0	0.01	0.01	0.5	0.02	3	0.02	6	15	*	0.4
33	377	928	42	3	0.5	1100	12	0.16	0.16	1	0.68	28	0.14	96	130	*	16
46	567	415	28	1.2	1.7	740	24	0.34	0.24	2.2	0.21	46	0.47	227	251	19	0.7
67	1395	521	40	3.7	2	30	2	0.47	0.42	7.7	0.34	39	0.2	128	207	*	5.6
1	2	15	1	t	t	7	3	0.01	0.01	t	0.01	2	0	4	3	*	0.4
69	487	260	26	0.6	2.8	9	2	0.06	0.06	1.3	0.12	35	4.74	38	129	*	1.4
0	13	288	21	0.6	0.4	149	8	0.03	0.04	0.9	0.07	6	0	28	36	1	*
0	7	191	12	0.7	0.2	108	5	0.04	0.05	0.9	0.08	6	0	17	22	1	*
0	53	356	22	1.3	0.4	235	48	0.06	0.1	1.2	0.16	77	0	26	80	1	0.5
1	148	21	3	0.3	0.1	4	1	0.03	0.02	0.2	0.02	2	0.01	5	12	*	0.2
0	14	9	*	*	*	*	*	*	*	*	*	*	*	*	*	*	*
171	1323	635	39	1.6	0.8	82	25	0.19	0.15	2.2	0.35	17	0.39	48	130	*	5.9
44	763	416	52	2.3	2.7	78	4	0.1	0.35	2.5	0.21	40	0.64	192	143	*	2.3
*	107	63	*	*	*	*	*	*	*	*	*	*	*	*	*	*	*
0	101	38	6	0.3	0.1	8	1	0.01	0.01	0.1	0.01	10	0.01	10	16	*	0.3
0	16	14	5	0.1	0.1	5	1	0.01	0.01	t	0.02	2	0.01	5	10	*	0.3
44	1222	274	27	1.5	1.8	174	13	0.16	0.14	1.6	0.23	26	0.55	53	89	*	1.9
9	75	27	6	0.3	0.3	11	t	0.02	0.04	0.8	0.05	5	0.03	7	26	*	0.8
93	2601	583	58	4.3	3.9	350	27	0.38	0.41	10.2	0.5	55	1.17	103	394	*	4.1
58	772	290	16	3.3	1.4	77	3	0.31	0.49	2.7	0.2	71	0.54	130	152	*	1.1
52	792	316	31	4.2	3.4	21	2	0.38	0.31	5.9	0.27	40	1.22	54	239	*	0.2
77	1634	345	40	5.1	5.4	46	0	0.38	0.46	5.9	0.34	41	2.05	183	401	*	0.4
73	798	525	49	5.2	4.5	44	6	0.4	0.37	7.3	0.37	89	1.57	91	297	*	0.4
73	845	330	67	2.8	4.4	50	6	0.42	0.42	6	0.32	45	1.82	41	193	*	5.2
35	1650	394	68	2.5	2.6	79	12	1	0.8	5.5	0.13	54	1.09	189	287	*	5.4
3	93	31	5	1.4	0.1	11	t	0.02	0.04	0.9	0.03	6	0.21	10	34	*	0.7
*	114	*	*	0.2	*	11	0	0.03	0.02	0.3	*	*	*	3	*	*	*
4	955	303	28	2.8	*	186	10	0.35	0.28	4.5	*	*	*	40	88	25	*
4	955	408	*	2.3	*	216	13	0.25	0.18	2.3	*	*	*	80	135	*	*
39	1220	245	28	3.3	*	200	5	0.15	0.18	2.3	*	*	*	53	113	*	*
75	1009	665	*	3.7	*	1590	22	0.25	0.3	4	*	*	*	124	236	22	*
184	763	201	38	1.3	1.3	675	3	0.09	0.31	0.5	0.12	62	1.36	230	231	*	1.8
57	802	473	71	2.4	3.9	147	2	0.15	0.45	3.2	0.24	23	1.04	221	203	*	1.7
68	434	*	*	2.7	*	118	2	0.08	0.23	10.3	*	*	*	41	291	*	0
0	243	474	26	1.7	0.7	1899	8	0.08	0.08	0.9	0.13	39	0	44	69	1	1
0	64	308	40	1.5	0.9	778	6	0.13	0.22	1.6	0.14	35	0	46	93	1	*
18	337	79	9	0.2	0.9	78	0	0.01	0.13	t	0.04	2	0.32	163	130	6	0.2
16	381	69	8	0.1	0.7	67	0	0.01	0.12	t	0.03	2	0.11	159	202	6	0.2
27	406	46	6	0.1	0.9	103	0	0.01	0.1	t	0.02	2	0.2	174	211	3	0.2
21	396	73	7	0.1	0.8	61	0	0.01	0.11	0.3	0.05	10	0.35	150	110	6	0.2
102	1884	346	31	0.4	3.6	292	0	0.04	0.52	1.4	0.22	49	1.64	712	523	27	0.9
27	159	38	7	0.1	0.7	92	0	t	0.1	t	0.02	6	0.36	191	128	3	0.2
28	178	43	6	0.1	0.7	57	0	0.02	0.15	0.1	0.07	18	0.47	52	53	*	0.2
27	320	71	8	0.1	0.9	105	0	0.01	0.19	0.2	0.09	24	0.49	147	132	8	0.2
26	196	26	6	0.2	0.8	90	0	0.01	0.13	0.1	0.02	5	0.08	191	139	*	0.2

WT, weight; **KCAL**, kcalories; **PROT**, protein; **CARB**, carbohydrate; **FIBR**, fiber; **FAT**, fat; **SATF**, saturated fat;

MONO, monosaturated fat; **POLY**, polyunsaturated fat; **CHOR**, cholesterol; **SOD**, sodium; **POT**, potassium;

Food Name	Portion	WT (Gm)	KCAL	PROT (Gm)	CARB (Gm)	FIBR (Gm)	FAT (Gm)	SATF (Gm)	MONO (Gm)	POLY (Gm)
CHEESE-CHEDDAR-CUT PIECES	OUNCE	28.4	114	7	t	0	9	6	2.7	0.3
CHEESE-CHEDDAR-INCH CUBES	ITEM	17.2	69	5	t	0	6	3.6	1.6	0.2
CHEESE-CHEDDAR-LOWFAT-LOW SODIUM-PAULY	OUNCE	28.4	83	9	1	0	5	1.3	0.6	0.1
CHEESE-CHEDDAR-SHREDDED	CUP	113	455	28	1	0	38	23.8	10.6	1.1
CHEESE-CHESHIRE	OUNCE	28.4	110	7	1	0	9	5.5	2.5	0.2
CHEESE-COLBY	OUNCE	28.4	112	7	1	0	9	5.7	2.6	0.3
CHEESE-COTTAGE-1% LOWFAT-UNPACKED	CUP	226	164	28	6	0	2	1.5	0.7	0.1
CHEESE-COTTAGE-2% LOWFAT-UNPACKED	CUP	226	203	31	8	0	4	2.8	1.2	0.1
CHEESE-COTTAGE-4% FAT-LARGE CURD-UNPACK	CUP	225	232	28	6	0	10	6.4	2.9	0.3
CHEESE-COTTAGE-4% FAT-SMALL CURD-UNPACK	CUP	210	217	26	6	0	9	6	2.7	0.3
CHEESE-COTTAGE-DRY CURD-UNCREAMED	CUP	145	123	25	3	0	1	0.4	0.2	t
CHEESE-COTTAGE-WITH FRUIT-UNPACKED	CUP	226	279	22	30	0	8	4.9	2.2	0.2
CHEESE-CREAM	OUNCE	28.4	100	2	1	0	10	6.3	2.8	0.4
CHEESE-EDAM	OUNCE	28.4	101	7	t	0	8	5	2.3	0.2
CHEESE-FETA	OUNCE	28.4	75	4	1	0	6	4.2	1.3	0.2
CHEESE-FONTINA	OUNCE	28.4	110	7	t	0	9	5.4	2.5	0.5
CHEESE-GARLIC-LOWFAT-LOW SODIUM-PAULY	OUNCE	28.4	80	8	0	0	6	3	*	2.5
CHEESE-GJETOST	OUNCE	28.4	132	3	12	0	8	5.4	2.2	0.3
CHEESE-GOUDA	OUNCE	28.4	101	7	1	0	8	5	2.2	0.2
CHEESE-GRUYERE	OUNCE	28.4	117	8	t	0	9	5.4	2.9	0.5
CHEESE-LIMBURGER	OUNCE	28.4	93	6	t	0	8	4.8	2.4	0.1
CHEESE-MONTEREY JACK	OUNCE	28.4	106	7	t	0	9	5.4	2.5	0.3
CHEESE-MONTEREY JACK-LOWFAT-LOW SODIUM	OUNCE	28.4	80	8	0	0	6	3	*	2.5
CHEESE-MOZZARELLA-MADE FROM SKIM MILK	OUNCE	28.4	72	7	1	0	5	2.9	1.3	0.1
CHEESE-MOZZARELLA-MADE FROM WHOLE MILK	OUNCE	28.4	80	6	1	0	6	3.7	1.9	0.2
CHEESE-MUENSTER	OUNCE	28.4	104	7	t	0	9	5.4	2.5	0.2
CHEESE-NEUFCHATEL	OUNCE	28.4	74	3	1	0	7	4.2	1.9	0.2
CHEESE-PARMESAN-GRATED	CUP	100	456	42	4	0	30	19.1	8.7	0.7
CHEESE-PIMENTO-PROCESSED	OUNCE	28.4	106	6	t	0	9	5.6	2.5	0.3
CHEESE-PORT DU SALUT	OUNCE	28.4	100	7	t	0	8	4.7	2.7	0.2
CHEESE-PROVOLONE	OUNCE	28.4	100	7	1	0	8	4.8	2.1	0.2
CHEESE-RICOTTA-MADE WITH PART SKIM MILK	CUP	246	340	28	13	0	20	12.1	5.7	0.6
CHEESE-RICOTTA-MADE WITH WHOLE MILK	CUP	246	428	28	7	0	32	20.4	8.9	1
CHEESE-ROMANO	OUNCE	28.4	110	9	1	0	8	4.9	2.2	0.2
CHEESE-ROQUEFORT	OUNCE	28.4	105	6	1	0	9	5.5	2.4	0.4
CHEESE-SWISS	OUNCE	28.4	107	8	1	0	8	5	2.1	0.3
CHEESE-SWISS-LOWFAT-LOW SODIUM-PAULY	OUNCE	28.4	97	9	1	0	7	5.1	2.1	0.3
CHEESE-SWISS-PASTEURIZED PROCESS	OUNCE	28.4	95	7	1	0	7	4.6	2	0.2
CHEESE-TILSIT	OUNCE	28.4	96	7	1	0	7	4.8	2	0.2
CREAM-COFFEE-TABLE-LIGHT-FLUID	CUP	240	469	6	9	0	46	28.9	13.4	1.7
CREAM-HALF & HALF-MILK AND CREAM-FLUID	CUP	242	315	7	10	0	28	17.3	8	1
CREAM-IMITATION-LIQUID-NON DAIRY-FROZEN	CUP	245	333	2	28	0	24	4.8	18.5	0.1
CREAM-IMITATION-NON DAIRY-POWDERED	CUP	94	514	5	52	0	33	30.6	0.9	t
CREAM-MOCHA MIX-NON DAIRY	TBSP	15	20	1	1	t	2	0.8	0.8	0.8
CREAM-SOUR-CULTURED	CUP	230	493	7	10	0	48	30	13.9	1.8
CREAM-SOUR-HALF & HALF	TBSP	15	20	t	1	0	2	1.1	0.5	0.1
CREAM-SOUR-IMITATION	OUNCE	28.4	59	1	2	0	6	5	0.2	t
CREAM-SOUR-IMITATION-NONFAT DRY MILK	CUP	235	415	8	11	0	39	31.2	5	1.2
CREAM-WHIPPED-IMITATION-NON DAIRY-FROZEN	CUP	75	239	1	17	0	19	16.3	1.2	0.4
CREAM-WHIPPED-IMITATION-NON DAIRY-POWDER	CUP	80	151	3	13	0	10	8.6	0.7	0.2
CREAM-WHIPPED-IMITATION-PRESSURIZED	CUP	60	154	2	7	0	13	8.3	3.9	0.5
CREAM-WHIPPED-IMITATION-PRESSURIZED	CUP	70	184	1	11	0	16	13.2	1.4	0.2
CREAM-WHIPPING-HEAVY-UNWHIPPED-FLUID	CUP	238	821	5	7	0	88	54.8	25.4	3.3
CREAM-WHIPPING-LIGHT-UNWHIPPED-FLUID	CUP	239	699	5	7	0	74	46.2	21.7	2.1
MILK-1% FAT-LOWFAT-FLUID	CUP	244	102	8	12	0	3	1.6	0.8	0.1
MILK-1% FAT-NONFAT MILK SOLIDS ADDED	CUP	245	104	9	12	0	2	1.5	0.7	0.1
MILK-1% FAT-PROTEIN FORTIFIED	CUP	246	119	10	14	0	3	1.8	0.8	0.1
MILK-2% FAT-FLUID-PROTEIN FORTIFIED	CUP	246	137	10	14	0	5	3	1.4	0.2
MILK-2% FAT-LOWFAT-FLUID	CUP	244	121	8	12	0	5	2.9	1.4	0.2
MILK-2% FAT-NONFAT MILK SOLIDS ADDED	CUP	245	125	9	12	0	5	2.9	1.4	0.2
MILK-BUTTERMILK-CULTURED-FLUID	CUP	245	99	8	12	0	2	1.3	0.6	0.1
MILK-BUTTERMILK-DRIED-SWEET CREAM	CUP	120	464	41	59	0	7	4.3	2	0.3
MILK-CHOCOLATE-1% FAT-FLUID	CUP	250	158	8	26	0.2	3	1.5	0.8	0.1
MILK-CHOCOLATE-2% FAT-FLUID	CUP	250	179	8	26	0.2	5	3.1	1.5	0.2

t = Trace of nutrient present   * = Not available

MAG, magnesium; IRON, iron; ZINC, zinc; VITA, vitamin A; VITC, vitamin C; THIA, thiamin; RIBO, riboflavin; NIAC, niacin; VB6, vitamin B-6; FOL, folate; VB12, vitamin B-12; CALC, calcium; PHOS, phosphorus; SEL, selenium; VE-a, alpha tocopherol equivalents.

CHOL (mg)	SOD (mg)	POT (mg)	MAG (mg)	IRON (mg)	ZINC (mg)	VITA (RE)	VITC (mg)	THIA (mg)	RIBO (mg)	NIAC (mg)	VB6 (mg)	FOL (µg)	VB12 (µg)	CALC (mg)	PHOS (mg)	SEL (µg)	VE-a (mg)
30	176	28	8	0.2	0.9	90	0	0.01	0.11	t	0.02	5	0.23	204	145	5	0.2
18	107	17	5	0.1	0.5	55	0	0.01	0.07	t	0.01	3	0.14	124	88	3	0.1
14	68	32	8	0.2	0.9	18	0	0.01	0.01	t	0.02	5	0.24	200	137	*	0.1
119	701	111	31	0.8	3.5	359	0	0.03	0.42	0.1	0.08	21	0.94	815	579	18	0.7
29	198	27	6	0.1	0.8	84	0	0.01	0.08	t	0.02	5	0.23	182	131	*	0.2
27	171	36	7	0.2	0.9	88	0	t	0.11	t	0.02	5	0.23	194	129	16	0.2
10	918	193	12	0.3	0.9	25	0	0.05	0.37	0.3	0.15	28	1.43	138	302	52	1.5
19	918	217	14	0.4	1	47	0	0.05	0.42	0.3	0.17	30	1.61	155	340	52	1.5
34	911	189	11	0.3	0.8	110	0	0.05	0.37	0.3	0.15	27	1.4	135	297	52	1.4
31	850	177	11	0.3	0.8	103	0	0.04	0.34	0.3	0.14	26	1.31	126	277	48	1.3
10	19	47	6	0.3	0.7	13	0	0.04	0.21	0.2	0.12	21	1.2	46	151	34	0.9
25	915	151	9	0.3	0.7	84	0	0.04	0.29	0.2	0.12	22	1.12	108	236	4	*
31	85	34	2	0.3	0.2	122	0	0.01	0.06	t	0.01	4	0.12	23	30	1	0.2
25	274	53	8	0.1	1.1	78	0	0.01	0.11	t	0.02	5	0.44	207	152	1	0.2
25	316	18	5	0.2	0.8	36	0	0.04	0.24	0.1	0.12	9	0.48	140	96	*	0.2
33	227	18	4	0.1	1	100	0	0.01	0.06	t	0.02	2	0.48	156	98	*	0.2
20	95	*	*	*	*	*	*	*	*	*	*	*	*	*	*	*	*
27	170	399	20	0.1	0.3	78	0	0.09	0.39	0.2	0.08	1	0.69	113	126	*	0.2
32	232	34	8	0.1	1.1	55	0	0.01	0.1	t	0.02	6	0.44	198	155	0	0.2
31	95	23	10	t	1.1	104	0	0.02	0.08	t	0.02	3	0.45	287	172	1	0.2
26	227	36	6	t	0.6	109	0	0.02	0.14	t	0.02	16	0.3	141	111	*	0.2
25	152	23	8	0.2	0.9	81	0	t	0.11	t	0.02	5	0.23	212	126	13	0.2
20	95	*	*	*	*	*	*	*	*	*	*	*	*	*	*	*	*
16	132	24	7	0.1	0.8	50	0	0.01	0.09	t	0.02	2	0.23	183	131	3	0.2
22	106	19	5	0.1	0.6	68	0	t	0.07	t	0.02	2	0.19	147	105	3	0.2
27	178	38	8	0.1	0.8	96	0	t	0.09	t	0.02	3	0.42	203	133	*	0.2
22	113	32	2	0.1	0.2	96	0	t	0.06	t	0.01	3	0.08	21	39	*	0.2
79	1862	107	51	1	3.2	211	0	0.05	0.39	0.3	0.11	8	1.4	1376	807	24	0.6
27	405	46	6	0.1	0.8	108	1	0.01	0.1	t	0.02	2	0.2	174	211	6	0.2
35	151	39	7	0.1	0.7	114	0	t	0.07	t	0.02	5	0.43	184	102	*	0.2
20	248	39	8	0.2	0.9	69	0	0.01	0.09	t	0.02	3	0.42	214	141	*	0.2
76	307	308	36	1.1	3.3	319	0	0.05	0.46	0.2	0.05	32	0.72	669	449	*	1.6
124	207	257	28	0.9	2.9	362	0	0.03	0.48	0.3	0.11	30	0.83	509	389	*	1.6
29	340	25	12	0.2	0.7	49	0	0.01	0.11	t	0.02	2	0.32	302	215	*	0.2
26	513	26	8	0.2	0.6	89	0	0.01	0.17	0.2	0.04	14	0.18	188	111	*	0.2
26	74	31	10	0.1	1.1	72	0	0.01	0.1	t	0.02	2	0.48	272	171	2	0.2
19	32	32	10	t	1.1	72	0	0.01	0.11	t	0.02	2	0.48	273	172	*	0.2
24	388	61	8	0.2	1	69	0	t	0.08	t	0.01	2	0.35	219	216	2	0.2
29	213	18	4	0.1	1	89	0	0.02	0.1	0.1	0.02	6	0.6	198	142	*	0.2
159	95	292	21	0.1	0.7	519	2	0.08	0.36	0.1	0.08	6	0.53	231	192	1	2
89	98	314	25	0.2	1.2	315	2	0.09	0.36	0.2	0.09	6	0.8	254	230	1	2
0	194	466	0	0.1	t	66	0	0	0	0	0	0	0	22	157	*	*
0	170	763	4	1.1	0.5	57	0	0	0.16	0	0	0	0	21	397	*	*
0	5	20	*	*	*	*	*	*	*	*	*	*	*	*	*	*	*
102	123	331	26	0.1	0.6	546	2	0.08	0.34	0.2	0.04	25	0.69	268	195	*	*
6	6	19	2	t	0.1	20	t	0.01	0.02	t	t	2	0.05	16	14	*	t
0	29	46	2	0.1	0.3	0	0	0	0	0	0	0	0	1	13	*	0
0	240	380	*	0.1	*	6	2	0.09	0.38	0.2	*	*	*	266	205	*	*
0	19	14	1	0.1	t	194	0	0	0	0	0	0	0	5	6	*	*
8	53	121	8	t	0.2	87	1	0.02	0.09	t	0.02	3	0.21	72	69	*	*
46	78	88	6	t	0.2	165	0	0.02	0.04	t	0.03	2	0.18	61	54	*	*
0	43	13	1	t	t	99	0	0	0	0	0	0	0	4	13	*	*
326	89	179	17	0.1	0.6	1051	1	0.05	0.26	0.1	0.06	9	0.43	154	149	*	2
265	82	231	17	0.1	0.6	809	1	0.06	0.3	0.1	0.07	9	0.47	166	146	*	2
10	123	381	34	0.1	1	150	2	0.1	0.41	0.2	0.11	12	0.9	300	235	3	0.1
10	128	397	35	0.1	1	150	2	0.1	0.42	0.2	0.11	13	0.94	313	245	3	0.1
10	143	444	39	0.2	1.1	150	3	0.11	0.47	0.2	0.12	15	1.05	349	273	3	0.1
19	145	447	40	0.2	1.1	150	3	0.11	0.48	0.2	0.13	15	1.05	352	276	6	0.1
18	122	377	33	0.1	1	150	2	0.1	0.4	0.2	0.11	12	0.89	297	232	7	0.1
18	128	397	35	0.1	1	150	2	0.1	0.42	0.2	0.11	13	0.94	313	245	7	0.1
9	257	371	27	0.1	1	24	2	0.08	0.38	0.1	0.08	12	0.54	285	219	3	1
83	621	1910	131	0.4	4.8	79	7	0.47	1.9	1.1	0.41	57	4.59	1421	1119	*	0
7	152	426	33	0.6	1	150	2	0.1	0.42	0.3	0.1	12	0.86	287	256	3	0.2
17	150	422	33	0.6	1	150	2	0.09	0.41	0.3	0.1	12	0.85	284	254	3	0.2

WT, weight; **KCAL,** kcalories; **PROT,** protein; **CARB,** carbohydrate; **FIBR,** fiber; **FAT,** fat; **SATF,** saturated fat;
MONO, monosaturated fat; **POLY,** polyunsaturated fat; **CHOR,** cholesterol; **SOD,** sodium; **POT,** potassium;

Food Name	Portion	WT (Gm)	KCAL	PROT (Gm)	CARB (Gm)	FIBR (Gm)	FAT (Gm)	SATF (Gm)	MONO (Gm)	POLY (Gm)
MILK-CHOCOLATE-WHOLE-FLUID	CUP	250	208	8	26	0.2	8	5.3	2.5	0.3
MILK-CONDENSED-SWEETENED-CANNED	CUP	306	982	24	166	0	27	16.8	7.4	1
MILK-EGGNOG-COMMERCIAL	CUP	254	342	10	34	0	19	11.3	5.7	0.9
MILK-EVAPORATED-SKIM-CANNED	CUP	255	199	19	29	0	1	0.3	0.2	t
MILK-EVAPORATED-WHOLE-CANNED	CUP	252	338	17	25	0	19	11.6	5.9	0.6
MILK-GOAT-WHOLE-FLUID	CUP	244	168	9	11	0	10	6.5	2.7	0.4
MILK-HUMAN-WHOLE-MATURE	CUP	246	171	3	17	0	11	4.9	4.1	1.2
MILK-IMITATION	CUP	244	150	4	15	0	8	1.9	4.9	1.2
MILK-INDIAN BUFFALO-WHOLE	CUP	244	236	9	13	0	17	11.2	4.4	0.4
MILK-MALTED-CHOCOLATE FLAVOR-PREPARED	CUP	265	229	9	30	0.1	9	5.5	2.6	0.4
MILK-MALTED-NATURAL FLAVOR-PREPARED	CUP	265	237	10	27	0.2	10	6	2.8	0.6
MILK-NONFAT/SKIM-FLUID	CUP	245	86	8	12	0	t	0.3	0.1	t
MILK-NONFAT/SKIM-INSTANTIZED-DRIED	CUP	68	244	24	36	0	t	0.3	0.1	t
MILK-NONFAT/SKIM-INSTANTIZED-ENVELOPE	ITEM	91	326	32	48	0	1	0.4	0.2	t
MILK-NONFAT/SKIM-MILK SOLIDS ADDED	CUP	245	90	9	12	0	1	0.4	0.2	t
MILK-NONFAT/SKIM-PROTEIN FORTIFIED	CUP	246	100	10	14	0	1	0.4	0.2	t
MILK-SHEEP-WHOLE-FLUID	CUP	245	264	15	13	0	17	11.3	4.2	0.8
MILK-SOY-FLUID	CUP	240	79	7	4	3.1	5	0.5	0.8	2
MILK-WHOLE-DRY	CUP	128	635	34	49	0	34	21.4	10.1	0.9
MILK-WHOLE-LOW SODIUM	CUP	244	149	8	11	0	8	5.3	2.4	0.3
MILK-WHOLE-REGULAR-3.3% FAT-FLUID	CUP	244	150	8	11	0	8	5.1	2.4	0.3
MILKSHAKE-CHOCOLATE-THICK	ITEM	300	356	9	64	0.8	8	5	2.3	0.3
MILKSHAKE-VANILLA-THICK	ITEM	313	350	12	56	0.2	9	5.9	2.7	0.4
WHEY-ACID-DRY	TBSP	2.9	10	t	2	0	t	t	t	t
WHEY-ACID-FLUID	CUP	246	59	2	13	0	t	0.1	0.1	t
WHEY-SWEET-DRY	TBSP	7.5	26	1	6	0	t	0.1	t	t
WHEY-SWEET-FLUID	CUP	246	66	2	13	0	1	0.6	0.2	t
YOGURT-FRUIT FLAVORS-LOWFAT-ADDED SOLIDS	CUP	227	231	10	43	0.8	2	1.6	0.7	0.1
YOGURT-ORIGINAL COFFEE-LOWFAT-DANNON	SERVING	227	200	10	34	0	3	1.8	0.8	0.1
YOGURT-PLAIN-LOWFAT-MILK SOLIDS ADDED	CUP	227	144	12	16	0	4	2.3	1	0.1
YOGURT-PLAIN-NONFAT-MILK SOLIDS ADDED	CUP	227	127	13	17	0	t	0.3	0.1	t
YOGURT-PLAIN-WHOLE MILK-NO SOLIDS	CUP	227	139	8	11	0	7	4.8	2	0.2

Desserts

Food Name	Portion	WT (Gm)	KCAL	PROT (Gm)	CARB (Gm)	FIBR (Gm)	FAT (Gm)	SATF (Gm)	MONO (Gm)	POLY (Gm)
BROWNIES WITH NUTS-HOME RECIPE	ITEM	20	95	1	10	0.5	6	1.5	3	1.2
BROWNIES-COMMERCIALLY PREPARED	ITEM	60	243	3	39	1.3	10	3.1	3.8	2.6
CAKE-ANGEL FOOD-PREPARED FROM MIX	SLICE	53	142	4	32	t	t	*	*	*
CAKE-CHEESECAKE-COMMERCIAL	SLICE	85	257	5	24	1.8	16	6.7	6	2.9
CAKE-COFFEE-PREPARED FROM MIX	SLICE	72	230	5	38	2.4	7	2	2.7	1.5
CAKE-DEVILS FOOD WITH ICING-FROM MIX	SLICE	69	235	3	40	1.5	8	3.1	2.8	1.1
CAKE-GINGERBREAD-PREPARED FROM MIX	SLICE	63	175	2	32	1.8	4	1.1	1.8	1.1
CAKE-PINEAPPLE UPSIDE DOWN-HOME RECIPE	SLICE	70	221	2	35	1.2	9	1.9	3.9	2.1
CAKE-POUND-HOME RECIPE	SLICE	33	160	2	16	0.1	10	5.9	3	0.6
CAKE-SHEET-NO ICING-HOME RECIPE	SLICE	86	315	4	48	1	12	3.3	4.9	2.6
CAKE-SPONGE-HOME RECIPE	SLICE	66	188	5	36	0	3	1.1	1.3	0.5
CAKE-STRAWBERRY SHORTCAKE	SERVING	175	344	5	61	2.1	9	*	*	*
CAKE-STREUSEL TYPE-WITH ICING-FROM MIX	SLICE	50	172	2	25	0.9	8	*	*	*
CAKE-WHITE/CHOCOLATE ICING-HOME RECIPE	SLICE	71	271	3	42	0.8	11	3	2.9	1.3
CAKE-YELLOW/CHOCOLATE ICING-HOME RECIPE	SLICE	69	268	3	40	0.6	11	3	3	1.4
COOKIE-CHOCOLATE CHIP-BAKED FROM MIX	ITEM	10.5	50	1	7	0.3	2	0.7	0.9	0.6
COOKIE-CHOCOLATE CHIP-FROM HOME RECIPE	ITEM	10	46	1	6	0.3	3	0.6	1.2	0.8
COOKIE-FIG BAR-COMMERCIAL	ITEM	14	53	1	11	0.6	1	0.2	0.3	0.2
COOKIE-GINGERSNAP-FROM HOME RECIPE	ITEM	7	34	t	5	0.3	2	*	*	*
COOKIE-MACAROON	ITEM	19	90	1	13	0.4	5	*	*	*
COOKIE-OATMEAL/RAISIN-PREPARED FROM MIX	ITEM	13	62	1	9	0.4	3	0.5	0.8	0.5
COOKIE-PEANUT BUTTER-FROM MIX	ITEM	10	50	1	6	0.2	3	0.6	1.2	0.7
COOKIE-SANDWICH-CHOCOLATE/VANILLA	ITEM	10	50	1	7	0.2	2	0.6	1	0.6
COOKIE-SUGAR-FROM MIX	ITEM	20	99	1	13	0.3	5	*	*	*
COOKIE-VANILLA WAFER	ITEM	4	19	t	3	t	1	0.1	0.2	0.1
CUPCAKE WITH CHOCOLATE ICING	ITEM	36	130	2	21	0.4	5	2	1.7	0.7
CUPCAKE-NO ICING	ITEM	25	90	1	14	0.3	3	0.8	1.2	0.7
CUSTARD-BAKED	CUP	265	305	14	29	1	15	6.8	5.4	0.7
DANISH PASTRY-CHEESE	ITEM	91	353	6	29	0.6	25	5.1	15.6	2.4
DANISH PASTRY-FRUIT	ITEM	94	335	5	45	1.8	16	3.3	10.1	1.6

*t = Trace of nutrient present   * = Not available*

MAG, magnesium; IRON, iron; ZINC, zinc; VITA, vitamin A; VITC, vitamin C; THIA, thiamin; RIBO, riboflavin; NIAC, niacin; VB6, vitamin B-6; FOL, folate; VB12, vitamin B-12; CALC, calcium; PHOS, phosphorus; SEL, selenium; VE-a, alpha tocopherol equivalents.

CHOL (mg)	SOD (mg)	POT (mg)	MAG (mg)	IRON (mg)	ZINC (mg)	VITA (RE)	VITC (mg)	THIA (mg)	RIBO (mg)	NIAC (mg)	VB6 (mg)	FOL (μg)	VB12 (μg)	CALC (mg)	PHOS (mg)	SEL (μg)	VE-a (mg)
30	149	417	33	0.6	1	91	2	0.09	0.41	0.3	0.1	12	0.84	280	251	3	0.2
104	389	1136	78	0.6	2.9	302	8	0.28	1.27	0.6	0.16	34	1.36	868	775	3	0
149	138	420	47	0.5	1.2	268	4	0.09	0.48	0.3	0.13	2	1.14	330	278	3	*
10	293	847	69	0.7	2.3	300	3	0.12	0.79	0.4	0.14	23	0.61	740	497	3	0
73	267	764	61	0.5	1.9	184	5	0.12	0.8	0.5	0.13	20	0.41	658	509	3	0
28	122	499	34	0.1	0.7	135	3	0.12	0.34	0.7	0.11	1	0.16	326	270	*	0
34	42	126	8	0.1	0.4	178	12	0.03	0.09	0.4	0.03	13	0.11	79	34	4	2.2
0	191	279	16	1	2.9	0	0	0.03	0.22	0	0	0	0	79	181	*	2.6
46	127	434	76	0.3	0.5	130	5	0.13	0.33	0.2	0.06	14	0.89	412	286	*	*
34	172	499	47	0.5	1.1	80	3	0.13	0.44	0.6	0.14	16	0.91	304	265	3	0.2
37	223	529	52	0.3	1.1	94	3	0.2	0.59	1.3	0.19	22	1.03	354	303	3	*
4	126	406	28	0.1	1	150	2	0.09	0.34	0.2	0.1	13	0.93	302	247	7	0.1
12	373	1160	80	0.2	3	484	4	0.28	1.19	0.6	0.24	34	2.72	837	670	*	*
17	499	1552	107	0.3	4	648	5	0.38	1.59	0.8	0.31	45	3.63	1120	896	22	*
5	130	418	36	0.1	1	150	2	0.1	0.43	0.2	0.11	13	0.95	316	255	3	0.1
5	144	446	40	0.2	1.1	150	3	0.11	0.48	0.2	0.12	15	1.05	352	275	3	0.1
66	108	334	45	0.2	1.3	108	10	0.16	0.87	1	0.15	17	1.74	474	387	*	0
0	29	338	46	1.4	0.6	7	0	0.39	0.17	0.4	0.1	4	0	10	118	*	t
124	475	1702	108	0.6	4.3	354	11	0.36	1.54	0.8	0.39	47	4.16	1168	993	*	0.2
33	6	617	12	0.1	0.9	95	2	0.05	0.26	0.1	0.08	12	0.88	246	209	3	0.1
33	120	370	33	0.1	0.9	92	2	0.09	0.4	0.2	0.1	12	0.87	291	228	3	0.1
32	333	672	48	0.9	1.4	78	0	0.14	0.67	0.4	0.08	15	0.95	396	378	5	*
37	299	572	37	0.3	1.2	107	0	0.09	0.61	0.5	0.13	21	1.63	457	361	5	*
t	28	66	6	t	0.2	1	t	0.02	0.06	t	0.02	1	0.07	59	39	*	t
1	118	352	24	0.2	1.1	5	t	0.1	0.34	0.2	0.1	5	0.44	253	191	*	*
t	80	155	13	0.1	0.2	1	t	0.04	0.17	0.1	0.04	1	0.18	59	70	*	t
5	132	396	20	0.2	0.3	12	t	0.09	0.39	0.2	0.08	2	0.68	115	112	*	*
10	133	442	33	0.2	1.7	31	2	0.08	0.4	0.2	0.09	21	1.06	345	271	11	*
11	140	498	37	0.2	1.9	30	2	0.1	0.46	0.2	0.1	24	1.2	389	306	*	0.1
14	159	531	40	0.2	2	45	2	0.1	0.49	0.3	0.11	25	1.28	415	326	11	*
4	174	579	43	0.2	2.2	5	2	0.11	0.53	0.3	0.12	28	1.39	452	355	11	*
29	105	351	26	0.1	1.3	84	1	0.07	0.32	0.2	0.07	17	0.84	274	215	11	*
0	50	38	3	0.4	*	7	0	0.04	0.03	0.2	*	*	*	8	30	1	0.5
9	153	83	16	1.3	0.6	3	3	0.07	0.13	0.6	0.03	4	0.15	25	87	3	*
0	142	52	6	0.5	0.1	0	0	0.06	0.12	0.6	0.01	5	0.02	50	63	3	1.4
57	189	83	9	0.4	0.4	43	4	0.03	0.11	0.4	0.05	15	0.42	48	75	*	1.5
*	310	78	*	1.2	*	24	0	0.14	0.15	1.3	*	*	*	44	125	5	1.9
33	180	90	*	1	*	20	0	0.07	0.1	0.6	*	4	*	41	72	4	1.9
1	90	173	14	0.9	0.3	0	0	0.09	0.11	0.8	0.05	5	0.07	57	63	4	*
20	167	119	12	1.1	0.4	54	4	0.11	0.08	0.7	0.04	8	0.06	50	44	*	0.6
68	58	20	*	0.5	*	16	0	0.05	0.06	0.4	*	2	*	6	24	2	0.9
1	382	68	12	0.9	0.3	30	0	0.13	0.15	1.1	0.02	6	0.09	55	88	6	2.3
162	164	59	7	1.1	0.8	25	0	0.09	0.13	0.7	0.04	15	0.33	25	65	4	1.8
*	*	*	*	2	*	86	89	0.17	0.21	1.3	*	*	*	73	84	*	*
*	214	55	7	0.7	0.2	6	0	0.06	0.06	0.5	0.02	5	0.1	27	99	*	0.4
3	200	77	14	0.7	0.3	4	0	0.07	0.11	0.7	0.02	4	0.06	70	127	5	1.9
36	191	73	13	0.8	0.3	10	0	0.08	0.1	0.7	0.02	6	0.12	57	61	4	1.9
6	38	14	3	0.2	0.1	6	0	0.01	0.02	0.2	t	1	*	3	7	1	0.3
5	21	21	4	0.2	t	1	0	0.02	0.02	0.1	t	1	0.01	3	8	1	0.3
0	45	41	4	0.3	0.1	3	0	0.02	0.02	0.2	0.02	1	0	10	8	1	0.4
0	20	14	1	0.2	t	1	0	0.01	0.01	0.1	t	1	0.01	3	4	1	0.2
0	6	88	*	0.2	*	0	0	0.01	0.03	0.1	*	*	*	5	16	1	0.5
0	37	23	4	0.3	0.1	2	0	0.02	0.02	0.2	0.01	2	*	4	14	1	0.3
3	57	19	4	0.2	0.8	3	0	0.02	0.02	0.4	0.01	2	0.01	12	24	1	0.3
0	63	4	5	0.2	0.1	0	0	0.02	0.03	0.2	t	t	0	3	24	1	0.3
*	109	14	2	0.4	0.1	3	0	0.04	0.02	0.5	0.01	2	*	21	38	1	0.5
3	10	3	1	0.1	*	1	0	0.01	0.01	0.1	*	*	*	2	3	0	0.1
15	120	42	*	0.4	*	12	0	0.05	0.06	0.4	*	*	*	47	71	3	0.1
0	113	21	*	0.3	*	8	0	0.05	0.05	0.4	*	*	*	40	59	2	0.7
278	209	387	*	1.1	*	87	1	0.11	0.5	0.3	*	*	*	297	310	3	*
20	320	116	16	1.9	0.6	43	3	0.27	0.21	2.6	0.06	15	0.23	70	80	*	3.2
19	333	110	14	1.4	0.5	24	2	0.29	0.21	1.8	0.06	15	0.23	22	69	*	2.3

WT, weight; **KCAL**, kcalories; **PROT**, protein; **CARB**, carbohydrate; **FIBR**, fiber; **FAT**, fat; **SATF**, saturated fat;

MONO, monosaturated fat; **POLY**, polyunsaturated fat; **CHOR**, cholesterol; **SOD**, sodium; **POT**, potassium;

Food Name	Portion	WT (Gm)	KCAL	PROT (Gm)	CARB (Gm)	FIBR (Gm)	FAT (Gm)	SATF (Gm)	MONO (Gm)	POLY (Gm)
DANISH PASTRY-PLAIN	ITEM	65	250	4	29	0.6	14	4.7	6.1	3.2
DOUGHNUTS-CAKE-PLAIN	ITEM	25	104	1	12	0.3	6	1.2	1.2	2
DOUGHNUTS-YEAST-GLAZED	ITEM	50	205	3	22	1.1	11	3	5.8	3.3
ECLAIR-CUSTARD WITH CHOCOLATE ICING	ITEM	100	239	6	23	0.5	14	*	*	*
FROZEN YOGURT-FRUIT VARIETIES	CUP	226	216	7	42	*	2	*	*	*
FRUIT BAR-OAT BRAN-NUTS-HEALTH VALLEY	ITEM	43	150	4	28	2.9	4	*	*	*
GRANOLA BAR	ITEM	24	109	2	16	1	4	*	*	*
ICE CREAM SUNDAE-CARAMEL	ITEM	165	323	8	53	*	10	4.8	3.2	1.1
ICE CREAM SUNDAE-HOT FUDGE	ITEM	165	297	6	50	1.2	9	5.3	2.4	0.8
ICE CREAM SUNDAE-STRAWBERRY	ITEM	165	289	7	48	0.7	8	4	2.9	1.1
ICE CREAM-FRENCH VANILLA-SOFT SERVE	CUP	173	377	7	38	0	23	13.5	5.9	0.7
ICE CREAM-VANILLA-HARDENED-10% FAT	CUP	133	269	5	32	0	14	8.9	3.6	0.3
ICE CREAM-VANILLA-RICH-HARDENED-16% FAT	CUP	148	349	4	32	0	24	14.7	6.8	0.9
ICE MILK-VANILLA-HARDENED-4.3% FAT	CUP	131	184	5	29	0	6	3.5	1.4	0.1
ICE MILK-VANILLA-SOFT SERVE-2.6% FAT	CUP	175	223	8	38	0	5	2.9	1.2	0.1
PIE-APPLE-FROM HOME RECIPE	SLICE	135	323	3	49	2.2	14	3.9	6.4	3.6
PIE-BANANA CREAM-FROM HOME RECIPE	SLICE	130	285	6	40	1.4	12	3.8	4.7	2.3
PIE-BLUEBERRY-FROM HOME RECIPE	SLICE	135	325	3	47	1.7	15	3.5	6.2	3.6
PIE-BOSTON CREAM-HOME RECIPE	SLICE	69	210	3	34	1	6	1.9	2.5	1.3
PIE-CHERRY-FROM HOME RECIPE	SLICE	135	350	4	52	1.1	15	4	6.4	3.6
PIE-CUSTARD-FROM HOME RECIPE	SLICE	130	285	7	30	2.1	14	4.8	5.5	2.5
PIE-LEMON MERINGUE-FROM HOME RECIPE	SLICE	120	300	4	47	1.4	11	3.7	4.8	2.3
PIE-MINCE-FROM HOME RECIPE	SLICE	135	365	3	56	2	16	4	6.6	3.6
PIE-PEACH-FROM HOME RECIPE	SLICE	135	345	3	52	1.8	14	3.5	6.2	3.6
PIE-PECAN-FROM HOME RECIPE	SLICE	118	495	6	61	4.1	27	4	14.4	6.3
PIE-PUMPKIN-FROM HOME RECIPE	SLICE	130	275	5	32	3.5	15	5.4	5.4	2.4
PUDDING-BANANA CREAM-INSTANT MIX-JELLO	OUNCE	28.4	106	0	27	0	0	0	0	0
PUDDING-BUTTERSCOTCH-INSTANT MIX-JELLO	OUNCE	28.4	105	0	27	0	0	0	0	0
PUDDING-CHOCOLATE-COOKED-FROM MIX & MILK	CUP	260	320	9	59	0	8	4.3	2.6	2
PUDDING-CHOCOLATE-INSTANT-FROM MIX	CUP	260	325	8	63	0	7	3.6	2.2	0.3
PUDDING-CHOCOLATE-SUGAR FREE-2% MILK	SERVING	133	100	5	14	0.3	3	*	*	*
PUDDING-LEMON-INSTANT MIX-JELLO	OUNCE	28.4	105	t	27	0.3	t	0	0	0
PUDDING-RICE WITH RAISINS	CUP	265	387	10	71	1.4	8	*	*	*
PUDDING-TAPIOCA CREAM-HOME RECIPE-STARCH	CUP	165	220	8	28	0.6	8	4.1	2.5	0.5
PUDDING-VANILLA (BLANCMANGE)-HOME RECIPE	CUP	255	285	9	41	0	10	6.2	2.5	0.2
PUDDING-VANILLA-SUGAR FREE-WITH 2% MILK	SERVING	133	90	4	12	0.2	2	*	*	*
SHERBET-ORANGE-2% FAT	CUP	193	270	2	59	0	4	2.4	1	0.1
TURNOVER-APPLE	OUNCE	28.4	85	1	11	0.2	5	1.3	2.3	1.4
TURNOVER-CHERRY	OUNCE	28.4	84	1	11	0.2	5	1.1	1.9	1.1
TWINKIE-HOSTESS	ITEM	42	143	1	26	*	4	*	*	*

Eggs

Food Name	Portion	WT (Gm)	KCAL	PROT (Gm)	CARB (Gm)	FIBR (Gm)	FAT (Gm)	SATF (Gm)	MONO (Gm)	POLY (Gm)
EGG SUBSTITUTE-FROZEN	CUP	240	384	27	8	0	27	4.6	5.8	15
EGG SUBSTITUTE-LIQUID	CUP	251	211	30	2	0	8	1.7	2.3	4
EGG SUBSTITUTE-POWDER	SERVING	28.4	126	16	6	0	4	1.1	1.5	0.5
EGG-DUCK-WHOLE-FRESH-RAW	ITEM	70	130	9	1	0	10	2.6	4.6	0.9
EGG-FRIED IN BUTTER-WHOLE-LARGE-CHICKEN	ITEM	46	92	6	1	0	7	1.9	2.8	1.3
EGG-HARD COOKED-NO SHELL-LARGE-CHICKEN	ITEM	50	77	6	1	0	5	1.6	2	0.7
EGG-POACHED-WHOLE-LARGE-CHICKEN	ITEM	50	74	6	1	0	5	1.5	1.9	0.7
EGG-RAW-WHITE-LARGE-CHICKEN	ITEM	33.4	17	4	t	0	0	0	0	0
EGG-RAW-WHOLE-LARGE-CHICKEN	ITEM	50	75	6	1	0	5	1.6	1.9	0.7
EGG-RAW-YOLK-LARGE-CHICKEN	ITEM	16.6	59	3	t	0	5	1.6	2	0.7
EGG-SCRAMBLED-WITH MILK & BUTTER-CHICKEN	ITEM	61	101	7	1	0	7	2.2	2.9	1.3
OMELET-TWO EGG-HAM AND CHEESE	ITEM	120	266	19	2	0	20	7.3	7.5	2.9

Fast Foods

Food Name	Portion	WT (Gm)	KCAL	PROT (Gm)	CARB (Gm)	FIBR (Gm)	FAT (Gm)	SATF (Gm)	MONO (Gm)	POLY (Gm)
ARBY'S-BEEF AND CHEESE SANDWCH	ITEM	176	402	32	27	1.1	18	9	3.7	3.5
ARBY'S-CHICKEN BREAST SANDWICH	ITEM	184	493	23	48	1.6	25	5.1	9.6	10.3
ARBY'S-CLUB SANDWICH	ITEM	252	560	30	43	2.3	30	11.6	9.3	8.4
ARBY'S-HAM AND CHEESE SANDWICH	ITEM	146	353	21	33	1	16	6.4	6.7	1.4
ARBY'S-ROAST BEEF SANDWICH	ITEM	139	346	22	34	1	14	3.6	6.8	1.7
ARBY'S-SUPER ROAST BEEF SANDWICH	ITEM	234	501	25	50	1.6	22	8.5	8.2	5.4
ARBY'S-TURKEY DELUXE	ITEM	236	510	28	46	*	24	*	*	*

t = Trace of nutrient present   * = Not available

MAG, magnesium; **IRON**, iron; **ZINC**, zinc; **VITA**, vitamin A; **VITC**, vitamin C; **THIA**, thiamin; **RIBO**, riboflavin; **NIAC**, niacin; **VB6**, vitamin B-6; **FOL**, folate; **VB12**, vitamin B-12; **CALC**, calcium; **PHOS**, phosphorus; **SEL**, selenium; **VE-a**, alpha tocopherol equivalents.

CHOL (mg)	SOD (mg)	POT (mg)	MAG (mg)	IRON (mg)	ZINC (mg)	VITA (RE)	VITC (mg)	THIA (mg)	RIBO (mg)	NIAC (mg)	VB6 (mg)	FOL (µg)	VB12 (µg)	CALC (mg)	PHOS (mg)	SEL (µg)	VE-a (mg)
0	249	61	10	1.2	0.5	11	0	0.16	0.15	1.5	*	*	*	69	66	*	*
10	139	27	6	0.4	0.1	2	0	0.06	0.05	0.4	0.01	2	*	11	55	2	0.2
13	117	34	10	0.6	*	5	0	0.1	0.1	0.8	*	11	*	16	33	4	0.4
*	82	122	*	0.7	*	68	0	0.04	0.16	0.1	*	*	*	80	112	*	*
*	*	*	24	0	*	0	0	0.01	0.26	0	*	*	*	200	200	*	*
0	5	230	40	1.4	0.8	0	10	0.19	0.06	0.7	0.06	19	0	25	134	*	3
*	67	78	*	0.8	*	*	*	0.07	0.03	*	*	*	0	14	67	*	*
26	208	338	30	0.2	0.9	56	4	0.07	0.31	1	0.05	13	0.64	201	231	*	1
22	190	413	35	0.6	1	46	2	0.07	0.31	1.1	0.13	10	0.68	216	238	*	0.7
23	99	292	26	0.3	0.7	48	2	0.07	0.3	1	0.08	20	0.69	173	167	*	0.8
153	153	338	25	0.4	2	199	1	0.08	0.45	0.2	0.1	9	1	236	199	2	0.1
59	116	257	18	0.1	1.4	133	1	0.05	0.33	0.1	0.06	3	0.63	176	134	2	0.1
88	108	221	16	0.1	1.2	207	1	0.04	0.28	0.1	0.05	2	0.54	151	115	3	0.1
18	105	265	19	0.2	0.6	52	1	0.08	0.35	0.1	0.09	3	0.88	176	129	2	0.1
13	163	412	29	0.3	0.9	44	1	0.12	0.54	0.2	0.13	5	1.37	274	202	3	1
0	207	115	11	1.2	0.2	5	2	0.15	0.11	1.2	0.04	7	0	12	31	15	2.2
40	252	264	*	1	*	66	1	0.11	0.22	1	*	*	*	86	107	15	*
0	361	88	9	1.4	*	8	4	0.15	0.11	1.4	*	*	0	15	31	15	2.2
0	128	61	*	0.7	*	28	0	0.09	0.11	0.8	*	*	*	46	70	5	*
0	410	142	9	0.9	*	118	0	0.16	0.12	1.4	*	*	0	19	34	15	2.2
*	373	178	*	1.2	*	60	0	0.11	0.27	0.8	*	*	*	125	147	15	2.1
0	223	53	7	0.9	0.3	33	4	0.1	0.12	0.7	0.03	11	0.19	16	48	13	1.9
0	604	240	24	1.9	*	0	1	0.14	0.12	1.4	*	*	*	38	51	15	2.2
0	361	21	9	1.2	*	198	0	0.15	0.14	2	*	*	0	14	39	15	2.2
0	260	145	*	3.7	*	40	0	0.26	0.14	1	*	*	*	55	122	12	*
0	278	208	17	1	*	320	0	0.11	0.18	1	*	*	*	66	90	15	2.1
0	190	1	*	t	*	0	0	0	0	0	*	*	*	1	111	*	*
0	244	1	*	t	*	0	0	0	0	0	*	*	*	1	102	*	*
32	335	354	*	0.8	*	68	2	0.05	0.39	0.3	*	*	*	265	247	*	*
28	322	335	*	1.3	*	68	2	0.08	0.39	0.3	*	*	*	374	237	*	*
*	310	*	*	0.7	*	40	*	0.06	0.26	*	*	*	*	150	300	*	*
0	190	1	*	t	*	0	0	0	0	0	*	*	*	1	111	*	*
*	188	469	*	1.1	*	35	0	0.08	0.37	0.5	*	*	*	260	249	*	*
80	257	223	*	0.7	*	60	2	0.07	0.3	0.2	*	*	*	173	180	*	*
36	165	352	*	0	*	82	2	0.08	0.41	0.3	*	*	*	298	232	*	*
*	380	*	*	*	*	40	*	0.03	0.17	*	*	*	*	150	200	*	*
14	88	198	15	0.3	1.3	39	4	0.03	0.09	0.1	0.03	14	0.16	103	74	*	*
1	109	14	3	0.3	0.1	2	t	0.03	0.02	0.3	0.01	1	0.03	4	11	*	0.5
4	124	20	3	0.2	0.1	12	t	0.02	0.02	0.2	0.01	1	0	4	14	*	0.5
21	189	*	*	0.5	*	8	0	0.06	0.06	0.5	*	*	*	19	*	*	*
5	479	512	36	4.8	2.4	324	1	0.29	0.93	0.3	0.32	39	0.81	175	172	*	1.3
3	444	828	22	5.3	3.3	542	0	0.28	0.75	0.3	0.01	37	0.75	133	304	*	1.4
162	227	211	18	0.9	0.5	105	t	0.06	0.5	0.2	0.04	35	1	92	136	*	0.2
619	102	156	12	2.7	1	279	0	0.11	0.28	0.1	0.18	56	3.78	45	154	*	0.6
211	162	61	5	0.7	0.5	114	0	0.03	0.24	t	0.07	18	0.42	25	89	12	*
213	62	63	5	0.6	0.5	84	0	0.03	0.26	t	0.06	22	0.56	25	86	12	0.4
212	140	60	5	0.7	0.6	95	0	0.03	0.22	t	0.06	18	0.4	25	89	12	0.4
0	55	48	4	t	0	0	0	t	0.15	t	t	1	0.07	2	4	5	0
213	63	60	5	0.7	0.6	95	0	0.03	0.25	t	0.07	23	0.5	25	89	22	0.4
213	7	16	1	0.6	0.5	323	0	0.03	0.11	t	0.07	24	0.52	23	81	7	0.3
215	171	84	7	0.7	0.6	119	t	0.03	0.27	t	0.07	18	0.47	44	104	*	1.3
445	598	182	17	1.7	1.8	273	4	0.18	0.57	0.8	0.19	38	1.08	153	286	33	0.1
77	1634	345	40	5.1	5.4	58	0	0.38	0.46	5.9	0.34	41	2.05	183	401	*	0.4
91	1019	330	46	3.5	1.7	15	0	0.45	0.39	14.8	0.65	32	0.34	111	290	*	2.6
100	1610	466	46	3.6	3.1	127	28	0.68	0.43	7	0.4	44	0.94	200	433	*	3.3
58	772	290	16	3.3	1.4	96	3	0.31	0.49	2.7	0.2	71	0.54	130	152	*	1.1
52	792	316	31	4.2	3.4	63	2	0.38	0.31	5.9	0.27	40	1.22	54	239	*	0.2
40	798	503	58	6.4	10.7	0	0	0.53	0.6	9.4	0.48	41	4.29	115	402	*	0.4
70	1220	*	*	2.7	*	*	*	0.45	0.34	8	*	*	*	80	*	*	*

WT, weight; **KCAL,** kcalories; **PROT,** protein; **CARB,** carbohydrate; **FIBR,** fiber; **FAT,** fat; **SATF,** saturated fat;

MONO, monosaturated fat; **POLY,** polyunsaturated fat; **CHOR,** cholesterol; **SOD,** sodium; **POT,** potassium;

Food Name	Portion	WT (Gm)	KCAL	PROT (Gm)	CARB (Gm)	FIBR (Gm)	FAT (Gm)	SATF (Gm)	MONO (Gm)	POLY (Gm)
ARBYS-SOUP-BOSTON CLAM CHOWDER	SERVING	227	207	10	18	1.4	11	4	5	2
ARBYS-SOUP-CREAM OF BROCCOLI	SERVING	227	180	9	19	1.8	8	5	2	1
ARBYS-SOUP-FRENCH ONION	SERVING	227	67	2	7	0.9	3	1	2	1
ARBYS-SOUP-LUMBERJACK MIXED VEGETABLE	SERVING	227	89	2	13	1.3	4	2	1	1
ARBYS-SOUP-OLD FASHIONED CHICKEN NOODLE	SERVING	227	99	6	15	0.7	2	1	1	1
ARBYS-SOUP-PILGRIM CLAM CHOWDER	SERVING	227	193	10	18	1.9	11	4	5	2
ARBYS-SOUP-ROAST BEEF AND VEGETABLE	SERVING	227	96	5	14	0.5	3	1	1	1
ARBYS-SOUP-SPLIT PEA AND HAM	SERVING	227	200	8	21	3.9	10	5	1	1
ARBYS-SOUP-TOMATO FLORENTINE	SERVING	227	84	3	15	0.5	2	1	1	1
ARBYS-SOUP-WISCONSIN CHEESE	SERVING	227	287	9	19	1.8	19	8	8	3
ARTHUR TREACHER-CHICKEN SANDWICH	ITEM	156	413	16	44	*	19	*	*	6.7
BEEF BURGER-FAST FOOD	OUNCE	28.3	72	5	7	t	3	*	*	*
BUN-HAMBURGER/HOTDOG-FAST FOOD	OUNCE	28.3	98	3	16	0	2	*	*	*
BURGER KING-BACON DOUBLE CHEESE-DELUXE	SERVING	195	592	33	28	1.1	39	16	14	6
BURGER KING-BARBECUE BACON DOUBLE CHEESE	ITEM	174	536	32	31	0.8	31	14	13	2
BURGER KING-BK BROILER	ITEM	168	379	24	31	1.8	18	3	8	3.8
BURGER KING-BK BROILER SAUCE	SERVING	14	90	0	0	0	10	1	2	5
BURGER KING-CHICKEN TENDERS	PIECE	90	39	3	2	0.3	2	0.5	0.8	0.5
BURGER KING-CROISSANT-EGG AND CHEESE	ITEM	127	369	13	24	2.1	25	14.1	7.5	1.4
BURGER KING-CROISSANT-EGG/CHEESE/HAM	ITEM	152	475	19	24	*	34	17.5	11.4	2.4
BURGER KING-DOUBLE CHEESEBURGER	ITEM	172	483	30	29	1.4	27	13	11	2
BURGER KING-FISH TENDERS	SERVING	99	267	12	18	1.1	16	3	7	4
BURGER KING-MUSHROOM SWISS DOUBLE CHEESE	ITEM	176	473	31	27	*	27	12	11	2
BURGER KING-RANCH DIP SAUCE	SERVING	28	171	0	2	*	18	3	4	10
BURGER KING-SWEET & SOUR SAUCE	SERVING	28	45	0	11	t	0	0	0	0
BURGER KING-TARTAR DIP SAUCE	SERVING	28	174	0	3	t	18	3	4	11
BURGER KING-TATER TENDERS	SERVING	71	213	2	25	*	12	3	6	3
BURGER KING-WHOPPER HAMBURGER	ITEM	261	630	26	50	2.5	36	16.5	13.8	2.2
CHEESE BURGER-FAST FOOD	OUNCE	28.3	78	6	7	0.1	3	1.7	1.7	0.2
CHICKEN-BREAST AND WING-BREADED-FRIED	SERVING	163	494	36	20	0.3	30	7.8	12.2	6.8
CHICKEN-BREAST-FAST FOOD	OUNCE	28.3	73	8	3	0	4	0.6	0.9	0.5
CHICKEN-DRUMSTICK & THIGH-BREADED-FRIED	SERVING	148	430	30	16	0.2	27	7.1	10.9	6.3
CHICKEN-DRUMSTICK-FAST FOOD	OUNCE	28.3	59	7	4	0	2	0.9	1.2	0.7
CHICKEN-FRIED-FAST FOOD-VARIOUS PORTIONS	OUNCE	28.3	82	5	6	0	5	1.1	1.7	1
CHICKEN-MEAT-SHAPED-FRIED-FAST FOOD	OUNCE	28.3	82	5	5	0	5	*	*	*
CHICKEN-SHOULDER-FAST FOOD	OUNCE	28.3	92	5	3	0	6	*	*	*
CHICKEN-THIGH-FAST FOOD	OUNCE	28.3	104	7	3	0	7	1.2	1.7	1
CHICKEN-WING-FAST FOOD	OUNCE	28.3	92	8	3	0	5	*	*	*
CHURCHS CHICKEN-WHITE MEAT	ITEM	100	327	21	10	*	23	*	*	*
COLESLAW-FAST FOOD	OUNCE	28.3	24	1	3	0	1	0.2	0.4	0.8
DAIRY QUEEN-BANANA SPLIT	ITEM	383	540	10	91	*	15	*	*	*
DAIRY QUEEN-DIP ICE CREAM CONE-REGULAR	ITEM	156	300	7	40	*	13	*	*	*
DAIRY QUEEN-FLOAT	ITEM	397	330	6	59	*	8	*	*	*
DAIRY QUEEN-ICE CREAM CONE-REGULAR	ITEM	142	226	5	33	*	8	4.9	2.5	0.5
DAIRY QUEEN-ICE CREAM SUNDAE-REGULAR	ITEM	177	319	6	53	2.2	10	5.6	2.6	0.9
DAIRY QUEEN-MALT-REGULAR	ITEM	418	600	15	89	*	20	*	*	*
DOUBLE CHEESE BURGER-FAST FOOD	OUNCE	28.3	66	4	7	0.1	3	2.2	1.9	0.2
FAST FOOD-PIZZA WITH CHEESE	OUNCE	28.4	63	3	9	0.6	1	0.7	0.4	0.2
FAST FOOD-PIZZA WITH PEPPERONI	OUNCE	28.4	72	4	8	0.6	3	0.9	1.3	0.5
FISH CAKE-FRIED-WITH BUN-FAST FOOD	OUNCE	28.3	85	3	8	0	5	0.4	0.8	0.5
FRANKFURTER-CONEY DOG-FAST FOOD	OUNCE	28.3	69	3	7	0	3	3.1	4	0.8
FRANKFURTER-HOT DOG-FAST FOOD	OUNCE	28.3	78	3	7	0	4	3.1	4	0.8
HAMBURGER-DOUBLE PATTY-EVERYTHING ON IT	OUNCE	28.4	68	4	5	0.3	3	1.3	1.3	0.4
HARDEE-BACON AND EGG BISCUIT	SERVING	124	410	15	35	0.6	24	5	14	5
HARDEE-BACON EGG AND CHEESE BISCUIT	SERVING	137	460	17	35	0.7	28	8	15	5
HARDEE-BIG COUNTRY BREAKFAST-COUNTRY HAM	SERVING	254	670	29	52	*	38	9	21	8
HARDEE-BIG COUNTRY BREAKFAST-SAUSAGE	SERVING	274	850	33	51	*	57	16	31	11
HARDEE-BIG COUNTRY BREAKFAST-WITH BACON	SERVING	217	660	24	51	0	40	10	22	8
HARDEE-BIG COUNTRY BREAKFAST-WITH HAM	SERVING	251	620	28	51	*	33	7	19	8
HARDEE-BIG ROAST BEEF SANDWICH	SERVING	134	300	18	32	0.9	11	5	5	2
HARDEE-BIG TWIN HAMBURGER	SERVING	173	450	23	34	1.7	25	11	9	5
HARDEE-BISCUIT N GRAVY	SERVING	221	440	9	45	*	24	6	14	5
HARDEE-CHICKEN N PASTA SALAD	SERVING	414	230	27	23	*	3	1	1	1

t = Trace of nutrient present   ** = Not available*

MAG, magnesium; **IRON**, iron; **ZINC**, zinc; **VITA**, vitamin A; **VITC**, vitamin C; **THIA**, thiamin; **RIBO**, riboflavin; **NIAC**, niacin; **VB6**, vitamin B-6; **FOL**, folate; **VB12**, vitamin B-12; **CALC**, calcium; **PHOS**, phosphorus; **SEL**, selenium; **VE-a**, alpha tocopherol equivalents.

CHOL (mg)	SOD (mg)	POT (mg)	MAG (mg)	IRON (mg)	ZINC (mg)	VITA (RE)	VITC (mg)	THIA (mg)	RIBO (mg)	NIAC (mg)	VB6 (mg)	FOL (μg)	VB12 (μg)	CALC (mg)	PHOS (mg)	SEL (μg)	VE-a (mg)
28	1157	319	20	1.4	0.7	100	4	0.06	0.22	0.9	0.12	9	9.38	170	143	*	0.1
3	1113	455	55	0.8	0.7	50	9	0.11	0.42	0.8	0.18	46	0.59	237	193	*	1.4
0	1248	106	2	0.6	0.6	10	2	0.03	0.02	0.6	0.05	14	0	25	11	*	0.3
4	1075	268	6	1.9	2.7	250	9	0.06	0.1	1.9	0.15	14	0.3	41	91	*	0.4
25	929	78	5	0.7	0.4	200	1	0.05	0.06	1.3	0.03	2	0.14	16	34	*	0.1
28	1157	379	19	2	1.1	350	4	0.06	0.16	1.3	0.15	9	9.67	134	126	*	0.2
10	996	211	5	1	1.4	300	5	0.03	0.05	1	0.07	10	0.3	16	39	*	0.3
30	1029	272	36	2	3	300	1	0.11	0.09	2.4	0.2	4	0.23	32	168	*	0.1
2	910	221	10	1.6	0.2	100	12	0.09	0.09	1.3	0.12	15	0.1	45	58	*	2.3
31	1129	441	7	1.3	1.1	90	2	0.03	0.24	0.7	0.05	7	0	252	241	*	0.4
*	708	279	27	1.7	*	37	19	0.17	0.24	8.1	*	*	*	59	147	*	*
*	55	46	*	0.3	*	8	t	0.02	0.04	0.8	*	*	*	3	25	*	*
*	22	31	*	0.2	*	0	t	0.07	0.02	0.4	*	*	*	9	13	*	*
111	804	463	38	4	6.4	71	8	0.3	0.39	8.1	0.37	31	3.24	156	373	*	1.5
105	795	429	36	4	6.5	49	4	0.29	0.39	8.3	0.35	27	3.34	158	379	*	0.6
53	764	324	29	3.2	3.2	44	6	0.27	0.26	5.2	0.24	38	1.52	74	153	*	2.6
7	95	*	*	*	*	*	*	*	*	*	*	*	*	*	*	*	*
8	90	249	22	1	0.7	25	0	0.14	0.12	6.2	0.32	9	0.3	9	234	*	0.3
216	551	174	22	2.2	1.8	300	t	0.19	0.38	1.5	0.1	36	0.78	244	349	*	0.7
213	1080	272	26	2.1	2.2	135	11	0.52	0.3	3.2	0.23	36	1.01	144	336	*	*
100	851	344	31	3	4	100	6	0.22	0.31	4.9	0.24	31	1.81	189	305	*	1.8
28	870	176	33	1.7	0.6	20	t	0.23	0.17	2.3	0.06	23	1.05	60	191	*	1.3
95	746	*	*	4.1	*	*	*	*	*	*	*	*	*	*	*	*	*
0	208	*	*	*	*	*	*	*	*	*	*	*	*	*	*	*	*
0	52	9	2	0.1	t	0	0	t	t	0.1	t	t	0	1	3	*	0
16	302	14	1	0.3	0.1	26	t	t	0.01	t	0.08	2	0.06	7	8	*	3.9
3	318	*	*	*	*	*	*	*	*	*	*	*	*	*	*	*	*
104	990	520	50	6	5.3	192	13	0.02	0.03	5.2	0.31	31	2.81	104	312	*	3.9
12	198	68	6	0.6	0.7	9	t	0.02	0.05	0.6	0.04	7	0.31	25	33	*	0.1
149	975	566	38	1.5	1.6	58	0	0.14	0.3	12	0.57	9	0.67	60	307	*	1
24	142	85	8	0.2	0.3	9	1	0.02	0.05	2	0.16	1	0.09	4	52	*	0.1
165	756	446	37	1.6	3.2	67	0	0.14	0.43	7.2	0.33	10	0.83	36	240	*	1.3
26	133	74	6	0.3	0.8	7	t	0.02	0.06	1.4	0.1	2	0.09	4	41	*	0.1
25	153	71	7	0.3	0.6	7	t	0.02	0.05	1.6	0.12	2	0.09	4	39	*	0.2
*	141	40	*	0.3	*	6	t	0.01	0.01	0.8	*	*	*	4	34	*	*
*	150	74	*	0.1	*	4	t	0.02	0.04	1.9	*	*	*	4	32	*	*
26	139	68	6	0.1	0.7	6	t	0.02	0.07	1.4	0.09	2	0.08	4	37	*	0.1
*	198	54	*	0.2	*	7	1	0.02	0.04	1.5	*	*	*	5	31	*	*
*	498	186	*	1	*	48	1	0.1	0.18	7.2	*	*	*	94	*	*	*
1	77	45	4	0.5	t	8	t	0.01	t	t	0.02	9	0.01	10	9	*	0.4
30	*	*	*	1.8	*	225	18	0.6	0.6	0.8	*	*	0.9	350	250	*	*
20	*	*	*	0.4	*	90	0	0.09	0.34	0	*	*	0.6	200	150	*	*
20	*	*	*	0	*	30	0	0.12	0.17	0	*	*	0.6	200	200	*	*
38	126	233	21	0.2	0.8	87	2	0.07	0.36	0.4	0.09	7	0.28	212	192	*	*
23	204	443	37	0.7	1.1	75	3	0.07	0.34	1.2	0.14	11	0.73	232	255	*	1.6
50	*	*	*	3.6	*	225	4	0.12	0.6	0.8	*	*	1.8	500	400	*	*
17	50	85	6	0.6	0.9	8	t	0.02	0.04	0.8	0.05	5	0.42	3	31	*	0.1
4	151	49	7	0.3	0.4	33	1	0.08	0.07	1.1	0.02	26	0.15	52	51	*	0.3
6	107	61	3	0.4	0.2	22	1	0.05	0.09	1.2	0.02	21	0.07	26	30	*	*
20	167	52	8	0.5	0.7	6	t	0.02	0.04	1.4	0.03	12	0.85	14	34	*	0.3
15	242	49	3	1	0.6	7	1	0.07	0.07	1.1	0.03	1	0.33	12	30	*	0.1
15	219	48	3	0.6	0.6	5	t	0.01	0.01	0.6	0.03	1	0.33	6	33	*	0.1
15	99	71	6	0.7	0.7	1	t	0.05	0.05	1	0.07	6	0.51	13	39	*	0.1
155	990	180	25	2.2	1.4	116	3	0.33	0.45	3	0.14	14	0.47	253	358	*	1.2
165	1220	200	27	2.4	1.5	129	3	0.37	0.49	3.3	0.15	15	0.52	279	396	*	1.3
345	2870	710	*	*	*	*	*	*	*	*	*	*	*	*	*	*	*
340	1980	670	*	*	*	*	*	*	*	*	*	*	*	*	*	*	*
305	1540	530	23	2.5	2.5	333	0	0.31	0.8	1.8	0.34	53	1.5	78	347	*	4.7
325	1780	620	*	*	*	*	*	*	*	*	*	*	*	*	*	*	*
45	880	320	33	3.7	6.1	0	0	0.3	0.34	5.4	0.28	24	2.45	66	230	*	0.2
55	580	280	35	4	4.6	17	3	0.28	0.31	6.7	0.27	34	2.27	80	197	*	0.9
15	1250	210	*	*	*	*	*	*	*	*	*	*	*	*	*	*	*
55	380	620	*	9	*	*	*	*	*	*	*	*	*	*	*	*	*

WT, weight; **KCAL**, kcalories; **PROT**, protein; **CARB**, carbohydrate; **FIBR**, fiber; **FAT**, fat; **SATF**, saturated fat;

MONO, monosaturated fat; **POLY**, polyunsaturated fat; **CHOR**, cholesterol; **SOD**, sodium; **POT**, potassium;

Food Name	Portion	WT (Gm)	KCAL	PROT (Gm)	CARB (Gm)	FIBR (Gm)	FAT (Gm)	SATF (Gm)	MONO (Gm)	POLY (Gm)
HARDEE-CRISPY CURLS	SERVING	85	300	4	36	*	16	3	8	5
HARDEE-GRILLED CHICKEN SANDWICH	SERVING	192	310	24	34	2.2	9	1	3	5
HARDEE-HAM & EGG BISCUIT	SERVING	138	370	15	35	1.1	19	4	12	4
HARDEE-HAM EGG & CHEESE BISCUIT	SERVING	151	420	18	35	0.8	23	6	13	4
HARDEE-MUSHROOM N SWISS HAMBURGER	SERVING	186	490	30	33	*	27	13	12	2
HARDEE-REGULAR ROAST BEEF SANDWICH	SERVING	114	260	15	31	0.8	9	4	4	2
HARDEE-THE LEAN ONE SANDWICH	ITEM	220	420	27	37	*	18	8	8	2
HARDEE-THREE PANCAKES	SERVING	137	280	8	56	1.4	2	1	1	1
JACK IN THE BOX-BREAKFAST JACK SANDWICH	ITEM	121	301	18	28	*	13	*	*	*
JACK IN THE BOX-JUMBO JACK CHEESEBURGER	ITEM	272	628	32	45	*	35	15	12.6	2
JACK IN THE BOX-JUMBO JACK HAMBURGER	ITEM	246	551	28	45	*	29	11.4	12.6	2.4
JACK IN THE BOX-MOBY JACK SANDWICH	ITEM	141	455	17	38	*	26	*	*	*
JACK IN THE BOX-ONION RINGS-BAG	ITEM	83	275	4	31	1.3	16	7	6.7	0.7
KFC-CHICKEN HOT WINGS	PIECE	119	63	4	3	0.1	4	0.8	10.3	0.7
KFC-CHICKEN SANDWICH	SERVING	166	482	21	39	1.4	27	6	3.9	9
KFC-CRISPY CHICKEN-BREAST	PIECE	135	342	33	12	0.1	20	5	4.7	2
KFC-CRISPY CHICKEN-DRUMSTICK	PIECE	69	204	14	6	t	14	3	3.7	2
KFC-CRISPY CHICKEN-THIGH	PIECE	119	406	20	14	0.1	30	8	7	4
KFC-CRISPY CHICKEN-WING	PIECE	65	254	12	9	0.1	19	4	5.7	3
LONG JOHN SILVER-BATTERED SHRIMP-9 PIECE	PIECE	357	95	3	10	1.8	5	1.1	3.2	0.6
LONG JOHN SILVER-BREADED SHRIMP	PIECE	420	51	1	6	2.1	2	0.5	1.6	0.3
LONG JOHN SILVER-CATFISH FILLET	SERVING	373	860	28	90	0.1	42	10	26	6
LONG JOHN SILVER-CHICKEN PLANK-4 PIECE	SERVING	415	940	39	94	*	44	10	29	5
LONG JOHN SILVER-CHICKEN-LIGHT HERB	SERVING	498	630	35	85	0	17	3	5	7
LONG JOHN SILVER-CLAM CHOWDER WITH COD	SERVING	198	140	11	10	1.7	6	2	3	2
LONG JOHN SILVER-CLAM DINNER	SERVING	363	980	21	122	0	45	10	30	6
LONG JOHN SILVER-COLE SLAW	SERVING	98	140	1	20	2.3	6	1	2	4
LONG JOHN SILVER-FISH & CHICKEN ENTREE	SERVING	398	870	35	91	*	40	9	26	5
LONG JOHN SILVER-FISH & MORE ENTREE	SERVING	381	800	31	88	1.7	37	8	23	5
LONG JOHN SILVER-FISH AND FRYES-3 PIECE	SERVING	358	810	42	77	*	38	9	27	2
LONG JOHN SILVER-FISH SANDWICH PLATTER	SERVING	379	870	26	108	4.1	38	8	22	7
LONG JOHN SILVER-FRIES	SERVING	85	220	3	30	2.9	10	3	7	1
LONG JOHN SILVER-GARDEN SALAD	SERVING	246	170	9	13	2.1	9	0.8	1	0.8
LONG JOHN SILVER-GUMBO-COD & SHRIMP BOBS	SERVING	198	120	9	4	3	8	2	3	3
LONG JOHN SILVER-HOMESTYLE FISH SANDWICH	SERVING	196	510	22	58	2.1	22	5	13	3
LONG JOHN SILVER-HOMESTYLE FISH-3 PIECE	SERVING	456	960	43	97	2	44	10	29	5
LONG JOHN SILVER-HOMESTYLE FISH-6 PIECE	SERVING	513	1260	49	124	2.3	64	14	43	6
LONG JOHN SILVER-HUSHPUPPIES	PIECE	24	70	2	10	*	2	1	1	1
LONG JOHN SILVER-LIGHT FISH-LEMON	SERVING	291	320	24	49	2.4	4	1	1	1
LONG JOHN SILVER-LIGHT FISH-PAPRIKA	SERVING	284	300	24	45	1.3	2	1	1	1
LONG JOHN SILVER-MIXED VEGETABLES	SERVING	113	60	2	9	5.9	2	1	1	1
LONG JOHN SILVER-OCEAN CHEF SALAD	SERVING	321	250	24	19	*	9	2	2	2
LONG JOHN SILVER-RICE PILAF	SERVING	142	210	5	43	0.8	2	1	1	1
LONG JOHN SILVER-SEAFOOD PLATTER	SERVING	400	970	30	109	5.3	46	10	30	6
LONG JOHN SILVER-SEAFOOD SALAD	SERVING	337	270	16	36	1.3	7	1	2	3
LONG JOHN SILVER-SEAFOOD SALAD-SCOOP	SERVING	142	210	14	26	0.6	5	1	2	3
LONG JOHN SILVER-SHRIMP & FISH DINNER	SERVING	348	770	25	85	7.3	37	8	23	5
LONG JOHN SILVER-SHRIMP FISH & CHICKEN	SERVING	380	840	31	89	*	40	9	26	5
LONG JOHN SILVER-SHRIMP SCAMPI	SERVING	529	610	25	87	0	18	3	6	7
MCDONALDS-APPLE BRAN MUFFIN	SERVING	85	190	5	46	4.5	0	0	0	0
MCDONALDS-APPLE DANISH	SLICE	115	390	6	51	1.6	18	3.5	10.8	2
MCDONALDS-APPLE PIE	SERVING	83	260	2	30	1.1	15	4.8	9.1	0.9
MCDONALDS-BACON AND EGG BISCUIT	SERVING	156	440	18	33	0.8	26	8.2	16.1	2
MCDONALDS-BACON BITS	SERVING	3	16	1	t		0	0	1.2	0
MCDONALDS-BARBEQUE (BARBECUE) SAUCE	SERVING	32	50	t	12	1.9	1	0.1	0.2	0.2
MCDONALDS-BIG MAC HAMBURGER	ITEM	215	560	25	43	*	32	10.1	20.1	1.5
MCDONALDS-BISCUIT WITH SPREAD	SERVING	75	260	5	32	1	13	3.4	8.6	0.6
MCDONALDS-CHEESEBURGER	ITEM	116	310	15	31	*	14	5.2	7.7	0.9
MCDONALDS-CHEF SALAD	SERVING	283	230	21	8	*	13	5.9	6.5	0.9
MCDONALDS-CHICKEN MCNUGGETS-6 PIECE	SERVING	113	290	19	17	*	16	4.1	10.4	1.8
MCDONALDS-CHOCOLATE MILKSHAKE-LOWFAT	SERVING	293	320	12	66	*	2	0.8	0.9	0.1
MCDONALDS-CHUNKY CHICKEN SALAD	SERVING	250	140	23	5	1	3	0.9	2	0.5
MCDONALDS-CINNAMON AND RAISIN DANISH	ITEM	110	440	6	58	*	21	4.2	13	1.6
MCDONALDS-COOKIE-CHOCOLATY	SERVING	56	330	4	42	1.1	16	5	10.2	0.4

*t = Trace of nutrient present   * = Not available*

MAG, magnesium; IRON, iron; ZINC, zinc; VITA, vitamin A; VITC, vitamin C; THIA, thiamin; RIBO, riboflavin; NIAC, niacin; VB6, vitamin B-6; FOL, folate; VB12, vitamin B-12; CALC, calcium; PHOS, phosphorus; SEL, selenium; VE-a, alpha tocopherol equivalents.

CHOL (mg)	SOD (mg)	POT (mg)	MAG (mg)	IRON (mg)	ZINC (mg)	VITA (RE)	VITC (mg)	THIA (mg)	RIBO (mg)	NIAC (mg)	VB6 (mg)	FOL (µg)	VB12 (µg)	CALC (mg)	PHOS (mg)	SEL (µg)	VE-a (mg)
0	840	370	*	*	*	*	*	*	*	*	*	*	*	*	*	*	*
60	890	410	44	3	2.7	413	t	0.43	0.59	4.2	0.1	31	0.47	542	611	*	3.4
160	1050	210	26	2.8	1.6	127	9	0.56	0.54	3.9	0.21	39	0.73	95	234	*	1.9
170	1270	230	30	2.7	1.7	142	4	0.4	0.54	3.7	0.17	17	0.57	308	436	*	1.5
70	940	370	*	*	*	*	*	*	*	*	*	*	*	*	*	*	*
35	730	260	28	3.1	5.2	0	0	0.26	0.29	4.6	0.24	20	2.09	56	196	*	0.2
85	760	510	*	*	*	*	*	*	*	*	*	*	*	*	*	*	*
15	890	240	25	1.9	0.9	63	1	0.22	0.39	1.4	0.1	14	0.42	341	411	*	1.6
182	1037	190	24	2.5	1.8	133	3	0.41	0.47	5.1	0.14	*	1.1	177	310	*	*
110	1666	499	49	4.6	4.8	220	5	0.52	0.38	11.3	0.31	*	3.05	273	411	*	*
80	1134	492	44	4.5	4.2	74	4	0.47	0.34	11.6	0.3	*	2.68	134	261	*	*
56	837	246	30	1.7	1.1	72	1	0.3	0.21	4.5	0.12	*	1.1	167	263	*	*
14	430	129	15	0.9	0.4	2	1	0.09	0.1	0.9	0.06	11	0.12	73	86	*	0.6
25	113	218	22	1.5	2.1	63	t	0.05	0.15	7.7	0.49	4	0.33	18	175	*	0.9
47	1060	297	41	3.1	1.5	14	0	0.4	0.35	13.4	0.59	29	0.31	100	261	*	2.3
114	790	347	40	1.6	1.5	20	0	0.11	0.17	18.4	0.77	5	0.46	21	312	*	0.6
71	324	157	16	0.9	2	17	0	0.06	0.16	4.1	0.24	6	0.22	8	120	*	0.5
129	688	280	29	1.8	3	35	0	0.11	0.29	8.2	0.4	10	0.36	16	221	*	0.6
67	422	115	12	0.8	1.1	25	0	0.04	0.09	4.3	0.27	2	0.18	10	97	*	0.6
14	163	94	132	10.3	4.2	242	5	0.3	0.5	9.9	0.36	34	3.4	214	764	*	14.1
6	85	41	156	12.1	5	285	6	0.35	0.58	11.6	0.43	39	3.99	252	899	*	16.6
65	990	1180	121	4.6	3.4	317	11	0.2	0.49	9.7	0.87	67	9.41	200	1017	*	5.7
70	1660	1320	*	*	*	*	*	*	*	*	*	*	*	*	*	*	*
85	2170	790	95	4.8	3.6	120	0	0.32	0.65	26.3	1.05	10	0.75	214	782	*	1.3
20	590	380	17	1.7	0.9	74	4	0.05	0.14	1.2	0.13	8	8.44	117	110	*	0.2
15	1200	870	41	56.7	6.2	365	47	0.34	0.91	7.2	0.26	54	201	209	572	*	4.5
15	260	190	13	0.5	0.1	225	30	0.04	0.03	0.3	0.13	37	0.03	36	23	*	4.4
70	1520	1290	*	*	*	*	*	*	*	*	*	*	*	*	*	*	*
70	1390	1260	131	3.3	2.1	71	5	0.39	0.5	12.3	0.72	46	5.17	133	769	*	7.7
85	1630	1340	*	*	*	*	*	*	*	*	*	*	*	*	*	*	*
55	1110	1050	94	6.4	2.3	65	2	0.87	0.65	11.1	0.42	89	2.29	238	488	*	5.7
5	60	390	29	0.6	0.3	0	9	0.15	0.02	2.8	0.2	25	0	16	79	*	0.2
5	380	20	40	1.7	1.1	239	26	0.14	0.15	11.4	0.56	66	0.27	42	217	*	0.9
25	740	310	41	2.3	0.8	300	21	0.12	0.08	2	0.17	47	0.24	100	105	*	1.7
45	780	470	48	18	1.2	33	1	0.45	0.34	5.7	0.22	46	1.19	123	252	*	2.9
100	1890	1540	157	3.9	2.6	85	6	0.47	0.59	14.7	0.87	56	6.19	159	920	*	9.3
130	1590	1660	177	4.4	2.9	96	7	0.53	0.67	16.6	0.98	62	6.97	179	1035	*	10.4
5	25	65	*	*	*	*	*	*	*	*	*	*	*	*	*	*	*
75	900	470	56	2.3	1.4	80	10	0.29	0.15	3.4	0.34	46	0.58	40	238	*	3.1
70	650	460	98	2.4	1.6	53	4	0.29	0.37	9.2	0.54	35	3.86	99	573	*	5.8
0	330	120	24	0.9	0.5	75	4	0.08	0.13	0.9	0.08	21	t	29	56	*	0.8
80	1340	160	*	*	*	*	*	*	*	*	*	*	*	*	*	*	*
0	570	140	17	1.8	0.6	60	1	0.15	0.02	1.5	0.08	5	0.01	17	45	*	0.8
70	1540	1100	114	4.1	2.2	59	13	0.42	0.37	8.2	0.88	37	1.68	109	484	*	4.3
90	670	100	86	3.2	5.2	129	20	0.13	0.16	3.7	0.27	47	2.89	148	444	*	7.4
90	570	100	36	1.4	2.2	250	8	0.05	0.07	1.6	0.11	20	1.22	63	187	*	3.1
80	1250	1030	82	3.5	1.6	28	17	0.37	0.21	6.6	0.64	35	1.06	54	422	*	4.4
80	1450	1170	*	*	*	*	*	*	*	*	*	*	*	*	*	*	*
220	2120	560	203	13.6	6.2	364	11	0.13	0.2	13.6	0.55	10	5.57	299	1156	*	12.9
0	230	202	55	0.6	1.2	1	1	0.02	0.08	0.4	0.37	77	0.78	31	178	*	0.4
26	370	69	8	1.4	0.2	35	16	0.28	0.2	2.2	0.03	3	0	14	31	*	3.8
0	240	50	6	0.7	0.2	0	11	0.06	0.02	0.3	0.02	2	0	11	22	*	2.7
253	1230	237	31	2.6	1.7	160	0	0.36	0.33	2.5	0.17	18	0.59	185	451	*	1.5
0	95	4	3	0	0.1	0	0	0	0	0	t	4	0.04	0	7	*	0.2
0	340	56	6	0.3	0.1	30	2	0.01	0.01	0.2	0.02	1	0	13	6	*	1.8
103	950	237	38	4	4.7	106	2	0.48	0.41	6.8	0.27	21	1.8	256	314	*	*
1	730	100	14	1.3	0.7	0	0	0.23	0.11	1.7	0.03	6	0.1	75	168	*	1.8
53	750	223	21	2.3	2.1	118	2	0.29	0.21	3.9	0.12	18	0.94	199	177	*	0.5
128	490	*	*	1.5	*	411	14	0.31	0.29	3.6	*	*	*	256	*	*	*
65	520	*	*	1	*	0	0	0.11	0.12	9	*	*	*	13	*	*	*
10	240	*	*	0.8	*	92	0	0.13	0.5	0.4	*	*	*	332	*	*	*
78	230	436	37	1	2.9	366	20	0.22	0.17	8.5	0.6	27	0.63	34	257	*	10.8
35	430	*	*	1.8	*	33	3	0.32	0.24	2.8	*	*	*	35	*	*	*
4	280	72	20	2.2	0.5	0	0	0.18	0.21	2.5	0.03	5	0.07	24	71	*	1.4

WT, weight; **KCAL**, kcalories; **PROT**, protein; **CARB**, carbohydrate; **FIBR**, fiber; **FAT**, fat; **SATF**, saturated fat;

MONO, monosaturated fat; **POLY**, polyunsaturated fat; **CHOR**, cholesterol; **SOD**, sodium; **POT**, potassium;

Food Name	Portion	WT (Gm)	KCAL	PROT (Gm)	CARB (Gm)	FIBR (Gm)	FAT (Gm)	SATF (Gm)	MONO (Gm)	POLY (Gm)
MCDONALDS-COOKIE-MCDONALDLAND	SERVING	56	290	4	47	0.6	9	1.9	6.8	0.5
MCDONALDS-CROUTONS	SERVING	11	50	1	7	0.5	2	0.5	1.3	0.1
MCDONALDS-EGG MCMUFFIN	ITEM	138	290	18	28	1.4	11	3.8	6.1	1.3
MCDONALDS-ENGLISH MUFFIN	SERVING	59	170	5	27	1.6	5	2.4	1.7	0.5
MCDONALDS-FILET O FISH	ITEM	142	440	14	38	1.1	26	5.2	10.2	10.8
MCDONALDS-FRENCH FRIES-LARGE	SERVING	122	400	6	46	4.2	22	9.1	11.6	0.9
MCDONALDS-FRENCH FRIES-MEDIUM	SERVING	97	320	4	36	3.4	17	7.2	9.2	0.7
MCDONALDS-FRENCH FRIES-REGULAR ORDER	SERVING	68	220	3	26	*	12	5.1	6.5	0.5
MCDONALDS-GARDEN SALAD	SERVING	213	110	7	6	1.8	7	2.9	3.2	0.5
MCDONALDS-HAMBURGER	ITEM	102	260	12	31	*	10	3.6	5.1	0.8
MCDONALDS-HASHBROWN POTATO	SERVING	55	130	1	15	1.1	7	3.2	3.7	0.4
MCDONALDS-HONEY SAUCE	SERVING	14	45	0	12	*	0	0	0	0
MCDONALDS-HOT CAKES WITH SYRUP	SERVING	176	410	8	74	*	9	3.7	3.1	2.5
MCDONALDS-HOT CARAMEL SUNDAE	SERVING	174	270	7	59	1	3	1.5	1.2	0.1
MCDONALDS-HOT FUDGE SUNDAE	SERVING	169	240	7	51	1.3	3	2.4	0.8	0.1
MCDONALDS-HOT MUSTARD SAUCE	SERVING	30	70	1	8	0.3	4	0.5	1.2	1.9
MCDONALDS-ICED CHEESE DANISH	SERVING	110	390	7	42	*	22	6	12.1	1.8
MCDONALDS-McCHICKEN SANDWICH	SERVING	190	490	19	40	1.6	29	5.4	11.5	11.6
MCDONALDS-McDLT HAMBURGER	ITEM	234	580	26	36	*	37	11.5	16.7	8.5
MCDONALDS-MCLEAN DELUXE HAMBURGER	SERVING	206	320	22	35	2.4	10	4	5	1
MCDONALDS-MILKSHAKE-CHOCOLATE-LOWFAT	SERVING	293	320	12	66	*	2	1	1	0
MCDONALDS-MILKSHAKE-STRAWBERRY-LOWFAT	SERVING	293	320	11	67	*	1	1	1	0
MCDONALDS-MILKSHAKE-VANILLA-LOWFAT	SERVING	293	290	11	60	0	1	1	1	0
MCDONALDS-PORK SAUSAGE	SERVING	48	180	8	0	0	16	5.9	8.5	1.9
MCDONALDS-QUARTER POUND CHEESEBURGER	ITEM	194	520	29	35	*	29	11.2	16.5	1.5
MCDONALDS-QUARTER POUNDER HAMBURGER	ITEM	166	410	23	34	*	21	8.1	11.4	1.2
MCDONALDS-RASPBERRY DANISH	ITEM	117	410	6	62	*	16	3.1	10.2	1.1
MCDONALDS-SALAD DRESSING-PEPPERCORN	OUNCE	28.4	160	0	2	0	18	2	4	10
MCDONALDS-SALAD DRESSING-RED FRENCH	OUNCE	28.4	80	0	10	0	4	0	2	2
MCDONALDS-SAUSAGE AND EGG BISCUIT	ITEM	180	520	20	33	*	35	11.2	20	2.5
MCDONALDS-SAUSAGE BISCUIT	ITEM	123	440	13	32	1.4	29	9.3	17.2	2.5
MCDONALDS-SAUSAGE MCMUFFIN	ITEM	117	370	17	27	1.1	22	7.8	11.7	2.4
MCDONALDS-SAUSAGE MCMUFFIN WITH EGG	ITEM	167	440	23	28	1.6	27	9.5	14.2	3.2
MCDONALDS-SCRAMBLED EGGS	SERVING	98	140	12	1	0	10	3.3	5	1.4
MCDONALDS-SIDE SALAD	SERVING	115	60	4	3	1.2	3	1.5	1.6	0.3
MCDONALDS-STRAWBERRY MILKSHAKE-LOWFAT	SERVING	293	320	11	67	*	1	0.6	0.6	0.1
MCDONALDS-STRAWBERRY SUNDAE	SERVING	171	210	6	49	0.7	1	0.6	0.4	t
MCDONALDS-SWEET AND SOUR SAUCE	SERVING	32	60	t	14	t	t	t	0.1	0.1
MCDONALDS-VANILLA MILKSHAKE-LOWFAT	SERVING	293	290	11	60	*	1	0.6	0.7	0.1
MCDONALDS-VANILLA-FROZEN YOGURT	SERVING	80	100	4	22	*	1	0.4	0.3	0.1
PIZZA-BEEF/CHICKEN/ONION	OUNCE	28.3	73	6	7	t	2	*	*	*
PIZZA-BEEF/ONION	OUNCE	28.3	73	4	8	0.1	3	*	*	*
PIZZA-CHICKEN CURRY/PEAS	OUNCE	28.3	82	4	9	0.2	3	*	*	*
PIZZA-CHICKEN/MUSHROOM/TOMATO	OUNCE	28.3	61	5	7	0.1	1	*	*	*
PIZZA-CHICKEN/PINEAPPLE	OUNCE	28.3	81	4	6	0.1	4	*	*	*
PIZZA-COMBINATION SUPREME	OUNCE	28.3	51	4	7	0.2	1	1.3	1.5	0.4
PIZZA-CURRY BEEF/PEAS	OUNCE	28.3	71	5	7	0.2	3	0.9	1.6	1
PIZZA-ONION/TOMATO/GREEN PEPPER/MUSHROOM	OUNCE	28.3	45	3	7	0.2	1	*	*	*
PIZZA-PEPPERONI/BEEF/SALAMI/MUSHROOM/ETC	OUNCE	28.3	83	5	5	0.1	5	*	*	*
PIZZA-SHRIMP/CUCUMBER	OUNCE	28.3	69	4	7	0.1	3	*	*	*
PIZZA-SHRIMP/SQUID/MUSHROOM	OUNCE	28.3	70	5	7	0.1	2	*	*	*
POTATOES-FRENCH FRIED-FAST FOOD	OUNCE	28.3	91	1	10	0	5	1.8	1.9	0.8
POTATOES-MASHED-FAST FOOD	OUNCE	28.3	26	1	5	0	t	0.3	0.5	0.3
RAX-GRILLED CHICKEN SANDWICH	ITEM	190	440	24	36	1.6	19	2.9	4.5	5.4
SALAD-FAST FOOD	OUNCE	28.3	34	t	3	0	2	*	*	*
SPAGHETTI-VEGETABLES/SAUCE/CHEESE	OUNCE	28.3	28	4	3	0.3	t	*	*	*
SUBWAY SANDWICH-HAM AND CHEESE-ON WHEAT	ITEM	194	673	39	86	6	22	7	8	4
SUBWAY-BMT SANDWICH-ON HONEY WHEAT ROLL	ITEM	220	1011	45	88	6	57	20	25	7
SUBWAY-BMT SANDWICH-ON ITALIAN ROLL	ITEM	213	982	44	83	5	55	20	24	7
SUBWAY-CLUB SANDWICH-ON HONEY WHEAT	ITEM	220	722	47	89	6	23	7	9	4
SUBWAY-CLUB SANDWICH-ON ITALIAN ROLL	ITEM	213	693	46	83	5	22	7	8	4
SUBWAY-COLD CUT COMBO SANDWICH-ITALIAN	ITEM	184	853	46	83	5	40	12	15	10
SUBWAY-COLD CUT COMBO SANDWICH-ON WHEAT	ITEM	191	883	48	88	6	41	12	15	10

t = Trace of nutrient present   * = Not available

MAG, magnesium; IRON, iron; ZINC, zinc; VITA, vitamin A; VITC, vitamin C; THIA, thiamin; RIBO, riboflavin; NIAC, niacin; VB6, vitamin B-6; FOL, folate; VB12, vitamin B-12; CALC, calcium; PHOS, phosphorus; SEL, selenium; VE-a, alpha tocopherol equivalents.

CHOL (mg)	SOD (mg)	POT (mg)	MAG (mg)	IRON (mg)	ZINC (mg)	VITA (RE)	VITC (mg)	THIA (mg)	RIBO (mg)	NIAC (mg)	VB6 (mg)	FOL (µg)	VB12 (µg)	CALC (mg)	PHOS (mg)	SEL (µg)	VE-a (mg)
0	300	38	13	2.1	0.3	0	0	0.25	0.18	2.5	0.03	4	0.07	9	91	*	1.4
0	140	20	5	0.4	0.1	0	t	0.05	0.03	0.4	0.01	3	0	6	15	*	0.1
226	740	213	33	2.8	1.8	150	1	0.47	0.33	3.7	0.16	44	0.8	256	319	*	1.8
9	270	74	12	1.6	0.4	37	0	0.33	0.14	2.5	0.1	51	t	151	60	*	0.1
50	1030	150	27	1.8	0.9	44	t	0.3	0.15	2.7	0.1	20	0.82	165	229	*	*
16	200	866	40	0.9	0.6	0	15	0.24	0	3.3	0.32	40	0.15	18	162	*	0.3
12	150	692	32	0.7	0.5	0	12	0.19	0	2.6	0.25	32	0.12	14	129	*	0.2
9	110	484	22	0.5	0.4	0	8	0.14	0	1.8	0.18	22	0.08	10	90	*	*
83	160	450	35	1.3	1	391	14	0.1	0.16	0.6	0.49	57	0.23	149	188	*	0.8
37	500	215	23	2.3	2.1	46	2	0.28	0.16	3.8	0.12	17	0.84	122	110	*	0.4
9	330	238	9	0.3	0.2	0	2	0.06	0.02	0.9	0.07	4	0	6	39	*	0.1
0	0	*	*	0.1	*	0	t	0	0.01	t	*	*	*	*	*	*	*
21	640	187	25	2.1	0.6	52	5	0.32	0.33	2.8	0.12	9	0.19	114	501	*	*
13	180	414	51	0.1	1.1	87	0	0.08	0.35	0.3	0.38	19	0.66	222	198	*	1.2
6	170	274	32	0.5	1.3	64	0	0.08	0.35	0.3	0.07	7	0.6	235	178	*	1.1
5	250	26	5	0.2	0.1	2	t	0.01	0.01	0.2	0.01	1	0	15	7	*	1.2
47	420	*	*	1.4	*	38	1	0.29	0.23	2.1	*	*	*	33	*	*	*
43	780	340	47	2.6	1.7	31	2	0.96	0.21	8.9	0.67	33	0.35	143	299	*	2.7
109	990	*	*	3.9	*	226	7	0.39	0.36	6.9	*	*	*	225	*	*	*
60	670	290	35	3.8	3.2	67	10	0.35	0.31	5.8	0.26	48	1.48	93	170	*	2.7
10	240	*	*	*	*	*	*	*	*	*	*	*	*	332	*	*	*
10	170	*	*	*	*	*	*	*	*	*	*	*	*	327	*	*	*
10	170	643	48	0.2	2.4	38	2	0.12	0.59	0.3	0.13	31	1.54	327	394	*	0.1
48	350	*	*	0.7	*	0	0	0.27	0.1	2.3	*	*	*	8	*	*	*
118	1150	341	41	3.7	5.7	211	3	0.37	0.39	6.7	0.23	23	2.15	295	382	*	*
86	660	322	37	3.7	5.1	67	3	0.36	0.29	6.7	0.27	23	1.88	142	249	*	*
26	310	*	*	1.5	*	35	3	0.33	0.21	2.1	*	*	*	14	*	*	*
14	170	22	0	0.1	t	6	0	t	0.01	t	t	1	0.04	3	4	*	2.4
0	220	22	0	0.1	t	6	0	t	0.01	t	t	1	0.04	3	4	*	2.4
275	1250	319	25	3.2	2.2	88	t	0.53	0.35	4	0.2	40	1.37	116	490	*	*
49	1080	196	20	2	1.5	0	0	0.49	0.21	4	0.11	9	0.5	83	443	*	3.1
64	830	179	20	2.3	1.7	72	1	0.6	0.29	4.8	0.13	48	0.5	235	273	*	1.6
263	980	255	29	3.3	2.4	150	0	0.64	0.42	4.8	0.19	68	0.72	263	390	*	2.3
399	290	102	10	2.1	1.1	156	1	0.07	0.26	0.1	0.08	27	1.68	57	136	*	2.9
41	85	219	12	0.7	0.3	217	7	0.05	0.08	0.3	0.06	40	0	76	26	*	0.4
10	170	*	*	0.1	*	92	0	0.13	0.48	0.3	*	*	*	327	*	*	*
5	95	263	19	0.2	1.2	64	1	0.07	0.29	0.3	0.07	9	0.54	190	127	*	0.6
0	190	10	2	0.2	t	65	1	0	0.01	0.1	t	t	0	11	3	*	0
10	170	*	*	0.1	*	92	0	0.13	0.48	0.3	*	*	*	327	*	*	*
3	80	*	*	0.2	*	38	0	0.04	0.18	0.4	*	*	*	112	*	*	*
*	267	49	*	0.7	*	23	1	0.03	0.02	1.3	*	*	*	73	53	*	*
*	132	50	*	0.2	*	23	t	0.01	0.02	0.9	*	*	*	21	36	*	*
*	146	45	*	0.2	*	30	t	0.02	0.03	1.7	*	*	*	19	37	*	*
*	167	44	*	0.2	*	23	t	0.01	0.01	0.8	*	*	*	24	37	*	*
*	267	37	*	0.4	*	25	1	0.03	0.03	2.1	*	*	*	86	114	*	*
6	165	45	6	0.2	0.3	10	1	0.02	0.02	1.8	0.04	7	0.08	27	39	*	0.3
8	130	47	7	0.2	0.7	29	1	0.02	0.02	3.6	0.06	2	0.37	24	38	*	0.7
*	136	43	*	0.2	*	9	t	0.01	0.02	1.6	*	*	*	25	33	*	*
*	367	61	*	0.2	*	22	t	0.02	t	3.1	*	*	*	76	59	*	*
*	143	46	*	0.2	*	12	t	0.01	0.01	2.3	*	*	*	25	48	*	*
*	160	33	*	0.2	*	13	t	0.01	0.01	0.9	*	*	*	22	38	*	*
3	17	130	10	0.6	0.1	6	t	0.02	0.01	0.4	0.07	8	0	2	20	*	0.1
1	82	48	5	0.8	0.1	15	t	0.02	0.01	0.2	0.06	2	0.02	3	14	*	0.2
88	1050	340	47	3.6	1.7	16	0	0.46	0.4	15.3	0.67	33	0.35	114	299	*	2.7
*	128	40	*	0.7	*	4	1	0.02	0.01	t	*	*	*	5	14	*	*
*	84	52	*	0.3	*	4	t	0.01	0.01	0.2	*	*	*	4	10	*	*
73	2508	918	*	*	*	*	*	*	*	*	*	*	*	*	*	*	*
133	3199	1002	*	*	*	*	*	*	*	*	*	*	*	*	*	*	*
133	3139	917	66	4.3	6.1	67	5	0.27	0.34	5.1	0.48	63	2.33	64	308	*	5.1
84	2777	1055	40	3.2	1.4	83	15	0.49	0.35	9.3	0.46	43	0.44	96	247	*	4.2
84	2717	971	66	3.1	2.5	74	20	0.48	0.33	12.5	0.58	47	0.95	58	384	*	1.3
166	2218	876	28	2.9	2.7	87	17	0.36	0.33	3.8	0.2	39	1.23	227	315	*	0.9
166	2278	1010	29	3	2.8	90	18	0.37	0.35	3.9	0.21	41	1.28	235	327	*	0.9

WT, weight; **KCAL**, kcalories; **PROT**, protein; **CARB**, carbohydrate; **FIBR**, fiber; **FAT**, fat; **SATF**, saturated fat;

MONO, monosaturated fat; **POLY**, polyunsaturated fat; **CHOR**, cholesterol; **SOD**, sodium; **POT**, potassium;

Food Name	Portion	WT (Gm)	KCAL	PROT (Gm)	CARB (Gm)	FIBR (Gm)	FAT (Gm)	SATF (Gm)	MONO (Gm)	POLY (Gm)
SUBWAY-HAM & CHEESE SANDWICH-ON ITALIAN	ITEM	184	643	38	81	5	18	7	8	4
SUBWAY-MEATBALL SANDWICH-ON ITALIAN ROLL	ITEM	215	918	42	96	3	44	17	17	4
SUBWAY-MEATBALL-ON HONEY WHEAT ROLL	ITEM	224	947	44	101	*	45	17	18	4
SUBWAY-ROAST BEEF SANDWICH-ITALIAN ROLL	ITEM	184	689	42	84	5	23	8	9	4
SUBWAY-ROAST BEEF SANDWICH-ON WHEAT ROLL	ITEM	189	717	41	89	6	24	8	9	4
SUBWAY-SALAD DRESSING-BUTTERMILK RANCH	SERVING	56.7	348	1	2	0	37	5	7	24
SUBWAY-SALAD DRESSING-LITE ITALIAN	SERVING	56.7	23	1	4	0	1	4	6.4	15.9
SUBWAY-SEAFOOD/CRAB SANDWICH-ON ITALIAN	ITEM	210	986	29	94	*	57	11	15	28
SUBWAY-SEAFOOD/CRAB SANDWICH-ON WHEAT	ITEM	219	1015	31	100	2.5	58	11	16	28
SUBWAY-SPICY ITALIAN SANDWICH-ON ITALIAN	ITEM	213	1043	42	83	5	63	23	28	7
SUBWAY-STEAK & CHEESE SANDWICH-ITALIAN	ITEM	213	765	43	83	6	32	12	12	4
SUBWAY-TURKEY BREAST SANDWICH-WHEAT ROLL	ITEM	192	674	42	88	7	20	6	7	7
TACO BELL-BEAN BURRITO	ITEM	168	332	17	43	6.4	12	5.6	4.2	0.6
TACO BELL-BEEF BURRITO	ITEM	110	262	13	29	1.3	10	5.2	3.7	0.4
TACO BELL-BEEFY TOSTADA	ITEM	225	334	16	30	5.2	17	11.5	3.5	0.5
TACO BELL-BURRITO SUPREME	ITEM	225	457	21	43	5	22	7.7	7.4	1.7
TACO BELL-DOUBLE BEEF BURRITO SUPREME	ITEM	255	457	24	42	5.7	22	10.1	15.4	2.1
TACO BELL-ENCHIRITO	ITEM	213	382	20	31	*	20	9.3	*	1.5
TACO BELL-MEXICAN PIZZA	SERVING	223	575	21	40	5.8	37	11.4	8.2	9.7
TACO BELL-NACHOS	SERVING	106	346	7	38	1.4	19	5.7	10	1.6
TACO BELL-NACHOS BELLGRANDE	SERVING	287	649	22	61	*	35	12.3	*	2.6
TACO BELL-PINTOS & CHEESE	SERVING	128	190	9	19	4.9	9	3.6	4.9	0.8
TACO BELL-SOFT TACO	ITEM	92.1	228	12	18	2.6	12	5.4	3.7	1.2
TACO BELL-TACO BELLGRANDE	ITEM	163	355	18	18	4.5	23	10.9	6.6	1.3
TACO BELL-TACO LIGHT	ITEM	170	410	19	18	*	29	11.6	*	5.4
TACO BELL-TACO SALAD WITH SALSA/NO SHELL	SERVING	530	520	31	30	7	31	14.4	19.2	1.7
TACO BELL-TACO SALAD WITH SALSA/SHELL	SERVING	595	941	36	63	7.9	61	18.7	21.6	12.1
TACO BELL-TACO SALAD-NO SALSA-NO SHELL	SERVING	530	502	30	26	7	31	14.4	19.2	1.7
TACO BELL-TACO-REGULAR	ITEM	171	370	21	27	1.2	21	11.4	6.6	1
TACO BELL-TOSTADA-REGULAR	ITEM	144	223	10	27	4	10	5.4	3.1	0.7
WENDYS-BACON AND CHEESE POTATO	SERVING	347	450	15	57	9.9	18	37.1	38.2	14.1
WENDYS-BIG CLASSIC-QUARTER POUND BURGER	SERVING	277	570	27	46	2.3	33	15.9	14.8	4.3
WENDYS-BROCCOLI AND CHEESE POTATO	SERVING	377	400	9	59	*	16	*	*	*
WENDYS-CHEESE POTATO	SERVING	348	470	13	57	3.6	21	12.1	9.3	4
WENDYS-CHEESE SAUCE	SERVING	56	40	1	5	0.2	2	1.9	1.1	0.3
WENDYS-CHEESE TORTELLINI/SPAGHETTI SAUCE	SERVING	112	120	4	24	1	1	2.8	2.2	0.9
WENDYS-CHICKEN CLUB SANDWICH	SERVING	231	500	30	42	2.3	24	5.5	8.5	8
WENDYS-CHICKEN SALAD	SERVING	56	120	7	4	0.2	8	3	2.8	3
WENDYS-CHILI	SERVING	255	220	21	23	6	7	3	5.7	1.1
WENDYS-DOUBLE HAMBURGER	ITEM	226	540	34	40	2.3	27	10.5	10.3	2.8
WENDYS-FRENCH FRIES-REGULAR SIZE	SERVING	134	440	5	53	4.6	23	8.5	9.1	3.6
WENDYS-KIDS MEAL HAMBURGER	SERVING	104	260	14	30	1.3	9	3.5	4.8	0.8
WENDYS-REFRIED BEANS	SERVING	56	70	4	10	3	3	1	2.2	1
WENDYS-SEAFOOD SALAD	SERVING	56	110	4	7	0.2	7	1	4.5	4
WENDYS-SINGLE CHEESEBURGER/EVERYTHING	SERVING	252	490	29	35	2.7	27	10.8	11.2	4.6
WENDYS-SINGLE HAMBURGER	ITEM	218	511	26	40	2.8	27	10.4	11.4	2.2
WENDYS-SINGLE HAMBURGER/EVERYTHING	SERVING	234	420	25	35	2.7	21	6.7	9.4	4.4
WENDYS-SPANISH RICE	SERVING	56	70	2	13	0.7	1	0.1	0.3	1
WENDYS-TACO SALAD WITH TACO CHIPS	SERVING	791	660	40	46	10.5	37	28.8	28.7	15.4
WENDYS-TRIPLE HAMBURGER	ITEM	259	693	50	29	*	42	15.9	18.2	2.7
WENDYS-TUNA SALAD	SERVING	56	100	8	4	0.3	6	1	0.8	3

Fats & Oils

Food Name	Portion	WT (Gm)	KCAL	PROT (Gm)	CARB (Gm)	FIBR (Gm)	FAT (Gm)	SATF (Gm)	MONO (Gm)	POLY (Gm)
BUTTER-REGULAR-PAT	ITEM	5	36	t	t	0	4	2.5	1.2	0.2
BUTTER-REGULAR-STICK	ITEM	113	813	1	t	0	92	57.3	26.6	3.4
BUTTER-REGULAR-TABLESPOON	TBSP	14	100	t	t	0	11	7.1	3.3	0.4
BUTTER-UNSALTED-PAT	ITEM	5	36	t	t	0.1	4	2.5	1.2	0.2
FAT-ANIMAL-CHICKEN-FOR COOKING	TBSP	12.8	115	0	0	0	13	3.8	5.7	2.7
FAT-ANIMAL-LARD (PORK)	CUP	205	1849	0	0	0	205	80.4	92.5	23
MARGARINE-DIET/LOW CALORIE-MAZOLA	TBSP	14	50	0	0	0	6	1	2.1	2.6
MARGARINE-IMITATION-40% FAT	TSP	4.8	17	0	0	0	2	0.4	0.8	0.7
MARGARINE-IMITATION-SPREAD-60% FAT	TSP	4.8	26	0	0	0	3	0.6	1.5	0.7
MARGARINE-NO STICK-SPRAY-MAZOLA	SERVING	0.72	6	0	0	0	1	0.1	0.2	0.4

t = Trace of nutrient present   * = Not available

MAG, magnesium; **IRON,** iron; **ZINC,** zinc; **VITA,** vitamin A; **VITC,** vitamin C; **THIA,** thiamin; **RIBO,** riboflavin; **NIAC,** niacin; **VB6,** vitamin B-6; **FOL,** folate; **VB12,** vitamin B-12; **CALC,** calcium; **PHOS,** phosphorus; **SEL,** selenium; **VE-a,** alpha tocopherol equivalents.

CHOL (mg)	SOD (mg)	POT (mg)	MAG (mg)	IRON (mg)	ZINC (mg)	VITA (RE)	VITC (mg)	THIA (mg)	RIBO (mg)	NIAC (mg)	VB6 (mg)	FOL (µg)	VB12 (µg)	CALC (mg)	PHOS (mg)	SEL (µg)	VE-a (mg)
73	1710	834	50	2.2	2.8	174	17	0.53	0.39	3.6	0.34	45	0.76	304	527	*	3.8
88	2022	1210	47	5	6.2	72	19	0.33	0.39	9.4	0.4	35	3.21	78	263	*	1
88	2082	1498	*	*	*	*	*	*	*	*	*	*	*	*	*	*	*
83	2288	910	57	3.7	5.3	58	5	0.23	0.29	4.4	0.42	54	2.01	55	266	*	4.4
75	2348	994	59	3.8	5.4	59	5	0.24	0.3	4.5	0.43	56	2.07	56	273	*	4.5
6	492	17	1	0.1	0.1	48	0	0.01	0.01	t	0.01	4	0.12	8	15	*	2.3
0	952	13	t	0.1	0.1	14	0	0.01	0.01	t	0.01	3	0.09	6	3	*	4.9
56	2027	641	62	4.4	5.3	107	5	0.51	0.38	7	0.26	91	6.54	230	336	*	2.5
56	1967	557	*	*	*	*	*	*	*	*	*	*	*	*	*	*	*
137	2282	880	*	*	*	*	*	*	*	*	*	*	*	*	*	*	*
82	1556	909	43	4.2	6.8	119	6	0.33	0.46	5.1	0.38	36	2.54	231	456	*	0.8
67	2520	605	*	*	*	*	*	*	*	*	*	*	*	*	*	*	*
79	1030	405	t	3.8	3	240	3	0.28	0.6	3.9	0.21	73	1	144	143	*	1.9
33	746	370	41	3.1	2.4	42	1	0.12	0.46	3.2	0.16	20	0.99	42	88	*	0.9
75	870	490	68	2.5	3.2	383	4	0.09	0.5	2.9	0.26	t	1.13	190	173	*	2
126	367	350	52	3.8	5.9	216	8	0.45	0.92	6.2	0.27	43	1.53	146	245	*	2.1
57	1053	431	87	4	5.9	286	9	0.43	2.19	3.7	0.35	132	2.18	145	548	*	2.3
54	1243	*	*	2.8	*	290	28	0.26	0.42	2.3	*	*	*	269	*	*	*
52	1031	408	63	3.7	2.3	295	31	0.32	0.33	3	0.27	113	0.2	257	360	*	2.5
9	399	159	43	0.9	2.6	169	2	0.01	0.16	0.7	0.12	16	0.62	191	439	*	2.8
36	997	674	*	3.5	*	341	58	0.1	0.34	2.2	*	*	*	297	*	*	*
16	642	399	50	1.4	1.1	132	51	0.05	0.15	0.4	0.19	98	0.08	156	175	*	1.4
32	516	178	31	2.3	1.4	64	1	0.39	0.22	2.7	0.16	40	0.31	116	132	*	0.9
56	472	334	54	1.9	2.4	254	5	0.11	0.29	2	0.28	71	0.55	182	234	*	1.6
56	594	316	*	2.4	*	199	5	0.2	0.33	2.5	*	*	*	155	*	*	*
80	1431	1151	111	5.1	9.1	908	76	0.26	0.64	3.2	0.78	99	4.29	367	567	*	6
80	1662	1212	125	7.1	10.3	888	77	0.51	0.75	4.8	0.88	111	4.82	398	637	*	6.8
80	1056	988	111	4.5	9.1	572	74	0.25	0.5	3.2	0.78	99	4.29	331	567	*	6
57	802	473	71	2.4	3.9	257	2	0.15	0.45	3.2	0.24	23	1.04	221	203	*	0.8
30	543	403	59	1.9	1.9	187	1	0.1	0.33	1.3	0.17	75	0.68	211	116	*	1.4
10	1125	1580	167	15.3	7	266	77	1.04	0.81	14.5	1.94	75	2.26	713	1015	*	4.9
85	1075	590	49	4.8	6.4	162	9	0.35	0.5	8	0.38	51	2.92	304	491	*	2.9
0	470	1555	*	*	*	*	*	*	*	*	*	*	*	*	*	*	*
0	580	1435	72	2.3	2.4	288	34	0.22	0.43	3.5	0.57	31	0.3	417	398	*	2.3
0	300	70	10	0.1	0.2	24	t	0.03	0.11	0.1	0.03	3	0.22	114	88	*	0.1
5	280	110	14	1.3	0.6	110	4	0.12	0.18	1.2	0.09	12	0.17	75	92	*	0.9
75	950	515	42	14.4	1.5	87	16	0.51	0.37	16	0.48	45	0.46	101	259	*	4.4
0	215	60	8	0.5	0.7	22	1	0.02	0.08	1.8	0.13	6	0.14	13	58	*	2.4
45	750	495	53	6.3	4.1	146	19	0.16	0.26	4.8	0.23	41	1.46	55	228	*	1.8
122	791	569	49	6	5.7	31	1	0.36	0.39	7.6	0.54	27	4.07	102	314	*	1.1
25	265	855	46	1	0.5	0	14	0.24	0.04	4.4	0.32	39	0	26	125	*	0.3
35	545	205	22	2.5	2.2	7	1	0.23	0.2	3.8	0.14	25	1	63	110	*	0.5
0	215	210	25	1.2	0.5	0	2	0.08	0.04	0.2	0.09	71	0	25	72	*	0.5
0	455	40	14	0.5	0.9	21	3	0.02	0.03	0.6	0.05	8	0.48	25	74	*	1.2
90	1155	495	44	4.3	4.3	136	11	0.4	0.42	6.5	0.3	55	1.8	234	348	*	3.2
86	825	479	43	4.9	4.9	93	3	0.42	0.38	7.3	0.33	36	2.38	96	233	*	1.1
70	865	495	40	4.3	3.7	76	11	0.4	0.35	6.6	0.29	54	1.68	105	193	*	3
0	440	130	9	0.7	0.2	24	9	0.05	0.02	0.6	0.06	4	0	15	17	*	0.3
35	1110	1330	166	9.2	13.6	1478	67	0.4	0.93	15.2	1.16	147	6.41	532	847	*	9
142	713	785	55	8.3	10.8	47	1	0.31	0.56	11	0.62	31	4.92	65	393	*	*
0	290	90	10	0.6	0.2	15	1	0.02	0.04	3.8	0.05	4	0.68	9	62	*	0.5
11	41	1	t	t	t	8	0	0	t	t	0	t	0.01	1	1	0	0.1
248	937	29	2	0.2	0.1	855	0	0.01	0.04	t	t	3	0.14	27	26	3	1.8
31	116	4	t	t	t	105	0	t	0.01	t	0	t	0.02	3	3	0	0.2
11	1	1	t	t	t	38	0	0	t	t	0	t	0.01	1	1	*	0.1
11	0	0	0	0	0	0	0	0	0	0	0	0	0	0	0	*	2.7
195	t	t	t	0	0.2	0	0	0	0	0	0	0	0	t	0	86	2.5
0	130	1	t	0	t	130	0	0	0	0	0	0	0	0	t	0	0.1
0	46	1	t	0	0	48	t	0	t	t	0	t	t	1	1	*	0.4
0	48	1	t	*	0	48	t	0	t	t	0	t	t	1	1	*	0.4
0	0	0	*	0	*	0	0	0	0	0	0	*	*	0	0	*	

WT, weight; **KCAL**, kcalories; **PROT**, protein; **CARB**, carbohydrate; **FIBR**, fiber; **FAT**, fat; **SATF**, saturated fat;
MONO, monosaturated fat; **POLY**, polyunsaturated fat; **CHOR**, cholesterol; **SOD**, sodium; **POT**, potassium;

Food Name	Portion	WT (Gm)	KCAL	PROT (Gm)	CARB (Gm)	FIBR (Gm)	FAT (Gm)	SATF (Gm)	MONO (Gm)	POLY (Gm)
MARGARINE-REGULAR-HARD-UNSALTED	TSP	4.7	34	0	0	0	4	0.7	1.7	1.2
MARGARINE-REGULAR-SOFT-UNSALTED	TSP	4.7	34	0	0	0	4	0.6	1.8	1.2
MARGARINE-SOYBEAN-SOFT-TUB-UNSALTED	TSP	4.7	34	0	0	0	4	0.6	1.7	1.3
MARGARINE-WHIPPED	TBSP	9	70	0	0	0	8	1.4	2.5	3.1
MAYONNAISE-IMITATION-MILK CREAM	TBSP	15	15	t	2	0	1	0.4	0.3	0.1
MAYONNAISE-LIGHT-LOW CALORIE-KRAFT	TBSP	14	40	0	1	0	4	0.5	0.6	1.4
MAYONNAISE-SOYBEAN-COMMERCIAL	TBSP	14	99	t	t	0	11	1.6	3.1	5.7
OIL-VEGETABLE-CORN	CUP	218	1927	0	0	0	218	27.7	52.7	128
OIL-VEGETABLE-OLIVE	CUP	216	1909	0	0	0	216	30.7	159	18.2
OIL-VEGETABLE-PEANUT	CUP	216	1909	0	0	0	216	36.4	99.9	69.2
OIL-VEGETABLE-SAFFLOWER	CUP	218	1927	0	0	0	218	20.5	26.3	162
OIL-VEGETABLE-SESAME	TBSP	13.6	120	0	0	0	14	1.9	5.4	5.7
OIL-VEGETABLE SOYBEAN	CUP	218	1927	0	0	0	218	31.8	93.8	82
SALAD DRESSING-BLUE CHEESE	TBSP	15.3	77	1	1	0.1	8	1.5	1.9	4.3
SALAD DRESSING-BLUE CHEESE-LOW CALORIE	TBSP	16	10	0	1	0	1	0.5	0.3	0
SALAD DRESSING-CAESAR	TBSP	15	70	0	1	t	7	*	*	*
SALAD DRESSING-FRENCH	TBSP	15.6	67	t	3	0.1	6	1.5	1.2	3.4
SALAD DRESSING-FRENCH-LOW CALORIE	TBSP	16.3	22	0	4	0.1	1	0.1	0.2	0.5
SALAD DRESSING-ITALIAN	TBSP	14.7	69	0	2	0.1	7	1	1.7	4.1
SALAD DRESSING-ITALIAN-LOW CALORIE	TBSP	15	16	0	1	0.1	2	0.2	0.3	0.9
SALAD DRESSING-MAYONNAISE TYPE	TBSP	14.7	57	0	4	0	5	0.7	1.3	2.6
SALAD DRESSING-MAYONNAISE-LOW CALORIE	TBSP	16	20	0	2	0	2	0.4	0.4	1
SALAD DRESSING-MIRACLE WHIP LIGHT	TBSP	14	45	0	2	0	4	*	*	*
SALAD DRESSING-OIL/VINEGAR-HOME RECIPE	TBSP	15.6	70	0	t	0	8	1.4	2.3	3.8
SALAD DRESSING-RANCH STYLE	TBSP	15	54	t	1	0	6	0.7	1.4	2.7
SALAD DRESSING-RUSSIAN	TBSP	15.3	76	t	2	0	8	1.1	1.8	4.5
SALAD DRESSING-RUSSIAN-LOW CALORIE	TBSP	16.3	23	t	5	0.2	1	0.1	0.2	0.4
SALAD DRESSING-THOUSAND ISLAND	TBSP	15.6	59	0	2	0.6	6	0.9	1.3	3.1
SALAD DRESSING-THOUSAND-LOW CALORIE	TBSP	15.3	24	t	3	0.3	2	0.2	0.4	1
SANDWICH SPREAD-COMMERCIAL	TBSP	15.3	60	t	3	t	5	0.8	1.1	3.1
SHORTENING-VEGETABLE-SOYBEAN/COTTONSEED	CUP	205	1812	0	0	0	205	51.2	89	52.2
VEGETABLE SPRAY-PAM-BUTTER FLAVORED	SERVING	0.9	7	0	0	0	1	0.1	0.2	0.5
VEGETABLE SPRAY-PAM-UNFLAVORED	SERVING	0.9	7	0	0	0	1	0.1	0.2	0.5

Fish

Food Name	Portion	WT (Gm)	KCAL	PROT (Gm)	CARB (Gm)	FIBR (Gm)	FAT (Gm)	SATF (Gm)	MONO (Gm)	POLY (Gm)
FISH STICKS-BREADED-FROZEN-COOKED	OUNCE	28.4	77	4	7	0.7	3	0.9	1.4	0.9
FISH-ANCHOVY-FILLET-CANNED	ITEM	4	8	1	0	0	t	0.1	0.2	0.1
FISH-BLUEFISH-BAKED WITH BUTTER	ITEM	155	246	41	0	0	8	1.8	1.8	3.9
FISH-CARP-COOKED-DRY HEAT	SERVING	85	138	19	0	0	6	1.2	2.5	1.6
FISH-CATFISH-BREADED-FRIED	SERVING	85	195	15	7	0.8	11	2.8	4.8	2.8
FISH-CLAMS-BREADED-FRIED	SERVING	85	172	12	9	0.3	9	2.3	3.9	2.4
FISH-CLAMS-CANNED-SOLIDS AND LIQUIDS	OUNCE	28.4	13	2	1	0	t	0.1	0	0
FISH-CLAMS-COOKED-MOIST HEAT	SERVING	85	126	22	4	0	2	0.2	0.1	0.5
FISH-CLAMS-RAW-MEAT ONLY	SERVING	85	63	11	2	0	1	0.1	0.1	0.2
FISH-COD-ATLANTIC-COOKED-DRY HEAT	PIECE	180	189	41	0	0	2	0.3	0.2	0.5
FISH-CRAB CAKE	ITEM	60	93	12	t	t	5	0.9	1.7	1.4
FISH-CRAB MEAT-KING-CANNED-UNPACKED	CUP	135	135	24	1	0	3	0.6	0.6	2
FISH-CRAB-ALASKA KING-RAW	SERVING	85	71	16	0	0	1	0.1	0.1	0.1
FISH-CRAB-BLUE-CANNED	CUP	135	134	28	0	0	2	0.3	0.3	0.6
FISH-CRAB-BLUE-COOKED-MOIST HEAT	CUP	135	138	27	0	0	2	0.3	0.4	0.9
FISH-CRAB-DEVILED	CUP	240	451	27	32	2.3	23	4.8	9.6	7.1
FISH-CRAB-IMITATION-SURIMI	SERVING	85	87	10	9	0	1	0.2	0.2	0.6
FISH-CRAB-IMPERIAL	CUP	220	323	32	9	0	17	4.2	6.7	4.8
FISH-CRAB-STEAMED-PIECES	CUP	155	150	30	0	0	2	0.2	0.3	0.8
FISH-CRAYFISH-COOKED-MOIST HEAT	SERVING	85	97	20	0	0	1	0.2	0.3	0.3
FISH-CROAKER-BREADED-FRIED	SERVING	85	188	16	6	0.3	11	3	4.5	2.5
FISH-EEL-COOKED-DRY HEAT	SERVING	85	201	20	0	0	13	2.6	7.8	1
FISH-FLATFISH-COOKED-DRY HEAT	SERVING	85	100	21	0	0	1	0.3	0.3	0.4
FISH-GEFILTEFISH-COMMERCIAL-WITH BROTH	PIECE	42	35	4	3	t	1	0.2	0.3	0.1
FISH-GROUPER-COOKED-DRY HEAT	SERVING	85	100	21	0	0	1	0.3	0.2	0.3
FISH-HADDOCK-BREADED-FRIED	PIECE	85	140	17	5	0.3	5	1.4	2.2	1.2
FISH-HADDOCK-BROILED	SERVING	85	95	21	0	0	1	0.1	0.1	0.3
FISH-HALIBUT-ALL TYPES-BROILED IN BUTTER	PIECE	125	214	32	0	0	9	*	*	*
FISH-HALIBUT-COOKED-BROILED	SERVING	85	119	23	0	0	2	0.4	0.8	0.8

t = Trace of nutrient present   ** = Not available*

MAG, magnesium; IRON, iron; ZINC, zinc; VITA, vitamin A; VITC, vitamin C; THIA, thiamin; RIBO, riboflavin; NIAC, niacin; VB6, vitamin B-6; FOL, folate; VB12, vitamin B-12; CALC, calcium; PHOS, phosphorus; SEL, selenium; VE-a, alpha tocopherol equivalents.

CHOL (mg)	SOD (mg)	POT (mg)	MAG (mg)	IRON (mg)	ZINC (mg)	VITA (RE)	VITC (mg)	THIA (mg)	RIBO (mg)	NIAC (mg)	VB6 (mg)	FOL (µg)	VB12 (µg)	CALC (mg)	PHOS (mg)	SEL (µg)	VE-a (mg)
0	t	1	t	0	0	47	t	0	t	t	0	t	t	1	1	0	0.6
0	1	2	t	0	0	47	t	0	t	t	0	t	t	1	1	0	0.5
0	1	2	t	0	0	47	t	0	t	t	0	t	t	1	1	0	0.1
0	97	2	t	0	0	310	0	0	0	0	t	t	0.01	2	2	0	1.1
6	76	15	1	0.1	t	t	t	t	0.02	t	t	t	0.04	11	9	*	0.1
5	15	1	0	0	t	1	0	0	t	0	0	t	0.01	0	0	*	2.9
8	78	5	t	0.1	t	12	0	0	0	0	0.08	1	0.04	2	4	*	2.9
0	0	0	0	0	0	0	0	0	0	0	0	0	0	0	0	*	31.1
0	t	0	t	0.8	0.1	0	0	0	0	0	0	0	0	0	t	3	*
0	t	t	t	0.1	t	0	0	0	0	0	0	0	0	t	0	*	25.1
0	0	0	0	0	0	0	0	0	0	0	0	0	0	0	0	*	74.2
0	0	0	0	0	0	0	0	0	0	0	0	0	0	0	0	*	0.2
0	0	0	0	0	0	0	0	0	0	0	0	0	0	0	0	*	17.7
9	167	6	0	0	0	10	t	0	0.02	0	0.01	1	0.04	12	11	*	0.9
4	177	5	*	0	*	9	0	0	0.01	0	*	*	*	10	8	*	8
*	*	*	*	*	*	*	*	*	*	*	*	*	*	*	*	*	7
2	214	12	0	0.1	t	3	0	t	t	0	t	1	0.02	2	2	*	0.8
1	128	13	0	0.1	t	0	0	0	0	0	0	1	*	2	2	*	0.2
0	116	2	t	0	t	4	0	0	0	0	t	1	0.02	1	1	*	0.7
1	118	2	0	0	t	0	0	0	0	0	0	0	0	0	1	*	0
4	104	1	t	0	t	10	0	0	0	0	t	1	0.03	2	4	*	0.6
2	44	1	*	0	*	12	*	0	0	0	*	*	*	3	4	*	5
5	95	*	*	*	*	*	*	*	*	*	*	*	*	*	*	*	4
0	t	1	0	0	0	0	0	0	0	0	0	0	0	2	1	*	0.6
4	97	1	t	t	t	13	0	t	t	t	t	1	0.03	2	4	*	0.6
0	133	24	t	0.1	0.1	32	1	0.01	0.01	0.1	0.01	2	0.05	3	6	*	0.9
1	141	26	t	0.1	t	3	1	t	t	0	t	1	0.02	3	6	*	0.1
5	109	18	t	0.1	t	15	0	0	0	0	t	1	0.03	2	3	*	0.6
2	153	17	t	0.1	t	15	0	0	0	0	t	1	0.03	2	3	*	0.2
12	153	5	0	0	0	0	0	0	0	0	0	0	0	0	0	*	0.6
0	0	0	0	0	0	0	0	0	0	0	0	0	0	0	0	*	27.9
0	0	0	*	0	*	0	0	0	*	*	*	*	*	0	0	*	*
0	0	0	*	0	*	0	0	0	*	*	*	*	*	0	0	*	*
32	165	74	7	0.2	0.2	9	0	0.04	0.05	0.6	0.02	5	0.51	6	51	3	*
3	147	22	3	0.2	0.1	1	0	t	0.02	0.8	0.01	1	0.04	9	10	2	t
108	161	*	43	1.1	*	24	*	0.17	0.16	2.9	*	*	1.64	45	445	47	*
72	54	363	32	1.4	1.6	8	1	0.12	0.06	1.8	0.19	15	1.25	44	451	26	1.8
69	238	289	23	1.2	0.7	7	0	0.06	0.11	1.9	0.16	14	1.62	37	184	*	1.8
52	309	277	12	11.8	1.2	77	9	0.09	0.21	1.8	0.05	16	34.2	54	160	*	1.7
18	15	40	*	1.2	0.3	*	*	t	0.03	0.3	*	*	5.4	16	39	46	0.6
57	95	534	16	23.8	2.3	145	19	0.13	0.36	2.9	0.09	16	84.1	78	287	*	1.7
29	48	267	8	11.9	1.2	77	11	0.07	0.18	1.5	0.05	14	42	39	144	16	0.2
99	141	440	76	0.9	1	25	2	0.16	0.14	4.5	0.51	15	1.89	25	248	81	0.1
90	198	195	20	0.7	2.5	49	2	0.05	0.05	1.7	0.1	25	3.56	63	128	13	1.2
135	675	149	29	1.1	5.8	*	*	0.11	0.11	2.6	*	*	13.5	61	246	30	1.7
36	711	173	42	0.5	5.1	6	6	0.04	0.04	0.9	0.13	37	7.65	39	186	19	*
120	450	505	53	1.1	5.4	3	4	0.11	0.11	1.9	0.2	57	0.62	136	351	30	1.4
135	376	437	45	1.2	5.7	3	4	0.14	0.07	4.5	0.24	69	9.86	140	278	30	1.4
223	2081	398	64	2.9	5.5	330	14	0.19	0.26	3.6	0.31	88	8.69	113	329	53	5.3
17	715	77	37	0.3	0.3	17	0	0.03	0.02	0.2	0.03	1	1.36	11	240	19	0.1
275	1602	288	57	2	6.4	211	11	0.13	0.26	2.4	0.31	83	10.6	132	365	48	3.5
82	1662	406	53	1.2	11.8	14	12	0.08	0.09	2.1	0.28	79	17.8	92	434	34	1.5
151	58	298	26	2.7	1.4	19	3	0.15	0.07	2.5	0.15	3	2.94	26	281	*	1.3
71	296	289	35	0.7	0.4	19	0	0.08	0.11	3.7	0.22	15	1.79	27	184	*	2.3
137	55	297	22	0.5	1.8	966	2	0.16	0.04	3.8	0.07	15	2.45	22	235	43	4.5
58	89	292	49	0.3	0.5	9	0	0.07	0.1	1.9	0.2	8	2.13	15	246	*	*
13	220	38	4	1	0.3	11	t	0.03	0.03	0.4	0.03	1	0.35	10	31	*	0
40	45	403	32	1	0.4	43	0	0.07	0.01	0.3	0.3	9	0.59	18	121	*	*
42	150	296	*	1	*	*	2	0.03	0.06	2.7	*	*	1.1	34	210	41	0.5
63	74	339	43	1.2	0.4	16	0	0.03	0.04	3.9	0.29	11	1.18	36	205	25	0.5
75	168	656	*	1	*	255	*	0.06	0.09	10.4	*	*	*	20	310	41	0.5
35	59	490	91	0.9	0.5	46	0	0.06	0.08	6.1	0.34	12	1.16	51	242	51	*

WT, weight; **KCAL**, kcalories; **PROT**, protein; **CARB**, carbohydrate; **FIBR**, fiber; **FAT**, fat; **SATF**, saturated fat;
MONO, monosaturated fat; **POLY**, polyunsaturated fat; **CHOR**, cholesterol; **SOD**, sodium; **POT**, potassium;

Food Name	Portion	WT (Gm)	KCAL	PROT (Gm)	CARB (Gm)	FIBR (Gm)	FAT (Gm)	SATF (Gm)	MONO (Gm)	POLY (Gm)
FISH-HERRING-ATLANTIC-BROILED	SERVING	85	173	20	0	0	10	2.2	4.1	2.3
FISH-HERRING-ATLANTIC-RAW	SERVING	85	134	15	0	0	8	1.7	3.2	1.8
FISH-HERRING-CANNED-SOLIDS AND LIQUIDS	SERVING	100	208	20	0	0	14	*	*	2
FISH-HERRING-PICKLED-BISMARCK TYPE	ITEM	50	131	7	5	0	9	1.2	6	0.8
FISH-LOBSTER NEWBURG	CUP	250	485	46	13	0	27	30.1	14.9	2.3
FISH-LOBSTER THERMIDOR	SERVING	157	405	29	15	0	27	18.9	9.4	1.5
FISH-LOBSTER-COOKED-MOIST HEAT	OUNCE	28.4	28	6	t	0	t	t	t	t
FISH-LOBSTER-NORTHERN-RAW	OUNCE	28.4	26	5	t	0	t	0.1	0.1	t
FISH-MACKEREL-ATLANTIC-CANNED	CUP	190	296	44	0	0	12	3.4	5.2	0.2
FISH-MACKEREL-ATLANTIC-RAW	OUNCE	28.4	58	5	0	0	4	0.9	1.2	1.4
FISH-MACKEREL-COOKED-DRY HEAT	SERVING	85	223	20	0	0	15	3.6	6	3.7
FISH-MULLET-COOKED-DRY HEAT	SERVING	85	128	21	0	0	4	1.2	1.2	0.8
FISH-MUSSELS-BLUE-RAW	CUP	150	129	18	6	0	3	0.6	0.8	0.9
FISH-OCEAN PERCH-BREADED-FRIED	PIECE	85	195	16	6	0.1	11	2.7	4.4	2.3
FISH-OCEAN PERCH-COOKED-DRY HEAT	SERVING	85	103	20	0	0	2	0.3	0.7	0.5
FISH-OYSTER-EASTERN-CANNED	CUP	248	171	18	10	0	6	1.6	0.6	1.8
FISH-OYSTER-EASTERN-COOKED-MOIST HEAT	SERVING	85	117	12	7	0	4	1.1	0.4	1.3
FISH-OYSTERS-BREADED-FRIED	SERVING	85	167	7	10	0.1	11	2.7	4	2.8
FISH-OYSTERS-EASTERN-RAW-MEAT ONLY	CUP	248	171	18	10	0	6	1.6	0.6	1.8
FISH-OYSTERS-PACIFIC-RAW	SERVING	85	69	8	4	0	2	0.4	0.3	0.8
FISH-PERCH-COOKED-DRY HEAT	SERVING	85	100	21	0	0	1	0.2	0.2	0.4
FISH-PIKE-COOKED-DRY HEAT	SERVING	85	96	21	0	0	1	0.1	0.2	0.2
FISH-POLLOCK-ATLANTIC-RAW	SERVING	85	78	17	0	0	1	0.1	0.1	0.4
FISH-POLLOCK-COOKED-DRY HEAT	SERVING	85	96	20	0	0	1	0.2	0.1	0.4
FISH-POMPANO-COOKED-DRY HEAT	SERVING	85	179	20	0	0	10	3.8	2.8	1.2
FISH-RED SNAPPER-COOKED-DRY HEAT	SERVING	85	109	22	0	0	1	0.3	0.3	0.5
FISH-RED SNAPPER-RAW	SERVING	85	85	17	0	0	1	0.2	0.2	0.4
FISH-ROCKFISH-COOKED-DRY HEAT	SERVING	100	121	24	0	0	2	0.5	0.4	0.6
FISH-SALMON PATTY	SERVING	100	239	16	16	1	12	3.5	5.3	3.6
FISH-SALMON-BROILED OR BAKED-WITH BUTTER	SERVING	100	182	27	0	0	7	1.4	2.7	2.7
FISH-SALMON-COOKED-MOIST HEAT	SERVING	85	157	23	0	0	6	1.2	2.2	1.9
FISH-SALMON-PINK-CANNED-SOLIDS & LIQUIDS	SERVING	85	118	17	0	0	5	1.3	1.5	1.7
FISH-SALMON-SMOKED	SERVING	100	117	18	0	0	4	0.9	2	1
FISH-SARDINES-ATLANTIC-CANNED IN OIL	ITEM	12	25	3	0	0	1	0.2	0.5	0.6
FISH-SARDINES-CANNED IN TOMATO SAUCE	ITEM	38	68	6	0	0.1	5	1.2	1.4	1.6
FISH-SCALLOPS-BAY AND SEA-STEAMED	OUNCE	28.4	32	7	1	0	t	*	*	*
FISH-SCALLOPS-FROZEN-BREADED-FRIED	ITEM	15	32	3	2	0.1	2	0.4	0.7	0.4
FISH-SCALLOPS-RAW	SERVING	85	75	14	2	0	1	0.1	t	0.2
FISH-SEA BASS-COOKED-DRY HEAT	SERVING	85	105	20	0	0	2	0.6	0.5	0.8
FISH-SHAD-BAKED-BUTTER/MARGARINE & BACON	SERVING	100	201	23	0	0	11	2.5	2.2	5.9
FISH-SHRIMP-CANNED MEAT	CUP	128	154	30	1	0	3	0.5	0.4	1
FISH-SHRIMP-COOKED-MOIST HEAT	SERVING	85	84	18	0	0	1	0.2	0.2	0.4
FISH-SHRIMP-FRENCH FRIED	SERVING	85	206	18	10	0.5	10	1.8	3.2	3.8
FISH-SMELT-ATLANTIC-CANNED	ITEM	20	40	4	0	0	3	*	*	*
FISH-SMELT-COOKED-DRY HEAT	SERVING	85	105	19	0	0	3	0.5	0.7	1
FISH-SOLE/FLOUNDER-BAKED	SERVING	127	148	31	0	0	2	0.5	0.4	0.5
FISH-SQUID-COOKED-FRIED	SERVING	85	149	15	7	0.3	6	1.6	2.3	1.8
FISH-SQUID-RAW	SERVING	85	78	13	3	0	1	0.3	0.1	0.4
FISH-STURGEON-STEAMED	SERVING	100	135	21	0	0	5	1.2	2.5	0.9
FISH-SURIMI	SERVING	85	84	13	6	0	1	0.2	0.1	0.4
FISH-SWORDFISH-BROILED-BUTTER/MARGARINE	SERVING	100	174	28	0	0	6	2	3.4	2.2
FISH-SWORDFISH-COOKED-DRY HEAT	SERVING	85	132	22	0	0	4	1.2	1.7	1
FISH-TILEFISH-COOKED-DRY HEAT	SERVING	85	125	21	0	0	4	0.7	1.1	1.1
FISH-TROUT-BROOK-COOKED	SERVING	100	196	24	t	0	11	1.5	2.8	2.6
FISH-TROUT-RAINBOW-COOKED-DRY HEAT	SERVING	85	128	22	0	0	4	0.7	1.1	1.3
FISH-TUNA-BLUEFIN-COOKED-DRY HEAT	SERVING	85	156	25	0	0	5	1.4	1.8	1.6
FISH-TUNA-CANNED IN OIL-DRAINED SOLIDS	SERVING	85	168	25	0	0	7	1.3	2.5	2.5
FISH-TUNA-DIETETIC-LOW SODIUM-DRAINED	OUNCE	28.4	36	8	t	0	1	0.1	0.2	0.2
FISH-TUNA-LIGHT-CANNED IN WATER-DRAINED	SERVING	85	111	25	0	0	t	0.1	0.1	0.1
FISH-TUNA-WHITE-ALBACORE-CANNED IN WATER	SERVING	85	116	23	0	0	2	0.6	0.6	0.8
FISH-TUNA-YELLOWFIN-RAW	SERVING	85	92	20	0	0	1	0.2	0.1	0.2
FISH-WHITE PERCH-FRIED FILET	ITEM	65	108	13	0	0	5	*	*	*
FISH-WHITEFISH-LAKE-BAKED-STUFFED	SERVING	100	215	15	6	0.6	14	*	*	*
FISH-WHITING-COOKED-DRY HEAT	SERVING	85	98	20	0	0	1	0.3	0.3	0.5

*t = Trace of nutrient present   * = Not available*

MAG, magnesium; IRON, iron; ZINC, zinc; VITA, vitamin A; VITC, vitamin C; THIA, thiamin; RIBO, riboflavin; NIAC, niacin; VB6, vitamin B-6;
FOL, folate; VB12, vitamin B-12; CALC, calcium; PHOS, phosphorus; SEL, selenium; VE-a, alpha tocopherol equivalents.

CHOL (mg)	SOD (mg)	POT (mg)	MAG (mg)	IRON (mg)	ZINC (mg)	VITA (RE)	VITC (mg)	THIA (mg)	RIBO (mg)	NIAC (mg)	VB6 (mg)	FOL (µg)	VB12 (µg)	CALC (mg)	PHOS (mg)	SEL (µg)	VE-a (mg)
66	98	356	35	1.2	1.1	26	1	0.1	0.25	3.5	0.3	10	11.2	63	258	52	0.9
51	76	278	27	0.9	0.8	24	1	0.08	0.2	2.7	0.26	9	11.6	49	201	85	0.9
98	*	*	*	1.8	*	*	*	0.18	*	*	*	*	*	147	297	58	*
7	435	35	4	0.6	0.3	129	0	0.02	0.07	1.7	0.09	1	2.14	39	45	50	0.5
376	573	428	56	2.3	4.2	530	1	0.18	0.28	1.6	0.17	32	4.11	218	480	188	2.6
236	360	388	35	1.9	2.6	295	0	0.15	0.51	4.8	0.11	20	2.58	290	451	118	1.7
20	108	100	10	0.1	0.8	7	0	t	0.02	0.3	0.02	3	0.88	17	53	23	0.3
27	84	78	8	0.1	0.9	6	0	t	0.01	0.4	0.02	3	0.26	14	41	21	*
150	720	369	70	3.9	1.9	248	2	0.08	0.4	11.7	0.4	10	13.2	458	572	89	3.2
20	26	89	22	0.5	0.2	14	t	0.05	0.09	2.6	0.11	t	2.47	3	62	*	0.4
64	71	341	83	1.3	0.8	46	t	0.14	0.35	5.8	0.39	1	16.2	13	236	30	1.9
54	60	389	28	1.2	0.7	36	1	0.09	0.09	5.4	0.42	8	0.21	26	207	*	2.1
42	429	479	51	5.9	2.4	72	12	0.24	0.32	2.4	0.08	63	18	39	296	84	1.1
32	128	242	*	1.1	*	*	*	0.1	0.1	1.6	*	*	0.85	28	192	20	1.1
46	82	298	33	1	0.5	12	1	0.11	0.11	2.1	0.23	9	0.98	117	235	30	1.6
136	278	568	134	16.6	226	223	12	0.37	0.41	3.1	0.24	22	47.5	112	344	149	2.6
93	190	389	93	11.4	155	145	7	0.25	0.28	2.1	0.08	15	32.5	76	236	51	*
69	355	208	49	5.9	74.1	77	3	0.13	0.17	1.4	0.05	12	13.3	53	135	*	1.9
136	277	568	135	16.6	226	222	12	0.34	0.41	3.3	0.12	25	47.5	111	344	141	2
43	90	143	19	4.3	14.1	69	7	0.06	0.2	1.7	0.04	9	13.6	7	138	56	0.7
98	67	292	32	1	1.2	9	1	0.07	0.1	1.6	0.12	5	1.87	87	218	30	1.6
43	42	281	34	0.6	0.7	20	3	0.06	0.07	2.4	0.12	15	1.96	62	239	32	1.4
60	73	303	57	0.4	0.4	9	0	0.04	0.16	2.8	0.24	3	2.71	51	188	*	*
82	99	329	62	0.2	0.5	20	0	0.06	0.07	1.4	0.06	3	3.57	5	410	*	*
54	65	541	27	0.6	0.6	31	0	0.58	0.13	3.2	0.2	15	1.02	36	290	*	0.9
40	48	444	31	0.2	0.4	30	1	0.05	t	0.3	0.39	5	2.98	34	171	*	*
31	54	355	27	0.2	0.3	26	1	0.04	t	0.2	0.34	4	2.55	27	169	*	*
44	77	520	34	0.5	0.5	66	1	0.04	0.08	3.9	0.27	10	1.2	12	228	39	*
64	96	89	34	1.2	0.8	20	4	0.12	0.22	4	0.07	13	3	78	104	*	2.1
47	116	443	32	1.2	0.7	48	2	0.16	0.06	9.8	0.22	5	2.71	18	418	48	1.4
42	50	454	32	0.8	0.4	15	1	0.16	0.17	7.1	0.39	4	3.06	39	248	26	1.2
47	471	277	29	0.7	0.8	14	0	0.02	0.16	5.6	0.26	13	5.85	181	279	45	1.2
23	784	175	18	0.9	0.3	26	0	0.02	0.1	4.7	0.28	2	3.26	11	164	61	1.4
17	61	48	5	0.4	0.2	8	0	0.01	0.03	0.6	0.02	1	1.07	46	59	6	*
23	157	130	13	0.9	0.5	27	t	0.02	0.09	1.6	0.05	9	3.42	91	139	*	0.2
15	75	135	*	0.9	*	*	*	*	*	*	*	*	*	33	96	15	*
9	70	50	9	0.1	0.2	3	t	0.01	0.02	0.2	0.02	3	0.2	6	35	12	0.1
28	137	274	48	0.2	0.8	13	3	0.01	0.06	1	0.13	14	1.3	20	186	65	*
45	74	279	45	0.3	0.4	54	0	0.11	0.13	1.6	0.39	5	0.26	11	211	*	1
69	79	377	*	0.6	*	9	*	0.13	0.26	8.6	*	*	*	24	313	*	2
222	216	269	53	3.5	1.6	23	3	0.04	0.05	3.5	0.14	2	1.44	75	299	41	3.6
166	190	155	29	2.6	1.3	56	2	0.03	0.03	2.2	0.11	3	1.26	33	116	54	3.2
150	292	191	34	1.1	1.2	48	1	0.11	0.12	2.6	0.08	7	1.59	57	185	27	0.8
*	*	*	*	0.3	*	*	*	*	*	*	*	*	*	72	74	10	0.1
77	66	316	32	1	1.8	15	0	0.63	0.12	1.5	0.15	4	3.37	66	251	105	1.7
86	133	436	74	0.4	0.8	14	4	0.1	0.15	2.8	0.31	11	3.19	23	368	160	1.5
221	260	237	33	0.9	1.5	9	4	0.05	0.39	2.2	0.05	5	1.04	33	213	*	1.9
198	37	209	28	0.6	1.3	9	4	0.02	0.35	1.9	0.05	4	1.1	27	188	*	1
75	108	364	35	2	0.5	243	0	0.08	0.09	9.8	0.22	17	2.6	40	263	49	0.6
26	122	95	37	0.2	0.3	17	0	0.02	0.02	0.2	0.03	1	1.36	8	240	*	*
4	478	354	33	1.3	1.4	616	3	0.04	0.05	10.9	0.36	3	1.9	7	275	47	1.2
43	98	314	29	0.9	1.3	35	1	0.04	0.1	10	0.32	2	1.72	5	287	*	1
54	50	435	28	0.3	0.5	18	0	0.12	0.16	3	0.26	15	2.13	22	201	*	*
69	79	602	35	1.1	1.3	96	1	0.12	0.06	2.5	0.44	17	3.25	218	272	*	0.8
62	29	539	33	2.1	1.2	19	3	0.07	0.19	5.9	0.39	15	2.98	73	273	*	0.7
42	43	275	54	1.1	0.7	643	0	0.24	0.26	9	0.45	2	9.25	9	277	85	0.9
15	301	176	26	1.2	0.8	20	0	0.03	0.1	10.5	0.09	5	1.87	11	264	61	1.4
10	11	74	9	0.3	0.1	7	*	0.01	0.01	3.5	0.11	0	0.4	1	63	33	1
15	303	267	25	2.7	0.4	20	0	0.03	0.1	10.5	0.32	4	1.87	10	158	61	*
35	333	241	29	0.5	0.4	20	0	t	0.04	4.9	0.37	4	1.87	3	227	61	*
38	32	377	43	0.6	0.4	15	1	0.37	0.04	8.3	0.77	2	0.44	14	162	85	0.4
*	*	*	*	0.7	*	0	0	0.04	0.05	2.7	*	*	*	9	113	16	0.8
*	195	291	*	0.5	*	601	0	0.11	0.11	2.3	*	*	*	*	246	*	*
71	113	369	23	0.4	0.5	29	0	0.06	0.05	1.4	0.15	13	2.21	53	242	*	*

WT, weight; KCAL, kcalories; PROT, protein; CARB, carbohydrate; FIBR, fiber; FAT, fat; SATF, saturated fat;
MONO, monosaturated fat; POLY, polyunsaturated fat; CHOR, cholesterol; SOD, sodium; POT, potassium;

Food Name	Portion	WT (Gm)	KCAL	PROT (Gm)	CARB (Gm)	FIBR (Gm)	FAT (Gm)	SATF (Gm)	MONO (Gm)	POLY (Gm)
Frozen Dinners										
BEEF AND GREEN PEPPERS-STOUFFER DINNER	ITEM	220	225	10	18	*	11	*	*	*
BEEF AND SPINACH PASTA SHELLS-STOUFFER	ITEM	255	290	19	28	*	11	*	*	*
BEEF BURGUNDY-FROZEN DINNER-EFFICIENC	ITEM	142	144	17	6	*	5	*	*	*
BEEF CUBES IN WINE SAUCE-HORMEL ENTREE	OUNCE	28.4	52	4	1	*	4	1.9	1.6	0.1
BEEF DINNER-SWANSON FROZEN DINNER	ITEM	326	320	25	34	3.3	9	9.6	12.7	4.1
BEEF SHORT RIBS IN BARBECUE SAUCE-HORMEL	OUNCE	28.4	54	5	1	0.8	3	1.7	1.4	0.2
BEEF SIRLOIN TIPS-LE MENU FROZEN DINNER	ITEM	326	400	29	27	*	19	*	*	*
BEEF STEW-HORMEL ENTREE	OUNCE	28.4	29	2	2	*	1	0.5	0.5	t
BEEF STROGANOFF-FROZEN DINNER-EFFICIENC	ITEM	170	192	20	8	*	8	*	*	*
BEEF TERIYAKI-LIGHT AND ELEGANT	ITEM	227	240	18	37	*	3	*	*	*
CHICKEN AND BROCCOLI-LIGHT AND ELEGANT	ITEM	270	290	19	30	*	11	*	*	*
CHICKEN AND DUMPLINGS WITH GRAVY-HORMEL	OUNCE	28.4	31	3	2	0.3	1	0.4	0.6	0.2
CHICKEN BURGUNDY-CLASSIC LITE DINNER	ITEM	319	240	23	24	*	5	*	*	*
CHICKEN CACCIATORE-STOUFFER DINNER	ITEM	319	310	25	29	2.9	11	8.4	12.2	9.7
CHICKEN CHOW MEIN-LEAN CUISINE DINNER	ITEM	319	250	14	36	*	5	*	*	*
CHICKEN CREPES/MUSHROOM SAUCE-STOUFFER	ITEM	234	390	30	19	2.3	22	7.3	3.8	0.9
CHICKEN DINNER-SWANSON FROZEN DINNER	ITEM	326	660	26	64	6.2	33	7.4	10.5	6.9
CHICKEN DIVAN-STOUFFER FROZEN DINNER	ITEM	241	335	21	14	1	22	9.2	8.2	3.3
CHICKEN FLORENTINE-LE MENU FROZEN DINNER	ITEM	354	510	28	35	6.7	28	8	11.4	7.5
CHICKEN KIEV-LE MENU FROZEN DINNER	ITEM	234	500	21	35	4.4	30	5.3	7.6	5
CHICKEN PARMIGIANA-LE MENU FROZEN DINNER	ITEM	333	390	26	28	*	19	*	*	*
CHICKEN PASTA SHELLS-STOUFFER DINNER	ITEM	255	400	26	24	3	22	2.5	3.2	2
CHICKEN-GLAZED-WITH RICE-LEAN CUISINE	ITEM	241	270	26	23	*	8	*	*	*
CHICKEN-SWEET AND SOUR-BUDGET GOURMET	SERVING	284	350	18	53	1.7	7	1.3	1.7	3.3
CORN SOUFFLE-STOUFFER FROZEN SIDE DISH	ITEM	113	155	4	19	*	7	*	*	*
EGG ROLL-BEEF AND SHRIMP-FROZEN-LA CHOY	ITEM	12	27	1	4	0.1	1	0.1	0.2	0.1
FETTUCINI ALFREDO-STOUFFER FROZEN DINNER	ITEM	142	270	8	19	*	18	*	*	*
FETTUCINI-CHICKEN-BUDGET GOURMET	SERVING	284	400	23	29	*	21	*	*	*
FILET OF FISH DIVAN-LEAN CUISINE DINNER	ITEM	351	270	31	16	*	10	*	*	*
FILET OF FISH FLORENTINE-LEAN CUISINE	ITEM	255	240	26	13	*	9	*	*	*
FISH AND CHIPS-VAN DE KAMPS DINNER	ITEM	224	500	16	45	4.7	30	6.2	7	6.9
FLOUNDER FILET-LE MENU FROZEN DINNER	ITEM	298	350	22	27	*	17	*	*	*
GLAZED CHICKEN-LIGHT AND ELEGANT	ITEM	227	230	24	25	*	4	*	*	*
HAM-BANQUET FROZEN DINNER	ITEM	284	369	17	48	2.6	12	2	3.4	3.1
LASAGNA-SAUSAGE-BUDGET GOURMET	SERVING	284	284	20	38	3.8	20	9	5.8	0.9
LINGUINI WITH CLAM SAUCE-STOUFFER DINNER	ITEM	298	285	17	36	*	8	*	*	*
MACARONI AND CHEESE-LIGHT AND ELEGANT	ITEM	255	300	15	37	*	9	*	*	*
MANICOTTI-CHEESE/MEAT-BUDGET GOURMET	SERVING	284	450	20	33	2.4	26	11.1	6	1.3
MEATBALLS AND NOODLES-STOUFFER DINNER	ITEM	312	475	25	33	*	27	*	*	*
MEATLOAF-BANQUET FROZEN DINNER	ITEM	312	412	21	29	5.4	24	7.5	9.1	2.9
MEXICAN DINNER-SWANSON FROZEN DINNER	ITEM	454	590	20	64	6.7	29	9.5	13	8.5
NOODLES ROMANOFF-STOUFFER FROZEN DINNER	ITEM	113	170	6	16	*	9	*	*	*
OCEAN FISH WITH LEMON SAUCE-EFFICIENC	SERVING	113	262	14	3	0.9	21	1.6	0.9	1.5
ORIENTAL BEEF-LEAN CUISINE FROZEN DINNER	ITEM	245	250	18	28	*	7	*	*	*
PEPPER STEAK WITH RICE-BUDGET GOURMET	SERVING	284	300	15	39	1.4	9	5.8	8.2	11.8
PORK LOIN AND GRAVY-HORMEL ENTREE	OUNCE	28.4	40	5	1	*	2	0.9	0.7	0.3
QUICHE LORRAINE-FROZEN DINNER-MRS SMITHS	ITEM	269	720	34	54	0.8	41	*	*	*
SALISBURY STEAK-LEAN CUISINE	ITEM	269	280	25	11	*	15	*	*	*
SCALLOPED POTATOES AND HAM-HORMEL ENTREE	OUNCE	28.4	28	2	3	0.6	1	0.6	0.4	0.1
SCALLOPS/VEGETABLES/RICE-LEAN CUISINE	ITEM	312	220	17	32	*	3	*	*	*
SEAFOOD GUMBO-HORMEL ENTREE	OUNCE	28.4	10	1	1	*	t	t	t	t
SHRIMP CREOLE-LIGHT AND ELEGANT	ITEM	283	200	11	31	2.2	2	2.9	5.6	5.1
SIRLOIN TIP/VEGETABLES-BUDGET GOURMET	SERVING	284	310	16	21	2.6	18	1.9	2	0.4
SOLE-LIGHT-VAN DE KAMP'S FROZEN DINNER	ITEM	142	293	16	17	1.9	18	0.4	0.3	0.5
SPAGHETTI-BEEF AND MUSHROOM-LEAN CUISINE	ITEM	326	280	15	38	*	7	*	*	*
SPAGHETTI-LIGHT AND ELEGANT	ITEM	290	290	16	40	*	8	*	*	*
SWEDISH MEATBALLS IN SAUCE-HORMEL ENTREE	SERVING	28.4	44	3	2	0.1	3	1.7	1.1	0.2
SWISS STEAK IN GRAVY-HORMEL ENTREE	OUNCE	28.4	34	4	1	0.4	2	0.7	1	0.2
TUNA NOODLE CASSEROLE-STOUFFER DINNER	ITEM	163	200	10	18	0.5	9	*	*	*
TURKEY & GRAVY-FROZEN	CUP	240	160	14	11	2.7	6	2	2.3	1.1
TURKEY BREAST-LE MENU FROZEN DINNER	ITEM	319	470	27	36	*	24	*	*	*
TURKEY PIE-STOUFFER FROZEN DINNER	ITEM	284	460	20	35	*	26	*	*	*

t = Trace of nutrient present   * = Not available

MAG, magnesium; **IRON**, iron; **ZINC**, zinc; **VITA**, vitamin A; **VITC**, vitamin C; **THIA**, thiamin; **RIBO**, riboflavin; **NIAC**, niacin; **VB6**, vitamin B-6; **FOL**, folate; **VB12**, vitamin B-12; **CALC**, calcium; **PHOS**, phosphorus; **SEL**, selenium; **VE-a**, alpha tocopherol equivalents.

CHOL (mg)	SOD (mg)	POT (mg)	MAG (mg)	IRON (mg)	ZINC (mg)	VITA (RE)	VITC (mg)	THIA (mg)	RIBO (mg)	NIAC (mg)	VB6 (mg)	FOL (µg)	VB12 (µg)	CALC (mg)	PHOS (mg)	SEL (µg)	VE-a (mg)
*	960	420	*	2.3	*	136	0	0.08	0.16	3.9	*	*	*	0	*	*	*
*	1315	485	*	*	*	*	*	*	*	*	*	*	*	*	*	*	*
411	147	*	0.6	*	449	0	0.04	0.24	4.1	*	*	*	5	*	*	*	*
15	106	71	4	0.5	1.3	*	t	0.77	0.05	0.5	0.02	4	0.41	3	23	*	*
84	1085	616	42	4	4.7	1140	6	0.14	0.27	4.9	0.52	24	2.1	36	283	*	2
15	176	92	5	0.7	1.7	11	t	0.01	0.07	0.7	0.03	11	0.52	3	28	*	0.8
*	1100	*	*	*	*	*	*	*	*	*	*	*	*	*	*	*	*
7	106	51	3	0.2	0.5	*	t	0.01	0.02	0.3	0.01	6	0.15	4	15	*	t
*	785	316	*	2.9	*	68	2	0.05	0.32	2.9	*	*	*	23	*	*	*
*	625	215	*	5.6	*	24	2	0.4	0.1	2.5	*	*	*	30	152	*	*
*	805	180	*	1.6	*	75	1	0.11	0.21	1.8	*	*	*	204	240	*	*
9	116	45	3	0.2	0.2	65	t	0.01	0.03	0.6	0.04	11	0.06	5	29	*	0
*	*	*	*	*	*	*	*	*	*	*	*	*	*	*	*	*	*
166	1135	300	73	3.9	4.1	176	33	0.24	0.42	18.2	0.95	22	0.57	75	398	*	2.9
25	1030	270	*	*	*	*	*	*	*	*	*	*	*	*	*	*	*
76	1040	420	50	2.6	1.1	910	33	0.15	0.19	8	0.46	28	0.19	54	192	*	0.9
111	1610	602	60	2.7	2.6	323	12	0.33	0.39	10.3	0.45	30	0.36	112	295	*	2.8
86	830	415	52	1.7	2	221	20	0.13	0.44	4.6	0.29	41	0.74	269	295	*	0.9
121	985	653	66	2.9	2.9	351	13	0.36	0.42	11.2	0.49	33	0.39	122	320	*	3.1
80	745	432	43	1.9	1.9	232	9	0.24	0.28	7.4	0.33	22	0.26	80	212	*	2
*	900	*	*	*	*	*	*	*	*	*	*	*	*	*	*	*	*
165	1060	350	47	3.7	2.2	177	28	0.3	0.43	7.5	0.35	28	0.39	59	226	*	1.3
55	810	380	*	*	*	*	*	*	*	*	*	*	*	*	*	*	*
40	640	429	45	0.7	1.4	80	2	0.12	0.34	3	0.38	13	0.17	60	163	*	1.3
*	510	190	*	0.4	*	94	0	0.08	0.16	0.8	*	34	*	48	*	*	*
2	81	15	1	0.1	0.1	12	2	0.01	0.01	0.1	0.01	1	0.02	2	5	*	0.1
*	1195	240	*	*	*	*	*	*	*	*	*	*	*	*	*	*	*
100	740	*	*	1.8	*	350	2	0.15	0.43	6	*	*	*	200	*	*	*
85	780	850	*	*	*	*	*	*	*	*	*	*	*	*	*	*	*
100	700	540	*	*	*	*	*	*	*	*	*	*	*	*	*	*	*
33	551	785	53	2.2	1	18	11	0.24	0.14	4.3	0.41	23	0.68	35	271	*	2.8
*	1125	*	*	*	*	*	*	*	*	*	*	*	*	*	*	*	*
*	655	300	*	4.8	*	31	*	0.21	0.07	7.7	*	*	*	18	348	*	*
36	1590	125	38	2.5	2.5	1311	57	0.57	0.23	3.4	0.48	21	0.45	151	278	*	4.4
80	950	591	54	2.7	3.7	183	18	0.45	0.43	4	0.28	23	0.91	400	348	*	1.1
*	1010	115	*	*	*	*	*	*	*	*	*	*	*	*	*	*	*
*	1015	210	*	2	*	60	t	0.34	0.43	1.5	*	*	*	238	334	*	*
50	920	484	45	2.7	2.3	280	10	0.45	0.51	4	0.23	31	0.72	450	376	*	2
*	1620	395	*	*	*	*	*	*	*	*	*	*	*	*	*	*	*
79	1991	468	64	4.3	3.4	427	8	0.16	0.22	4.2	0.36	48	1.21	84	243	*	1.7
44	1865	603	75	5.1	3.6	93	7	0.35	0.3	3.8	0.3	135	0.83	198	340	*	4
*	675	95	*	0.8	*	61	*	0.08	0.16	0.8	*	*	*	88	*	*	*
16	370	224	22	0.7	0.5	0	0	0.17	0.18	2.8	0.13	18	0.22	15	93	*	1.2
35	1150	270	*	*	*	*	*	*	*	*	*	*	*	*	*	*	*
25	800	729	49	0.7	6	60	2	0.15	0.17	3	0.59	22	3.9	40	350	*	4
9	133	82	5	0.2	0.4	*	t	2.61	0.04	0.9	0.06	10	0.07	2	32	*	*
95	1965	610	*	2.7	*	67	0	0.33	1.01	6	*	*	*	97	*	*	*
95	800	650	*	*	*	*	*	*	*	*	*	*	*	*	*	*	*
4	146	68	4	0.1	0.2	8	1	0.05	0.03	0.4	0.02	6	0.06	8	23	*	0.4
20	1200	360	*	*	*	*	*	*	*	*	*	*	*	*	*	*	*
6	146	82	5	0.2	0.1	*	t	0.01	0.02	0.2	0.03	6	0.09z	8	16	*	*
293	1045	200	88	2.5	2.4	889	1	0.22	0.03	3.3	0.32	14	1.91Z	54	225	*	6.5
40	570	504	35	0.4	4.4	150	2	0.15	0.17	4	0.44	16	1.87	60	195	*	0.4
45	412	453	39	0.9	0.6	10	21	0.13	0.13	3.3	0.25	36	1.35	39	200	*	0.7
20	1450	580	*	*	*	*	*	*	*	*	*	*	*	*	*	*	*
*	700	273	*	6	*	157	10	0.25	0.15	3.4	*	*	*	100	252	*	*
8	165	87	6	0.5	0.4	11	t	1.07	0.06	0.5	0.03	9	0.18	15	39	*	0.1
8	110	86	5	0.5	0.6	76	t	0.02	0.05	0.9	0.04	27	0.32	5	15	*	0.1
*	670	210	*	1.2	*	54	*	0.17	0.23	3.5	*	*	*	98	*	*	*
43	1328	146	20	2.2	1.7	20	0	0.06	0.31	4.3	0.23	10	0.58	33	194	*	2
*	1165	*	*	*	*	*	*	*	*	*	*	*	*	*	*	*	*
*	1735	270	*	*	*	*	*	*	*	*	*	*	*	*	*	*	*

WT, weight; **KCAL**, kcalories; **PROT**, protein; **CARB**, carbohydrate; **FIBR**, fiber; **FAT**, fat; **SATF**, saturated fat;

MONO, monosaturated fat; **POLY**, polyunsaturated fat; **CHOR**, cholesterol; **SOD**, sodium; **POT**, potassium;

Food Name	Portion	WT (Gm)	KCAL	PROT (Gm)	CARB (Gm)	FIBR (Gm)	FAT (Gm)	SATF (Gm)	MONO (Gm)	POLY (Gm)
TURKEY TETRAZZINI-STOUFFER FROZEN DINNER	ITEM	170	240	12	17	*	14	*	*	*
TURKEY-SLICED-LIGHT AND ELEGANT	ITEM	227	230	20	25	*	5	*	*	*
VEAL PARMIGIANA-EFFICIENC ENTREE	ITEM	213	296	24	17	1.6	14	9	7.6	4.8
VEAL STEAK-CLASSIC LITE FROZEN DINNER	ITEM	312	280	25	27	5.8	8	5.9	6.9	3.6
VEGETABLE LASAGNA-LE MENU FROZEN DINNER	ITEM	312	400	15	30	5.1	24	9.4	6.7	4.2

Fruits

Food Name	Portion	WT (Gm)	KCAL	PROT (Gm)	CARB (Gm)	FIBR (Gm)	FAT (Gm)	SATF (Gm)	MONO (Gm)	POLY (Gm)
APPLES-RAW-PEELED	ITEM	128	73	t	19	2.4	t	0.1	t	0.1
APPLES-RAW-PEELED-BOILED	CUP	171	91	t	23	4.1	1	0.1	t	0.2
APPLES-RAW-SLICED-WITH SKIN	CUP	110	65	t	17	2.4	t	0.1	t	0.1
APPLESAUCE-CANNED-SWEETENED	CUP	255	194	t	51	3.1	t	0.1	t	0.1
APPLESAUCE-CANNED-UNSWEETENED	CUP	244	105	t	28	3.7	t	t	t	t
APRICOT-RAW-WITHOUT PIT	ITEM	35.3	17	t	4	0.7	t	t	0.1	t
APRICOTS-CANNED-JUICE PACK	CUP	248	119	2	31	2.8	t	t	t	t
APRICOTS-DRIED-SULFURED-COOKED-NO SUGAR	CUP	250	213	3	55	19.5	t	t	0.2	0.1
APRICOTS-DRIED-SULFURED-UNCOOKED	CUP	130	309	5	80	10.1	1	t	0.3	0.1
AVOCADO-RAW-CALIFORNIA	ITEM	173	306	4	12	6.1	30	4.5	19.4	3.5
BANANAS-RAW-PEELED	ITEM	114	105	1	27	1.8	1	0.2	t	0.1
BLACKBERRIES-FROZEN-UNSWEETENED	CUP	151	97	2	24	7.6	1	t	0.1	0.4
BLACKBERRIES-RAW	CUP	144	75	1	18	8.9	1	0.1	0.2	0.3
BLUEBERRIES-CANNED-HEAVY SYRUP PACK	CUP	256	225	2	57	2.8	1	0.1	0.1	0.3
BLUEBERRIES-FROZEN-UNSWEETENED	CUP	155	79	1	19	4.9	1	t	0.1	0.6
BLUEBERRIES-RAW	CUP	145	81	1	21	3.3	1	0.1	0.2	0.3
BOYSENBERRIES-FROZEN-UNSWEETENED	CUP	132	66	1	16	5.2	t	t	t	0.2
CHERRIES-SWEET-RAW	ITEM	6.8	5	t	1	0.1	t	t	t	t
CRANAPPLE JUICE-CANNED	CUP	253	170	t	43	0	0	0	0	0
CRANBERRY JUICE COCKTAIL-BOTTLED	CUP	253	144	0	36	0	t	0	0	0
CRANBERRY SAUCE-CANNED-SWEETENED	CUP	277	418	1	108	3.2	t	0.1	0.1	0.2
DATES-DOMESTIC-NATURAL AND DRY-WHOLE	ITEM	8.3	23	t	6	0.7	t	0	0	0
FIGS-DRIED-UNCOOKED	CUP	199	507	6	130	18.5	2	0.5	0.5	1.1
FRUIT COCKTAIL-CANNED-JUICE PACK	CUP	248	114	1	29	1.5	t	t	t	t
FRUIT ROLL UP-CHERRY	ITEM	14.4	50	0	12	*	1	*	*	*
GRAPE DRINK-CANNED	CUP	253	154	1	38	0	t	0.1	t	0.1
GRAPEFRUIT-CANNED-JUICE PACK	CUP	249	92	2	23	1.6	t	t	t	0.1
GRAPEFRUIT-PINK & RED-RAW	ITEM	246	74	1	19	3.2	t	t	t	0.1
GRAPEFRUIT-WHITE-RAW	ITEM	236	78	2	20	2.5	t	t	t	0.1
GRAPES-RAW-SLIP SKIN (AMERICAN) TYPE	CUP	92	58	1	16	1.5	t	0.1	t	0.1
JUICE APPLE-CANNED OR BOTTLED	CUP	248	116	t	29	0.5	t	t	t	0.1
JUICE-APPLE-FROZEN-DILUTED	CUP	239	112	t	28	0.6	t	t	t	0.1
JUICE-GRAPE-CANNED & BOTTLED	CUP	253	154	1	38	0	t	0.1	t	0.1
JUICE-GRAPE-FROZEN CONCENTRATE	ITEM	216	387	1	96	0.6	1	0.2	t	0.2
JUICE-GRAPEFRUIT-CANNED-SWEETENED	CUP	250	115	1	28	0	t	t	t	0.1
JUICE-GRAPEFRUIT-CANNED-UNSWEETENED	CUP	247	94	1	22	0.4	t	t	t	0.1
JUICE-GRAPEFRUIT-FROZEN CONCENTRATE	ITEM	207	302	4	72	0	1	0.1	0.1	0.2
JUICE-LEMON-CANNED & BOTTLED	CUP	244	51	1	16	0.7	1	0.1	t	0.2
JUICE-LEMON-FROZEN-SINGLE STRENGTH	CUP	244	54	1	16	0.7	1	0.1	t	0.2
JUICE-LEMON-RAW	CUP	244	61	1	21	0.7	0	0	0	0
JUICE-ORANGE GRAPEFRUIT-CANNED	CUP	247	106	1	25	0.5	t	t	t	t
JUICE-ORANGE GRAPEFRUIT-FROZEN-DILUTED	CUP	248	110	1	26	0	0	0	0	0
JUICE-ORANGE-CANNED	CUP	249	104	1	25	0.3	t	t	0.1	0.1
JUICE-ORANGE-CANNED-FROZEN CONCENTRATE	ITEM	213	339	5	81	1.7	t	0.1	0.1	0.1
JUICE-PINEAPPLE-CANNED	CUP	250	140	1	35	0.3	t	t	t	0.1
JUICE-PINEAPPLE-FROZEN-DILUTED	CUP	250	130	1	32	0.3	t	t	t	t
JUICE-PRUNE-CANNED & BOTTLED	CUP	256	182	2	45	2.6	t	t	0.1	t
LEMONADE-CANNED-FROZEN CONCENTRATE	ITEM	219	425	0	112	5.6	0	0	0	0
LEMONADE-FROZEN CONCENTRATE-DILUTED	CUP	248	105	0	28	0.6	0	0	0	0
LEMONS-RAW-UNPEELED	ITEM	108	22	1	12	1	t	t	t	0.1
MELONS-CANTALOUPE-RAW-CUBED PIECES	CUP	160	56	1	13	1.3	t	0	0	0
MELONS-CASABA-RAW	CUP	170	44	2	11	2	t	0	0	0
MELONS-HONEYDEW-RAW-CUBED PIECES	CUP	170	60	1	16	1.5	t	0	0	0
NECTARINES-RAW	ITEM	136	67	1	16	2.2	1	0.1	0.2	0.3
ORANGES-RAW-ALL COMMON VARIETIES-WHOLE	ITEM	131	62	1	15	3.1	t	t	t	t
PAPAYA NECTAR-CANNED	CUP	250	143	t	36	1.2	t	0.1	0.1	0.1
PAPAYAS-RAW	CUP	140	55	1	14	1.3	t	0.1	0.1	t

t = Trace of nutrient present   * = Not available

MAG, magnesium; **IRON**, iron; **ZINC**, zinc; **VITA**, vitamin A; **VITC**, vitamin C; **THIA**, thiamin; **RIBO**, riboflavin; **NIAC**, niacin; **VB6**, vitamin B-6;

FOL, folate; **VB12**, vitamin B-12; **CALC**, calcium; **PHOS**, phosphorus; **SEL**, selenium; **VE-a**, alpha tocopherol equivalents.

CHOL (mg)	SOD (mg)	POT (mg)	MAG (mg)	IRON (mg)	ZINC (mg)	VITA (RE)	VITC (mg)	THIA (mg)	RIBO (mg)	NIAC (mg)	VB6 (mg)	FOL (μg)	VB12 (μg)	CALC (mg)	PHOS (mg)	SEL (μg)	VE-a (mg)
*	620	200	*	0.6	*	41	*	0.12	0.24	2.4	*	*	*	72	*	*	*
*	1020	280	*	1	*	171	1	0.12	0.14	4.6	*	*	*	18	121	*	*
162	973	466	49	2.3	3.6	123	6	0.3	0.38	6.8	0.43	25	1.21	97	401	*	2.6
60	1738	932	81	3.6	4.2	241	33	0.36	0.43	6.5	0.53	62	0.85	171	299	*	2.7
39	1135	519	82	3.2	1.5	723	62	0.23	0.47	3.3	0.34	78	0.2	296	274	*	2.5
0	0	144	4	0.1	0.1	6	5	0.02	0.01	0.1	0.06	1	0	5	9	1	0.3
0	2	150	5	0.3	0.1	8	t	0.03	0.02	0.2	0.08	1	0	9	13	1	0.1
0	0	126	5	0.2	t	6	6	0.02	0.02	0.1	0.05	3	0	8	8	1	0.6
0	8	156	7	0.9	0.1	3	4	0.03	0.07	0.5	0.07	2	0	9	17	1	0.2
0	5	183	7	0.3	0.1	7	3	0.03	0.06	0.5	0.06	1	0	7	17	1	0.2
0	t	104	3	0.2	0.1	92	4	0.01	0.01	0.2	0.02	3	0	5	7	0	0.3
0	9	409	24	0.7	0.3	420	12	0.05	0.05	0.9	0.13	4	0	30	50	1	2.2
0	9	1222	42	4.2	0.7	591	4	0.02	0.08	2.4	0.29	0	0	40	104	*	*
0	13	1791	61	6.1	1	941	3	0.01	0.2	3.9	0.2	13	0	59	152	*	*
0	21	1097	70	2	0.7	106	14	0.19	0.21	3.3	0.48	113	0	19	73	*	3.7
0	1	451	33	0.4	0.2	9	10	0.05	0.11	0.6	0.66	22	0	7	22	1	0.3
0	2	211	33	1.2	0.4	17	5	0.04	0.07	1.8	0.09	51	0	44	45	1	1.1
0	0	282	29	0.8	0.4	24	30	0.04	0.06	0.6	0.08	49	0	46	30	1	0.9
0	9	102	9	0.8	0.2	16	3	0.09	0.14	0.3	0.09	4	0	14	26	2	1.7
0	2	84	8	0.3	0.1	13	4	0.05	0.06	0.8	0.09	10	0	12	17	1	1.6
0	9	129	7	0.2	0.2	15	19	0.07	0.07	0.5	0.05	9	0	9	15	1	*
0	2	183	21	1.1	0.3	9	4	0.07	0.05	1	0.07	84	0	36	36	1	0.6
0	0	15	1	t	t	1	t	t	t	t	t	t	0	1	1	0	t
0	5	68	5	0.2	0.1	0	81	0.01	0.05	0.2	0.05	1	0	18	8	1	*
0	10	46	5	0.4	0.2	0	90	0.02	0.02	0.1	0.05	1	0	8	5	1	*
0	80	72	8	0.6	0.1	6	11	0.04	0.06	0.3	0.04	*	0	11	17	1	*
0	t	54	3	0.1	t	t	0	0.01	0.01	0.2	0.02	1	0	3	3	*	*
0	22	1417	117	4.4	1	26	2	0.14	0.18	1.4	0.45	15	0	287	135	*	0
0	10	236	17	0.5	0.2	76	7	0.03	0.04	1	0.13	6	0	20	35	1	0.5
0	5	45	*	*	*	*	*	*	*	*	*	*	0	*	*	*	*
0	8	334	25	0.6	0.1	2	t	0.07	0.09	0.7	0.16	7	0	23	28	*	*
0	19	420	26	0.5	0.2	0	84	0.07	0.05	0.6	0.05	22	0	37	30	1	0.6
0	0	312	20	0.3	0.2	64	91	0.1	0.05	0.5	0.1	23	0	36	22	1	0.6
0	0	350	21	0.1	0.2	2	79	0.09	0.05	0.6	0.1	24	0	28	18	1	0.6
0	2	176	5	0.3	t	9	4	0.09	0.05	0.3	0.1	4	0	13	9	1	0.6
0	7	296	8	0.9	0.1	t	2	0.05	0.04	0.2	0.07	t	0	16	18	2	t
0	17	301	12	0.6	0.1	*	1	0.01	0.04	0.1	0.08	1	0	14	17	2	t
0	8	334	25	0.6	0.1	2	t	0.07	0.09	0.7	0.16	7	0	23	28	1	*
0	15	160	32	0.8	0.3	6	179	0.11	0.2	0.9	0.32	10	0	28	32	2	*
0	5	405	25	0.9	0.2	0	67	0.1	0.06	0.8	0.05	26	0	20	28	1	0.1
0	2	378	25	0.5	0.2	2	72	0.1	0.05	0.6	0.05	26	0	17	27	1	0.1
0	6	1002	78	1	0.4	7	248	0.3	0.16	1.6	0.32	26	0	56	101	1	0.1
0	51	249	20	0.3	0.1	4	61	0.1	0.02	0.5	0.11	25	0	27	22	1	*
0	2	217	20	0.3	0.1	3	77	0.14	0.03	0.3	0.15	23	0	20	20	1	*
0	2	303	15	0.1	0.1	5	112	0.07	0.02	0.2	0.12	32	0	17	15	1	*
0	7	390	25	1.1	0.2	29	72	0.14	0.07	0.8	0.06	35	0	20	35	1	0.1
0	2	439	24	0.2	0.2	27	102	0.15	0.02	0.7	0.06	*	0	20	32	1	0.1
0	6	436	27	1.1	0.2	44	86	0.15	0.07	0.8	0.22	136	0	21	36	1	0.1
0	7	1435	73	0.7	0.4	59	294	0.6	0.14	1.5	0.33	331	0	67	122	1	*
0	3	335	33	0.7	0.3	1	27	0.14	0.06	0.6	0.24	58	0	43	20	2	*
0	3	340	23	0.8	0.3	3	30	0.18	0.05	0.5	0.19	27	0	28	20	2	0.1
0	10	707	36	3	0.5	1	11	0.04	0.18	2	0.56	1	0	31	64	1	*
0	4	153	*	0.4	*	4	66	0.05	0.06	0.7	*	*	0	9	13	1	*
0	0	40	*	0.1	*	1	17	0.01	0.02	0.2	*	12	0	2	3	1	*
0	3	157	13	0.8	0.1	3	83	0.05	0.04	0.2	0.12	11	0	66	16	1	0.3
0	14	494	18	0.3	0.3	516	68	0.06	0.03	0.9	0.18	27	0	18	27	1	0.2
0	20	357	14	0.7	0.3	5	27	0.1	0.03	0.7	0.2	29	0	9	12	1	0.2
0	17	461	12	0.1	*	7	42	0.13	0.03	1	0.1	*	0	10	17	1	0.2
0	0	288	11	0.2	0.1	100	7	0.02	0.06	1.4	0.03	5	0	7	22	1	1.2
0	0	237	13	0.1	0.1	27	70	0.11	0.05	0.4	0.08	40	0	52	18	2	0.3
0	13	78	8	0.9	0.4	28	8	0.02	0.01	0.4	0.02	5	0	25	0	1	1.9
0	4	359	14	0.1	0.1	282	87	0.04	0.05	0.5	0.03	53	0	34	7	1	

WT, weight; KCAL, kcalories; PROT, protein; CARB, carbohydrate; FIBR, fiber; FAT, fat; SATF, saturated fat;
MONO, monosaturated fat; POLY, polyunsaturated fat; CHOR, cholesterol; SOD, sodium; POT, potassium;

Food Name	Portion	WT (Gm)	KCAL	PROT (Gm)	CARB (Gm)	FIBR (Gm)	FAT (Gm)	SATF (Gm)	MONO (Gm)	POLY (Gm)
PEACHES-CANNED-HEAVY SYRUP PACK	CUP	256	189	1	51	1.1	t	t	0.1	0.1
PEACHES-RAW-SLICED	CUP	170	73	1	19	2.7	t	t	0.1	0.1
PEACHES-RAW-WHOLE	ITEM	87	37	1	10	1.4	t	t	t	t
PEAR NECTAR-CANNED	CUP	250	150	t	39	1.6	t	t	t	t
PEARS-CANNED-HEAVY SYRUP PACK	CUP	255	189	1	49	2.4	t	t	0.1	0.1
PEARS-RAW-BARTLETT WITH SKIN	ITEM	166	98	1	25	4.3	1	t	0.1	0.2
PINEAPPLE GRAPEFRUIT DRINK	CUP	253	129	1	32	0	t	t	t	0.1
PINEAPPLE ORANGE DRINK	CUP	253	134	1	32	0	0	0	0	0
PINEAPPLE-BITS-CANNED IN SYRUP	CUP	252	131	1	34	1.9	t	t	t	0.1
PINEAPPLE-FROZEN-SWEETENED	CUP	245	208	1	54	5.4	t	t	t	0.1
PINEAPPLE-RAW-DICED	CUP	155	76	1	19	1.9	1	0.1	0.1	0.2
PLUMS-PURPLE-CANNED-HEAVY SYRUP PACK	CUP	258	230	1	60	1.1	t	t	0.2	0.1
PLUMS-RAW JAPANESE & HYBRID	ITEM	66	36	1	9	1.4	t	t	0.3	0.1
PLUMS-RAW-PRUNE TYPE	ITEM	28.4	20	0	6	0.6	0	0	0	0
POMEGRANATES-RAW	ITEM	154	105	1	26	1.1	t	0.1	t	0.1
PRUNES-CANNED-HEAVY SYRUP PACK	CUP	234	246	2	65	8.6	t	t	0.3	0.1
PRUNES-DRIED-COOKED-WITH SUGAR	CUP	238	295	3	78	7.6	1	t	0.3	0.1
PRUNES-DRIED-COOKED-WITHOUT SUGAR	CUP	212	227	2	60	7.5	t	t	0.3	0.1
PRUNES-DRIED-UNCOOKED	CUP	161	385	4	101	11	1	0.1	0.5	0.2
RAISINS-SEEDLESS	CUP	145	435	5	115	7.7	1	0.2	t	0.2
RAISINS-SEEDLESS-PACKET	ITEM	14	42	t	11	0.7	t	t	t	t
RASPBERRIES-CANNED-HEAVY SYRUP PACK	CUP	256	234	2	60	6.5	t	t	t	0.2
RASPBERRIES-FROZEN-SWEETENED	CUP	250	258	2	65	11	t	t	t	0.2
RASPBERRIES-RAW	CUP	123	60	1	14	5.5	1	t	0.1	0.4
RHUBARB-COOKED FROM RAW-ADDED SUGAR	CUP	270	380	1	97	5.4	0	0	0	0
STRAWBERRIES-CANNED-HEAVY SYRUP PACK	CUP	254	234	1	60	3.1	1	t	0.1	0.3
STRAWBERRIES-FROZEN-SWEETENED-SLICED	CUP	255	245	1	66	19.8	t	t	t	0.2
STRAWBERRIES-FROZEN-SWEETENED-WHOLE	CUP	255	199	1	54	5.6	t	t	t	0.2
STRAWBERRIES-FROZEN-UNSWEETENED	CUP	149	52	1	14	3.9	t	t	t	0.1
STRAWBERRIES-RAW-WHOLE	CUP	149	45	1	11	3.9	1	t	0.1	0.3
TANGERINES-CANNED-LIGHT SYRUP PACK	CUP	252	154	1	41	1.4	t	t	t	0.1
TANGERINES-RAW-PEELED	ITEM	84	37	1	9	1.7	t	t	t	t
WATERMELON-RAW	CUP	160	51	1	12	0.6	1	*	*	*

Grains

Food Name	Portion	WT (Gm)	KCAL	PROT (Gm)	CARB (Gm)	FIBR (Gm)	FAT (Gm)	SATF (Gm)	MONO (Gm)	POLY (Gm)
BISQUICK MIX-DRY	CUP	112	480	8	76	3	16	*	*	*
CORN CHIPS	OUNCE	28.4	155	2	17	1.7	9	1.5	3.4	4.3
CORN GRITS-DRY	CUP	156	579	14	124	18.6	2	0.3	0.5	0.8
CORNMEAL-DEGERMED-ENRICHED-COOKED	CUP	240	878	20	186	1.9	4	0.5	1	1.7
CROUTONS-HERB SEASONED	CUP	30	100	4	20	1.4	0	0	0	0
FLOUR-WHEAT-ENRICHED-SIFTED	CUP	115	419	12	88	3.1	1	0.2	0.1	0.5
FLOUR-WHEAT-WHITE-FOR BREAD	CUP	137	495	16	99	4.5	2	0.3	0.2	1
MACARONI-COOKED-FIRM STAGE-HOT	CUP	130	183	6	37	2.1	1	0.1	0.1	0.4
NOODLES-EGG-COOKED	CUP	160	213	8	40	3	2	0.5	0.7	0.7
NOODLES-EGG-SPINACH-COOKED	CUP	160	211	8	39	0.4	3	0.6	0.8	0.6
NOODLES-RAMEN-ORIENTAL	CUP	227	207	6	31	2	9	0.4	0.4	0.4
OAT BRAN-RAW	CUP	94	231	16	62	12.5	7	1.3	2.2	2.6
OATS-WHOLE GRAIN-UNCOOKED	CUP	156	607	26	104	20.8	11	1.9	3.4	4
PASTA-FRESH-PLAIN-COOKED	OUNCE	28.4	38	1	7	0.3	t	t	t	0.1
POPCORN-POPPED-OIL & SALT	CUP	9	40	1	5	0.4	2	1.5	0.2	0.2
POPCORN-POPPED-PLAIN	CUP	6	25	1	5	0.4	0	0	0	0
POPCORN-POPPED-SUGAR COATED	CUP	35	135	2	30	1.4	1	0.5	0.2	0.4
PRETZEL-DUTCH-TWISTED	ITEM	16	60	2	12	*	1	*	*	*
PRETZEL-THIN-STICK	ITEM	0.3	1	t	t	*	t	0	0	0
PRETZEL-THIN-TWISTED	ITEM	6	24	1	5	*	t	*	*	*
RICE CAKE-LOW SODIUM	ITEM	9.31	35	1	8	0.2	t	1.2	0.1	t
RICE CAKE-REGULAR	ITEM	9.31	35	1	8	0.2	t	1.2	0.1	t
RICE-BROWN-LONG GRAIN-COOKED	CUP	195	216	5	45	3.3	2	0.4	0.6	0.6
RICE-BROWN-LONG GRAIN-RAW	CUP	185	685	15	143	10.7	5	1.1	2	1.9
RICE-WHITE-INSTANT-HOT	CUP	165	162	3	35	1.3	t	0.1	0.1	0.1
RICE-WHITE-LONG GRAIN-COOKED	CUP	205	264	6	57	2.1	1	0.2	0.2	0.2
RICE-WHITE-LONG GRAIN-RAW	CUP	185	675	13	148	1.9	1	0.3	0.4	0.3
RICE-WILD-COOKED	CUP	164	166	7	35	2.6	1	0.1	0.1	0.4
RYE-WHOLE-DRY	CUP	169	566	25	118	8.9	4	0.5	0.5	0.9

t = Trace of nutrient present   * = Not available

MAG, magnesium; **IRON**, iron; **ZINC**, zinc; **VITA**, vitamin A; **VITC**, vitamin C; **THIA**, thiamin; **RIBO**, riboflavin; **NIAC**, niacin; **VB6**, vitamin B-6; **FOL**, folate; **VB12**, vitamin B-12; **CALC**, calcium; **PHOS**, phosphorus; **SEL**, selenium; **VE-a**, alpha tocopherol equivalents.

CHOL (mg)	SOD (mg)	POT (mg)	MAG (mg)	IRON (mg)	ZINC (mg)	VITA (RE)	VITC (mg)	THIA (mg)	RIBO (mg)	NIAC (mg)	VB6 (mg)	FOL (µg)	VB12 (µg)	CALC (mg)	PHOS (mg)	SEL (µg)	VE-a (mg)
0	15	235	13	0.7	0.1	85	7	0.03	0.06	1.6	0.05	8	0	8	28	1	*
0	0	335	12	0.2	0.2	91	11	0.03	0.07	1.7	0.03	6	0	9	20	1	0.2
0	0	171	6	0.1	0.1	47	6	0.02	0.04	0.9	0.02	3	0	4	10	1	0.1
0	10	33	8	0.7	0.2	t	3	0.01	0.03	0.3	0.04	3	0	13	8	1	t
0	13	166	10	0.6	0.2	0	3	0.03	0.06	0.6	0.04	3	0	13	18	1	0.3
0	0	208	10	0.4	0.2	3	7	0.03	0.07	0.2	0.03	12	0	18	18	1	0.8
0	56	139	15	0.8	0.1	0	68	0.05	0.05	0.6	2.02	25	0	15	10	2	0.2
0	8	121	15	0.7	0.2	134	63	0.08	0.05	0.5	0.12	28	0	13	10	2	0
0	3	266	40	1	0.3	4	19	0.23	0.06	0.7	0.19	12	0	36	17	3	0.3
0	5	245	25	1	0.3	7	20	0.25	0.07	0.7	0.18	26	0	22	10	2	0.2
0	2	175	22	0.6	0.1	4	24	0.14	0.06	0.7	0.14	16	0	11	11	1	0.2
0	50	234	13	2.2	0.2	67	1	0.04	0.1	0.8	0.07	7	0	24	33	1	*
0	0	114	5	0.1	0.1	21	6	0.03	0.06	0.3	0.05	1	0	3	7	0	0.5
0	0	48	2	0.1	t	8	1	0.01	0.01	0.1	0.02	1	0	3	5	0	0.2
0	5	399	5	0.5	0.2	0	9	0.05	0.05	0.5	0.16	9	0	5	12	1	0.8
0	7	529	35	1	0.4	187	7	0.08	0.29	2	0.48	t	0	40	61	1	*
0	4	741	45	2.5	0.5	68	6	0.05	0.22	1.6	0.48	t	0	51	78	1	*
0	4	708	43	2.4	0.5	65	6	0.05	0.21	1.5	0.46	t	0	48	75	1	*
0	6	1200	73	4	0.9	320	5	0.13	0.26	3.2	0.43	6	0	82	127	1	*
0	17	1089	48	3	0.4	1	5	0.23	0.13	1.2	0.36	5	0	71	141	1	1
0	2	105	5	0.3	t	t	t	0.02	0.01	0.1	0.04	t	0	7	14	0	0.1
0	9	241	31	1.1	0.4	9	22	0.05	0.08	1.1	0.11	27	0	27	23	1	1.2
0	3	285	33	1.6	0.5	15	41	0.05	0.11	0.6	0.09	65	0	38	43	1	0.8
0	0	187	22	0.7	0.6	16	31	0.04	0.11	1.1	0.07	32	0	27	15	1	0.4
0	5	548	32	1.6	0.2	22	16	0.05	0.14	0.8	0.05	14	0	211	41	1	0.5
0	9	218	22	1.2	0.2	7	80	0.05	0.09	0.1	0.12	01	0	33	29	1	0.4
0	8	249	18	1.5	0.1	6	106	0.04	0.13	1	0.08	38	0	28	32	1	0.5
0	3	250	15	1.2	0.1	7	101	0.04	0.2	0.7	0.07	10	0	28	31	1	0.5
0	3	221	16	1.1	0.2	7	61	0.03	0.06	0.7	0.04	25	0	24	19	1	0.3
0	1	247	15	0.6	0.2	4	85	0.03	0.1	0.3	0.09	26	0	21	28	1	0.2
0	15	197	20	0.9	0.6	212	50	0.13	0.11	1.1	0.11	12	0	18	25	1	*
0	1	132	10	0.1	0.2	77	26	0.09	0.02	0.1	0.06	17	0	12	8	1	*
0	3	186	18	0.3	0.1	59	15	0.13	0.03	0.3	0.23	4	0	13	14	1	*
*	1400	*	*	*	*	*	*	*	*	*	*	*	*	*	*	*	0.3
0	164	43	22	0.4	0.4	11	1	0.05	0.03	0.6	0.05	2	0	37	55	2	1.9
0	1	213	42	6.1	0.6	0	0	1	0.59	7.7	0.23	7	0	3	114	*	0.2
0	7	389	96	9.9	1.7	98	0	1.72	0.98	12.1	0.62	115	0	12	202	6	0.4
0	372	39	11	1.5	0.3	0	0	0.13	0.2	1.7	0	0	0	29	42	*	0.3
0	2	123	25	5.3	0.8	0	0	0.9	0.57	6.8	0.05	30	0	17	124	5	t
0	2	136	34	6	1.2	0	0	1.11	0.7	10.4	0.05	40	0	21	133	*	*
0	1	41	23	1.8	0.7	0	0	0.27	0.13	2.2	0.05	1	0	1	71	32	t
53	11	45	30	2.5	1	10	0	0.3	0.13	2.4	0.06	11	0.14	19	110	*	*
52	20	59	38	1.7	1	17	0	0.39	0.2	2.4	0.18	34	0.22	30	91	*	12.7
36	829	69	17	1.8	0.6	221	t	0.16	0.1	1.4	0.07	8	0.01	18	70	*	0.2
0	4	532	221	5.1	2.9	0	0	1.1	0.21	0.9	0.16	49	0	55	690	*	1.6
0	3	669	276	7.4	6.2	0	0	1.19	0.22	1.5	0.19	87	0	84	816	*	1.7
10	2	7	5	0.3	0.2	2	0	0.06	0.04	0.3	0.01	2	0.04	2	18	*	0.1
0	174	*	16	0.2	0.4	*	0	*	0.01	0.2	*	*	*	1	19	2	*
0	0	*	*	0.2	0.5	*	0	*	0.01	0.1	0.01	*	0	1	17	1	*
0	0	*	*	0.5	*	*	0	*	0.02	0.4	*	*	*	2	47	7	*
0	258	21	4	0.2	0.2	0	0	0.05	0.04	0.7	t	3	0	4	21	*	t
0	5	t	t	t	t	0	0	t	t	t	0	t	0	t	t	*	0
0	97	6	1	0.1	0.1	0	0	0.02	0.02	0.3	t	1	0	2	5	*	t
0	t	26	3	0.2	0.1	0	t	t	t	0.1	0.01	1	0	7	10	*	t
0	11	27	3	0.2	0.1	0	t	t	t	0.1	0.01	1	0	7	10	*	t
0	9	83	83	0.8	1.2	0	0	0.19	0.05	3	0.28	8	0	20	161	76	1.3
0	13	413	265	2.7	3.7	0	0	0.74	0.17	9.4	0.94	36	0	43	616	*	1.3
0	5	7	8	1	0.4	0	0	0.12	0.08	1.5	0.02	6	0	13	23	33	0.2
0	4	80	26	2.3	0.9	0	0	0.33	0.03	3	0.19	7	0	23	95	41	0.2
0	9	213	46	2	8	0	0	1.07	0.09	7.8	0.3	16	0	52	213	37	0.2
0	6	166	53	1	2.2	0	0	0.09	0.14	2.1	0.22	43	0	5	134	*	0.3
0	10	4462	204	4.5	6.3	0	0	0.53	0.42	7.2	0.5	101	0	56	632	*	2.2

WT, weight; **KCAL**, kcalories; **PROT**, protein; **CARB**, carbohydrate; **FIBR**, fiber; **FAT**, fat; **SATF**, saturated fat;

MONO, monosaturated fat; **POLY**, polyunsaturated fat; **CHOR**, cholesterol; **SOD**, sodium; **POT**, potassium;

Food Name	Portion	WT (Gm)	KCAL	PROT (Gm)	CARB (Gm)	FIBR (Gm)	FAT (Gm)	SATF (Gm)	MONO (Gm)	POLY (Gm)
SHAKE 'N BAKE-PACKAGE-GENERAL FOODS	OUNCE	28.4	116	2	18	*	4	*	*	*
SORGHUM-WHOLE-DRY	CUP	192	651	22	143	28.6	6	0.9	1.9	2.6
SPAGHETTI-COOKED-TENDER STAGE-HOT	CUP	140	155	5	32	2.2	1	*	*	*
STUFFING MIX-DRY FORM	CUP	30	111	4	22	*	1	*	*	*
STUFFING MIX-PREPARED	CUP	140	501	9	50	*	31	*	*	*
TACO SHELLS	ITEM	11	50	1	7	0.9	2	0.3	1.2	0.5
TORTILLA CHIPS-DORITOS	OUNCE	28.4	139	2	19	1.9	7	1.4	3.2	1.8

Meats

Food Name	Portion	WT (Gm)	KCAL	PROT (Gm)	CARB (Gm)	FIBR (Gm)	FAT (Gm)	SATF (Gm)	MONO (Gm)	POLY (Gm)
BACON BITS	TBSP	6	27	2	2	0.6	2	0.2	0.4	0.8
BACON-PORK-BROILED/PAN-FRIED/ROASTED	SLICE	6.3	36	2	t	0	3	1.1	1.5	0.4
BARBECUE LOAF-PORK AND BEEF	SLICE	23	40	4	1	*	2	0.7	1	0.2
BEEF CUTS-LEAN AND FAT-SIMMERED/ROASTED	SLICE	85	297	21	0	0	23	9.5	10.2	0.9
BEEF CUTS-LEAN ONLY-SIMMERED/ROASTED	SLICE	85	347	19	0	0	30	12.3	13.7	1
BEEF-DRIED-CURED-CHIPPED	SERVING	71	117	21	1	0	3	1.1	1.1	0.1
BEEF-HEART-COOKED-SIMMERED	SLICE	85	149	25	t	0	5	1.4	1.1	1.2
BEEF-LIVER-FRIED IN MARGARINE	SLICE	85	184	23	7	0	7	2.4	1.5	1.5
BEEF-POT ROAST-CHUCK-ARM CUT-COOKED	SLICE	100	231	33	0	0	10	3.8	4.4	0.4
BEEF-POT ROAST-CHUCK-BLADE CUT-COOKED	SLICE	100	270	31	0	0	15	6.2	6.8	0.5
BEEF-RIB STEAK-COOKED	ITEM	100	221	28	0	0	11	4.8	4.9	0.3
BEEF-STEAK-CHICKEN FRIED	ITEM	100	389	18	12	0	30	6.6	7.4	1.1
BEEF-TENDERLOIN STEAK-BROILED	ITEM	100	204	28	0	0	9	3.6	3.6	0.4
BEERWURST-BEER SALAMI-BEEF	SLICE	6	20	1	t	0	2	0.8	0.8	0.1
BEERWURST-BEER SALAMI-PORK	SLICE	6	14	1	t	0	1	0.4	0.5	0.1
BOCKWURST-RAW-PORK-LINK	ITEM	65	200	9	t	0	18	6.6	8.5	1.9
BOLOGNA-CURED PORK-4 BY 1/8 INCH SLICE	SLICE	23	57	4	t	0	5	1.6	2.3	0.5
BRATWURST-PORK-COOKED-LINK	ITEM	85	256	12	2	0	22	7.9	10.4	2.3
BRAUNSCHWEIGER-LIVER SAUSAGE-CURED PORK	SLICE	18	65	2	1	0	6	2	2.7	0.7
BRISKET-LEAN-COOKED	SLICE	100	241	29	0	0	13	4.6	5.8	0.4
CANADIAN BACON-PORK-GRILLED	SLICE	23.3	43	6	t	0	2	0.7	0.9	0.2
CHEESEFURTER-PORK AND BEEF	ITEM	43	141	6	1	0	13	4.5	5.9	1.3
CHITTERLINGS-PORK-SIMMERED	OUNCE	28.4	86	3	0	0	8	2.9	2.8	2.1
CHORIZO-PORK AND BEEF-LINK	ITEM	60	273	15	1	0	23	8.6	11	2.1
CORNED BEEF HASH-CANNED	CUP	220	400	19	24	*	25	11.9	10.9	0.5
CORNED BEEF LOAF-JELLIED	SLICE	28.4	44	7	0	0	2	0.7	0.8	0.1
CORNED BEEF-CANNED	SERVING	85	213	23	1	0	13	5.3	5.1	0.5
FRANKFURTER (HOT DOG)-NO BUN-BEEF & PORK	ITEM	57	183	6	1	0	17	6.1	7.8	1.6
FROG LEGS-FRIED-FLOUR COATED	ITEM	24	70	4	2	0.2	5	0.7	1.2	0.7
HAM AND CHEESE LOAF/ROLL	SLICE	28.4	74	5	t	0.5	6	2.1	2.6	0.6
HAM AND CHEESE SPREAD	TBSP	15	37	2	t	*	3	1.3	1.1	0.2
HAM SALAD SPREAD	TBSP	15	32	1	2	0	2	0.8	1.1	0.4
HAM-BOILED-REGULAR-11% FAT-LUNCHEON MEAT	SLICE	28.4	52	5	1	0	3	1	1.4	0.3
HAM-CANNED-CHOPPED-LUNCHEON MEAT	SLICE	21	50	3	t	0	4	1.3	1.9	0.4
HAM-CANNED-EXTRA LEAN-4% FAT	CUP	140	190	30	1	0	7	2.2	3.5	0.6
HAM-CANNED-PORK-ROASTED-13% FAT	CUP	140	316	29	1	0	21	7.1	9.9	2.5
HAM-DEVILED-CANNED-LUNCHEON MEAT	TBSP	13	45	2	0	0	4	1.5	1.8	0.4
HAM-EXTRA LEAN-5% FAT-ROASTED	CUP	140	203	29	2	0	8	2.5	3.7	0.8
HAM-LEAN ONLY-ROASTED	CUP	140	220	35	0	0	8	2.6	3.5	0.9
HAM-MINCED-PORK	SLICE	21	55	3	t	0	4	1.5	2	0.5
HAM-ROASTED-REGULAR-11% FAT-BONELESS	CUP	140	249	32	0	0	13	4.4	6.2	2
HAMBURGER PATTY-BROILED-EXTRA LEAN BEEF	ITEM	85	218	22	0	0	14	5.5	6.1	0.5
HAMBURGER PATTY-BROILED-MEDIUM-LEAN BEEF	ITEM	85	231	21	0	0	16	6.2	6.9	0.6
HAMBURGER-GROUND-REGULAR-BAKED	SERVING	85	244	20	0	0	18	7	7.8	0.7
HAMBURGER-GROUND-REGULAR-FRIED	SERVING	85	260	20	0	0	19	7.5	8.4	0.7
HEADCHEESE-PORK	SLICE	28.4	60	5	t	0	4	1.4	2.3	0.5
ITALIAN SAUSAGE-PORK-LINK	ITEM	67	216	13	1	0	17	6.1	8	2.2
KIELBASA-PORK AND BEEF	SLICE	26	81	3	1	0	7	2.6	3.4	0.8
KNOCKWURST-PORK AND BEEF-LINK	ITEM	68	209	8	1	0	19	6.9	8.7	2
LAMB CHOP-RIB-BROILED-LEAN AND FAT	SERVING	85	307	19	0	0	25	10.8	10.3	2
LAMB CHOP-RIB-BROILED-LEAN ONLY	SERVING	57	134	16	0	0	7	2.7	3	0.7
LAMB-LEG-ROASTED-LEAN AND FAT	SLICE	85	219	22	0	0	14	5.9	5.9	1
LAMB-LEG-ROASTED-LEAN ONLY	SLICE	71	136	20	0	0	6	2	2.4	0.4
LAMB-SHOULDER-ROASTED-LEAN AND FAT	SLICE	85	235	19	0	0	17	7.2	6.9	1.4
LAMB-SHOULDER-ROASTED-LEAN ONLY	SLICE	64	131	16	0	0	7	2.6	2.8	0.6

t = Trace of nutrient present   * = Not available

MAG, magnesium; **IRON**, iron; **ZINC**, zinc; **VITA**, vitamin A; **VITC**, vitamin C; **THIA**, thiamin; **RIBO**, riboflavin; **NIAC**, niacin; **VB6**, vitamin B-6;

FOL, folate; **VB12**, vitamin B-12; **CALC**, calcium; **PHOS**, phosphorus; **SEL**, selenium; **VE-a**, alpha tocopherol equivalents.

CHOL (mg)	SOD (mg)	POT (mg)	MAG (mg)	IRON (mg)	ZINC (mg)	VITA (RE)	VITC (mg)	THIA (mg)	RIBO (mg)	NIAC (mg)	VB6 (mg)	FOL (µg)	VB12 (µg)	CALC (mg)	PHOS (mg)	SEL (µg)	VE-a (mg)
*	984	57	*	0.7	*	62	t	0.16	0.18	2.2	*	*	*	14	44	*	*
0	12	672	*	8.5	*	0	0	0.46	0.27	5.6	*	*	0	54	551	*	*
0	1	85	24	1.3	0.7	0	0	0.2	0.11	1.5	0.09	17	0	11	70	85	0.1
*	399	52	*	1	*	0	0	0.07	0.08	1	*	*	*	37	57	*	*
*	1254	126	*	2.2	*	91	0	0.13	0.17	2.1	*	*	*	92	136	*	*
0	20	27	11	0.3	0.1	5	0	0.03	0.02	0.2	0.04	3	0	16	25	*	0.5
0	180	51	21	0.5	0.2	5	0	0.03	0.03	t	0.1	4	0	30	59	*	1.2
0	165	9	6	0.3	0.1	0	t	0.03	0.02	0.1	0.01	8	0.07	8	18	*	0.4
5	101	31	2	0.1	0.2	0	2	0.04	0.02	0.5	0.02	t	0.11	1	21	1	t
9	307	76	4	0.3	0.6	2	4	0.08	0.06	0.5	0.06	2	0.39	13	30	3	*
78	50	244	18	2.2	4.7	0	0	0.07	0.18	2.9	0.26	6	2.03	8	164	25	0.1
78	55	186	14	1.9	4.5	0	0	0.05	0.15	2.4	0.2	5	1.91	8	147	25	0.1
65	2464	315	23	3.2	3.7	*	0	0.05	0.23	2.7	*	*	1.31	4	124	38	*
164	54	198	21	6.4	2.7	0	1	0.12	1.31	3.5	0.18	2	12.2	5	213	48	0.5
410	90	309	20	5.3	4.6	9216	19	0.18	3.52	12.3	1.22	187	95	9	392	48	0.5
101	66	289	24	3.8	8.7	0	0	0.08	0.29	3.7	0.33	11	3.4	9	268	6	0.1
106	71	263	23	3.7	10.3	0	0	0.08	0.28	2.7	0.29	6	2.47	13	235	6	0.1
80	69	394	27	2.6	7	0	0	0.11	0.22	4.8	0.4	8	3.32	13	208	6	0.1
97	815	126	30	2.3	4.9	8	0	0.11	0.14	2.7	0.5	11	3.27	11	110	*	0.1
84	63	419	30	3.6	5.6	0	0	0.13	0.3	3.9	0.38	8	0.44	7	238	*	0.2
4	62	10	1	0.1	0.1	0	1	t	0.01	0.2	0.01	t	0.12	1	6	2	t
4	74	15	1	t	0.1	0	2	0.03	0.01	0.2	0.02	t	0.05	t	6	2	t
38	718	176	12	0.4	1	4	0	0.27	0.11	2.7	0.15	4	0.53	10	95	10	*
14	272	65	3	0.2	0.5	0	8	0.12	0.04	0.9	0.06	1	0.21	3	32	4	t
51	473	180	12	1.1	2	0	1	0.43	0.16	2.7	0.18	2	0.81	38	126	25	*
28	206	36	2	1.7	0.5	759	2	0.05	0.28	1.5	0.06	8	3.62	2	30	2	0.1
93	72	287	23	2.8	6.9	0	0	0.07	0.22	3.8	0.3	8	2.55	6	239	5	0.1
14	360	91	5	0.2	0.4	0	5	0.19	0.05	1.6	0.11	1	0.18	3	69	3	0.1
29	465	89	5	0.5	1	16	8	0.11	0.07	1.3	0.05	1	0.74	25	76	10	0.1
41	11	2	3	1.1	1.4	0	0	0	0.02	t	t	1	0.29	8	13	*	0.1
53	741	239	11	1	2.1	0	0	0.38	0.18	3.1	0.32	1	1.2	5	90	10	0.1
50	1188	440	*	4.4	*	*	*	0.02	0.2	4.6	*	*	*	29	147	*	0.1
13	270	29	3	0.6	1.2	0	2	0	0.03	0.5	0.03	2	0.36	3	21	7	0.1
73	855	116	12	1.8	3	0	t	0.02	0.2	2.9	0.11	3	1.38	17	94	21	0.1
29	639	95	6	0.7	1.1	0	15	0.11	0.07	1.5	0.08	2	0.74	6	49	5	0.1
32	119	65	6	0.3	0.3	0	1	0.03	0.06	0.3	0.03	6	0.11	5	39	*	0.5
16	381	84	5	0.3	0.6	7	7	0.17	0.05	1	0.07	1	0.23	17	72	*	t
9	179	24	3	0.1	0.3	14	1	0.05	0.03	0.3	0.02	t	0.11	33	74	*	0
6	137	23	2	0.1	0.2	0	1	0.07	0.02	0.3	0.02	t	0.11	1	18	*	0
16	373	94	5	0.3	0.6	0	8	0.24	0.07	1.5	0.1	1	0.24	2	70	13	0
10	287	60	3	0.2	0.4	0	0	0.11	0.04	0.7	0.07	1	0.15	1	29	10	0
42	1589	487	29	1.3	3.1	0	39	1.45	0.35	6.9	0.63	7	0.99	8	293	66	0.4
87	1317	500	24	1.9	3.5	0	20	1.15	0.36	7.4	0.42	7	1.48	11	340	66	0.4
10	160	*	2	0.3	0.2	0	*	0.02	0.01	0.2	0.04	*	0.09	1	12	2	0
74	1684	402	20	2.1	4	0	29	1.06	0.28	5.6	0.56	5	0.91	11	275	66	0.4
77	1858	442	31	1.3	3.6	0	t	0.95	0.36	7	0.66	6	0.98	10	318	66	0.4
15	261	65	3	0.2	0.4	0	6	0.15	0.04	0.9	0.06	t	0.2	2	33	10	*
83	2100	573	30	1.9	3.5	0	32	1.02	0.46	8.6	0.43	4	0.98	12	393	66	0.4
71	60	266	18	2	4.6	6	0	0.05	0.23	4.2	0.23	8	1.84	6	137	20	0.3
74	65	256	18	1.8	4.6	9	0	0.04	0.18	4.4	0.22	8	2	9	134	20	0.3
74	51	188	13	2.1	4.2	0	0	0.03	0.14	4	0.2	7	1.99	8	117	*	0.3
75	71	255	17	2.1	4.3	0	0	0.03	0.17	5	0.2	8	2.3	10	145	*	0.3
23	357	9	3	0.3	0.4	*	6	0.01	0.05	0.3	0.05	1	0.3	5	17	5	*
52	618	204	12	1	1.6	0	1	0.42	0.16	2.8	0.22	3	0.87	16	114	22	0.1
17	280	71	4	0.4	0.5	0	5	0.06	0.06	0.7	0.05	1	0.42	11	39	4	t
39	687	136	8	0.6	1.1	0	18	0.23	0.1	1.9	0.11	1	0.8	7	67	10	0
84	64	230	20	1.6	3.4	0	0	0.08	0.19	6	0.09	12	2.16	16	151	14	0.1
52	49	178	17	1.3	3	0	0	0.06	0.14	3.7	0.09	12	1.5	9	121	10	0.1
79	56	266	20	1.7	3.7	*	*	0.09	0.23	5.6	0.13	17	2.2	9	162	14	t
63	48	240	19	1.5	3.5	*	*	0.08	0.21	4.5	0.12	16	1.87	6	146	12	t
78	56	214	19	1.7	4.4	*	*	0.08	0.2	5.2	0.11	18	2.24	17	156	14	0.1
56	44	170	16	1.4	3.9	*	*	0.06	0.17	3.7	0.1	16	1.73	12	128	11	0.1

WT, weight; **KCAL**, kcalories; **PROT**, protein; **CARB**, carbohydrate; **FIBR**, fiber; **FAT**, fat; **SATF**, saturated fat;

MONO, monosaturated fat; **POLY**, polyunsaturated fat; **CHOR**, cholesterol; **SOD**, sodium; **POT**, potassium;

Food Name	Portion	WT (Gm)	KCAL	PROT (Gm)	CARB (Gm)	FIBR (Gm)	FAT (Gm)	SATF (Gm)	MONO (Gm)	POLY (Gm)
LIVER CHEESE-PORK	SLICE	38	116	6	1	0	10	3.4	4.7	1.3
LIVERWURST-LIVER SAUSAGE-PORK	SLICE	18	59	3	t	0	5	1.9	2.4	0.5
MORTADELLA-PORK AND BEEF	SLICE	15	47	2	t	0	4	1.4	1.7	0.5
OLIVE LOAF-PORK	SLICE	28.4	67	3	3	0	5	1.7	2.2	0.6
PEPPERONI-PORK AND BEEF	SLICE	5.5	27	1	t	0	2	0.9	1.2	0.2
PIMENTO/PICKLE LOAF-PORK	SLICE	28.4	74	3	2	*	6	2.2	2.7	0.7
POLISH SAUSAGE-PORK	ITEM	227	740	32	4	0	65	23.4	30.6	7
PORK CHOP-LOIN-BROILED-LEAN AND FAT	ITEM	82	284	19	0	0	22	8.1	10.2	2.5
PORK CHOP-LOIN-BROILED-LEAN ONLY	ITEM	66	169	18	0	0	10	3.5	4.5	1.2
PORK-CENTER LOIN-ROASTED-LEAN AND FAT	ITEM	88	268	22	0	0	19	6.9	8.8	2.2
PORK-CENTER LOIN-ROASTED-LEAN ONLY	SLICE	72	173	21	0	0	9	3.3	4.2	1.1
PORK-FEET-PICKLED	OUNCE	28.4	58	4	t	0	5	1.6	2.2	0.5
PORK-FEET-SIMMERED	OUNCE	28.4	55	5	0	0	4	1.2	1.7	0.4
PORK-KIDNEYS-BRAISED	CUP	140	211	36	0	0	7	2.1	2.2	0.5
PORK-LIVER-BRAISED	OUNCE	28.4	47	7	1	0	1	0.4	0.2	0.3
PORK-SHOULDER-ROASTED-LEAN ONLY	CUP	140	342	36	0	0	21	7.2	9.4	2.6
PORK-SPARERIBS-BRAISED	OUNCE	28.4	113	8	0	0	9	3.3	4	1
PORK-TENDERLOIN-ROASTED-LEAN ONLY	OUNCE	28.4	47	8	0	0	1	0.5	0.6	0.2
PORK-TONGUE-BRAISED	SERVING	85	230	21	0	0	16	5.5	7.5	1.6
POTTED MEAT-CANNED-BEEF/CHICKEN/TURKEY	TBSP	13	30	2	0	0	2	0.8	0.9	0.1
RABBIT-STEWED-BONELESS-SKINLESS	SERVING	85	175	26	0	0	7	2.1	1.9	1.4
ROAST BEEF-BOTTOM ROUND-COOKED-LEAN ONLY	SLICE	78	173	25	0	0	8	2.7	3.4	0.3
ROAST BEEF-BOTTOM ROUND-LEAN AND FAT	SLICE	85	222	25	0	0	13	4.8	5.7	0.5
ROAST BEEF-RIB-BROILED-LEAN AND FAT	SLICE	85	308	18	0	0	26	10.8	11.4	0.9
ROAST BEEF-RIB-BROILED-LEAN ONLY	SLICE	51	122	14	0	0	7	3	3.1	0.2
SALAMI-COOKED-BEEF-4 BY 1/8 INCH SLICE	SLICE	23	60	3	1	0	5	2.1	2.2	0.2
SALAMI-DRY OR HARD-PORK-SLICE	SLICE	10	41	2	t	0	3	1.2	1.6	0.4
SAUSAGE-LINK-COOKED-PORK	ITEM	13	48	3	t	0	4	1.4	1.8	0.5
SAUSAGE-PATTY-COOKED-FRESH PORK	ITEM	27	100	5	t	0	8	2.9	3.8	1
SAUSAGE-VIENNA-CANNED-BEEF AND PORK	ITEM	16	45	2	t	0	4	1.5	2	0.3
STEAK-SIRLOIN-BROILED-LEAN AND FAT	ITEM	85	238	23	0	0	15	6.4	6.9	0.6
STEAK-SIRLOIN-BROILED-LEAN ONLY	ITEM	56	116	17	0	0	5	2	2.2	0.2
STEAK-TOP ROUND-BROILED-LEAN AND FAT	SLICE	85	179	26	0	0	7	2.8	3.1	0.3
STEAK-TOP ROUND-BROILED-LEAN ONLY	SLICE	68	130	22	0	0	4	1.5	1.7	0.2
SWEETBREADS-CALF-BRAISED	SERVING	85	143	28	0	0	3	*	*	*
THURINGER/CERVELAT-PORK	SLICE	23	77	4	t	0	7	2.8	3	0.3
VEAL-LEG-TOP ROUND-PAN FRIED	SERVING	85	179	27	0	0	7	2.7	2.8	0.5
VEAL-RIB-SEPARABLE LEAN ONLY-BRAISED	SERVING	85	185	29	0	0	7	2.2	2.2	0.6
VEAL-SHOULDER-ARM-LEAN ONLY-ROASTED	SERVING	85	139	22	0	0	5	2	1.8	0.4
VENISON-DRIED-SALTED	SERVING	100	142	31	0	0	1	*	*	0.1
VENISON-ROASTED	SLICE	100	146	30	0	0	2	2.1	1.1	1.9

Miscellaneous

Food Name	Portion	WT (Gm)	KCAL	PROT (Gm)	CARB (Gm)	FIBR (Gm)	FAT (Gm)	SATF (Gm)	MONO (Gm)	POLY (Gm)
BAKING POWDER-LOW SODIUM	TSP	4.3	7	t	2	*	0	0	0	0
BAKING POWDER-NO CALCIUM SULFATE	TSP	3	4	t	1	*	0	0	0	0
BAKING POWDER-STRAIGHT PHOSPHATE	TSP	3.8	5	t	1	*	0	0	0	0
BAKING POWDER-WITH CALCIUM SULFATE	TSP	2.9	3	t	1	*	0	0	0	0
BAKING SODA	TSP	3	0	0	0	0	0	0	0	0
CHEWING GUM-CANDY COATED	ITEM	1.7	5	0	2	0	t	0	0	0
CHEWING GUM-WRIGLEYS	ITEM	3	10	0	2	0	0	0	0	0
GELATIN DESSERT-PREPARED	CUP	240	140	4	34	0	0	0	0	0
GELATIN-D ZERTA-LOW CALORIE-PREPARED	CUP	240	16	4	0	0	0	0	0	0
GELATIN-DRY-ENVELOPE	ITEM	7	25	6	0	0	0	0	0	0
GELATIN-JELLO-SUGAR FREE-PREPARED	CUP	240	16	2	0	0	0	0	0	0
OLIVES-GREEN-PICKLED-CANNED	ITEM	4	4	t	t	0.1	1	0.1	0.4	t
OLIVES-MISSION-RIPE-CANNED	ITEM	3	5	t	t	0.1	1	0.1	0.4	t
PICKLE RELISH-HAMBURGER-HEINZ	OUNCE	28.4	30	0	7	*	0	0	0	0
PICKLE RELISH-HOT DOG-HEINZ	OUNCE	28.4	35	0	8	*	0	0	0	0
PICKLE RELISH-SWEET-CHOPPED	TBSP	15	20	0	5	0.3	0	0	0	0
PICKLE-DILL-CUCUMBER-MEDIUM SIZED	ITEM	65	5	0	1	0.8	0	0	0	0
PICKLE-FRESH PACK-CUCUMBER-SLICED	ITEM	7.5	5	0	2	0.1	0	0	0	0
PICKLE-SWEET/GHERKIN-SMALL-WHOLE	ITEM	15	20	0	5	0.2	0	0	0	0
POPSICLE	ITEM	95	70	0	18	0	0	0	0	0

t = Trace of nutrient present   * = Not available

MAG, magnesium; **IRON**, iron; **ZINC**, zinc; **VITA**, vitamin A; **VITC**, vitamin C; **THIA**, thiamin; **RIBO**, riboflavin; **NIAC**, niacin; **VB6**, vitamin B-6; **FOL**, folate; **VB12**, vitamin B-12; **CALC**, calcium; **PHOS**, phosphorus; **SEL**, selenium; **VE-a**, alpha tocopherol equivalents.

CHOL (mg)	SOD (mg)	POT (mg)	MAG (mg)	IRON (mg)	ZINC (mg)	VITA (RE)	VITC (mg)	THIA (mg)	RIBO (mg)	NIAC (mg)	VB6 (mg)	FOL (µg)	VB12 (µg)	CALC (mg)	PHOS (mg)	SEL (µg)	VE-a (mg)
66	466	86	5	4.1	1.4	1996	1	0.08	0.85	4.5	0.18	40	9.33	3	79	6	0.1
28	215	36	2	1.2	0.5	760	2	0.05	0.19	1.5	0.03	5	2.42	5	41	3	0.1
8	187	25	2	0.2	0.3	0	4	0.02	0.02	0.4	0.02	t	0.22	3	15	2	t
11	421	84	5	0.2	0.4	6	3	0.08	0.07	0.5	0.07	1	0.36	31	36	4	0.1
4	112	19	1	0.1	0.1	0	0	0.02	0.01	0.3	0.01	t	0.14	1	7	1	t
11	394	97	5	0.3	0.4	2	4	0.08	0.07	0.6	0.05	1	0.34	27	40	4	*
159	1989	538	32	3.3	4.4	0	2	1.14	0.34	7.8	0.43	5	2.22	27	309	66	0.4
77	54	287	20	0.7	2	2	t	0.69	0.29	4.3	0.31	4	0.81	5	193	14	0.1
63	49	276	19	0.6	1.9	2	t	0.64	0.28	3.9	0.3	4	0.71	5	184	11	0.1
80	56	284	17	0.9	1.8	2	t	0.73	0.21	4.4	0.35	1	0.53	5	173	28	0.1
66	50	261	15	0.8	1.6	2	t	0.65	0.19	3.9	0.32	1	0.43	4	158	23	0.1
26	262	67	1	0.2	0.4	0	0	t	0.01	0.1	0.11	1	0.18	9	10	*	0.1
28	9	42	1	0.1	0.3	0	0	t	0.02	0.1	0.03	t	0.05	13	14	*	0.1
673	111	200	25	7.4	5.8	109	15	0.55	2.22	8.1	0.65	57	10.9	18	337	294	0.6
101	14	43	4	5.1	1.9	1531	7	0.07	0.62	2.4	0.16	46	5.3	3	68	20	0.1
136	106	493	28	2.1	5.9	3	t	0.82	0.51	6	0.56	7	1.23	11	323	43	0.2
34	26	91	7	0.5	1.3	1	0	0.12	0.11	1.6	0.1	1	0.31	13	74	5	t
26	19	153	7	0.4	0.9	1	t	0.27	0.11	1.3	0.12	2	0.16	3	82	9	0.1
124	93	201	17	4.2	3.9	0	1	0.27	0.43	4.5	0.2	3	2.03	16	148	*	0.3
15	156	*	*	*	*	*	*	0	0.03	0.2	*	*	*	*	*	2	0
73	32	255	17	2	2	0	0	0.05	0.15	6.1	0.29	8	5.53	17	192	*	1.6
75	40	240	20	2.7	4.3	0	0	0.06	0.2	3.2	0.28	9	1.93	4	212	19	0.1
81	43	248	20	2.8	4.4	0	0	0.06	0.21	3.3	0.29	9	2.04	5	217	20	0.1
73	52	257	17	1.8	4.3	0	0	0.07	0.15	2.7	0.25	5	2.37	10	140	20	0.1
41	38	192	13	1.3	3.5	0	0	0.04	0.11	2.1	0.15	4	1.49	5	109	12	0.1
15	270	52	3	0.5	0.5	0	4	0.02	0.04	0.7	0.05	t	1.11	2	26	4	t
8	226	38	2	0.1	0.4	0	0	0.09	0.03	0.6	0.06	t	0.28	1	23	2	t
11	168	47	2	0.2	0.3	0	0	0.1	0.03	0.6	0.04	t	0.22	4	24	4	t
22	349	97	5	0.3	0.7	0	0	0.2	0.07	1.2	0.09	1	0.47	9	50	3	t
8	152	16	1	0.1	0.3	0	0	0.01	0.02	0.3	0.02	1	0.16	2	8	8	0
77	54	306	24	2.6	4.9	15	0	0.1	0.22	3.3	0.34	8	2.26	9	185	29	0.1
50	37	226	18	1.9	3.7	3	0	0.07	0.17	2.4	0.25	6	1.6	6	137	19	0.1
72	51	365	26	2.4	4.6	0	0	0.1	0.22	5	0.46	10	2.08	5	203	29	0.1
57	42	301	21	2	3.8	0	0	0.08	0.18	4.1	0.38	8	1.69	4	167	23	0.1
*	*	*	*	*	*	*	*	0.05	0.14	2.5	*	*	*	*	*	*	*
17	286	62	3	0.6	0.6	0	5	0.04	0.08	1	0.06	t	1.27	3	26	3	t
89	64	362	26	0.8	2.8	0	t	0.06	0.3	1	0.41	13	1.23	5	237	10	t
123	84	270	22	1.2	5.1	0	0	0.05	0.26	6.7	0.29	14	1.3	20	186	10	t
93	77	302	23	1	3.7	0	0	0.06	0.28	7	0.25	15	1.33	23	192	*	0.3
*	*	*	*	1.9	*	*	*	0.09	0.34	10	*	*	*	60	298	*	*
82	70	336	29	3.5	4.5	0	0	0.37	0.28	7.4	0.26	7	6.22	20	264	*	t
0	t	471	*	0	*	0	0	0	0	0	*	*	*	207	314	*	*
0	329	5	*	0	*	0	0	0	0	0	*	*	*	58	87	*	*
0	312	6	*	0	*	0	0	0	0	0	*	*	*	239	359	*	*
0	290	4	*	0	*	0	0	0	0	0	*	*	*	183	45	*	*
0	821	*	*	*	*	0	0	0	0	0	0	0	0	*	*	*	0
0	t	0	0	0	0	0	0	0	0	0	0	0	0	t	0	*	0
0	0	0	0	0	0	0	0	0	0	0	0	0	0	3	0	*	0
0	0	0	0	0	0	0	0	0	0	0	0	0	0	5	46	16	0
0	20	3	2	t	0.1	0	0	0	0	0	0	t	0	6	0	*	0
0	8	180	*	0.4	0	0	4	0	0	0	0	0	0	0	0	2	0
0	120	*	*	*	*	*	*	*	*	*	*	*	*	*	*	*	*
0	81	2	1	0.1	t	1	0	0	0	t	0	t	0	2	1	0	0.1
0	19	1	1	t	t	1	0	0	0	t	0	t	0	3	t	0	0.1
0	325	*	*	0.2	*	*	*	*	*	*	*	*	*	6	4	0	*
0	200	*	*	0.2	*	*	*	*	*	*	*	*	*	6	4	0	*
0	124	30	1	0.1	t	2	1	0	t	0	t	1	0	3	2	0	t
0	928	130	8	0.7	0.2	7	4	0	0.01	0	0.01	1	0	17	14	0	0.1
0	50	15	t	0.2	t	1	1	0	0	0	t	t	0	3	2	0	t
0	128	30	t	0.2	t	1	1	0	0	0	t	t	0	2	2	0	t
0	0	4	0	0	0	0	0	0	0	0	0	0	0	0	0	*	0

WT, weight; **KCAL,** kcalories; **PROT,** protein; **CARB,** carbohydrate; **FIBR,** fiber; **FAT,** fat; **SATF,** saturated fat;
MONO, monosaturated fat; **POLY,** polyunsaturated fat; **CHOR,** cholesterol; **SOD,** sodium; **POT,** potassium;

Food Name	Portion	WT (Gm)	KCAL	PROT (Gm)	CARB (Gm)	FIBR (Gm)	FAT (Gm)	SATF (Gm)	MONO (Gm)	POLY (Gm)
VANILLA-PURE	TSP	4.7	14	0	1	0	0	0	0	0
VINEGAR-CIDER	TBSP	15	0	0	1	0	0	0	0	0
VINEGAR-DISTILLED	CUP	240	29	0	12	0	0	0	0	0
YEAST-BAKER'S-DRY-ACTIVE-PACKAGE	SERVING	7	20	3	3	2.2	0	0	0	0
YEAST-BREWER'S-DRY	TBSP	8	25	3	3	2.5	0	0	0	0

Nuts & Seeds

Food Name	Portion	WT (Gm)	KCAL	PROT (Gm)	CARB (Gm)	FIBR (Gm)	FAT (Gm)	SATF (Gm)	MONO (Gm)	POLY (Gm)
ALMOND BUTTER-PLAIN	TBSP	16	101	2	3	1.8	9	0.9	6.1	2
NUT-FILBERT/HAZEL-DRIED-CHOPPED	CUP	115	727	15	18	9.8	72	5.3	56.5	6.9
NUT-WALNUT-PERSIAN/ENGLISH	CUP	120	770	17	22	5.8	74	6.7	17	47
NUTS-ALMONDS-UNBLANCHED-SHELLED-CHOPPED	CUP	130	766	26	27	12.1	68	6.4	44.1	14.2
NUTS-ALMONDS-UNBLANCHED-SHELLED-SLIVERED	CUP	115	677	23	24	10.7	60	5.7	39	12.6
NUTS-BEECHNUTS-DRIED	OUNCE	28.4	164	2	10	2.6	14	1.6	6.2	5.7
NUTS-BRAZIL-DRIED-SHELLED	CUP	140	918	20	18	10.8	93	22.6	32.2	33.8
NUTS-BUTTERNUTS-DRIED	OUNCE	28.4	174	7	3	2.4	16	0.4	3	12.1
NUTS-CASHEWS-DRY ROASTED	CUP	137	786	21	45	10	64	12.5	37.4	10.7
NUTS-CASHEWS-OIL ROASTED	CUP	130	749	21	37	7.8	63	12.4	36.9	10.6
NUTS-HICKORY-DRIED	OUNCE	28.4	187	4	5	2.4	18	2	9.3	6.2
NUTS-MACADAMIA-DRIED	CUP	134	941	11	18	12.4	99	14.8	77.9	1.7
NUTS-MACADAMIA-OIL ROASTED	CUP	134	962	10	17	9.3	103	15.4	80.9	1.8
NUTS-MIXED-DRY ROASTED	CUP	137	814	24	35	11.6	71	9.5	43	14.8
NUTS-MIXED-OIL ROASTED	CUP	142	876	24	30	12.8	80	12.4	45	18.9
NUTS-PEANUTS-OIL ROASTED	CUP	144	837	38	27	12.8	71	9.9	35.2	22.4
NUTS-PEANUTS-OIL ROASTED-SALTED	CUP	144	837	38	27	12.8	71	9.9	35.2	22.4
NUTS-PEANUTS-SPANISH-DRIED	CUP	146	828	38	24	11.7	72	10	35.7	22.7
NUTS-PECANS-DRIED-HALVES	CUP	108	720	8	20	7	73	5.9	45.5	18.1
NUTS-PECANS-OIL ROASTED	CUP	110	754	8	18	8.5	78	6.3	48.8	19.4
NUTS-PISTACHIO-DRIED	CUP	128	739	26	32	13.8	62	7.8	41.8	9.4
NUTS-PISTACHIO-DRY ROASTED	CUP	128	776	19	35	13.8	68	8.6	45.6	10.2
NUTS-SOYBEAN KERNELS-ROASTED	CUP	108	489	40	33	9.2	26	3.4	6	13.8
NUTS-WALNUT-BLACK-DRIED-CHOPPED	CUP	125	759	30	15	8.1	71	4.5	15.9	46.9
NUTS-WALNUTS-FINELY GROUND	CUP	80	486	20	10	5.2	45	2.9	10.2	29.9
PEANUT BUTTER-CHUNK STYLE	TBSP	16.1	95	4	3	1.1	8	1.5	3.8	2.3
PEANUT BUTTER-LOW SODIUM-PETER PAN	TBSP	16	95	5	3	1.7	9	1.4	4	2.5
PEANUT BUTTER-OLD FASHIONED	TBSP	16	95	4	3	1.1	8	1.5	3.8	2.7
PEANUT BUTTER-SMOOTH TYPE	TBSP	16	94	4	3	1	8	1.5	3.8	2.3
SEEDS-BREADFRUIT-ROASTED	OUNCE	28.4	59	2	11	8	1	0.2	0.1	0.4
SEEDS-PUMPKIN/SQUASH-DRIED	CUP	138	747	34	25	14.8	63	12	19.7	28.8
SEEDS-PUMPKIN/SQUASH-ROASTED	CUP	64	285	12	34	29.4	12	2.4	3.9	5.7
SEEDS-SESAME-DRIED-WHOLE	CUP	144	825	26	34	21.6	72	10	27	31.4
SEEDS-SESAME-ROASTED-WHOLE	OUNCE	28.4	161	5	7	5.3	14	1.9	5.2	6
SEEDS-SUNFLOWER-DRIED	CUP	144	821	33	27	9.8	71	7.5	13.6	47.1
SEEDS-SUNFLOWER-OIL ROASTED	CUP	135	830	29	20	9.2	78	8.1	14.8	51.2

Poultry

Food Name	Portion	WT (Gm)	KCAL	PROT (Gm)	CARB (Gm)	FIBR (Gm)	FAT (Gm)	SATF (Gm)	MONO (Gm)	POLY (Gm)
CHICK-BREAST-NO SKIN-ROASTED	ITEM	172	284	53	0	0	6	1.7	2.1	1.3
CHICK-THIGH-NO SKIN-ROASTED	ITEM	52	109	14	0	0	6	1.6	2.2	1.3
CHICKEN FRANKFURTER	ITEM	45	116	6	3	0	9	2.5	3.8	1.8
CHICKEN ROLL-LIGHT	SLICE	28.4	45	6	1	0	2	0.6	0.8	0.5
CHICKEN SPREAD-CANNED	TBSP	13	25	2	1	0	2	1.7	0.8	0.1
CHICKEN-BACK-FRIED-FLOUR COATED	ITEM	144	477	40	9	0.2	30	8.1	11.8	6.9
CHICKEN-BACK-STEWED	ITEM	122	316	27	0	0	22	6.1	8.7	4.9
CHICKEN-BREAST-NO SKIN-FRIED	ITEM	172	322	58	1	0	8	2.2	3	1.8
CHICKEN-BREAST-ROASTED	ITEM	196	386	58	0	0	15	4.3	5.9	3.3
CHICKEN-BREAST-STEWED	ITEM	220	404	60	0	0	16	4.6	6.4	3.5
CHICKEN-BREAST-WITH SKIN-FRIED IN BATTER	ITEM	280	728	70	25	*	37	9.9	15.3	8.6
CHICKEN-BREAST-WITH SKIN-FRIED IN FLOUR	ITEM	196	436	62	3	0.1	17	4.8	6.9	3.8
CHICKEN-CANNED-BONELESS-WITH BROTH	ITEM	142	234	31	0	0	11	3.1	4.5	2.5
CHICKEN-CAPON-ROASTED	ITEM	1274	2914	369	0	0	148	41.6	60.5	32.1
CHICKEN-DRUMSTICK-WITH SKIN-FRIED/FLOUR	ITEM	49	120	13	1	0	7	1.8	2.7	1.6
CHICKEN-GIBLETS-FRIED-FLOUR COATED	CUP	145	402	47	6	*	20	5.5	6.4	4.9
CHICKEN-GIBLETS-SIMMERED	CUP	145	228	38	1	0	7	2.2	1.7	1.6
CHICKEN-GIZZARD-SIMMERED	CUP	145	222	39	2	0	5	1.5	1.4	1.5

t = Trace of nutrient present   ** = Not available*

MAG, magnesium; IRON, iron; ZINC, zinc; VITA, vitamin A; VITC, vitamin C; THIA, thiamin; RIBO, riboflavin; NIAC, niacin; VB6, vitamin B-6; FOL, folate; VB12, vitamin B-12; CALC, calcium; PHOS, phosphorus; SEL, selenium; VE-a, alpha tocopherol equivalents.

CHOL (mg)	SOD (mg)	POT (mg)	MAG (mg)	IRON (mg)	ZINC (mg)	VITA (RE)	VITC (mg)	THIA (mg)	RIBO (mg)	NIAC (mg)	VB6 (mg)	FOL (µg)	VB12 (µg)	CALC (mg)	PHOS (mg)	SEL (µg)	VE-a (mg)
0	0	0	*	0	*	0	0	0	0	0	*	*	0	0	*	*	*
0	t	15	3	0.1	t	0	0	0	0	0	0	0	0	1	1	13	0
0	2	36	0	1.4	0	0	0	0	0	0	0	0	0	14	22	74	0
0	1	140	4	1.1	*	0	0	0.16	0.38	2.6	0.14	286	0	3	90	0	t
0	9	152	18	1.4	0.6	0	0	1.25	0.34	3	0.2	313	0	17	140	0	t
0	2	121	48	0.6	0.5	0	t	0.02	0.1	0.5	0.01	10	0	43	84	*	1.5
0	3	512	328	3.8	2.8	8	1	0.58	0.13	1.3	0.7	83	0	216	359	2	27.3
0	12	602	203	2.9	3.3	15	4	0.46	0.18	1.3	0.67	79	0	113	380	23	3.1
0	14	952	385	4.8	3.8	0	1	0.27	1.01	4.4	0.15	76	0	346	676	5	31.1
0	13	842	340	4.2	3.4	0	1	0.24	0.9	3.9	0.13	68	0	306	598	5	27.6
0	11	289	0	0.7	0.1	0	4	0.09	0.11	0.2	0.19	32	0	t	0	2	*
0	3	840	315	4.8	6.4	0	1	1.4	0.17	2.3	0.35	6	0	246	840	2260	9
0	0	119	67	1.1	0.9	3	1	0.11	0.04	0.3	0.16	19	0	15	127	2	*
0	22	774	356	8.2	7.7	0	0	0.27	0.27	1.9	0.35	95	0	62	671	7	0.8
0	22	689	332	5.3	6.2	0	0	0.55	0.23	2.3	0.33	88	0	53	554	88	0.2
0	t	124	49	0.6	1.2	4	1	0.25	0.04	0.3	0.06	11	0	17	95	2	1.5
0	7	493	155	3.2	2.3	0	0	0.47	0.15	2.9	0.26	21	0	94	182	7	4.7
0	9	441	157	2.4	1.5	1	0	0.29	0.15	2.7	0.27	21	0	60	268	7	4.7
0	16	817	308	5.1	5.2	2	1	0.27	0.27	6.4	0.41	69	0	96	596	7	8.2
0	16	825	333	4.6	7.2	3	1	0.71	0.32	7.2	0.34	118	0	153	659	7	8.5
0	8	982	266	2.6	9.6	0	0	0.36	0.16	20.6	0.37	181	0	127	744	55	10
0	624	982	266	2.6	9.6	0	0	0.36	0.16	20.6	0.37	181	0	127	744	55	10
0	26	1029	245	6.7	4.8	0	0	0.93	0.2	17.6	0.51	350	0	134	549	7	12.2
0	1	423	138	2.3	5.9	14	2	0.92	0.14	1	0.2	42	0	39	314	3	3.4
0	1	395	142	2.3	6.1	*	2	0.34	0.11	1	0.21	43	0	37	324	6	1.4
0	7	1399	203	8.7	1.7	30	9	1.05	0.22	1.4	0.32	74	0	173	644	7	6.7
0	8	1242	166	4.1	1.7	31	9	0.54	0.32	1.8	0.33	76	0	90	609	7	6.7
0	4	1588	187	4.8	3.9	22	2	0.11	0.16	1.9	0.32	244	0	149	392	*	*
0	2	655	252	3.8	4.3	37	4	0.27	0.14	0.9	0.69	82	0	72	580	24	1.1
0	1	419	161	2.5	2.7	24	3	0.18	0.09	0.6	0.44	52	0	46	371	15	0.7
0	78	121	26	0.3	0.4	0	0	0.02	0.02	2.2	0.07	15	0	7	51	1	1
0	5	110	28	0.3	0.5	0	0	0.02	0.02	2.2	0.06	13	0	5	60	2	1.1
0	75	110	30	0.3	0.5	0	0	0.01	0.01	2.3	0.06	13	0	5	60	2	1
0	77	115	25	0.3	0.4	*	0	0.02	0.02	2.1	0.06	13	0	5	52	2	1.1
0	8	307	18	0.3	0.3	8	2	0.12	0.07	2.1	0.12	17	0	24	50	4	*
0	24	1114	738	20.7	10.3	53	3	0.29	0.44	2.4	0.12	79	0	59	1620	*	1.4
0	12	588	168	2.1	6.6	4	t	0.02	0.03	0.2	0.02	6	0	35	59	*	0.6
0	16	674	505	21	11.2	1	0	1.14	0.36	6.5	1.14	139	0	1404	906	*	3.3
0	3	135	101	4.2	2	t	0	0.23	0.07	1.3	0.23	28	0	281	181	*	0.6
0	4	992	509	9.8	7.3	7	2	3.29	0.36	6.5	1.81	327	0	168	1015	111	71.7
0	4	652	171	9.1	7	7	2	0.43	0.38	5.6	1.07	316	0	76	1538	104	66.8
146	126	440	50	1.8	1.7	11	0	0.12	0.2	23.6	1.02	6	0.58	26	392	46	0.6
49	46	124	12	0.7	1.3	10	0	0.04	0.12	3.4	0.18	4	0.16	6	95	21	0.2
45	617	38	5	0.9	0.5	17	0	0.03	0.05	1.4	0.14	2	0.11	43	48	10	0.1
14	166	65	5	0.3	0.2	7	0	0.02	0.04	1.5	0.06	1	0.04	12	45	*	0.1
7	50	14	2	0.3	0.2	3	0	t	0.02	0.4	0.02	t	0.02	16	12	*	t
128	130	325	33	2.3	3.6	53	0	0.15	0.34	10.5	0.44	12	0.4	35	239	25	0.5
96	78	178	20	1.5	2.4	113	0	0.05	0.18	5.3	0.18	6	0.22	22	146	25	0.4
156	136	474	54	2	1.9	12	0	0.14	0.22	25.4	1.1	8	0.62	28	424	31	0.6
166	138	480	54	2.1	2	55	0	0.13	0.23	24.9	1.08	6	0.64	28	420	53	0.7
166	136	390	48	2	2.1	54	0	0.09	0.25	17.2	0.64	6	0.46	28	344	53	0.8
238	770	564	68	3.5	2.7	57	0	0.32	0.41	29.5	1.2	16	0.82	56	516	30	1
176	150	506	58	2.3	2.1	29	0	0.16	0.26	26.9	1.14	8	0.68	32	456	21	0.7
78	714	196	17	2.3	2	100	3	0.02	0.18	9	0.5	6	0.42	20	350	20	0.4
1098	626	3252	308	18.9	22.1	260	0	0.89	2.17	114	5.5	70	4.14	182	3140	227	4.5
44	44	112	11	0.7	1.4	12	0	0.04	0.11	3	0.17	4	0.16	6	86	5	0.2
647	164	478	37	15	9.1	5195	13	0.14	2.21	15.9	0.88	550	19.3	26	414	25	2
570	85	229	30	9.3	6.6	3234	12	0.13	1.38	6	0.49	545	14.7	18	331	25	2
281	97	259	29	6	6.4	82	2	0.04	0.35	5.8	0.17	77	2.81	14	225	25	*

WT, weight; **KCAL**, kcalories; **PROT**, protein; **CARB**, carbohydrate; **FIBR**, fiber; **FAT**, fat; **SATF**, saturated fat;

MONO, monosaturated fat; **POLY**, polyunsaturated fat; **CHOR**, cholesterol; **SOD**, sodium; **POT**, potassium;

Food Name	Portion	WT (Gm)	KCAL	PROT (Gm)	CARB (Gm)	FIBR (Gm)	FAT (Gm)	SATF (Gm)	MONO (Gm)	POLY (Gm)
CHICKEN-HEART-SIMMERED	CUP	145	268	38	t	0	12	3.3	2.9	3.3
CHICKEN-LEG-NO SKIN-ROASTED	ITEM	95	182	26	0	0	8	2.2	2.9	1.9
CHICKEN-LEG-NO SKIN-STEWED	ITEM	101	187	27	0	0	8	2.2	3	1.9
CHICKEN-LEG-ROASTED	ITEM	114	265	30	0	0	15	4.2	6	3.4
CHICKEN-LIVER PATE-CANNED	TBSP	13	26	2	1	0	2	0.5	0.7	0.3
CHICKEN-LIVER-SIMMERED	CUP	140	219	34	1	0	8	2.6	1.9	1.3
CHICKEN-THIGH-FRIED-FLOUR COATED	ITEM	62	162	17	2	t	9	2.5	3.6	2.1
CHICKEN-THIN SLICED-SMOKED-LAND O FROST	SERVING	28.4	60	5	1	0	4	1	1.4	0.8
CHICKEN-WING-FRIED-FLOUR COATED	ITEM	32	103	8	1	0	7	1.9	2.8	1.6
CHICKEN-WING-ROASTED	ITEM	34	99	9	0	0	7	1.9	2.6	1.4
CHICKEN-WING-STEWED	ITEM	40	100	9	0	0	7	1.9	2.6	1.4
DUCK-FLESH & SKIN-ROASTED	ITEM	764	2574	145	0	0	217	73.9	98.6	27.9
DUCK-NO SKIN-ROASTED	ITEM	442	890	104	0	0	50	18.4	16.4	6.3
GOOSE-FLESH & SKIN-ROASTED	ITEM	1548	4721	389	0	0	339	106	159	39
GOOSE-LIVER PATE-SMOKED-CANNED	TBSP	13	60	1	1	0	6	*	*	*
GOOSE-NO SKIN-ROASTED	ITEM	1182	2813	342	0	0	150	53.9	51.3	18.3
TURKEY HAM-CURED THIGH MEAT	SLICE	28.4	37	5	t	0	1	0.5	0.3	0.4
TURKEY LOAF-BREAST	SERVING	28.4	31	6	0	0	t	0.1	0.1	0.1
TURKEY PASTRAMI	SLICE	28.4	40	5	t	0	2	1	0.6	0.5
TURKEY ROLL-LIGHT	OUNCE	28.4	42	5	t	0	2	0.6	0.7	0.5
TURKEY ROLL-LIGHT AND DARK	OUNCE	28.4	42	5	1	0	2	0.6	0.7	0.5
TURKEY-BREAST-NO SKIN-ROASTED	ITEM	612	826	184	0	0	5	1.4	0.8	1.2
TURKEY-DARK MEAT-NO SKIN-ROASTED	CUP	140	262	40	0	0	10	3.4	2.3	3
TURKEY-GIBLETS-SIMMERED	CUP	145	242	39	3	0	7	2.2	1.7	1.7
TURKEY-GIZZARD-SIMMERED	CUP	145	236	43	1	0	6	1.6	1.1	1.6
TURKEY-LIGHT MEAT-NO SKIN-ROASTED	CUP	140	219	42	0	0	5	1.4	0.8	1.2
TURKEY-LIGHT/DARK MEAT-NO SKIN-ROASTED	CUP	140	238	41	0	0	7	2.3	1.5	2
TURKEY-LIVER-SIMMERED	CUP	140	237	34	5	0	8	2.6	2.1	1.5
TURKEY-THIN SLICED-SMOKED-LAND O FROST	SERVING	28.4	50	5	1	0	3	0.8	0.9	0.7

Sauces & Dips

Food Name	Portion	WT (Gm)	KCAL	PROT (Gm)	CARB (Gm)	FIBR (Gm)	FAT (Gm)	SATF (Gm)	MONO (Gm)	POLY (Gm)
CATSUP-TOMATO-HEINZ LITE	TBSP	15	8	t	2	*	0	0	0	0
CATSUP-TOMATO-LOW SODIUM-HEINZ	TBSP	15	8	t	2	*	0	0	0	0
DIP-BACON AND HORSERADISH-KRAFT	TBSP	15	30	1	2	*	3	*	*	*
DIP-BUTTERMILK-KRAFT	TBSP	15	40	1	1	*	4	*	*	*
DIP-CLAM-KRAFT	TBSP	15	30	1	2	*	2	*	*	*
DIP-FRENCH ONION-KRAFT	TBSP	15	30	1	2	*	2	*	*	*
DIP-GARLIC-KRAFT	TBSP	15	30	1	2	*	2	*	*	*
DIP-GREEN ONION-KRAFT	TBSP	15	25	1	2	*	2	*	*	*
DIP-GUACAMOLE-KRAFT	TBSP	15	25	1	2	*	2	*	*	*
DIP-JALAPENO BEAN-FRITOS	OUNCE	28.4	33	2	3	1.9	1	0.2	0.4	0.9
DIP-JALAPENO PEPPER-KRAFT	TBSP	15	25	1	2	*	2	*	*	*
GRAVY-BEEF-CANNED	CUP	233	123	9	11	0.1	5	2.7	2.2	0.2
GRAVY-BROWN-FROM DRY-PREPARED WITH WATER	CUP	258	75	2	13	t	2	0.8	0.7	0.1
GRAVY-CHICKEN-CANNED	CUP	238	188	5	13	2.1	14	3.4	6.1	3.4
GRAVY-MUSHROOM-CANNED	CUP	238	119	3	13	1	6	1	2.8	2.4
GRAVY-PORK-FROM DRY-PREPARED WITH WATER	CUP	258	77	2	13	*	2	0.7	0.9	0.2
GRAVY-TURKEY-CANNED	CUP	238	121	6	12	*	5	1.5	2.1	1.2
HORSERADISH-PREPARED	TBSP	15	6	t	1	0.3	0	0	0	0
MUSTARD-BROWN-PREPARED	CUP	250	228	15	13	2.1	16	7.7	14	30.8
MUSTARD-LOW SODIUM-FEATHERWEIGHT	TSP	5	4	t	t	*	t	*	*	*
MUSTARD-YELLOW-PREPARED	TSP	5	5	t	t	0.1	t	0	0	0
SAUCE-BARBECUE-READY TO SERVE	CUP	250	188	5	32	2.3	5	0.7	1.9	1.7
SAUCE-BEARNAISE-FROM DRY MIX-MILK/BUTTER	CUP	255	701	8	18	0.1	68	41.8	19.9	3
SAUCE-CHEESE-FROM DRY MIX-MILK/BUTTER	CUP	279	307	16	23	0.1	17	9.3	5.3	1.6
SAUCE-CHILI-BOTTLED	TBSP	15	16	t	4	*	0	0	0	0
SAUCE-CHILI-LOW SODIUM	TBSP	14.2	8	0	2	*	0	0	0	0
SAUCE-CURRY-FROM DRY MIX-MADE WITH MILK	CUP	272	269	11	26	0.9	15	6	5.1	2.8
SAUCE-HOLLANDAISE-DRY MIX-MADE WITH MILK	CUP	255	703	8	18	0.1	68	41.9	20	2.9
SAUCE-MARINARA-CANNED	CUP	250	170	4	26	*	8	1.2	4.3	2.3
SAUCE-MUSHROOM-DRY MIX-MADE WITH MILK	CUP	267	227	11	24	0.5	10	5.4	3.3	1.1
SAUCE-PICANTE-CANNED	FL OZ	16	9	t	2	*	1	0	0	0
SAUCE-SALSA WITH GREEN CHILIES-CANNED	FL OZ	16	10	t	2	*	1	0	0	0
SAUCE-SOUR CREAM-FROM MIX-WITH MILK	CUP	314	509	19	45	*	30	16.1	9.9	2.8

t = Trace of nutrient present   * = Not available

MAG, magnesium; **IRON**, iron; **ZINC**, zinc; **VITA**, vitamin A; **VITC**, vitamin C; **THIA**, thiamin; **RIBO**, riboflavin; **NIAC**, niacin; **VB6**, vitamin B-6;

FOL, folate; **VB12**, vitamin B-12; **CALC**, calcium; **PHOS**, phosphorus; **SEL**, selenium; **VE-a**, alpha tocopherol equivalents.

CHOL (mg)	SOD (mg)	POT (mg)	MAG (mg)	IRON (mg)	ZINC (mg)	VITA (RE)	VITC (mg)	THIA (mg)	RIBO (mg)	NIAC (mg)	VB6 (mg)	FOL (µg)	VB12 (µg)	CALC (mg)	PHOS (mg)	SEL (µg)	VE-a (mg)
350	70	192	29	13.1	10.6	12	3	0.1	1.07	4.1	0.47	116	10.6	27	289	71	1.7
89	87	230	23	1.2	2.7	18	0	0.07	0.22	6	0.35	8	0.31	12	174	13	0.3
90	78	192	21	1.4	2.8	18	0	0.06	0.22	4.9	0.22	8	0.23	11	151	13	0.4
105	99	256	26	1.5	3	46	0	0.08	0.24	7.1	0.37	8	0.35	14	199	16	0.4
51	50	12	2	1.2	0.3	28	1	0.01	0.18	1	0.03	42	1.05	1	23	*	t
883	71	196	29	11.9	6.1	6886	22	0.21	2.45	6.2	0.82	1077	27.1	20	437	99	3.4
60	55	147	15	0.9	1.6	18	0	0.06	0.15	4.3	0.21	5	0.19	8	116	11	0.2
21	182	49	5	0.4	0.5	0	0	0	0.03	1.6	0.07	2	0.06	0	39	*	0.1
26	25	57	6	0.4	0.6	12	0	0.02	0.04	2.1	0.13	1	0.09	5	48	6	0.1
29	28	62	7	0.4	0.6	16	0	0.01	0.04	2.3	0.14	1	0.1	5	51	6	0.1
28	27	56	6	0.5	0.7	16	0	0.02	0.04	1.9	0.09	1	0.07	5	48	6	0.1
640	454	1560	124	20.6	14.2	483	0	1.33	2.06	36.9	1.4	50	2.26	86	1190	*	5.3
396	286	1114	88	11.9	11.5	103	0	1.15	2.08	22.5	1.1	44	1.76	52	898	*	3.1
1416	1084	5092	341	43.8	40.6	325	0	1.19	5	64.5	5.73	31	6.35	201	4180	*	26.8
20	91	18	2	0.7	0.1	130	t	0.01	0.04	0.3	0.01	8	1.22	9	26	*	0
1138	898	4586	296	33.9	499	142	0	1.09	4.61	48.2	5.5	142	5.56	165	3652	*	21
16	283	92	5	0.8	0.8	0	0	0.02	0.07	1	0.07	2	0.07	3	54	*	0.2
12	406	79	6	0.1	0.3	0	0	0.01	0.03	2.4	0.1	1	0.57	2	65	*	0.1
15	297	74	4	0.5	0.6	0	0	0.02	0.07	1	0.08	1	0.07	3	57	*	0.1
12	139	71	5	0.4	0.4	0	0	0.03	0.06	2	0.09	1	0.07	11	52	*	0.1
16	166	77	5	0.4	0.6	0	0	0.03	0.08	1.4	0.08	1	0.07	9	48	*	0.1
510	318	1784	178	9.4	10.6	0	0	0.26	0.8	45.9	3.42	38	2.36	76	1370	49	0.6
119	110	406	34	3.3	6.3	0	0	0.09	0.35	5.1	0.5	13	0.52	45	286	35	0.9
606	86	290	25	9.7	5.3	2629	3	0.07	1.31	6.5	0.47	501	34.8	19	296	*	0.2
336	79	306	27	7.9	6	81	2	0.05	0.47	4.5	0.17	75	2.76	22	186	*	3.4
97	89	426	39	1.9	2.9	0	0	0.09	0.18	9.6	0.75	8	0.52	27	307	*	0.1
107	99	418	37	2.5	4.3	0	0	0.09	0.26	7.6	0.64	10	0.52	35	298	35	0.9
876	89	272	21	10.9	4.3	5288	3	0.07	1.99	8.3	0.73	932	66.5	15	381	*	4
23	283	80	7	0.4	0.8	0	0	0	0.03	1.2	0.12	2	0.1	40	58	*	0.1
0	110	54	*	0.1	*	21	2	0.01	0.01	0.2	*	*	*	7	8	0	*
0	90	54	*	0.1	*	21	2	0.01	0.01	0.2	*	*	*	7	8	0	*
0	100	*	*	*	*	*	*	*	*	*	*	*	*	*	*	*	*
3	135	*	*	*	*	*	*	*	*	*	*	*	*	*	*	*	*
5	115	*	*	*	*	*	*	*	*	*	*	*	*	*	*	*	*
0	120	*	*	*	*	*	*	*	*	*	*	*	*	*	*	*	*
0	80	*	*	*	*	*	*	*	*	*	*	*	*	*	*	*	*
0	85	*	*	*	*	*	*	*	*	*	*	*	*	*	*	*	*
0	108	*	*	*	*	*	*	*	*	*	*	*	*	*	*	*	*
1	163	77	9	0.4	0.1	4	0	0.02	0.03	1.1	0.03	20	0	7	23	6	0.3
0	80	*	*	*	*	*	*	*	*	*	*	*	*	*	*	*	*
7	1305	189	5	1.6	2.3	0	0	0.08	0.08	1.5	0.02	5	0.23	14	70	*	*
3	1076	57	10	0.2	0.3	0	0	0.04	0.09	0.8	0	0	0	66	44	*	*
5	1373	260	5	1.1	1.9	264	0	0.04	0.1	1.1	0.02	5	0.24	48	69	*	1.7
0	1357	252	5	1.6	1.7	0	0	0.08	0.15	1.6	0.05	29	0	17	36	*	t
3	1235	57	10	0.3	0.3	0	2	0.05	0.06	0.8	0.03	3	0.16	31	44	*	*
5	1373	259	5	1.7	1.9	0	0	0.05	0.19	3.1	0.02	5	0	10	69	*	*
0	165	44	3	0.1	0.1	0	3	t	t	t	0.01	t	0	9	5	*	t
0	3268	325	46	4.5	0.8	0	2	0.07	0.02	0.4	0.09	11	0	310	335	*	4.4
0	1	7	*	0.1	*	*	*	*	*	*	*	*	*	4	4	3	0.1
0	65	7	2	0.1	*	*	*	*	*	*	*	*	*	4	4	0	0.1
0	2032	435	45	2.3	0.5	218	18	0.08	0.05	2.3	0.19	10	0	48	50	*	3.3
189	1265	298	26	0.3	0.8	757	2	0.08	0.26	0.3	0.08	10	0.51	230	186	*	*
53	1566	554	47	0.3	1	117	2	0.15	0.56	0.3	0.14	13	1.12	570	437	*	*
0	201	56	*	0.1	*	21	2	0.01	0.01	0.2	*	*	*	3	8	0	*
0	10	*	*	*	*	*	*	*	*	*	*	*	*	*	*	*	*
35	1276	495	46	1.1	1.1	41	3	0.11	0.54	0.5	0.11	16	1.09	484	280	*	*
189	1134	309	26	0.2	0.8	696	2	0.08	0.33	0.2	0.08	10	0.51	240	194	*	*
0	1573	1060	60	2	0.7	240	32	0.11	0.15	4	0.62	34	0	45	88	*	*
34	1535	494	37	0.5	1.3	94	2	0.19	0.8	4.8	0.19	40	0.8	302	166	*	0.7
0	218	77	*	0.3	*	23	9	0.02	0.01	0.2	*	*	*	4	8	*	*
0	111	87	*	0.3	*	39	9	0.02	0.01	0.3	*	*	*	4	9	*	*
91	1007	733	44	0.6	1.4	144	3	0.13	0.7	0.6	0.13	16	0.94	546	*	*	*

WT, weight; **KCAL**, kcalories; **PROT**, protein; **CARB**, carbohydrate; **FIBR**, fiber; **FAT**, fat; **SATF**, saturated fat;

MONO, monosaturated fat; **POLY**, polyunsaturated fat; **CHOR**, cholesterol; **SOD**, sodium; **POT**, potassium;

Food Name	Portion	WT (Gm)	KCAL	PROT (Gm)	CARB (Gm)	FIBR (Gm)	FAT (Gm)	SATF (Gm)	MONO (Gm)	POLY (Gm)
SAUCE-SOY	TBSP	18	10	1	2	0	t	t	t	t
SAUCE-SOY-TAMARI	TBSP	18	11	2	1	0	t	t	t	t
SAUCE-SPAGHETTI-TOMATO BASED-CANNED	CUP	249	271	5	40	*	12	1.7	6.1	3.3
SAUCE-STEAK-HEINZ 57	TBSP	15	15	t	3	*	t	0	0	0
SAUCE-STROGANOFF-FROM MIX-PREPARED	CUP	296	272	12	34	1.2	11	6.8	3	0.4
SAUCE-SWEET/SOUR-FROM MIX-PREPARED	CUP	313	294	1	73	1.9	t	t	t	t
SAUCE-TABASCO	TSP	5	0	t	t	0	0	0	0	0
SAUCE-TACO-CANNED	FL OZ	16	11	t	2	*	1	*	*	*
SAUCE-TARTAR-REGULAR	TBSP	14	75	0	1	*	8	1.5	1.8	4.1
SAUCE-TERIYAKI-BOTTLED-READY TO SERVE	TBSP	18	15	1	3	t	0	0	0	0
SAUCE-TERIYAKI-FROM MIX-PREPARED-WATER	CUP	283	130	4	28	0.1	1	0.1	0.2	0.5
SAUCE-TOMATO-CANNED-LOW SODIUM-S&W	CUP	226	90	4	18	3.4	0	0	0	0
SAUCE-TOMATO-CANNED-SALT ADDED	CUP	245	74	3	18	3.7	t	0.1	0.1	0.2
SAUCE-TOMATO-SPANISH-CANNED	CUP	244	81	4	18	3.7	1	0.1	0.1	0.3
SAUCE-TOMATO-WITH HERBS/CHEESE-CANNED	CUP	244	144	5	25	3.7	5	1.5	0.9	2
SAUCE-TOMATO-WITH MUSHROOMS-CANNED	CUP	245	86	4	21	3.7	t	t	t	0.1
SAUCE-TOMATO-WITH ONIONS-CANNED	CUP	245	103	4	24	3.7	t	0.1	0.1	0.2
SAUCE-WHITE-DEHYDRATED-PREPARED-MILK	CUP	264	240	10	21	0.1	14	6.4	4.7	1.7
SAUCE-WHITE-MEDIUM-WITH ENRICHED FLOUR	CUP	250	405	10	22	0.4	31	19.3	7.8	0.8
SAUCE-WORCESTERSHIRE	TBSP	15	12	t	3	0	0	0	0	0
TOMATO CATSUP	TBSP	15	15	0	4	0.2	0	0	0	0

Soups

Food Name	Portion	WT (Gm)	KCAL	PROT (Gm)	CARB (Gm)	FIBR (Gm)	FAT (Gm)	SATF (Gm)	MONO (Gm)	POLY (Gm)
SOUP-BEAN WITH BACON-CANNED-WITH WATER	CUP	253	173	8	23	3.2	6	1.5	2.2	1.8
SOUP-BEEF BROTH-CANNED-READY TO EAT	CUP	240	17	3	t	0	1	0.3	0.2	t
SOUP-BEEF BROTH-DEHYDRATED-CUBED	ITEM	3.6	6	1	1	0	t	0.1	0.1	t
SOUP-BEEF NOODLE-CANNED-PREPARED-WATER	CUP	244	84	5	9	1.5	3	1.2	1.2	0.5
SOUP-BEEF-CHUNKY-CANNED-READY TO SERVE	CUP	240	170	12	20	*	5	2.6	2.1	0.2
SOUP-BLACK BEAN-CANNED-PREPARED-WATER	CUP	247	116	6	20	*	2	0.4	0.5	0.5
SOUP-CHEESE-CANNED-PREPARED WITH MILK	CUP	251	230	9	16	2	15	9.1	4.1	0.4
SOUP-CHICKEN AND DUMPLINGS-CANNED-MILK	CUP	241	96	6	6	0.7	6	1.3	2.5	1.3
SOUP-CHICKEN BROTH-CANNED-PREPARED-WATER	CUP	244	39	5	1	0	1	0.4	0.6	0.3
SOUP-CHICKEN NOODLE-CANNED-WITH WATER	CUP	241	75	4	9	1.5	2	0.7	1.1	0.6
SOUP-CHICKEN NOODLE-LOW SODIUM	CUP	240	91	5	10	1.4	2	0.7	1.1	0.6
SOUP-CHICKEN NOODLE-PREPARED FROM DRY	CUP	252	53	3	7	0.2	1	0.3	0.5	0.4
SOUP-CHICKEN-CHUNKY-CANNED-READY TO EAT	CUP	251	178	13	17	0.8	7	2	3	1.4
SOUP-CHICKEN-CHUNKY-LOW SODIUM	CUP	251	173	13	15	*	5	*	*	*
SOUP-CHICKEN/RICE-CANNED-READY TO SERVE	CUP	240	127	12	13	1.4	3	1	1.4	0.7
SOUP-CHILI-BEEF-CANNED-PREPARED-WATER	CUP	250	170	7	22	*	7	3.4	2.8	0.3
SOUP-CLAM CHOWDER-MANHATTAN STYLE-WATER	CUP	244	78	2	12	2.1	2	0.4	0.4	1.3
SOUP-CLAM CHOWDER-NEW ENGLAND-WITH MILK	CUP	248	163	9	17	1.5	7	3	2.3	1.1
SOUP-CLAM CHOWDER-NEW ENGLAND-WITH WATER	CUP	244	95	5	12	1.5	3	0.4	1.2	1.1
SOUP-CONSOMME-CANNED-PREPARED WITH WATER	CUP	241	29	5	2	*	0	0	0	*
SOUP-CORN-CANNED-LOW SODIUM-CAMPBELLS	SERVING	305	191	3	31	*	5	*	*	*
SOUP-CRAB-CANNED-READY TO SERVE	CUP	244	76	5	10	*	2	0.4	0.7	0.4
SOUP-CREAM OF ASPARAGUS-CANNED-WITH MILK	CUP	248	161	6	16	0.8	8	3.3	2.1	2.2
SOUP-CREAM OF CELERY-CANNED-WITH MILK	CUP	248	164	6	15	0.8	10	3.9	2.5	2.7
SOUP-CREAM OF CHICKEN-CANNED-WITH MILK	CUP	248	191	7	15	0.5	12	4.6	4.5	1.6
SOUP-CREAM OF CHICKEN-CANNED-WITH WATER	CUP	244	117	3	9	0.5	7	2.1	3.3	1.5
SOUP-CREAM OF MUSHROOM-CANNED-WITH MILK	CUP	248	203	6	15	0.5	14	5.1	3	4.6
SOUP-CREAM OF MUSHROOM-CANNED-WITH WATER	CUP	244	129	2	9	0.9	9	2.4	1.7	4.2
SOUP-CREAM OF POTATO-CANNED-WITH MILK	CUP	248	148	6	17	0.5	6	3.8	1.7	0.6
SOUP-CREAM OF SHRIMP-CANNED-WITH MILK	CUP	248	164	7	14	0.2	9	5.8	2.7	0.3
SOUP-ESCAROLE-CANNED-READY TO SERVE	CUP	248	27	2	2	*	2	0.5	0.8	0.4
SOUP-GAZPACHO-CANNED-READY TO SERVE	CUP	244	57	9	1	*	2	0.3	0.5	1.3
SOUP-LENTIL WITH HAM-CANNED-READY TO EAT	CUP	248	139	9	20	*	3	1.1	1.3	0.3
SOUP-MINESTRONE-CANNED-PREPARED-WATER	CUP	241	82	4	11	1.9	3	0.6	0.7	1.1
SOUP-ONION-CANNED-PREPARED WITH WATER	CUP	241	58	4	8	*	2	0.3	0.7	0.7
SOUP-ONION-DEHYDRATED-PACKET	SERVING	39	115	5	21	2.2	2	0.5	1.4	0.3
SOUP-ONION-DEHYDRATED-PREPARED-WATER	CUP	246	27	1	5	0.4	1	0.1	0.3	0.1
SOUP-OYSTER STEW-CANNED-PREPARED-MILK	CUP	245	134	6	10	*	8	5.1	2.1	0.3
SOUP-OYSTER STEW-CANNED-PREPARED-WATER	CUP	241	58	2	4	*	4	2.5	0.9	0.2
SOUP-PEA GREEN-CANNED-PREPARED WITH MILK	CUP	254	239	13	32	2.8	7	4	2.2	0.5

*t = Trace of nutrient present   * = Not available*

MAG, magnesium; IRON, iron; ZINC, zinc; VITA, vitamin A; VITC, vitamin C; THIA, thiamin; RIBO, riboflavin; NIAC, niacin; VB6, vitamin B-6; FOL, folate; VB12, vitamin B-12; CALC, calcium; PHOS, phosphorus; SEL, selenium; VE-a, alpha tocopherol equivalents.

CHOL (mg)	SOD (mg)	POT (mg)	MAG (mg)	IRON (mg)	ZINC (mg)	VITA (RE)	VITC (mg)	THIA (mg)	RIBO (mg)	NIAC (mg)	VB6 (mg)	FOL (μg)	VB12 (μg)	CALC (mg)	PHOS (mg)	SEL (μg)	VE-a (mg)
0	1029	32	6	0.4	0.1	0	0	0.01	0.02	0.6	0.03	3	0	3	20	*	0
0	1005	38	7	0.4	0.1	0	0	0.01	0.03	0.7	0.04	3	0	4	23	*	0
0	1235	956	60	1.6	0.5	306	28	0.14	0.15	3.8	0.88	54	0	70	90	*	*
0	265	*	*	*	*	*	*	*	*	*	*	*	*	*	*	0	*
39	1829	672	39	1.3	1.1	127	1	0.86	0.77	0.8	0.12	9	0.59	521	302	*	*
0	779	66	9	1.6	0.1	0	0	0.01	0.1	0.9	0.31	2	0	41	188	*	1.4
0	22	3	1	t	t	3	3	0	0.01	0	0.01	1	0	t	1	*	t
0	128	88	*	0.3	*	4	6	0.02	0.01	0.3	*	*	*	6	10	*	*
9	98	11	*	0.1	*	3	0	0	0	0	*	*	*	3	4	*	7
0	690	41	11	0.3	t	0	0	0.01	0.01	0.2	0.02	4	0	5	28	*	0.1
0	4791	216	85	2.8	0.1	0	0	0.03	0.09	1.3	0.14	28	0	113	215	*	1.2
0	65	838	43	1.7	0.6	221	30	0.16	0.14	2.6	0.36	20	0	32	72	2	2.9
0	1482	908	47	1.9	0.6	240	32	0.16	0.14	2.8	0.38	23	0	34	78	*	*
0	1152	900	46	8.5	0.8	242	21	0.18	0.15	3.2	0.43	33	0	42	117	*	*
*	1325	869	46	2.1	0.9	240	25	0.19	0.3	3	0.05	20	0	90	132	*	*
0	1107	931	47	2.2	0.5	233	30	0.18	0.27	3.1	0.33	23	0	32	78	*	*
0	1350	1012	47	2.3	0.6	208	31	0.18	0.33	3	0.65	55	0	42	96	*	*
34	797	443	264	0.3	0.5	92	3	0.08	0.45	0.5	0.07	16	1.06	425	256	*	3.9
33	796	348	38	0.5	0.5	115	2	0.12	0.43	0.7	0.06	12	0.7	288	233	*	3.7
0	147	120	2	0.9	t	5	27	0	0.03	0	0	0	0	15	9	*	0
0	156	54	4	0.1	t	21	2	0.01	0.01	0.2	0.02	1	0	3	8	0	0.3
3	952	403	44	2.1	1	89	2	0.09	0.03	0.6	0.04	32	0.05	81	132	8	*
0	782	130	5	0.4	0	0	0	0.01	0.05	1.9	0.02	5	0.17	14	31	8	*
t	864	15	2	0.1	t	1	0	0.01	0.01	0.1	0.01	1	0.04	2	8	0	t
5	952	99	6	1.1	1.5	63	t	0.07	0.06	1.1	0.04	4	0.2	15	46	8	0.8
14	866	336	5	2.3	2.6	261	7	0.06	0.15	2.7	0.13	13	0.61	31	120	8	*
0	1198	273	42	2.2	1.4	49	1	0.08	0.05	0.5	0.09	25	0.02	45	107	8	*
48	1020	340	20	0.8	0.7	147	1	0.06	0.33	0.5	0.08	10	0.44	288	250	8	0.4
34	860	116	5	0.6	0.4	52	0	0.02	0.07	1.8	0.04	2	0.16	15	60	8	0
1	776	210	2	0.5	0.2	0	0	0.01	0.07	3.4	0.02	5	0.24	9	73	8	*
7	1106	55	5	0.8	0.4	72	t	0.05	0.06	1.4	0.03	2	0.15	17	36	8	0.1
7	36	106	5	1.2	0.4	109	t	0.17	0.14	2.6	0.03	2	0.14	17	36	8	0.1
3	1283	30	8	0.5	0.2	6	t	0.07	0.06	0.9	0.01	2	0	33	33	8	*
30	887	176	8	1.7	1	130	1	0.09	0.17	4.4	0.05	5	0.25	24	113	8	0.1
*	78	264	*	1.8	*	94	2	0.13	0.25	4.8	*	*	*	28	*	8	*
12	888	108	10	1.9	1	586	4	0.02	0.1	4.1	0.05	4	0.31	35	72	8	0.1
13	1035	525	30	2.1	1.4	151	4	0.06	0.08	1.1	0.16	18	0.32	43	148	8	*
2	578	188	12	1.6	1	96	4	0.03	0.04	0.8	0.1	10	4.05	27	42	8	0.2
22	992	300	23	1.5	0.8	40	4	0.07	0.24	1	0.13	10	10.3	187	157	8	0.1
5	915	146	7	1.5	0.8	1	2	0.02	0.04	1	0.08	4	8	44	54	8	0.1
0	636	154	0	0.5	0.4	0	1	0.02	0.03	0.7	0.02	3	0	10	31	8	*
*	33	164	*	0.8	*	93	6	0.1	0.15	1.9	*	*	*	28	*	8	*
10	1234	326	88	1.2	1.5	50	2	0.2	0.07	1.3	0.12	15	0.2	66	88	8	*
22	1041	359	20	0.9	0.9	83	4	0.1	0.28	0.9	0.06	30	0.5	175	153	8	0.8
32	1009	310	22	0.7	0.2	68	1	0.07	0.25	0.4	0.06	9	0.5	186	151	8	1
27	1046	273	18	0.7	0.7	94	1	0.07	0.26	0.9	0.07	8	0.55	180	152	8	0.2
10	986	88	2	0.6	0.6	56	t	0.03	0.06	0.8	0.02	2	0.1	34	37	8	0.2
20	1076	270	20	0.6	0.6	38	2	0.08	0.28	0.9	0.06	10	0.5	178	156	8	1.3
2	1031	101	5	0.5	0.6	0	1	0.05	0.09	0.7	0.02	5	0.05	46	50	*	1.2
22	1060	323	17	0.5	0.7	67	1	0.08	0.24	0.6	0.09	9	0.5	166	160	8	0.1
35	1036	248	22	0.6	0.8	54	1	0.06	0.23	0.5	0.45	10	1.04	164	337	8	3.3
2	3864	265	5	0.7	2.2	217	4	0.07	0.05	2.3	0.22	35	0.5	32	79	8	*
0	1183	224	7	1	0.2	20	3	0.05	0.02	0.9	0.15	10	0	24	37	8	*
7	1319	357	22	2.7	0.7	36	4	0.17	0.11	1.4	0.22	50	0.3	42	184	8	*
2	911	313	7	0.9	0.7	234	1	0.05	0.04	0.9	0.1	16	0	34	55	8	*
0	1053	68	2	0.7	0.6	0	1	0.03	0.02	0.6	0.05	15	0	27	12	8	*
2	3493	260	25	0.6	0.2	1	1	0.11	0.24	2	0.04	6	0	55	126	0	t
0	849	64	5	0.1	0.1	0	t	0.03	0.06	0.5	0	1	0	12	30	*	*
32	1040	235	21	1	10.3	45	4	0.07	0.23	0.3	0.06	10	2.63	167	162	8	*
15	981	48	5	1	10.3	7	3	0.02	0.04	0.2	0.01	2	2.19	22	48	8	*
18	1048	377	55	2	1.8	58	3	0.16	0.27	1.3	0.1	8	0.44	173	238	8	0.2

WT, weight; **KCAL**, kcalories; **PROT**, protein; **CARB**, carbohydrate; **FIBR**, fiber; **FAT**, fat; **SATF**, saturated fat;

MONO, monosaturated fat; **POLY**, polyunsaturated fat; **CHOR**, cholesterol; **SOD**, sodium; **POT**, potassium;

Food Name	Portion	WT (Gm)	KCAL	PROT (Gm)	CARB (Gm)	FIBR (Gm)	FAT (Gm)	SATF (Gm)	MONO (Gm)	POLY (Gm)
SOUP-PEA GREEN-CANNED-PREPARED/WATER	CUP	250	165	9	27	2.8	3	1.4	1	0.4
SOUP-PEA GREEN-LOW SODIUM-CANNED-WATER	CUP	250	165	9	27	0.8	3	1.4	1	0.4
SOUP-PEA-SPLIT-CANNED-PREPARED-WATER	CUP	253	189	10	28	2.8	4	1.8	1.8	0.6
SOUP-PEPPERPOT-CANNED-PREPARED/WATER	CUP	241	103	6	9	*	5	2.1	2	0.4
SOUP-TOMATO BEEF & NOODLE-CANNED/WATER	CUP	244	139	4	21	1.5	4	1.6	1.7	0.7
SOUP-TOMATO BISQUE-CANNED-PREPARED/MILK	CUP	251	198	6	29	*	7	3.1	1.9	1.2
SOUP-TOMATO BISQUE-LOW SODIUM-WITH WATER	CUP	247	123	2	24	*	3	0.5	0.7	1.1
SOUP-TOMATO RICE-CANNED-PREPARED/WATER	CUP	247	119	2	22	1.7	3	0.5	0.6	1.4
SOUP-TOMATO VEGETABLE-PREPARED FROM DRY	CUP	253	56	2	10	1.1	1	0.4	0.3	0.1
SOUP-TOMATO-CANNED-PREPARED WITH MILK	CUP	248	161	6	22	0.8	6	2.9	1.6	1.1
SOUP-TOMATO-CANNED-PREPARED WITH WATER	CUP	244	85	2	17	0.9	2	0.4	0.4	1
SOUP-TURKEY NOODLE-CANNED-PREPARED/WATER	CUP	244	68	4	9	0.7	2	0.6	0.8	0.5
SOUP-TURKEY NOODLE-LOW SODIUM-WITH WATER	CUP	244	68	4	9	*	2	0.6	0.8	0.5
SOUP-TURKEY VEGETABLE-CANNED-WATER	CUP	241	72	3	9	1	3	0.9	1.3	0.7
SOUP-TURKEY-CHUNKY-CANNED-READY TO SERVE	CUP	236	135	10	14	2.5	4	1.2	1.8	1.1
SOUP-VEGETABLE BEEF-CANNED-LOW SODIUM	SERVING	305	165	12	18	1.2	4	1.1	1	0.1
SOUP-VEGETABLE BEEF-CANNED-WITH WATER	CUP	245	78	6	10	1	2	0.9	0.8	0.1
SOUP-VEGETABLE-CANNED-LOW SODIUM	CUP	240	98	2	14	3.1	0	0	0	0
SOUP-VEGETARIAN-CANNED-PREPARED-WATER	CUP	241	72	2	12	1.2	2	0.3	0.8	0.7
SOUP-VICHYSSOISE-CANNED-PREPARED/MILK	CUP	248	148	6	17	*	6	3.8	1.7	0.6

Sugars & Sweets

Food Name	Portion	WT (Gm)	KCAL	PROT (Gm)	CARB (Gm)	FIBR (Gm)	FAT (Gm)	SATF (Gm)	MONO (Gm)	POLY (Gm)
APPLE BUTTER	TBSP	20	37	t	9	0.2	t	t	t	t
CANDY-ALMOND JOY	OUNCE	28.4	151	2	19	0.3	8	1.7	2.5	1.7
CANDY-BIT O HONEY	OUNCE	28.4	121	1	21	*	4	1.7	1.6	0.2
CANDY-CARAMELS-PLAIN/CHOCOLATE	OUNCE	28.4	115	1	22	0.8	3	1.6	1.1	0.1
CANDY-CHOCOLATE COATED PEANUTS	OUNCE	28.4	160	5	11	*	12	4	4.7	2.1
CANDY-CHOCOLATE-SEMISWEET	CUP	170	860	7	97	8.8	61	36.2	19.8	1.7
CANDY-FONDANT-UNCOATED	OUNCE	28.4	105	0	25	0	1	0.1	0.3	0.1
CANDY-FUDGE-CHOCOLATE-PLAIN	OUNCE	28.4	115	1	21	0.4	3	1.3	1.4	0.6
CANDY-GUM DROPS	OUNCE	28.4	100	0	25	0	0	0	0	0
CANDY-HARD	OUNCE	28.4	110	0	28	0	0	0	0	0
CANDY-JELLY BEANS	ITEM	2.8	7	0	3	0	0	0	0	0
CANDY-KIT KAT BAR	ITEM	43	210	3	25	0.6	11	5.6	3.8	0.4
CANDY-LIFE SAVERS	ITEM	2	8	0	2	0	t	0	0	0
CANDY-LOLLIPOP	ITEM	28.4	108	0	28	0	0	0	0	0
CANDY-M & M-PLAIN-PACKAGE	ITEM	45	220	3	31	*	10	*	*	*
CANDY-MILK CHOCOLATE BAR-NO SUGAR	ITEM	10.1	60	1	5	*	4	*	*	*
CANDY-MILK CHOCOLATE WITH ALMONDS	OUNCE	28.4	151	3	15	1.3	10	4.1	3.9	1.4
CANDY-MILK CHOCOLATE WITH PEANUTS	OUNCE	28.4	154	4	13	*	11	5.2	5	1.8
CANDY-MILK CHOCOLATE-PLAIN	OUNCE	28.4	145	2	16	*	9	5.5	3	0.3
CANDY-MILKY WAY BAR	ITEM	60	260	3	43	0.1	9	5.1	3.6	0.3
CANDY-PEANUT BRITTLE	OUNCE	28.4	123	2	20	0.5	4	1.9	1.8	0.6
CANDY-PEANUT BUTTER CUP	PIECE	17	92	2	9	0.8	5	2.8	1.8	0.8
CANDY-SNICKERS BAR	ITEM	57	270	6	33	1.4	13	4.7	5	2
CHOCOLATE-BITTER-FOR BAKING	OUNCE	28.4	145	3	8	4.3	15	8.9	4.9	0.4
COCONUT CREAM-RAW	CUP	240	792	9	16	1.6	83	73.8	3.5	0.9
COCONUT MILK-RAW	CUP	240	552	6	13	1.1	57	50.7	2.4	0.6
HONEY-STRAINED/EXTRACTED	TBSP	21	65	0	17	0.1	0	0	0	0
ICING-CAKE-CHOCOLATE-PREPARED FROM MIX	CUP	275	1035	9	185	*	38	23.4	11.7	1
ICING-CAKE-FUDGE-PREPARED FROM MIX/WATER	CUP	245	830	7	183	*	16	5.1	6.7	3.1
ICING-CAKE-WHITE-BOILED	CUP	94	295	1	75	0	0	0	0	0
ICING-CAKE-WHITE-UNCOOKED	CUP	319	1200	2	260	0	21	12.7	5.1	0.5
ICING-CAKE-WHITE/COCONUT-BOILED	CUP	166	605	3	124	*	13	11	0.9	0
JAM/PRESERVES-STRAWBERRY-LOW CALORIE	TSP	6	8	0	2	0.1	0	0	0	0
JAMS/PRESERVES-REGULAR	TBSP	20	55	0	14	0.2	0	0	0	0
JAMS/PRESERVES-REGULAR-PACKET SIZE	ITEM	14	40	0	10	0.1	0	0	0	0
JELLIES-REGULAR	TBSP	18	50	0	13	0	0	0	0	0
JELLIES-REGULAR-PACKET SIZE	ITEM	14	40	0	10	0	0	0	0	0
MARSHMALLOWS	OUNCE	28.4	90	1	23	0	0	0	0	0
MOLASSES-CANE-BLACKSTRAP	TBSP	20	45	0	11	0	0	0	0	0
MOLASSES-CANE-LIGHT	TBSP	20	50	0	13	0	0	0	0	0
NUTS-COCONUT-DRIED-FLAKED-CANNED	CUP	77	341	3	32	4.4	24	21.6	1	0.3

t = Trace of nutrient present   * = Not available

MAG, magnesium; **IRON**, iron; **ZINC**, zinc; **VITA**, vitamin A; **VITC**, vitamin C; **THIA**, thiamin; **RIBO**, riboflavin; **NIAC**, niacin; **VB6**, vitamin B-6; **FOL**, folate; **VB12**, vitamin B-12; **CALC**, calcium; **PHOS**, phosphorus; **SEL**, selenium; **VE-a**, alpha tocopherol equivalents.

CHOL (mg)	SOD (mg)	POT (mg)	MAG (mg)	IRON (mg)	ZINC (mg)	VITA (RE)	VITC (mg)	THIA (mg)	RIBO (mg)	NIAC (mg)	VB6 (mg)	FOL (µg)	VB12 (µg)	CALC (mg)	PHOS (mg)	SEL (µg)	VE-a (mg)
0	988	190	39	2	1.7	20	2	0.11	0.07	1.2	0.05	2	0	28	124	8	0.1
0	33	190	39	2	1.7	20	2	0.11	0.07	1.2	0.05	2	0	28	124	8	0.1
8	1008	399	48	2.3	1.3	44	1	0.15	0.08	1.5	0.07	3	0	22	213	8	0.1
10	970	152	5	0.9	1.2	87	1	0.05	0.05	1.2	0.06	10	0.17	23	42	8	*
5	917	221	8	1.1	0.8	53	0	0.08	0.09	1.9	0.09	7	0.19	17	56	8	0.8
22	1108	604	25	0.9	0.6	110	7	0.11	0.27	1.3	0.14	21	0.44	186	174	8	*
4	30	417	9	0.8	0.6	72	6	0.07	0.07	1.2	0.09	15	0	40	60	8	*
2	815	330	5	0.8	0.5	76	15	0.06	0.05	1.1	0.08	14	0	22	33	8	0.8
0	1146	103	20	0.6	0.2	20	6	0.06	0.05	0.8	0.05	10	0	8	29	*	t
17	932	449	22	1.8	0.3	108	68	0.13	0.25	1.5	0.16	21	0.44	159	149	8	*
0	871	263	8	1.8	0.2	69	66	0.09	0.05	1.4	0.11	15	0	12	34	8	2.5
5	815	75	5	0.9	0.6	29	t	0.07	0.06	1.4	0.04	2	0.15	12	48	8	*
5	42	75	5	0.9	0.6	29	t	0.07	0.06	1.4	0.04	2	0.15	12	48	8	*
2	905	175	4	0.8	0.6	244	0	0.03	0.04	1	0.05	5	0.17	17	40	8	0.2
9	923	361	24	1.9	2.1	716	6	0.04	0.11	3.6	0.31	11	2.12	50	104	8	*
6	57	455	8	1.4	1.9	553	11	0.24	0.33	4.2	0.1	13	0.39	49	50	8	5007
5	960	174	5	1.1	1.6	189	2	0.04	0.05	1	0.08	11	0.31	17	42	8	0.3
0	38	185	7	1	0.5	371	3	0.05	0.05	1.2	0.06	11	0	19	35	8	0.5
0	823	209	7	1.1	0.5	300	1	0.05	0.05	0.9	0.06	11	0	21	35	8	0.3
22	1060	323	17	0.5	0.7	67	1	0.08	0.24	0.6	0.09	9	0.5	166	160	8	*
0	0	50	2	0.1	t	0	t	t	t	t	0.01	t	0	3	4	*	t
1	22	114	13	0.3	0.4	3	t	0.02	0.1	0.2	0.02	4	0.18	60	68	1	0.3
*	*	*	*	0.3	*	*	*	0	0.13	1.4	*	*	*	13	*	1	t
0	74	54	1	0.4	0.2	0	0	0.01	0.05	0.1	0.01	2	0.04	42	35	1	t
0	16	143	*	0.4	*	0	0	0.1	0.05	2.1	*	*	*	33	84	1	0.2
0	3	553	192	4.4	2.6	9	0	0.02	0.14	0.9	0.07	5	0	51	255	6	1.2
0	60	1	t	0.3	0	0	0	0	0	0	0	0	0	4	2	1	0
0	54	42	13	0.3	0.1	0	0	0.01	0.03	0.1	0.01	1	0.06	22	24	1	0.2
0	10	1	t	0.1	t	0	0	0	0	0	0	0	0	2	0	1	t
0	9	1	*	0.5	*	0	0	0	0	0	*	*	*	6	2	1	t
0	t	0	*	t	*	0	0	0	*	*	*	*	*	t	t	0	*
3	38	129	19	0.6	0.4	9	0	0.03	0.11	0.1	0.02	3	0.07	65	78	2	0.3
0	1	0	*	t	*	0	0	0	0	0	*	*	*	t	t	0	*
0	*	*	*	0	*	0	0	0	0	0	*	*	*	0	0	1	*
																2	0.5
*	10	*	*	*	*	*	*	*	*	*	*	*	*	*	*	1	*
5	23	125	27	0.5	0.4	21	0	0.02	0.12	0.2	0.01	4	0.15	65	77	1	0.3
*	19	138	*	0.4	*	15	0	0.07	0.07	1.4	*	*	*	49	83	1	0.3
0	28	109	16	0.3	*	24	0	0.02	0.1	0.1	*	2	*	65	65	1	0.2
4	114	157	20	0.4	0.4	4	t	0.02	0.14	0.3	0.02	4	0.22	79	79	2	0.7
0	9	43	11	0.6	0.3	2	0	0.02	0.01	1.3	0.02	14	0	11	35	1	0.5
3	55	68	15	0.2	0.2	1	0	0.05	0.03	0.8	0.03	17	0.04	15	41	1	0.2
9	145	189	37	0.5	0.6	3	0	0.03	0.1	1.7	0.06	29	0.17	66	102	2	0.6
0	1	235	82	1.9	0.3	6	0	0.01	0.07	0.4	0.01	3	0	22	109	*	0.3
0	10	781	41	5.5	2.3	0	7	0.07	0	2.1	0.07	34	0	26	293	*	1.8
0	37	630	89	3.9	1.6	0	7	0.06	0	1.8	0.08	39	0	39	240	*	1.8
0	1	11	1	0.1	t	0	0	0	0.01	0.1	t	0	0	1	1	1	0
0	882	536	*	3.3	*	174	1	0.06	0.28	0.6	*	*	*	165	305	3	*
0	568	238	*	2.7	*	0	0	0.05	0.2	0.7	*	*	*	96	218	3	*
0	134	17	*	0	*	0	0	0	0.03	0	*	*	*	2	2	1	*
0	156	57	*	0	*	258	0	0	0.06	0	*	*	*	48	38	3	*
0	195	277	*	0.8	*	0	0	0.02	0.07	0.3	*	*	*	10	50	2	*
0	6	5	t	t	t	t	1	t	t	t	t	1	0	1	t	0	t
0	2	18	1	0.2	t	0	0	0	0.01	0	t	2	0	4	2	0	t
0	1	12	1	0.1	t	0	0	0	0	0	t	1	0	3	1	0	t
0	3	14	1	0.3	t	0	1	0	0.01	0	t	t	0	4	1	0	t
0	2	11	1	0.2	t	0	1	0	0	0	t	t	0	3	1	0	t
0	11	2	1	0.5	t	0	0	0	0	0	0	0	0	5	2	0	t
0	18	585	9	3.2	0.1	0	0	0.02	0.04	0.4	0.04	0	0	137	17	13	0.1
0	3	183	9	0.9	0.1	0	0	0.01	0.01	0	0.04	0	0	33	9	13	0.1
0	15	249	38	1.4	1.2	0	0	0.02	0.02	0.2	0.18	5	0	11	79	*	0.5

WT, weight; **KCAL,** kcalories; **PROT,** protein; **CARB,** carbohydrate; **FIBR,** fiber; **FAT,** fat; **SATF,** saturated fat;

MONO, monosaturated fat; **POLY,** polyunsaturated fat; **CHOR,** cholesterol; **SOD,** sodium; **POT,** potassium;

Food Name	Portion	WT (Gm)	KCAL	PROT (Gm)	CARB (Gm)	FIBR (Gm)	FAT (Gm)	SATF (Gm)	MONO (Gm)	POLY (Gm)
NUTS-COCONUT-DRIED-SHREDDED	CUP	93	466	3	44	3.9	33	29.3	1.4	0.4
NUTS-COCONUT-RAW-SHREDDED	CUP	80	283	3	12	7.2	27	23.8	1.1	0.3
SORGHUM	TBSP	21	55	0	14	0	0	0	0	0
SUGAR-BROWN-PRESSED DOWN	CUP	220	820	0	212	0	0	0	0	0
SUGAR-EQUAL-PACKET SIZE	ITEM	1	4	0	1	0	0	0	0	0
SUGAR-SWEET & LOW-PACKET SIZE	ITEM	1	4	0	1	0	0	0	0	0
SUGAR-WHITE-GRANULATED	TBSP	12	45	0	12	0	0	0	0	0
SUGAR-WHITE-POWDERED-SIFTED	CUP	100	385	0	100	0	0	0	0	0
SYRUP-CHOCOLATE FLAVORED-FUDGE-THICK	FL OZ	38	125	2	20	*	5	3.1	1.6	0.1
SYRUP-CHOCOLATE FLAVORED-THIN	FL OZ	38	83	1	22	0.1	t	0.2	0.1	t
SYRUP-CORN-TABLE BLENDS-LIGHT AND DARK	TBSP	21	60	0	15	0	0	0	0	0
SYRUP-PANCAKE-KARO	TBSP	20.5	60	0	15	0	0	0	0	0
SYRUP-PANCAKE-LIGHT-AUNT JEMIMA	FL OZ	39	60	0	15	0	0	0	0	0

Vegetables

Food Name	Portion	WT (Gm)	KCAL	PROT (Gm)	CARB (Gm)	FIBR (Gm)	FAT (Gm)	SATF (Gm)	MONO (Gm)	POLY (Gm)
ALFALFA SEEDS-SPROUTED-RAW	CUP	33	10	1	1	0.7	t	t	t	0.1
AMARANTH-BOILED-DRAINED	CUP	132	28	3	5	12.5	t	0.1	0.1	0.1
AMARANTH-RAW	CUP	28	7	1	1	2.7	t	t	t	t
ARTICHOKES-BOILED-DRAINED	ITEM	120	60	4	13	4	t	t	t	0.1
ASPARAGUS-CANNED-DIETARY PACK-LOW SODIUM	CUP	244	34	4	5	3.9	t	0.1	t	0.2
ASPARAGUS-CANNED-SPEARS-DRAINED SOLIDS	CUP	242	46	5	6	3.5	2	0.4	0.1	0.7
ASPARAGUS-FROZEN-BOILED-DRAINED-SPEARS	CUP	180	50	5	9	2.2	1	0.2	t	0.3
ASPARAGUS-FROZEN-BOILED-DRAINED-TIPS	CUP	180	50	5	9	2.2	1	0.2	t	0.3
ASPARAGUS-RAW-BOILED-DRAINED-SPEARS	CUP	180	45	5	8	2.2	1	0.1	t	0.2
ASPARAGUS-RAW-BOILED-DRAINED-TIPS	CUP	180	45	5	8	2.2	1	0.1	t	0.2
BALSAM PEAR-LEAFY TIPS-BOILED-DRAINED	CUP	58	20	2	4	1.2	t	t	t	t
BALSAM PEAR-PODS-BOILED-DRAINED	CUP	124	24	1	5	2.5	t	t	t	t
BAMBOO SHOOTS-BOILED-DRAINED	CUP	120	14	2	2	2.2	t	0.1	t	0.1
BAMBOO SHOOTS-CANNED-DRAINED	CUP	131	25	2	4	3.4	1	0.1	t	0.2
BAMBOO SHOOTS-RAW	CUP	151	41	4	8	3.9	t	0.1	t	0.2
BEANS-ADZUKI-BOILED	CUP	230	294	17	57	14.3	t	0.1	7.2	2.1
BEANS-ADZUKI-CANNED-SWEETENED	CUP	296	702	11	163	13.7	t	0	0	0
BEANS-BAKED BEANS-CANNED	CUP	254	236	12	52	19.6	1	0.3	0.1	0.5
BEANS-BAKED BEANS-HOME RECIPE	CUP	253	382	14	54	19.5	13	4.9	5.4	1.9
BEANS-BLACK-COOKED-BOILED	CUP	172	227	15	41	7.2	1	0.2	0.1	0.4
BEANS-FRENCH-COOKED-BOILED	CUP	177	228	13	43	14.9	1	0.1	0.1	0.8
BEANS-GARBANZO-CANNED-RECONSTITUTED	SERVING	28.4	28	1	5	1.4	1	0.1	0.2	0.3
BEANS-GARBANZO-DRY-RAW	CUP	200	720	41	122	*	10	*	*	*
BEANS-GREAT NORTHERN-DRY-COOKED-DRAINED	CUP	180	210	14	38	9.7	1	4.4	5.5	1.7
BEANS-GREEN-CANNED-DIETARY-LOW SODIUM	CUP	136	26	2	6	1.8	t	t	t	0.1
BEANS-GREEN-FROZEN-BOILED-FRENCH STYLE	CUP	135	35	2	8	2.2	t	t	t	0.1
BEANS-KIDNEY-CANNED-DIETARY-LOW SODIUM	CUP	255	230	15	42	12.5	1	0	0	0
BEANS-LIMA-BABY-FROZEN-BOILED-DRAINED	CUP	180	189	12	35	13	1	0.1	t	0.3
BEANS-LIMA-CANNED-DIETARY-LOW SODIUM	CUP	248	186	11	34	10.4	1	0.2	t	0.4
BEANS-LIMA-CANNED-SOLIDS & LIQUIDS	CUP	248	186	11	34	10.4	1	0.2	t	0.4
BEANS-LIMA-FROZEN-BOILED-DRAINED	CUP	170	170	10	32	8.3	1	0.1	t	0.3
BEANS-LIMA-RAW-BOILED-DRAINED	CUP	170	209	12	40	12.2	1	0.1	t	0.3
BEANS-MUNG-SPROUTED-BOILED	CUP	125	26	3	5	2.7	t	t	t	t
BEANS-MUNG-SPROUTED-RAW	CUP	104	31	3	6	1.6	t	t	t	0.1
BEANS-NAVY PEA-DRY-COOKED-DRAINED	CUP	190	225	15	40	9.3	1	0.2	0.1	0.3
BEANS-NAVY-SPROUTED-BOILED	OUNCE	28.4	22	2	4	1.4	t	t	t	0.1
BEANS-PINTO-FROZEN-BOILED	OUNCE	28.4	46	3	9	1.4	t	t	t	0.1
BEANS-RED KIDNEY-CANNED-SOLIDS & LIQUIDS	CUP	255	230	15	42	12.5	1	1.2	3.5	3.1
BEANS-REFRIED	CUP	253	271	16	47	11.6	3	1	1.2	0.3
BEANS-REFRIED-CANNED-SAUSAGE-OLD EL PASO	CUP	200	388	14	26	6	26	6.9	7.9	2.3
BEANS-SHELLIE-CANNED	CUP	245	74	4	15	12	t	0.1	t	0.3
BEANS-SMALL WHITE-BOILED	CUP	179	254	16	46	7.9	1	0.3	0.1	0.5
BEANS-SNAP-GREEN-CANNED-DRAINED-CUTS	CUP	135	27	2	6	1.8	t	t	t	0.1
BEANS-SNAP-GREEN-DIETETIC-LOW SODIUM	OUNCE	28.4	4	t	1	0.4	t	0	0	0
BEANS-SNAP-GREEN-FROZEN-BOILED-CUTS	CUP	135	35	2	8	2.2	t	t	t	0.1
BEANS-SNAP-GREEN-RAW-BOILED	CUP	125	44	2	10	2.3	t	0.1	t	0.2
BEANS-SNAP-YELLOW/WAX-CANNED	CUP	136	27	2	6	1.8	t	t	t	0.1
BEANS-SNAP-YELLOW/WAX-FROZEN-BOILED	CUP	135	35	2	8	2.2	t	t	t	0.1

t = Trace of nutrient present   * = Not available

MAG, magnesium; IRON, iron; ZINC, zinc; VITA, vitamin A; VITC, vitamin C; THIA, thiamin; RIBO, riboflavin; NIAC, niacin; VB6, vitamin B-6; FOL, folate; VB12, vitamin B-12; CALC, calcium; PHOS, phosphorus; SEL, selenium; VE-a, alpha tocopherol equivalents.

CHOL (mg)	SOD (mg)	POT (mg)	MAG (mg)	IRON (mg)	ZINC (mg)	VITA (RE)	VITC (mg)	THIA (mg)	RIBO (mg)	NIAC (mg)	VB6 (mg)	FOL (µg)	VB12 (µg)	CALC (mg)	PHOS (mg)	SEL (µg)	VE-a (mg)
0	244	313	47	1.8	1.7	0	1	0.03	0.02	0.4	0.25	8	0	14	99	16	0.7
0	16	285	26	1.9	0.9	0	3	0.05	0.02	0.4	0.04	21	0	12	90	11	0.6
0	2	37	t	2.6	t	0	0	0.03	0.02	0	0	0	0	35	5	26	0.1
0	66	757	44	7.5	0.6	0	0	0.02	0.07	0.4	0.09	0	0	187	42	3	0
0	0	0	0	0	0	0	0	0	0	0	0	0	0	0	0	0	0
0	4	3	0	0	0	0	0	0	0	0	0	0	0	0	0	0	0
0	t	0	0	0	t	0	0	0	0	0	0	0	0	0	0	0	0
0	1	3	0	0.1	0	0	0	0	0	0	0	0	0	0	0	1	0
0	27	107	*	0.5	0.3	18	0	0.02	0.08	0.2	*	*	*	48	60	*	*
0	20	106	21	0.6	0.3	0	0	0.01	0.03	0.2	t	2	0	6	35	*	t
0	15	1	t	0.8	t	0	0	0	0	0	0	0	0	9	3	3	0
0	35	1	t	0.8	t	0	0	0	0	0	0	0	0	9	3	0	0
0	18	7	1	0.1	t	0	0	t	0.01	0	0	0	0	1	4	0	0
0	2	26	9	0.3	0.3	5	3	0.03	0.04	0.2	0.01	12	0	11	23	*	t
0	28	846	73	3	1.2	366	54	0.03	0.18	0.7	0.23	75	0	276	95	*	11.2
0	5	171	15	0.7	0.3	82	12	0.01	0.04	0.2	0.05	24	0	60	14	*	2.4
0	114	425	72	1.6	0.6	22	12	0.08	0.08	1.2	0.13	61	0	54	103	*	0.2
0	849	373	22	1.4	1.2	115	40	0.13	0.22	2.1	0.24	208	0	34	93	3	0.9
0	944	416	24	4.4	1	128	45	0.15	0.24	2.3	0.27	231	0	39	104	9	0.9
0	7	392	23	1.2	1	147	44	0.12	0.19	1.9	0.04	242	0	41	99	7	2.5
0	7	392	23	1.2	1	148	44	0.12	0.19	1.9	0.04	242	0	41	99	7	2.5
0	7	558	34	1.2	0.9	149	49	0.18	0.22	1.9	0.25	177	0	43	110	7	3.6
0	7	558	34	1.2	0.9	149	49	0.18	0.22	1.9	0.25	177	0	43	110	7	3.6
0	8	349	55	0.6	0.2	100	32	0.09	0.16	0.6	0.44	51	0	24	45	*	0.3
0	7	396	20	0.5	1	14	41	0.06	0.07	0.3	0.05	63	0	11	45	*	0.6
0	5	640	4	0.3	0.6	0	0	0.02	0.06	0.4	0.12	3	0	14	24	*	1.2
0	9	105	5	0.4	0.9	1	1	0.03	0.03	0.2	0.18	4	0	11	33	*	1.3
0	6	805	5	0.8	1.7	3	6	0.23	0.11	0.9	0.36	11	0	20	89	*	1.6
0	18	1224	120	4.6	4.1	1	0	0.27	0.15	1.7	0.22	279	0	63	385	*	0.5
0	646	353	91	3.3	4.6	3	0	0.3	0.17	1.9	0.25	316	0	66	220	*	1.9
0	1008	752	81	0.7	3.6	43	8	0.39	0.15	1.1	0.34	61	0	127	264	*	*
13	1068	907	110	5	1.8	t	3	0.34	0.12	1	0.23	122	0.03	155	275	*	0.5
0	1	611	121	3.6	1.9	1	0	0.42	0.1	0.9	0.12	256	0	47	241	*	*
0	11	655	99	1.9	1.1	1	2	0.23	0.11	1	0.19	132	0	111	181	*	*
0	113	55	9	0.7	0.3	1	1	t	0.01	0.1	*	*	0	11	30	*	1
0	52	1594	*	13.8	*	10	*	0.62	0.3	4	*	*	0	300	662	4	6
0	12	749	86	4.9	1.8	0	0	0.25	0.13	1.3	1.01	63	0	90	266	23	0.4
0	3	148	18	1.2	0.4	*	6	0.02	0.08	0.3	*	43	0	32	26	1	t
0	18	151	28	1.1	0.8	72	11	0.07	0.1	0.6	0.08	11	0	61	32	1	0.2
0	10	673	10	4.6	1.9	1	8	0.13	0.1	1.5	1.12	36	0	74	278	5	0
0	52	740	101	3.5	1	31	10	0.13	0.1	1.4	0.21	28	0	50	202	1	0
0	10	668	84	3.9	1.6	43	22	0.07	0.11	1.3	0.15	40	0	70	176	3	1.6
0	618	668	84	3.9	1.6	43	22	0.07	0.11	1.3	0.15	40	0	70	176	4	0.7
0	90	694	58	2.3	0.7	32	22	0.12	0.1	1.8	0.21	111	0	38	153	1	0
0	29	969	126	4.2	1.3	63	17	0.24	0.16	1.8	0.33	45	0	54	221	9	0
0	13	126	18	0.8	0.6	1	14	0.06	0.13	1	0.07	37	0	15	35	*	t
0	6	155	22	0.9	0.4	2	14	0.09	0.13	0.8	0.09	63	0	14	56	*	t
0	13	790	97	5.1	1.8	0	0	0.27	0.13	1.3	1.06	67	0	95	281	21	0.6
0	4	90	32	0.6	0.3	t	5	0.11	0.07	0.4	0.06	30	0	5	29	4	0.1
0	24	183	15	0.8	0.2	0	t	0.08	0.03	0.2	0.06	10	0	15	28	*	t
0	833	673	10	4.6	1.9	1	8	0.13	0.1	1.5	1.12	36	0	74	278	9	0
0	1073	994	99	4.5	3.5	0	15	0.12	0.14	1.2	0.25	211	0	116	213	*	2.1
16	624	600	88	4.2	1.8	0	6	0.29	0.14	0.6	0.31	254	0	88	258	*	1.7
0	818	267	37	2.4	0.7	56	8	0.08	0.13	0.5	0.12	44	0	71	74	*	*
0	4	828	122	5.1	2	0	0	0.42	0.11	0.5	0.23	245	0	131	302	*	0.3
0	339	147	18	1.2	0.4	47	7	0.02	0.08	0.3	0.05	43	0	35	34	1	t
0	t	24	3	0.2	0.1	10	1	0.01	0.01	0.1	*	*	0	7	6	0	t
0	18	151	28	1.1	0.8	72	11	0.07	0.1	0.6	0.08	11	0	61	32	1	0.2
0	4	374	31	1.6	0.5	84	12	0.09	0.12	0.8	0.07	42	0	58	49	1	t
0	341	148	18	1.2	0.4	48	7	0.02	0.08	0.3	0.05	43	0	35	26	1	0.4
0	18	151	28	1.1	0.8	72	11	0.07	0.1	0.6	0.08	11	0	61	32	1	0.2

WT, weight; **KCAL**, kcalories; **PROT**, protein; **CARB**, carbohydrate; **FIBR**, fiber; **FAT**, fat; **SATF**, saturated fat;
MONO, monosaturated fat; **POLY**, polyunsaturated fat; **CHOR**, cholesterol; **SOD**, sodium; **POT**, potassium;

Food Name	Portion	WT (Gm)	KCAL	PROT (Gm)	CARB (Gm)	FIBR (Gm)	FAT (Gm)	SATF (Gm)	MONO (Gm)	POLY (Gm)
BEANS-SNAP-YELLOW/WAX-RAW-BOILED	CUP	125	44	2	10	2.3	t	0.1	t	0.2
BEET GREENS-BOILED-DRAINED	CUP	145	39	4	8	4.4	t	t	0.1	0.1
BEETS-CANNED-DIETARY PACK-LOW SODIUM	CUP	246	71	2	17	2.7	t	t	t	0.1
BEETS-SLICED-BOILED-DRAINED	CUP	170	53	2	11	3.4	t	t	t	t
BEETS-SLICED-CANNED-DRAINED	CUP	170	53	2	12	2.9	t	t	t	0.1
BEETS-WHOLE-BOILED-DRAINED	ITEM	50	16	1	3	1.1	t	t	t	t
BEETS-WHOLE-CANNED	CUP	246	71	2	17	2.7	t	t	t	0.1
BROCCOLI-FROZEN-BOILED-DRAINED	CUP	185	52	6	10	7.3	t	t	t	0.1
BROCCOLI-RAW	CUP	88	25	3	5	2.5	t	t	t	0.1
BROCCOLI-RAW-BOILED-DRAINED	CUP	155	43	5	8	4	1	0.1	t	0.3
BRUSSELS SPROUTS-FROZEN-BOILED	CUP	155	65	6	13	4.5	1	0.1	t	0.3
BRUSSELS SPROUTS-RAW-BOILED	CUP	156	61	4	14	6.7	1	0.2	0.1	0.4
BURDOCK ROOT-BOILED-DRAINED	ITEM	166	146	3	35	*	t	*	*	*
CABBAGE-CELERY-RAW	CUP	76	12	1	2	0.8	t	t	t	0.1
CABBAGE-COMMON-BOILED-DRAINED	CUP	145	31	1	7	4	t	t	t	0.2
CABBAGE-COMMON-RAW-SHREDDED	CUP	90	22	1	5	1.8	t	t	t	0.1
CABBAGE-COMMON-RAW-SLICED	CUP	70	17	1	4	1.5	t	t	t	0.1
CABBAGE-RED-RAW-SHREDDED	CUP	70	19	1	4	1.4	t	t	t	0.1
CABBAGE-SAVOY-RAW-SHREDDED	CUP	70	19	1	4	1.5	t	t	t	t
CABBAGE-WHITE MUSTARD-BOILED	CUP	170	20	3	3	2.7	t	t	t	0.1
CABBAGE-WHITE MUSTARD-RAW	CUP	70	9	1	2	0.7	t	t	t	0.1
CARROT JUICE-CANNED	CUP	246	98	2	23	5.9	t	0.1	t	0.2
CARROT-RAW-SCRAPED-SHREDDED	CUP	110	47	1	11	3.5	t	t	t	0.1
CARROT-RAW-SCRAPED-WHOLE	ITEM	72	31	1	7	2.3	t	t	t	0.1
CARROTS-BOILED-DRAINED-SLICED	CUP	156	70	2	16	5.8	t	0.1	t	0.1
CARROTS-CANNED-DIETARY PACK-LOW SODIUM	CUP	246	57	2	12	2.7	t	0.1	t	0.2
CARROTS-CANNED-SLICED-DRAINED	CUP	146	34	1	8	2.2	t	0.1	t	0.1
CARROTS-FROZEN-BOILED-DRAINED	CUP	146	53	2	12	5.4	t	t	t	0.1
CAULIFLOWER-FROZEN-BOILED	CUP	180	34	3	7	3.2	t	0.1	t	0.2
CAULIFLOWER-RAW-BOILED-DRAINED	CUP	124	30	2	6	2.7	t	t	t	0.1
CAULIFLOWER-RAW-CHOPPED	CUP	100	24	2	5	2.4	t	0	0	0
CELERY-PASCAL-RAW-DICED	CUP	120	19	1	4	1.9	t	t	t	0.1
CELERY-PASCAL-RAW-STALK	ITEM	40	6	t	1	0.6	t	t	t	t
CHARD-SWISS-BOILED-DRAINED	CUP	175	35	3	7	3.7	t	t	0	0.1
CHARD-SWISS-RAW	CUP	36	7	1	1	0.6	t	0	0	0
CHICORY GREENS-RAW-CHOPPED	CUP	180	41	3	8	4.3	1	0.1	t	0.2
CHICORY ROOTS-RAW	ITEM	60	44	1	11	1.4	t	t	t	0.1
CHIVES-FREEZE DRIED	TBSP	0.2	1	t	t	t	t	t	t	t
CHIVES-RAW-CHOPPED	TBSP	3	1	t	t	0.1	t	t	t	t
COLLARDS-FROZEN-BOILED-DRAINED	CUP	170	61	5	12	5.2	1	*	*	*
COLLARDS-RAW-BOILED-DRAINED	CUP	128	35	2	8	2.1	t	t	t	0.1
CORN FRITTER	ITEM	35	132	3	14	0.6	8	2	3.2	1.9
CORN-CREAMED-CANNED-DIETARY-LOW SODIUM	CUP	256	184	4	46	3.1	1	0.2	0.3	0.5
CORN-EAR-FROZEN-BOILED-DRAINED	ITEM	126	117	4	28	2.7	1	0.1	0.3	0.4
CORN-FROZEN-BOILED-DRAINED-KERNELS	CUP	165	134	5	34	3.5	t	t	t	0.1
CORN-KERNELS FROM ONE EAR-BOILED-DRAINED	ITEM	77	83	3	19	2.9	1	0.2	0.3	0.5
CORN-SWEET-CANNED-DRAINED	CUP	165	134	4	31	2.3	2	0.3	0.5	0.8
CORN-SWEET-CANNED-LOW SODIUM	CUP	256	156	5	38	2.1	1	0.2	0.3	0.5
CORN-SWEET-CANNED-VACUUM PACKED	CUP	210	166	5	41	9.5	1	0.2	0.3	0.5
CORN-SWEET-CREAM STYLE-CANNED	CUP	256	184	4	46	3.1	1	0.2	0.3	0.5
CORN-WITH RED AND GREEN PEPPERS-CANNED	CUP	227	170	5	41	5.1	1	0.2	0.4	0.6
CRESS-GARDEN-RAW	CUP	50	16	1	3	0.6	t	t	0.1	0.1
CUCUMBER-RAW-SLICED	CUP	104	14	1	3	1	t	t	t	0.1
CUCUMBER-RAW-WHOLE	ITEM	301	39	2	9	3	t	0.1	t	0.2
DANDELION GREENS-BOILED	CUP	105	35	2	7	4.1	1	0.1	t	0.4
EGGPLANT-BOILED-DRAINED	CUP	96	27	1	6	2.7	t	t	t	0.1
ENDIVE-RAW-CHOPPED	CUP	50	9	1	2	1.2	t	t	t	t
FRIJOLES-BEANS WITH CHEESE	CUP	167	226	11	29	*	8	4.1	2.6	0.7
GARLIC-RAW-CLOVE	ITEM	3	4	t	1	0.1	t	t	0	t
GINGER ROOT-RAW-SLICED	CUP	96	66	2	15	0.7	1	0.2	0.1	0.1
GOURD-WHITE FLOWERED-BOILED	CUP	146	22	1	5	1.6	t	t	t	t
HUMMUS	CUP	246	421	12	50	0	21	3.1	8.8	7.8
JERUSALEM ARTICHOKES-RAW	CUP	150	114	3	26	2	t	0	t	t

*t = Trace of nutrient present   * = Not available*

MAG, magnesium; **IRON**, iron; **ZINC**, zinc; **VITA**, vitamin A; **VITC**, vitamin C; **THIA**, thiamin; **RIBO**, riboflavin; **NIAC**, niacin; **VB6**, vitamin B-6; **FOL**, folate; **VB12**, vitamin B-12; **CALC**, calcium; **PHOS**, phosphorus; **SEL**, selenium; **VE-a**, alpha tocopherol equivalents.

CHOL (mg)	SOD (mg)	POT (mg)	MAG (mg)	IRON (mg)	ZINC (mg)	VITA (RE)	VITC (mg)	THIA (mg)	RIBO (mg)	NIAC (mg)	VB6 (mg)	FOL (µg)	VB12 (µg)	CALC (mg)	PHOS (mg)	SEL (µg)	VE-a (mg)
0	4	374	31	1.6	0.5	84	12	0.09	0.12	0.8	0.07	42	0	58	48	1	0.4
0	349	1318	99	2.8	0.7	740	36	0.17	0.42	0.7	0.19	21	0	165	60	*	2.2
0	113	349	39	1.7	0.6	2	10	0.03	0.09	0.4	0.14	71	0	34	39	3	0.1
0	83	530	63	1.1	0.4	2	9	0.05	0.02	0.5	0.05	90	0	19	53	1	0.1
0	466	252	29	3.1	0.4	2	7	0.02	0.07	0.3	0.1	51	0	26	29	1	0.1
0	25	156	19	0.3	0.1	1	3	0.02	0.01	0.1	0.02	27	0	6	12	1	t
0	647	349	39	1.7	0.6	2	10	0.03	0.09	0.4	0.14	71	0	34	39	1	0.1
0	44	333	37	1.1	0.6	350	74	0.1	0.15	0.8	0.24	104	0	94	102	3	0.9
0	24	286	22	0.8	0.4	136	82	0.06	0.11	0.6	0.14	63	0	42	58	1	0.4
0	40	453	37	1.3	0.6	215	116	0.09	0.18	0.9	0.22	78	0	71	92	3	0.7
0	36	504	37	1.2	0.6	92	71	0.16	0.18	0.8	0.45	157	0	37	84	1	1.3
0	33	495	31	1.9	0.5	112	97	0.17	0.12	0.9	0.28	94	0	56	87	1	1.3
0	7	597	65	1.3	0.6	0	4	0.07	0.1	0.5	0.46	32	0	82	154	*	*
0	7	181	10	0.2	0.2	91	21	0.03	0.04	0.3	0.18	60	0	59	22	2	0.1
0	28	297	22	0.6	0.2	13	35	0.08	0.08	0.3	0.09	29	0	48	36	3	2.4
0	16	221	14	0.5	0.2	11	43	0.05	0.03	0.3	0.09	51	0	42	21	2	1.5
0	13	172	11	0.4	0.1	9	33	0.04	0.02	0.2	0.07	40	0	33	16	2	1.2
0	8	144	11	0.3	0.1	3	40	0.04	0.02	0.2	0.15	15	0	36	29	2	0.1
0	20	161	20	0.3	0.2	70	22	0.05	0.02	0.2	0.13	56	0	25	29	2	0.1
0	58	631	19	1.8	0.3	437	44	0.05	0.11	0.7	0.28	69	0	158	49	4	1.2
0	46	176	13	0.6	0.1	210	32	0.03	0.05	0.4	0.14	46	0	74	26	2	0.1
0	71	718	34	1.1	0.4	6335	21	0.23	0.14	1	0.53	9	0	59	103	*	t
0	39	355	17	0.6	0.2	3094	10	0.11	0.06	1	0.16	15	0	30	48	2	0.5
0	25	233	11	0.4	0.1	2025	7	0.07	0.04	0.7	0.11	10	0	19	32	2	0.3
0	103	354	20	1	0.5	3830	4	0.05	0.09	0.8	0.38	22	0	48	47	2	0.7
0	96	426	22	1.5	0.7	3239	7	0.05	0.07	1	0.28	20	0	62	49	3	1
0	352	261	12	0.9	0.4	2010	4	0.03	0.04	0.8	0.16	13	0	37	35	2	0.6
0	86	231	15	0.7	0.4	2584	4	0.04	0.05	0.6	0.19	16	0	41	38	3	0.6
0	32	250	16	0.7	0.2	4	56	0.07	0.1	0.6	0.16	74	0	31	43	1	0.1
0	8	400	14	0.5	0.3	2	69	0.08	0.06	0.7	0.25	63	0	34	44	1	t
0	15	355	14	0.6	0.2	2	72	0.08	0.06	0.6	0.23	66	0	29	46	1	t
0	104	344	13	0.5	0.2	16	8	0.06	0.05	0.4	0.1	34	0	48	30	0	0.4
0	35	115	4	0.2	0.1	5	3	0.02	0.02	0.1	0.04	11	0	16	10	0	0.1
0	313	961	150	4	0.6	549	32	0.06	0.15	0.6	0.15	15	0	102	58	70	2.6
0	64	198	31	0.8	0.1	113	6	0.01	0.03	0.1	0.03	3	0	21	12	*	0.5
0	81	756	54	1.6	0.8	720	43	0.11	0.18	0.9	0.19	197	0	180	85	*	*
0	30	174	13	0.5	0.2	1	3	0.02	0.02	0.2	0.15	14	0	25	37	*	0.6
0	t	6	1	t	t	14	1	t	t	t	t	t	0	2	1	*	129
0	t	8	2	t	t	19	2	t	0.01	t	0.01	t	0	2	2	*	t
0	85	427	51	1.9	0.5	1017	45	0.08	0.2	1.1	0.19	129	0	357	46	1	*
0	21	168	9	0.2	0.1	349	16	0.03	0.07	0.4	0.07	8	0	29	10	1	2.9
25	167	47	8	0.6	0.2	14	1	0.06	0.07	0.6	0.02	11	0.06	22	54	*	1.1
0	8	343	44	1	1.4	26	12	0.06	0.14	2.5	0.16	115	0	8	131	1	0.1
0	5	316	37	0.8	0.8	27	6	0.22	0.09	1.9	0.28	38	0	4	95	1	0.1
0	8	228	30	0.5	0.6	41	4	0.11	0.12	2.1	0.16	33	0	4	78	1	0.1
0	13	192	25	0.5	0.4	17	5	0.17	0.06	1.2	0.05	36	0	2	79	1	0.1
0	533	322	33	1.4	0.6	26	14	0.05	0.13	2	0.08	80	0	8	107	1	0.1
0	8	392	41	0.9	0.9	31	17	0.07	0.16	2.4	0.1	98	0	10	131	1	0.1
0	572	390	48	0.9	1	51	17	0.09	0.15	2.5	0.12	104	0	10	134	1	0.1
0	730	343	44	1	1.4	26	12	0.06	0.14	2.5	0.16	115	0	8	131	1	0.1
0	788	347	57	1.8	0.8	52	20	0.05	0.18	2.2	0.22	77	0	11	141	1	0.1
0	8	304	19	0.7	0.1	465	35	0.04	0.13	0.5	0.12	40	0	40	38	*	0.4
0	2	155	11	0.3	0.2	5	5	0.03	0.02	0.3	0.05	15	0	15	18	1	0.2
0	6	448	33	0.8	0.7	15	14	0.09	0.06	0.9	0.16	42	0	42	51	1	0.5
0	46	244	25	1.9	0.3	1229	19	0.14	0.18	0.5	0.17	13	0	147	44	1	2.6
0	3	238	13	0.3	0.1	6	1	0.07	0.02	0.6	0.08	14	0	6	21	*	t
0	11	157	8	0.4	0.4	103	3	0.04	0.04	0.2	0.01	71	0	26	14	*	0.5
36	882	605	85	2.2	1.7	46	2	0.14	0.33	1.5	0.19	111	0.68	188	175	*	*
0	1	12	1	0.1	t	0	1	0.01	t	t	0.04	t	0	5	5	0	0
0	13	398	41	0.5	0.3	0	5	0.02	0.03	0.7	0.15	11	0	17	26	*	0.7
0	3	248	16	0.4	1	0	12	0.04	0.03	0.6	0.06	6	0	35	19	*	*
0	600	428	71	3.9	2.7	5	19	0.23	0.13	1	0.98	146	0	123	275	*	0
0	6	644	26	5.1	0.2	3	6	0.3	0.09	2	0.12	20	0	21	117	*	0.3

WT, weight; **KCAL**, kcalories; **PROT**, protein; **CARB**, carbohydrate; **FIBR**, fiber; **FAT**, fat; **SATF**, saturated fat;

MONO, monosaturated fat; **POLY**, polyunsaturated fat; **CHOR**, cholesterol; **SOD**, sodium; **POT**, potassium;

Food Name	Portion	WT (Gm)	KCAL	PROT (Gm)	CARB (Gm)	FIBR (Gm)	FAT (Gm)	SATF (Gm)	MONO (Gm)	POLY (Gm)
KALE-FROZEN-BOILED-DRAINED	CUP	130	39	4	7	3.8	1	0.1	t	0.3
KALE-RAW-BOILED-DRAINED	CUP	130	42	2	7	4.3	1	0.1	t	0.3
KOHLRABI-BOILED-DRAINED	CUP	165	48	3	11	3.3	t	t	t	0.1
KOHLRABI-RAW	CUP	140	38	2	9	2.5	t	t	t	0.1
LEEKS-BOILED-DRAINED	ITEM	124	38	1	9	4	t	t	t	0.1
LEEKS-RAW	ITEM	124	76	2	18	2.5	t	0.1	t	0.2
LENTILS-SPROUTED-RAW	CUP	77	82	7	17	6.2	t	t	0.1	0.2
LENTILS-WHOLE-COOKED	CUP	198	231	18	40	9.8	1	0.1	0.1	0.3
LETTUCE-BUTTERHEAD-HEAD	ITEM	163	21	2	4	1.6	t	t	t	0.2
LETTUCE-BUTTERHEAD-LEAVES	SLICE	15	2	t	t	0.2	t	t	t	t
LETTUCE-ICEBERG-RAW-CHOPPED	CUP	55	7	1	1	0.6	t	t	t	0.1
LETTUCE-ICEBERG-RAW-HEAD	ITEM	539	70	5	11	5.4	1	0.1	t	0.5
LETTUCE-ICEBERG-RAW-LEAVES	PIECE	20	3	t	t	0.2	t	t	t	t
LETTUCE-LOOSELEAF-RAW	CUP	55	10	1	2	0.8	t	t	t	0.1
LETTUCE-ROMAINE-RAW-SHREDDED	CUP	56	9	1	1	1	t	t	t	0.1
LOTUS ROOT-BOILED-DRAINED	OUNCE	28.4	19	t	5	0.9	t	t	t	t
LOTUS ROOT-RAW	ITEM	115	64	3	20	3.5	t	t	t	t
MISO-FERMENTED SOYBEANS	CUP	275	567	33	77	9.9	17	2.4	3.7	9.4
MUSHROOMS-BOILED-DRAINED	ITEM	12	3	t	1	0.3	t	t	t	t
MUSHROOMS-CANNED-DRAINED	ITEM	12	3	t	1	0.2	t	t	t	t
MUSHROOMS-RAW-CHOPPED	CUP	70	18	1	3	0.9	t	t	t	0.1
MUSTARD GREENS-BOILED-DRAINED	CUP	140	21	3	3	2.7	t	t	0.2	0.1
NATTO-FERMENTED SOYBEANS	CUP	280	468	47	32	9.7	21	4.5	6.8	17.4
NUTS-CHESTNUTS-CHINESE-DRIED	OUNCE	28.4	103	2	23	2.2	1	0.1	0.3	0.1
NUTS-CHESTNUTS-CHINESE-RAW	OUNCE	28.4	64	1	14	2.2	t	t	0.2	0.1
NUTS-CHESTNUTS-ROASTED	OUNCE	28.4	68	1	15	2.2	t	0.1	0.2	0.1
OKRA-RAW-BOILED-DRAINED	CUP	160	51	3	12	2	t	0.1	t	0.1
ONION RINGS-FROZEN-PREPARED-HEATED	ITEM	10	41	1	4	0.4	3	0.9	1.1	0.5
ONIONS-MATURE-BOILED-DRAINED	CUP	210	92	3	21	1.7	t	0.1	0.1	0.2
ONIONS-MATURE-RAW-CHOPPED	CUP	160	61	2	14	2.6	t	t	t	0.1
ONIONS-YOUNG GREEN	ITEM	5	1	t	t	0.1	t	t	0	0
PARSLEY-RAW-CHOPPED	TBSP	4	1	t	t	0.2	t	t	t	t
PARSNIPS-SLICED-BOILED-DRAINED	CUP	156	126	2	31	7.6	t	0.1	0.2	0.1
PEAS-BLACKEYE/COWPEAS-BOILED-DRAINED	CUP	165	179	13	30	15.8	1	0.3	0.1	0.4
PEAS-BLACKEYE/COWPEAS-FROZEN-BOILED	CUP	170	224	14	40	9.8	1	0.3	0.1	0.5
PEAS-BLACKEYE/COWPEAS-RAW-BOILED	CUP	165	160	5	34	11	1	0.2	0.1	0.3
PEAS-EDIBLE PODDED-RAW	CUP	145	61	4	11	3.8	t	0.1	t	0.1
PEAS-GREEN-CANNED-DIETARY-LOW SODIUM	CUP	170	117	8	21	5.8	1	0.1	0.1	0.3
PEAS-GREEN-CANNED-DRAINED	CUP	170	117	8	21	5.8	1	0.1	0.1	0.3
PEAS-GREEN-FROZEN-BOILED-DRAINED	CUP	160	125	8	23	6.1	t	0.1	t	0.2
PEAS-SPLIT-DRY-COOKED	CUP	200	230	16	42	10.5	1	0.1	0.2	0.3
PEAS-SWEET-CANNED IN WATER-DIETETIC	OUNCE	28.4	12	1	2	0.6	t	0	0	0
PEPPERS-HOT CHILI-CANNED	CUP	136	34	1	8	2.1	t	t	t	0.1
PEPPERS-HOT CHILI-RAW	CUP	150	60	3	14	3.6	t	t	t	0.2
PEPPERS-HOT-RED-DRIED	TSP	2	5	0	1	0.7	0	0	0	0
PEPPERS-JALAPENO-CANNED-CHOPPED	CUP	136	33	1	1	2	1	0.1	t	0.4
PEPPERS-SWEET-BOILED-DRAINED	ITEM	73	20	1	5	0.7	t	t	t	0.1
PEPPERS-SWEET-RAW	ITEM	74	20	1	5	1.2	t	t	t	0.1
PIMIENTOS-4 OUNCE CAN OR JAR	ITEM	113	31	1	7	2.6	1	0.1	t	0.4
POI-TARO ROOT PRODUCT	CUP	240	269	1	65	4.8	t	0.1	t	0.1
POTATO CHIPS-SALT ADDED	ITEM	2	11	t	1	t	1	0.2	0.1	0.4
POTATO PANCAKES-HOME RECIPE	ITEM	76	495	5	26	1.4	13	3.4	5.4	2.5
POTATO PUFFS-FROZEN-HEATED	ITEM	7	16	t	2	0.2	1	0.4	0.3	0.1
POTATO SKIN-BAKED	ITEM	58	115	2	27	3	t	t	t	t
POTATO-AU GRATIN-HOME RECIPE	CUP	245	323	12	28	4.4	19	11.6	5.3	0.7
POTATO-AU GRATIN-PREPARED FROM MIX	OUNCE	28.4	26	1	4	0.5	1	0.7	0.3	t
POTATO-BAKED-FLESH & SKIN-WHOLE	ITEM	202	220	5	51	4.9	t	0.1	t	0.1
POTATO-BAKED-PEELED AFTER BAKING	ITEM	156	145	3	34	3.7	t	t	t	0.1
POTATO-BOILED-PEELED AFTER BOILING	ITEM	136	118	3	27	2	t	t	t	0.1
POTATO-BOILED-PEELED BEFORE BOILING	ITEM	135	116	2	27	1.5	t	t	t	0.1
POTATO-CANNED-DRAINED	ITEM	35	21	t	5	0.9	t	t	t	t
POTATO-FRENCH FRIED-PREPARED FROM FROZEN	ITEM	5	11	t	2	0.2	t	0.2	0.2	t
POTATO-FRENCH FRIED-PREPARED FROM RAW	ITEM	5	14	t	2	0.2	1	0.2	0.2	t
POTATO-HASH BROWN-PREPARED FROM RAW	CUP	156	239	4	12	3.1	22	8.5	9.7	2.5

t = Trace of nutrient present   * = Not available

MAG, magnesium; IRON, iron; ZINC, zinc; VITA, vitamin A; VITC, vitamin C; THIA, thiamin; RIBO, riboflavin; NIAC, niacin; VB6, vitamin B-6; FOL, folate; VB12, vitamin B-12; CALC, calcium; PHOS, phosphorus; SEL, selenium; VE-a, alpha tocopherol equivalents.

CHOL (mg)	SOD (mg)	POT (mg)	MAG (mg)	IRON (mg)	ZINC (mg)	VITA (RE)	VITC (mg)	THIA (mg)	RIBO (mg)	NIAC (mg)	VB6 (mg)	FOL (μg)	VB12 (μg)	CALC (mg)	PHOS (mg)	SEL (μg)	VE-a (mg)
0	20	417	23	1.2	0.2	826	33	0.06	0.15	0.9	0.11	19	0	179	36	1	10.4
0	30	296	23	1.2	0.3	962	53	0.07	0.09	0.7	0.18	17	0	94	36	1	10.4
0	35	561	31	0.7	0.5	7	89	0.07	0.03	0.6	0.25	20	0	41	74	*	2.7
0	28	490	27	0.6	t	6	87	0.07	0.03	0.6	0.21	23	0	34	64	1	t
0	12	108	17	1.4	0.1	6	5	0.03	0.03	0.2	0.14	30	0	37	21	0	1.1
0	25	223	35	2.6	0.1	12	15	0.07	0.04	0.5	0.29	80	0	73	43	0	1.1
0	8	248	29	2.5	1.2	4	13	0.18	0.1	0.9	0.15	77	0	19	133	8	1
0	4	731	71	6.6	2.5	2	3	0.34	0.15	2.1	0.35	358	0	37	356	20	0.2
0	8	419	21	0.5	0.3	158	13	0.1	0.1	0.5	0.08	119	0	52	38	2	0.9
0	1	39	2	t	t	15	1	0.01	0.01	t	0.01	11	0	5	3	0	0.1
0	5	87	5	0.3	0.1	18	2	0.03	0.02	0.1	0.02	31	0	11	11	0	0.2
0	49	852	49	2.7	1.2	178	21	0.25	0.16	1	0.22	302	0	102	108	5	2.3
0	2	32	2	0.1	t	7	1	0.01	0.01	t	0.01	11	0	4	4	0	0.1
0	5	145	6	0.8	0.2	105	10	0.03	0.04	0.2	0.03	27	0	37	14	0	0.2
0	4	162	3	0.6	0.1	146	13	0.06	0.06	0.3	0.03	76	0	20	25	0	0.2
0	13	103	6	0.3	0.1	0	8	0.04	t	0.1	0.06	2	0	7	22	*	t
0	46	639	27	1.3	0.4	0	51	0.18	0.25	0.5	0.21	15	0	52	115	*	t
0	10030	451	116	7.5	9.1	25	0	0.27	0.69	2.4	0.59	91	0	182	421	*	*
0	t	43	1	0.2	0.1	0	t	0.01	0.04	0.5	0.01	2	0	1	10	1	t
0	51	16	2	0.1	0.1	0	0	0.01	t	0.2	0.01	1	0	1	8	5	t
0	3	259	7	0.9	0.5	0	2	0.07	0.31	2.9	0.07	15	0	4	73	9	0.1
0	22	283	21	1	0.2	424	35	0.06	0.09	0.6	0	103	0	103	58	1	2.8
0	20	697	322	10.4	8.5	0	0	0.07	0.5	1.1	0.36	22	0	103	182	*	t
0	2	206	39	0.7	0.4	9	17	0.07	0.08	0.4	0.19	31	0	8	44	2	0.1
0	1	127	24	0.4	0.2	6	10	0.05	0.05	0.2	0.12	19	0	5	27	2	0.1
0	1	135	26	0.4	0.3	t	11	0.04	0.03	0.4	0.12	21	0	5	29	2	0.1
0	8	515	91	0.7	0.9	92	26	0.21	0.09	1.4	0.3	73	0	101	90	1	1.1
0	38	13	2	0.2	t	2	t	0.03	0.01	0.4	0.01	1	0	3	8	*	0.1
0	6	349	23	0.5	0.4	0	11	0.09	0.05	0.3	0.27	32	0	46	74	7	0.3
0	5	251	16	0.4	0.3	0	10	0.07	0.03	0.2	0.19	30	0	32	53	3	0.5
0	t	13	1	0.1	t	25	2	t	0.01	t	t	1	0	3	2	0	t
0	2	21	2	0.2	t	21	4	t	t	0.1	t	7	0	5	2	0	0.1
0	16	574	46	0.9	0.4	0	20	0.13	0.08	1.1	0.15	91	0	58	108	1	1.6
0	7	693	83	2.4	1.3	105	3	0.11	0.18	1.8	0.08	173	0	46	197	0	0.2
0	9	638	85	3.6	2.4	13	5	0.44	0.11	1.2	0.16	240	0	40	208	*	0.2
0	7	690	86	1.9	1.7	130	4	0.17	0.24	2.3	0.11	210	0	211	84	*	0.2
0	6	290	35	3	0.4	20	87	0.22	0.12	0.9	0.23	61	0	62	77	1	0.2
0	3	294	29	1.6	1.2	131	16	0.21	0.13	1.2	0.11	75	0	34	114	2	t
0	372	294	29	1.6	1.2	131	16	0.21	0.13	1.2	0.11	75	0	34	114	1	t
0	139	269	46	2.5	1.5	107	16	0.45	0.16	2.4	0.18	94	0	38	144	1	0.2
0	8	592	72	3.4	2.1	8	1	0.3	0.18	1.8	0.1	129	0	22	178	3	0.2
0	1	27	5	0.6	0.2	16	3	0.02	0.02	0.2	*	*	0	6	17	0	1
0	1595	254	19	0.7	0.2	83	92	0.03	0.07	1.1	0.21	14	0	10	24	*	0.9
0	10	510	38	1.8	0.5	116	364	0.14	0.14	1.4	0.42	35	0	26	68	*	1
0	20	20	3	0.3	0.1	130	0	0	0.02	0.2	t	t	0	5	4	0	t
0	1990	185	16	3.8	0.3	231	18	0.04	0.07	0.7	0.28	18	0	35	23	0	0.9
0	1	121	7	0.3	0.1	43	54	0.04	0.02	0.3	0.17	11	0	7	13	0	0.5
0	1	131	7	0.3	0.1	47	66	0.05	0.02	0.4	0.18	16	0	7	14	0	0.5
0	35	311	6	1.7	0.2	260	107	0.02	0.07	0.5	0.19	14	0	8	19	*	1
0	28	439	58	2.1	0.5	5	10	0.31	0.1	2.6	0.66	51	0	37	94	*	0.5
0	9	26	1	t	t	0	1	t	0	0.1	0.01	1	0	1	3	0	0.1
93	388	538	24	1.2	0.7	9	t	0.1	0.1	1.6	0.29	22	0.22	21	78	*	1.1
0	52	27	1	0.1	t	t	t	0.01	0.01	0.2	0.02	1	0	2	3	*	0.3
0	12	332	25	4.1	0.3	0	8	0.07	0.06	1.8	0.36	13	0	20	59	*	t
56	1061	970	49	1.6	1.7	93	24	0.16	0.28	2.4	0.43	20	0.49	292	277	*	1.6
*	125	62	4	0.1	0.1	9	1	0.01	0.02	0.3	0.01	2	0	24	27	*	*
0	16	844	55	2.8	0.7	*	26	0.22	0.07	3.3	0.7	22	0	20	115	1	0.1
0	8	610	39	0.6	0.5	0	20	0.16	0.03	2.2	0.47	14	0	8	78	1	t
0	5	515	30	0.4	0.4	0	18	0.14	0.03	2	0.41	14	0	7	60	1	t
0	7	443	26	0.4	0.4	0	10	0.13	0.03	1.8	0.36	12	0	10	54	1	t
0	91	80	5	0.4	0.1	0	2	0.02	0.01	0.3	0.07	2	0	2	10	1	0.1
0	2	23	1	0.1	t	0	1	0.01	t	0.1	0.01	1	0	t	4	0	t
0	11	43	2	0.1	t	0	1	0.01	t	0.2	0.01	1	0	1	6	0	t
0	37	501	31	1.3	0.5	0	9	0.12	0.03	3.1	0.43	12	0	13	66	*	0.3

WT, weight; KCAL, kcalories; PROT, protein; CARB, carbohydrate; FIBR, fiber; FAT, fat; SATF, saturated fat;
MONO, monosaturated fat; POLY, polyunsaturated fat; CHOR, cholesterol; SOD, sodium; POT, potassium;

Food Name	Portion	WT (Gm)	KCAL	PROT (Gm)	CARB (Gm)	FIBR (Gm)	FAT (Gm)	SATF (Gm)	MONO (Gm)	POLY (Gm)
POTATO-HASH BROWN-PREPARED FROM FROZEN	CUP	156	340	5	44	1.5	18	7	8	2.1
POTATO-HUSH PUPPIES	SERVING	78	256	5	35	1.9	12	2.7	7.8	0.4
POTATO-MASHED-FROM DEHYDRATED-WITH MILK	CUP	210	166	4	28	1.2	5	1.4	1.4	1.3
POTATO-MASHED-FROM RAW-WITH MILK	CUP	210	162	4	37	1.2	1	0.7	0.3	0.1
POTATO-MASHED-HOME RECIPE-MILK/BUTTER	CUP	210	223	4	35	3.2	9	2.2	3.7	2.5
POTATO-O'BRIEN-HOME RECIPE	CUP	194	157	5	30	*	2	1.6	0.7	0.1
POTATO-SCALLOPED-HOME RECIPE	CUP	245	211	7	26	4.4	9	5.5	2.6	0.4
POTATO-SCALLOPED-PREPARED FROM MIX	OUNCE	28.4	26	1	4	0.5	1	0.7	0.3	0.1
PUMPKIN PIE MIX-CANNED	CUP	270	281	3	71	*	t	0.2	t	t
PUMPKIN-BOILED-DRAINED-MASHED	CUP	245	49	2	12	6.7	t	0.1	t	t
PUMPKIN-CANNED	CUP	245	83	3	20	5	1	0.4	0.1	t
PUMPKIN-RAW-CUBED	CUP	116	30	1	8	2	t	0.1	t	t
RADISH-DAIKON-SLICED-BOILED-DRAINED	CUP	147	25	1	5	2.9	t	0.1	0.1	0.2
RADISHES-RAW	ITEM	4.5	1	t	t	0.1	t	t	t	t
RUTABAGAS-BOILED-DRAINED	CUP	170	58	2	13	2.5	t	t	t	0.1
SAUERKRAUT-CANNED	CUP	236	45	2	10	6.1	t	0.1	t	0.1
SEAWEED-AGAR-DRIED	SERVING	28.4	87	2	23	0.9	t	t	t	t
SEAWEED-IRISHMOSS-RAW	OUNCE	28.4	14	t	3	1	t	t	t	t
SEAWEED-KELP (KOMBU)-RAW	OUNCE	28.4	12	t	3	1.2	t	0.1	t	t
SEAWEED-LAVER (NORI)-RAW	OUNCE	28.4	10	2	1	1	t	t	t	t
SEAWEED-SPIRULINA-DRIED	OUNCE	28.4	82	16	7	1.4	2	0.8	0.2	0.6
SEAWEED-WAKAME-RAW	OUNCE	28.4	13	1	3	1.2	t	t	t	0.1
SHALLOTS-FREEZE DRIED	TBSP	0.9	3	t	1	0.1	t	t	t	t
SHALLOTS-RAW	TBSP	10	7	t	2	*	t	t	t	t
SOYBEANS-DRY-COOKED	CUP	180	234	20	19	*	10	*	*	*
SOYBEANS-GREEN-BOILED-DRAINED	CUP	180	254	22	20	*	12	1.3	1.3	6.4
SOYBEANS-SPROUTED-STEAMED	CUP	94	76	8	6	1	4	0.5	0.5	2.3
SPINACH-CANNED-DIETARY PACK-LOW SODIUM	CUP	234	45	5	7	5.1	1	0.1	t	0.4
SPINACH-CANNED-DRAINED	CUP	214	50	6	7	6.8	1	0.2	t	0.4
SPINACH-CANNED-SOLIDS AND LIQUIDS	CUP	234	45	5	7	5.1	1	0.1	t	0.4
SPINACH-FROZEN-BOILED-CHOPPED	CUP	205	57	6	11	4.5	t	0.1	t	0.2
SPINACH-LEAF-FROZEN-BOILED-DRAINED	CUP	190	53	6	10	4	t	0.1	t	0.2
SPINACH-RAW-BOILED-DRAINED	CUP	180	41	5	7	4	t	0.1	t	0.2
SPINACH-RAW-CHOPPED	CUP	56	12	2	2	1.5	t	t	t	0.1
SQUASH-ACORN-BAKED	CUP	205	115	2	30	4.3	t	0.1	t	0.1
SQUASH-BUTTERNUT-BAKED	CUP	205	82	2	22	3.5	t	t	t	0.1
SQUASH-HUBBARD-BOILED-MASHED	CUP	236	71	3	15	4.2	1	0.2	0.1	0.4
SQUASH-SUMMER-BOILED-SLICED	CUP	180	36	2	8	2.5	1	0.1	t	0.2
SQUASH-WINTER-BAKE-MASHED	CUP	205	80	2	18	5.7	1	0.3	0.1	0.5
SQUASH-ZUCCHINI-FROZ-BOILED	CUP	223	38	3	8	3.2	t	0.1	t	0.1
SQUASH-ZUCCHINI-ITALIA-CANNED	CUP	227	66	2	16	7	t	0.1	t	0.1
SQUASH-ZUCCHINI-RAW-BOILED	CUP	180	29	1	7	2.3	t	t	t	t
SQUASH-ZUCCHINI-RAW-SLICED	CUP	130	18	2	4	2	t	t	t	0.1
SUCCOTASH-BOILED-DRAINED	CUP	192	221	10	47	14	2	0.3	0.3	0.7
SWEET POTATO-BAKED-PEELED	ITEM	114	117	2	28	3.4	t	t	t	0.1
SWEET POTATO-BOILED-MASHED	CUP	328	344	5	80	9.8	1	0.2	t	0.4
SWEET POTATO-CANDIED	PIECE	105	144	1	29	1.1	3	1.4	0.7	0.2
SWEET POTATO-CANNED-MASHED	CUP	255	258	5	59	4.6	1	0.1	t	0.2
SWEET POTATO-CANNED-VACUUM PACK	CUP	200	182	3	42	4.8	t	0.1	t	0.2
TARO ROOT-COOKED-SLICED	CUP	132	187	1	46	6	t	t	t	0.1
TARO ROOT-RAW-SLICED	CUP	104	111	2	28	*	t	t	t	0.1
TEMPEH-SOYBEAN PRODUCT	CUP	166	330	32	28	*	13	1.8	2.8	7.2
TOFU-FRIED	PIECE	13	35	2	1	0.2	3	0.4	0.6	1.5
TOFU-OKARA	CUP	122	94	4	15	5	2	0.2	0.4	0.9
TOFU-RAW-FIRM	CUP	252	365	40	11	3	22	3.2	4.9	12.4
TOFU-SOYBEAN CURD	PIECE	120	86	9	3	1.4	5	2.6	4.4	4.8
TOMATO JUICE-CANNED	CUP	244	42	2	10	2.9	t	t	t	0.1
TOMATO JUICE-LOW SODIUM	CUP	244	42	2	10	2.8	t	t	t	0.1
TOMATO PASTE-CANNED-LOW SODIUM	CUP	262	220	10	49	11.3	2	0.3	0.4	0.9
TOMATO PASTE-CANNED-SALT ADDED	CUP	262	220	10	49	11.3	2	0.3	0.4	0.9
TOMATO POWDER	OUNCE	28.4	86	4	21	0.7	t	t	t	0.1
TOMATO PUREE-CANNED-LOW SODIUM	CUP	250	103	4	25	5.8	t	t	t	0.1
TOMATO PUREE-CANNED-SALT ADDED	CUP	250	103	4	25	5.8	t	t	t	0.1

t = Trace of nutrient present   * = Not available

MAG, magnesium; **IRON**, iron; **ZINC**, zinc; **VITA**, vitamin A; **VITC**, vitamin C; **THIA**, thiamin; **RIBO**, riboflavin; **NIAC**, niacin; **VB6**, vitamin B-6; **FOL**, folate; **VB12**, vitamin B-12; **CALC**, calcium; **PHOS**, phosphorus; **SEL**, selenium; **VE-a**, alpha tocopherol equivalents.

CHOL (mg)	SOD (mg)	POT (mg)	MAG (mg)	IRON (mg)	ZINC (mg)	VITA (RE)	VITC (mg)	THIA (mg)	RIBO (mg)	NIAC (mg)	VB6 (mg)	FOL (µg)	VB12 (µg)	CALC (mg)	PHOS (mg)	SEL (µg)	VE-a (mg)
0	54	680	26	2.3	0.5	0	10	0.17	0.03	3.8	0.2	39	0	24	112	1	0.3
135	965	188	16	1.4	0.4	9	0	0	0.02	2	0.1	21	0.18	69	190	*	1.8
4	491	704	34	1.3	0.5	19	6	0.06	0.11	1.7	0.42	15	0	65	92	1	0.1
4	636	628	39	0.6	0.6	4	14	0.19	0.08	2.4	0.49	17	0.11	55	100	1	0.1
4	620	607	38	0.5	0.6	42	13	0.18	0.08	2.3	0.47	17	0	55	97	1	0.1
7	421	516	35	0.9	0.6	93	32	0.15	0.11	2	0.41	16	0.16	70	97	*	*
29	821	926	47	1.4	1	47	26	0.17	0.23	2.6	0.44	21	0	140	154	*	1.1
*	97	58	4	0.1	0.1	6	1	0.01	0.02	0.3	0.01	t	0	10	16	*	*
0	562	373	43	2.9	0.7	2241	9	0.04	0.32	1	0.43	95	0	100	122	*	*
0	3	564	22	1.4	0.6	265	12	0.08	0.19	1	0.11	21	0	37	74	*	2.5
0	12	505	56	3.4	0.4	5404	10	0.06	0.13	0.9	0.14	30	0	64	86	*	2.5
0	1	1	14	0.9	0.4	186	10	0.06	0.13	0.7	0.06	16	0	24	51	1	1.2
0	19	419	13	0.2	0.2	0	22	0	0.03	0.2	0.06	26	0	25	35	1	0.7
0	1	10	t	t	t	t	1	0	t	t	t	1	0	1	1	0	0
0	31	488	36	0.8	0.5	0	37	0.12	0.06	1.1	0.15	26	0	71	83	*	0.3
0	1560	401	31	3.5	0.4	5	35	0.05	0.05	0.3	0.31	56	0	71	47	24	3.9
0	29	320	219	6.1	1.7	0	0	t	0.06	0.1	0.09	165	0	178	15	2	1.6
0	19	18	41	2.5	0.6	3	3	t	0.13	0.2	0.02	52	0	20	45	*	0.3
0	66	25	34	0.8	0.3	3	1	0.01	0.04	0.1	t	51	0	48	12	2	0.2
0	14	101	1	0.5	0.3	148	11	0.03	0.13	0.4	0.05	42	0	20	17	1	0.3
0	298	387	55	8.1	0.6	16	3	0.68	1.04	3.6	0.1	27	0	34	34	2	1
0	248	14	30	0.6	0.1	10	1	0.02	0.07	0.5	t	56	0	43	23	1	0.3
0	1	15	1	0.1	t	51	t	t	t	t	0.02	1	0	2	3	*	*
0	1	33	2	0.1	t	125	1	0.01	t	t	0.04	3	0	4	6	*	t
0	4	972	*	4.9	*	5	0	0.38	0.16	1.1	*	*	0	131	322	*	*
0	25	970	108	4.5	1.6	29	31	0.47	0.28	2.3	0.11	201	0	261	284	90	0
0	9	334	56	1.2	1	8	8	0.19	0.05	1	0.1	75	0	56	127	47	t
0	746	538	131	3.7	1	1505	32	0.04	0.25	0.6	0.19	136	0	194	75	3	t
0	57	740	162	4.9	1	1878	31	0.03	0.3	0.8	0.21	209	0	271	94	2	t
0	746	538	131	3.7	1	1505	32	0.04	0.25	0.6	0.19	136	0	194	75	3	t
0	176	611	141	3.1	1.4	1596	25	0.12	0.34	0.9	0.3	220	0	299	98	2	3.9
0	164	566	131	2.9	1.3	1479	23	0.11	0.32	0.8	0.28	204	0	277	91	2	3.6
0	126	839	157	6.4	1.4	1474	18	0.17	0.43	0.9	0.44	262	0	245	101	2	3.4
0	44	312	44	1.5	0.3	376	16	0.04	0.11	0.4	0.11	108	0	55	27	1	0.2
0	9	896	87	1.9	0.4	88	22	0.34	0.03	1.8	0.4	38	0	90	93	2	0.2
0	8	582	60	1.2	0.3	1435	31	0.15	0.04	2	0.25	39	0	84	55	2	0.2
0	12	505	32	0.7	0.2	946	15	0.1	0.07	0.8	0.24	23	0	24	33	2	0.3
0	2	346	44	0.6	0.7	52	10	0.08	0.07	0.9	0.12	36	0	48	69	6	0.2
0	2	896	16	0.7	0.5	730	20	0.17	0.05	1.4	0.15	57	0	29	41	6	0.2
0	4	433	29	1.1	0.4	96	8	0.09	0.09	0.9	0.1	17	0	38	56	7	0.3
0	850	622	31	1.5	0.6	123	5	0.1	0.09	1.2	0.35	69	0	39	66	*	0.3
0	5	455	40	0.6	0.3	43	8	0.07	0.07	0.8	0.14	30	0	23	72	6	0.2
0	4	322	29	0.5	0.3	44	12	0.09	0.04	0.5	0.12	29	0	20	42	4	0.2
0	33	787	102	2.9	1.2	56	16	0.32	0.18	2.6	0.22	63	0	33	225	*	0.7
0	11	397	23	0.5	0.3	2487	28	0.08	0.15	0.7	0.28	26	0	32	63	1	5.2
0	42	602	32	1.8	0.9	5594	56	0.17	0.46	2.1	0.8	36	0	70	88	2	15
0	73	198	12	1.2	0.2	440	7	0.02	0.04	0.4	0.04	12	0.03	27	27	1	4.6
0	191	536	61	3.4	0.5	3857	13	0.07	0.23	2.4	0.17	27	0	76	133	2	1.1
0	106	624	44	1.8	0.4	1596	53	0.07	0.11	1.5	0.38	33	0	44	98	2	0.9
0	20	638	40	1	0.4	0	7	0.14	0.04	0.7	0.44	25	0	24	100	*	3.3
0	11	615	34	0.6	0.2	0	5	0.1	0.03	0.6	0.29	23	0	45	87	*	*
0	10	609	116	3.8	3	114	0	0.22	0.18	7.7	0.5	86	1.66	154	342	*	*
0	2	19	8	0.6	0.3	0	0	0.02	0.01	t	0.01	3	0	48	37	0	t
0	11	259	32	1.6	0.7	0	0	0.02	0.02	0.1	0.14	32	0	98	73	*	*
0	35	597	237	26.4	4	43	1	0.4	0.26	1	0.23	74	0	517	479	5	*
0	8	50	115	2.3	1	0	0	0.07	0.04	0.1	0.06	21	0.05	154	151	2	1.1
0	881	537	27	1.4	0.3	137	45	0.11	0.08	1.6	0.27	49	0	22	46	1	0.5
0	24	537	27	1.4	0.3	137	45	0.11	0.08	1.6	0.27	49	0	22	46	1	0.5
0	172	2442	134	7.8	2.1	647	111	0.41	0.5	8.4	1	59	0	92	207	3	*
0	2070	2442	134	7.8	2.1	647	111	0.41	0.5	8.4	1	59	0	92	207	3	4.4
0	38	547	51	1.3	0.5	490	33	0.26	0.22	2.6	0.13	34	0	47	84	*	0.2
0	50	1050	60	2.3	0.6	340	88	0.18	0.14	4.3	0.38	28	0	38	100	3	0.6
0	998	1050	60	2.3	0.6	340	88	0.18	0.14	4.3	0.38	28	0	38	100	3	0.6

WT, weight; **KCAL**, kcalories; **PROT**, protein; **CARB**, carbohydrate; **FIBR**, fiber; **FAT**, fat; **SATF**, saturated fat;

MONO, monosaturated fat; **POLY**, polyunsaturated fat; **CHOR**, cholesterol; **SOD**, sodium; **POT**, potassium;

Food Name	Portion	WT (Gm)	KCAL	PROT (Gm)	CARB (Gm)	FIBR (Gm)	FAT (Gm)	SATF (Gm)	MONO (Gm)	POLY (Gm)
TOMATO-CANNED-DIETARY PACK-LOW SODIUM	CUP	240	48	2	10	1.7	1	0.1	0.1	0.2
TOMATO-COOKED-STEWED-HOME RECIPE	CUP	101	80	2	13	1	3	0.5	1.1	0.9
TOMATO-RED-CANNED-STEWED	CUP	255	66	2	17	2	t	0.1	0.1	0.1
TOMATO-RED-CANNED-WHOLE	CUP	240	48	2	10	1.9	1	0.1	0.1	0.2
TOMATO-RED-CANNED-WITH GREEN CHILIES	CUP	241	36	2	9	0.9	t	t	t	0.1
TOMATO-RED-RAW-BOILED	CUP	240	65	3	14	2.1	1	0.1	0.2	0.4
TOMATO-RED-RIPE-RAW	ITEM	123	26	1	6	1.6	t	0.1	0.1	0.2
TOMATOES-GREEN-RAW	ITEM	123	30	1	6	0.6	t	t	t	0.1
TURNIP GREENS-FROZEN-BOILED	CUP	164	49	5	8	5.1	1	0.2	t	0.3
TURNIP GREENS-RAW-BOILED	CUP	144	29	2	6	4.5	t	0.1	t	0.1
TURNIPS-BOILED-DRAINED-DICED	CUP	156	28	1	8	3.1	t	t	t	0.1
VEGETABLE JUICE-CANNED	CUP	242	46	2	11	2.7	t	t	t	0.1
VEGETABLE JUICE-SNAP E TOM-TOMATO	CUP	243	46	2	9	1.9	0	0	0	0
VEGETABLE JUICE-V8 COCKTAIL-LOW SODIUM	CUP	243	51	0	10	2.7	0	0	0	0
VEGETABLE JUICE-V8-REGULAR	CUP	243	49	0	10	2.4	0	0	0	0
WATERCHESTNUTS-CHINESE-CANNED	CUP	140	70	1	17	*	t	t	t	t
WATERCHESTNUTS-CHINESE-RAW	CUP	124	131	2	30	*	t	t	t	t
WATERCRESS-RAW	CUP	34	4	1	t	0.4	t	t	t	t
YAM-MOUNTAIN-HAWAII-STEAMED	CUP	145	119	3	29	5.6	t	t	t	0.1
YAMS-BOILED OR BAKED-DRAINED	CUP	136	158	2	38	3.3	t	t	t	0.1

t = Trace of nutrient present   * = Not available

MAG, magnesium; **IRON**, iron; **ZINC**, zinc; **VITA**, vitamin A; **VITC**, vitamin C; **THIA**, thiamin; **RIBO**, riboflavin; **NIAC**, niacin; **VB6**, vitamin B-6; **FOL**, folate; **VB12**, vitamin B-12; **CALC**, calcium; **PHOS**, phosphorus; **SEL**, selenium; **VE-a**, alpha tocopherol equivalents.

CHOL (mg)	SOD (mg)	POT (mg)	MAG (mg)	IRON (mg)	ZINC (mg)	VITA (RE)	VITC (mg)	THIA (mg)	RIBO (mg)	NIAC (mg)	VB6 (mg)	FOL (μg)	VB12 (μg)	CALC (mg)	PHOS (mg)	SEL (μg)	VE-a (mg)
0	31	530	29	1.5	0.4	144	36	0.11	0.07	1.8	0.22	19	0	62	46	2	0.5
0	460	249	15	1.1	0.2	68	18	0.11	0.08	1.1	0.09	11	0	26	38	1	0.3
0	648	609	31	1.9	0.4	140	34	0.12	0.09	1.8	0.04	14	0	84	51	2	0.6
0	391	530	29	1.5	0.4	144	36	0.11	0.07	1.8	0.22	19	0	62	46	2	0.5
0	966	258	27	0.6	0.3	94	15	0.08	0.05	1.5	0.25	22	0	48	34	2	0.5
0	26	670	34	1.3	0.3	178	55	0.17	0.14	1.8	0.23	31	0	14	74	1	0.8
0	11	273	14	0.6	0.1	76	24	0.07	0.06	0.8	0.1	19	0	6	30	1	0.4
0	16	251	12	0.6	0.1	79	29	0.07	0.05	0.6	0.1	11	0	16	34	*	0.5
0	25	367	43	3.2	0.7	1309	36	0.09	0.12	0.8	0.11	65	0	249	56	1	3.7
0	42	292	32	1.2	0.2	792	40	0.07	0.1	0.6	0.26	171	0	197	42	1	3.3
0	78	211	13	0.3	0.3	0	18	0.04	0.04	0.5	0.11	14	0	34	30	1	t
0	883	467	27	1	0.5	283	67	0.1	0.07	1.8	0.34	51	0	27	41	1	0.8
0	1298	688	27	1.9	0.5	103	10	0.1	0.07	2.4	0.34	51	0	37	41	*	0.5
0	58	571	*	1.5	*	437	53	0.05	0.07	1.9	*	*	0	39	*	1	*
0	819	513	27	1.5	0.5	342	49	0.05	0.05	1.7	0.34	51	0	29	41	1	0.8
0	12	164	6	1.2	0.5	1	2	0.02	0.03	0.5	0.22	8	0	6	28	*	*
0	17	724	27	0.1	0.6	0	5	0.17	0.25	1.2	0.41	20	0	14	78	*	*
0	14	112	8	0.1	t	160	15	0.03	0.04	0.1	0.04	3	0	40	20	*	0.3
0	18	717	15	0.6	0.5	0	0	0.13	0.02	0.2	0.3	18	0	11	57	1	6.6
0	11	911	25	0.7	0.3	0	17	0.13	0.04	0.8	0.31	22	0	19	66	1	6.2

APPENDIX B

DIETARY ADVICE FOR CANADIANS

Canada has its own version of RDA, called Recommended Nutrient Intakes (RNI), published by the Minister of National Health and Welfare.

Age	Gender	Energy (kcal)	Thiamin (mg)	Riboflavin (mg)	Niacin (Ne)*	o-3 PUFA† (g)	o-6 PUFA* (g)
MONTHS							
0-4	Both	600	0.3	0.3	4	0.5	3
5-12	Both	900	0.4	0.5	7	0.5	3
YEARS							
1	Both	1100	0.5	0.6	8	0.6	4
2-3	Both	1300	0.6	0.7	9	0.7	4
4-6	Both	1800	0.7	0.9	13	1.0	6
7-9	M	2200	0.9	1.1	16	1.2	7
	F	1900	0.8	1.0	14	1.0	6
10-12	M	2500	1.0	1.3	18	1.4	8
	F	2200	0.9	1.1	16	1.2	7
13-15	M	2800	1.1	1.4	20	1.5	9
	F	2200	0.9	1.1	16	1.2	7
16-18	M	3200	1.3	1.6	23	1.8	11
	F	2100	0.8	1.1	15	1.2	7
19-24	M	3000	1.2	1.5	22	1.6	10
	F	2100	0.8	1.1	15	1.2	7
25-49	M	2700	1.1	1.4	19	1.5	9
	F	1900	0.8	1.0	14	1.1	7
50-74	M	2300	0.9	1.2	16	1.3	8
	F	1800	0.8‡	1.0‡	14‡	1.1‡	7‡
75+	M	200	0.8	1.0	14	1.1	7
	F§	1700	0.8‡	1.0‡	14‡	1.1‡	7‡
PREGNANCY (ADDITIONAL)							
1st Trimester		100	0.1	0.1	1	0.05	0.3
2nd Trimester		300	0.1	0.3	2	0.16	0.9
3rd Trimester		300	0.1	0.3	2	0.16	0.9
Lactation (additional)		450	0.2	0.4	3	0.25	1.5

Summary of Examples of Recommended Nutrients Based on Energy Expressed as Daily Rates

From Scientific Review Committee: Nutrition recommendation, Ottawa, Canada, 1990, Health and Welfare.
*Niacin equivalents.
†PUFA, polyunsaturated fatty acids.
‡Level below which intake should not fall.
§Assumes moderate physical activity.

Summary Examples of Recommended Nutrient Intake Based on Age and Body Weight Expressed as Daily Rates

Age	Gender	Weight (kg)	Protein (g)	Vit. A (RE)*	Vit. D (µg)	Vit. E (mg)	Vit. C (mg)	Folate (µg)	Vit. B$_{12}$ (µg)	Calcium (mg)	Phosphorus (mg)	Magnesium (mg)	Iron (mg)	Iodine (µg)	Zinc (mg)
MONTHS															
0-4	Both	6.0	12†	400	10	3	20	25	0.3	250‡	150	20	0.3§	30	2
5-12	Both	9.0	12	400	10	3	20	40	0.4	400	200	32	7	40	3
YEARS															
1	Both	11	13	400	10	3	20	40	0.5	500	300	40	6	55	4
2-3	Both	14	16	400	5	4	20	50	0.6	550	350	50	6	65	4
4-6	Both	18	19	500	5	5	25	70	0.8	600	400	65	8	85	5
7-9	M	25	26	700	2.5	7	25	90	1.0	700	500	100	8	110	7
	F	25	26	700	2.5	6	25	90	1.0	700	500	100	8	95	7
10-12	M	34	34	800	2.5	8	25	120	1.0	900	700	130	8	125	9
	F	36	36	800	2.5	7	25	130	1.0	1100	800	135	8	110	9
13-15	M	50	49	900	2.5	9	30	175	1.0	1100	900	185	10	160	12
	F	48	46	800	2.5	7	30	170	1.0	1000	850	180	13	160	9
16-18	M	62	58	1000	2.5	10	40‖	220	1.0	900	1000	230	10	160	12
	F	53	47	800	2.5	7	30‖	190	1.0	700	850	200	12	160	9
19-24	M	71	61	1000	2.5	10	40‖	220	1.0	800	1000	240	9	160	12
	F	58	50	800	2.5	7	30‖	180	1.0	700	850	200	13	160	9
25-49	M	74	64	1000	2.5	9	40‖	230	1.0	800	1000	250	9	160	12
	F	59	51	800	2.5	6	30‖	185	1.0	700	850	200	13	160	9
50-74	M	73	63	1000	5	7	40‖	230	1.0	800	1000	250	9	160	12
	F	63	54	800	5	6	30‖	195	1.0	800	850	210	8	160	9
75+	M	69	59	1000	5	6	40‖	215	1.0	800	1000	230	9	160	12
	F	64	55	800	5	5	30‖	200	1.0	800	850	210	8	160	9
PREGNANCY (ADDITIONAL)															
1st Trimester			5	0	2.5	2	0	200	1.2	500	200	15	0	25	6
2nd Trimester			20	0	2.5	2	10	200	1.2	500	200	45	5	25	6
3rd Trimester			24	0	2.5	2	10	200	1.2	500	200	45	10	25	6
Lactation (additional)			20	400	2.5	3	25	100	0.2	500	200	65	0	50	6

From Scientific Review Committee: Nutrition recommendations, Ottawa, Canada, 1990, Health and Welfare.
*Retinol equivalents.
†Protein is assumed to be from breast milk and must be adjusted for infant formula.
‡Infant formula with high phosphorus should contain 375 mg calcium.
§Breast milk is assumed to be the source of the mineral.
‖Smokers should increase vitamin C by 50%.

APPENDIX C

THE EXCHANGE SYSTEM

The exchange system is used to convert nutrient and food intake standards into practical meal plans. It was originally developed to help people with diabetes control their blood glucose levels. It proved so useful that the exchange system is now used to help people with a variety of medical conditions plan nutritious meals. It is even used by people with weight control problems to count fat and kcalories. You needn't have a special medical condition to use the exchange system. Because it is based on sound principles of nutrition, it is a useful meal planning tool for everyone. Using the exchange system to plan meals is a good way to familiarize yourself with low-fat and high-fiber alternatives.

How does the exchange system work? The exchange system divides food into six categories: starch/bread, milk, fruit, vegetables, meat and meat substitutes, and fat. Items in each category are organized into exchange lists. Every food on a given list contains approximately the same amount of carbohydrate, fat, protein, and kcalories, except as noted. This means any serving of food on a given list can be *exchanged* for one serving of any other food on the *same list*.

How can I put the exchange system into action? Suppose you decide you would like to eat less fat and more carbohydrates but you aren't sure how to make these changes part of your diet. You consult a dietitian, who tells you your goal should be a 2000-kcalorie-a-day diet that obtains of 55% its energy from carbohydrate, 30% from fat, and 15% from protein. To help you plan your diet, the dietitian gives you the following daily diet prescription: 11 servings of food from the starch/bread group, 5 servings of fruit, 3 servings of vegetables, 3 servings of medium-fat meat (note that 1 meat exchange is only 1 ounce compared with 3 ounces for a serving of meat using the Food Guide Pyramid), 2 servings of milk, and 8 servings of fat (Table C-1).

TABLE C-1 Exchange Patterns to Get You Started

Kcalories/day	1200	1600	2000	2400	2800	3200	3600
EXCHANGE GROUP							
Milk (low-fat)	2	2	2	2	2	2	2
Vegetables	2	2	3	3	3	3	3
Fruit	5	4	5	8	8	10	10
Starch/bread	4	8	11	11	15	17	20
Meat (medium-fat)	2	2	3	5	5	7	8
Fat	4	7	8	9	12	12	14

This is just one set of options. More meat could be included if less milk is used, for example. The breakdown is 55% energy as carbohydrate, 30% energy as fat, and 15% energy as protein.

Next the dietitian converts the diet prescription into a meal plan by dividing the total number of exchanges per day among three meals and a snack. You then can use the meal plan to develop a menu (Table C-2).

This menu is just one of many possible food combinations you can choose using the meal plan shown in Table C-2. You can use the six exchange lists plus the free foods list shown below to create other equally appropriate menus.

EXCHANGE LISTS*

List 1. Starch/Bread Exchanges

One exchange or equivalent of 1 slice of bread contains:

Carbohydrate	15 g	fat	trace
Protein	3 g	kcal	80
Dietary fiber	2 g (whole grains)		

Note: Bran cereals supply approximately 8 grams of dietary fiber.

½ cup pasta or barley
⅓ cup rice or cooked dried beans and peas
1 small potato (or ½ cup mashed)
½ cup starchy vegetables (corn, peas, or winter squash)
1 slice bread or 1 roll
½ English muffin, bagel, or hamburger/hot dog bun
½ cup cooked cereal
¾ cup dry cereal, unsweetened
4-6 crackers
3 cups popcorn, unbuttered, not cooked in oil

List 2. Meat Exchanges

One exchange or equivalent of meat is 1 oz. unless otherwise specified. One lean meat exchange contains:

Carbohydrate	0	fat	3 g
Protein	7 g	kcal	55 g

Lean meats:

Beef:	Flank filet mignon, sirloin, round (USDA Good or Choice)
Pork:	Ham, loin, Canadian bacon
Poultry:	Skinless chicken, turkey, Cornish hen

---

*Adapted from *Exchange Lists for Meal Planning.* © 1989, American Diabetes Association, American Dietetic Association; and Clamp B et al: *Problem solving exercises in nutrition,* Scottsdale, Ariz, 1994, Gorsuch.

TABLE C-2 Turning an Exchange System Plan into a Menu for 1 Day

BREAKFAST

1 low-fat milk exchange	1% milk (put some on cereal), 1 cup
2 fruit exchanges	Orange juice, 1 cup
3 bread exchanges	Cold cereal, ¾ cup Whole-wheat toast, 2 pieces
2 fat exchanges	Margarine on toast, 2 tsp.

LUNCH

4 bread exchanges	Whole-wheat bread, 2 slices Animal crackers, 16
3 fat exchanges	Bacon, 2 slices Mayonnaise, 1 tsp.
1 vegetable exchange	1 sliced tomato
2 fruit exchanges	1 banana (9 inches)
1 low-fat milk exchange	1% milk, 1 cup

DINNER

3 medium-fat meat exchanges	T-bone steak, broiled, 3 oz.
2 bread exchanges	Baked potato, 1 large
1 fat exchange	Margarine, 1 tsp.
2 vegetable exchanges	Broccoli, 1 cup
1 fruit exchange	1 kiwi fruit Coffee (if desired)

SNACK

2 bread exchanges	1 bagel
2 fat exchanges	Cream cheese, 2 tbsp.

PRESCRIPTION	Values calculated using a computer and nutrient analysis software

2000		Kcalories	2037
55%		Carbohydrate	55%
15%		Protein	16%
30%		Fat	29%

Fish:	Any fresh or frozen (except shellfish)	
	Shellfish except oysters	2 oz.
	Oysters	6 medium
	Sardines	2 medium
	Tuna, canned in water	¼ cup
Cheeses:	Diet (less than 55 kcal/oz.)	
	Cottage cheese, ¼ cup	
	Parmesan cheese	2 tbsp.
	Luncheon meats (95% fat free)	
	Legumes (**add 2 Starch/Bread**)	1 cup

1 medium-fat meat = 1 lean meat exchange + ½ fat exchange (2.5 g fat)

Beef:	Ground, roast, steak, meatloaf	
Pork:	Chops, loin roast, butt, cutlets	
Lamb:	Chops, leg, roasts	
Poultry:	Chicken with skin, ground turkey, skinless duck or goose	
Fish:	Salmon, canned	¼ cup
	Tuna, canned in oil	¼ cup

Organ meats

Cheeses:	Part-skim milk cheeses such as mozzarella or ricotta (56-80 kcal/oz.)	¼ cup
Egg		1
Tofu		4 oz.

1 high-fat meat = 1 lean meat exchange + 1 fat exchange (5 g)

Beef: Most USDA Prime cuts
Lamb: Ground lamb
Pork: Spareribs, ground pork
Poultry: duck or goose with skin
Cheese: Regular cheeses
Cold cuts (4 ½″ × ⅛″)

Sausage or hotdog (1.6 oz.)	1 lean meat exchange and 1 additional fat exchange
Peanut butter	1 tbsp.

List 3. Vegetable Exchanges

One exchange of vegetables contains:			
Carbohydrate	5 g	fat	trace
Protein	2 g	kcal	25
Fiber	2 g		

½ cup of cooked vegetables or 1 cup raw or ½ cup vegetable juice like V-8 equals 1 vegetable exchange.

Examples are: artichokes, asparagus, beans (green), bean sprouts, beets, broccoli, cabbage, carrots, cauliflower, collard greens, eggplant, kale, kohlrabi, mushrooms, okra, onions, peppers (bell), spinach, summer squash, tomato (large), turnips, water chestnuts, vegetable juices.

Exceptions:
• Some raw vegetables are found in the **Free Foods** list.
• Starchy vegetables are found in **List 1. Starch/Bread.**

List 4. Fruit Exchanges

One exchange of fruit contains:			
Carbohydrate	15 g	fat	0 g
Protein	0 g	kcal	60 g
Fiber	3 g		

1 fresh medium fruit
1 cup berries or melon

½ cup canned in juice or without sugar
½ cup fruit juice
¼ cup dried fruit
2 plums, figs, or tangerines
4 apricots

List 5. Milk Exchanges

One exchange or equivalent of 1 nonfat milk contains:			
Carbohydrate	12 g	fat	trace
Protein	8 g	kcal	90 g

1 cup skim or nonfat milk, buttermilk, yogurt
1 cup low-fat (2%) milk, buttermilk, yogurt = 1 nonfat milk + 1 fat exchange (5 g fat)
1 cup whole milk, buttermilk, yogurt = 1 nonfat milk + 2 fat exchanges (10 g fat)

List 6. Fat Exchanges

One exchange or equivalent of 1 tsp fat contains:			
Carbohydrate	0 g	fat	5 g
Protein	0 g	kcal	45 g

Fats/Oils	Amount	Other Foods	Amount
Butter, margarine	1 tsp.	Avocado	⅛
Mayonnaise	1 tsp.	Bacon	1 slice
Oil	1 tsp.	Olives	5 large
Cream, light, sour substitute	2 tbsp.	Almonds	6 whole
Cream, heavy	1 tbsp.	Coconut, flaked	2 tbsp.
Creamers, dry	4 tsp.	Pecans	2 large
Cream cheese	1 tbsp.	Peanuts, Spanish	20
Dressings		Peanuts, Virginia	10
French and Italian	1 tbsp.	Walnuts	2
mayonnaise type	2 tsp.	Seeds	1 tbsp.
Diet margarine, mayonnaise		1 tbsp. salt pork (¾″ cube)	1
Diet salad dressing	2 tbsp.		

Free Food List (foods or drinks that contain fewer than 20 kcal per serving)

Condiments: horseradish, mustard, dill pickles, taco sauce, vinegar
Drinks: bouillon or broth (no fat), sugar-free drinks, plain coffee/tea
Herbs and spices
Nonstick spray
Sugar substitutes: Nutrasweet™/Equal™ (aspartame), saccharin
Vegetables (raw): (up to 1 cup can be used 2 to 3 times per day): cabbage, celery, Chinese cabbage,

cucumber, endive, escarole, green onion, hot peppers, lettuce, mushrooms, parsley, radishes, romaine, spinach, zucchini

Pyramid Food Choices Charts

Another useful menu planning tool is the Pyramid Food Choices Charts. This system groups foods into six charts that correspond to the food groups used in the Food Guide Pyramid. Like the exchange lists, the food choices charts can help you identify and restrict your intake of high-fat foods. The food lists in these charts are not as extensive as the exchange lists. They do, however, supply useful information, such as the amount of added sugar and sodium in specific foods, that is not shown in the exchange lists.

How much is a gram of fat?   To help you visualize how much fat is in these foods, keep in mind that 1 teaspoon (1 pat) of butter or margarine has 5 grams of fat.

Bread, Cereal, Rice, and Pasta Group

Eat 6 to 11 servings daily.	Servings	Grams of fat	Added sodium, mg	Added sugar, tsp.
Breakfast cereal, 1 oz.	1	*	100-360	*
Rice, pasta, cooked, unsalted, ½ cup	1	0	Trace	
Bread, 1 slice	1	1	110-175	
Hamburger roll, bagel, English muffin, 1	2	2	50-200	0
Pancakes, 4" diameter, 2	2	3	500	
Plain crackers, small, 3-4	1	3	100-150	
Tortilla, 1	1	3		
Cookies, 2 medium	1	4	@100	1
Doughnut, 1 medium (2 oz.)	2	11	60	2
Croissant, 1 large (2 oz.)	2	12	@300	
Cake, frosted, 1/16 average	1	13	210-250	6
Danish, 1 medium (2 oz.)	2	13	150-250	1
Pie, fruit, 2-crust, 1/6 8" pie	2	19	@125	6
Muffin, 1 medium			200-300	1
Pound cake, no-fat, 1 oz.			90-100	2
Angelfood cake, ½ tube cake			130	5

*Check product label.

Vegetable Group

Eat 3 to 5 servings daily.	Servings	Grams of fat	Added sodium, mg	Added sugar, tsp.
Vegetables, cooked, unsalted, ½ cup	1	Trace	Less than 70	
Vegetables, leafy, raw, 1 cup	1	Trace		
Vegetables, nonleafy, raw, chopped, ½ cup	1	Trace		
Vegetables, canned or frozen with sauce, ½ cup	1	*	140-460	
Avocado, ¼ whole	1	9		
Tomato juice, canned ¾ cup	1	Trace	660	
Vegetable soup, canned, 1 cup	1	*	820	
Potatoes, scalloped, ½ cup	1	4		
Potato salad, ½ cup	1	8		
French fries, 10	1	8		

*Check product label.

Fruit Group

Eat 2 to 4 servings daily.	Servings	Grams of fat	Added sodium, mg	Added sugar, tsp.
Whole fruit: medium apple, orange, banana	1	Trace		
Fruit, raw or canned, in juice, ½ cup	1	Trace	Trace	0
Fruit, canned, in light syrup, ½ cup	1	Trace	Trace	2
Fruit, canned, in heavy syrup, ½ cup	1	9	Trace	4
Fruit juice, unsweetened, ¾ cup	1	Trace		

Milk Group

Eat 2 to 3 servings daily.	Servings	Grams of fat	Sodium, mg*	Added sugar, tsp.
Nonfat yogurt, plain, 8 oz.	1	Trace	160	0
Skim milk, 1 cup	1	Trace	120	0
Frozen yogurt, ½ cup	½	2		3
Ice milk, ½ cup	⅓	3	160	3
Lowfat yogurt, fruit, 8 oz.	1	3	140	7
Chocolate shake, 10 fl. oz.	1	†	Varies	10
Lowfat yogurt, plain, 8 oz.	1	4	170	0
Chocolate milk, 2%, 1 cup	1	5	140	3
Cottage cheese, 4% fat, ½ cup	¼	5	400	0
Lowfat milk, 2%, 1 cup	1	5	120	0
Ice cream, ½ cup	⅓	7	150	3
Mozzarella, part skim, 1½ oz.	1	7	220	
Whole milk, 1 cup	1	8	120	
Ricotta, part skim, ½ cup	1	10	300	
Natural cheddar cheese, 1½ oz.	1	14	300	
Process cheese, 2 oz.	1	18	800	

_____
*Natural and/or added.
†Depends on types of milk and ice cream.

Meat, Poultry, Fish, Dry Beans, Eggs, and Nuts Group

Eat 5 to 7 ounces daily.	Servings	Grams of fat	Sodium, mg*	Added sugar, tsp.
Dry beans and peas, cooked, ½ cup	1 oz.†	Trace	Trace	
Egg, 1	1 oz.†	5	69	
Fresh lean meat, poultry	3 oz.†	6	<90	
Chicken, with skin, fried	3 oz.†	13	750	
Bologna, 2 slices	1 oz.†	16	580‡	
Ground beef, lean, cooked	3 oz.†	16	<90	
Peanut butter, 2 tbsp.	1 oz.†	16	5, 150‡	
Nuts, ⅓ cup	1 oz.†	22	0-2, 120‡	
Ham, lean, roasted	3 oz.	5-6	1020‡	
Tuna, canned, water pack	3 oz.	0.5-2	300‡	

_____
*Natural and/or added.
†Equivalent in ounces of lean meat.
‡Added in processing.

Fats, Oils, Sweets

Use sparingly.	Servings	Grams of fat	Added sodium, mg	Added sugar, tsp.
Cola, 12 fl. oz.	1	0	25	9
Fruit drink, ade, 12 fl. oz.	1	0		12
Fruit sorbet, ½ cup	1	0		3
Gelatin dessert, ½ cup	1	0	60	4
Sugar, jam, jelly, 1 tsp.	1	0		1
Sherbet, ½ cup	1	2		5
Reduced-calorie salad dressing, 1 tbsp.	1	*	110-200	
Butter, margarine, 1 tsp.	1	4		
Sour cream, 2 tbsp.	1	6		
Salad dressing, 1 tbsp.	1	7	75-220	
Chocolate bar, 1 oz.	1	9		3
Cream cheese, 1 oz.	1	10	120	
Mayonnaise, 1 tbsp.	1	11	115	
Syrup or honey, 1 tbsp.				3
Salt, 1 tsp.			2,000	
Soy sauce, 1 tbsp.			1,030	
Dill pickle, 1 medium			930	
Ketchup, mustard, steak sauce, 1 tbsp.			130-230	
Corn chips, salted, 1 oz.	1		235	
Potato chips, salted, 1 oz.	1		130	

*Check product label.
Note: 4 grams of sugar = 1 teaspoon.

What About Alcoholic Beverages?

If adults choose to drink, they should have no more than one to two drinks a day. Alcoholic beverages provide calories, but little else nutritionally. These standard-size drinks each provide about the same amount of alcohol.

Alcoholic Beverages	Calories
Beer, 12 fl. oz. (1 regular can)	150
Wine, dry, 5 fl oz.	115
Liquor, 1-½ oz.*	105

*A mixer such as a soft drink will add more calories.

APPENDIX D

DIETARY INTAKE ASSESSMENT

Though it may seem overwhelming at first, it is actually very easy to track the foods you eat. One tip is to record foods and beverages consumed as close as possible to the actual time of consumption.

I. Fill in the food record form that follows. We supply a blank copy. Then, to estimate the nutrient values of the foods you are eating, consult food labels and the food composition table in Appendix A or use your Mosby Diet Simple II nutrition software package. If these resources do not have the serving size you need, adjust the value. If you drink ½ cup of orange juice, for example, but a table has values for only 1 cup, halve all values before you record them. Then consider pooling all the same food to save time: if you drink a cup of 1% milk three times throughout the day, enter your milk consumption only once as 3 cups. As you record your intake for use on the nutrient analysis form that follows, consider the following tips:

- Measure and record the amounts of food eaten in portion sizes of cups, teaspoons, tablespoons, ounces, slices, or inches (or convert metric units to these units).
- Record brand names of all food products, such as "Quick Quaker Oats."
- Measure and record all those little extras, such as gravies, salad dressings, taco sauces, pickles, jelly, sugar, ketchup, and margarine.
- For beverages
  —List the type of milk, such as whole, skim, 2%, evaporated, chocolate, or reconstituted dry.
  —Indicate whether fruit juice is fresh, frozen, or canned.
  —Indicate type for other beverages, such as fruit drink, fruit-flavored drink, Kool-Aid, or hot chocolate made with water or milk.
- For fruits
  —Indicate whether fresh, frozen, dried, or canned.
  —If whole, record number eaten and size with approximate measurements (such as 1 apple—3 inches in diameter).
  —Indicate whether processed in water, light syrup, heavy syrup, or other medium.

- For vegetables
  —Indicate whether fresh, frozen, dried, or canned.
  —Record as portion of cup, teaspoon, or tablespoon or as pieces (such as 2 carrot sticks—4 inches long, ½ inch thick).
  —Record preparation method.
- For cereals
  —Record cooked cereals in portions of tablespoon or cup (a level measurement after cooking).
  —Record dry cereal in level portions of tablespoon or cup.
  —If margarine, milk, sugar, fruit, or something else is added, measure and record amount and type.
- For breads
  —Indicate whether whole wheat, rye, white, and so on.
  —Measure and record number and size of portion (biscuit—2 inches across, 1 inch thick; slice of homemade rye bread—3 inches by 4 inches, ¼ inch thick).
  —Sandwiches: list ALL ingredients (lettuce, mayonnaise, tomato, and so on) with amounts.
- For meats, fish, poultry, cheese
  —Give size (length, width, thickness) in inches or weight in ounces after cooking for meats, fish, and poultry (such as cooked hamburger patty—3 inches across, ½ inch thick).
  —Give size (length, width, thickness) in inches or weight in ounces for cheese.
  —Record measurements only on the cooked edible part—without bone or fat that is left on the plate.
  —Describe how meat was prepared.
- For eggs
  —Record as soft or hard cooked, fried, scrambled, poached, or omelet.
  —If milk, butter, or drippings are used, specify kind and amount.
- For desserts
  —List commercial brand or "homemade" or "bakery" under brand.
  —Purchased candies, cookies, and cakes: Specify kind and size.
  —Measure and record portion size of cakes, pies, and cookies by specifying thickness, diameter, and width or length, depending on the item.

Time	Minutes Spent Eating	Meal (M) or Snack (S)	Hunger (H) 0 = none 3 = max.	Activity While Eating	Place of Eating	Food and Quantity	Others Present	Reason for Food Choice

II. Now complete the nutrient analysis form as shown using your food record. A blank copy of this form also follows for your use. Note that your Mosby Diet Simple II software will create this table for you if you simply enter all food eaten.

Nutrient Analysis Form (Sample)

Quantity	Name	Kcalories	Protein (grams)	Carbohydrate (grams)	Dietary fiber (grams)	Fat total (grams)	Saturated fat (grams)	Monounsaturated fat (grams)	Polyunsaturated fat (grams)	Cholesterol (milligrams)	Sodium (milligrams)	Potassium (milligrams)
1 ea.	Egg bagel, 3.5 inch diam.	180	7.45	34.7	0.748	1.00	0.171	0.286	0.400	44.0	300	65.0
1 tbsp.	Jelly	49.0	0.018	12.7	—	0.018	0.005	0.005	0.005	—	4.00	16.0
1½ cup	Orange juice, prepared fresh or frozen	165	2.52	40.2	1.49	0.210	0.025	0.037	0.045	—	3.00	711
2 ea.	Cheeseburger, McDonald's	636	30.2	57.0	0.460	32.0	13.3	12.2	2.18	80.0	1460	314
1 ea.	French fries, McDonald's	220	3.00	26.1	4.19	11.5	4.61	4.37	0.570	8.57	109	564
1½ cups	Cola beverage, regular	151	—	38.5	—	—	—	—	—	—	15.0	4.00
4 oz.	Pork loin chop, broiled, lean	261	36.2	—	—	11.9	4.09	5.35	1.43	112	88.2	476
1 ea.	Baked potato with skin	220	4.65	51.0	3.90	0.200	0.052	0.004	0.087	—	16.0	844
½ cup	Peas, frozen, cooked	63.0	4.12	11.4	3.61	0.220	0.039	0.019	0.103	—	70.0	134
20 g.	Margarine, regular or soft, 80% fat	143	0.160	0.100	—	16.1	2.76	5.70	6.92	—	216	7.54
2 cups	Iceberg lettuce, chopped	14.6	1.13	2.34	1.68	0.212	0.028	0.008	0.112	—	10.1	177
2 oz.	French dressing	300	0.318	3.63	0.431	32.0	4.94	14.2	12.4	—	666	7.03
1 cup	2% low-fat milk	121	8.12	11.7	—	4.78	2.92	1.35	0.170	22.0	122	377
2 ea.	Graham crackers	60.0	1.04	10.8	1.40	1.46	0.400	0.600	0.400	—	86.0	36.0
	Totals	2584	99.0	300	17.9	112	33.4	44.1	24.8	266	3165	3732
RDA or minimal requirement*		2900	58		—						500	2000
% of RDA		89	170		—						633	187

*Values from inside front cover. The values listed are for a male aged 19 to 24 years. Note that number of kcalories is just a rough estimate. It is better to base energy needs on actual energy output.

Nutrient Analysis Form (Sample)—cont'd

Magnesium (milligrams)	Iron (milligrams)	Zinc (milligrams)	Vitamin A (RE)	Vitamin C (milligrams)	Thiamin (milligrams)	Riboflavin (milligrams)	Niacin (milligrams)	Vitamin B-6 (milligrams)	Folate (micrograms)	Vitamin B-12 (micrograms)	Calcium (milligrams)	Phosphorus (milligrams)	Selenium (micrograms)	Vitamin E (milligrams)
18.0	2.10	0.612	7.00	—	2.58	0.197	2.40	0.030	16.3	0.065	20.0	61.0	5.00	1.80
0.720	0.120	—	0.200	0.710	0.002	0.005	0.036	0.005	2.00	—	2.00	1.00	0.360	0.016
36.0	0.411	0.192	28.5	145	0.300	0.060	0.750	0.165	163	—	33.0	60.0	0.735	0.714
45.8	5.68	5.20	134	4.10	0.600	0.480	8.66	0.230	42.0	1.82	338	410	58.0	0.560
26.7	0.605	0.320	5.00	12.5	0.122	0.020	2.26	0.218	19.0	0.027	9.10	101	0.600	0.203
3.00	0.120	0.049	—	—	—	—	—	—	—	—	9.00	46.0	—	—
34.0	1.04	2.54	3.15	0.454	1.30	0.350	6.28	0.535	6.77	0.839	5.67	277	20.6	0.405
55.0	2.75	0.650	—	26.1	0.216	0.067	3.32	0.701	22.2	—	20.0	115	1.80	0.100
23.0	1.25	0.750	53.4	7.90	0.226	0.140	1.18	0.090	46.9	—	19.0	72.0	3.20	0.400
0.467	—	0.041	199	0.028	0.002	0.006	0.004	0.002	0.211	0.017	5.29	4.06	0.199	2.19
10.1	0.560	0.246	37.0	4.36	0.052	0.034	0.210	0.044	62.8	—	21.2	22.4	0.448	0.120
5.81	0.227	0.045	0.023		—	—	—	0.006	—	—	7.10	3.63		15.9
33.0	0.120	0.963	140	2.32	0.095	0.403	0.210	0.105	12.0	0.888	297	232	5.66	0.080
6.00	0.367	0.113	—	—	0.020	0.030	0.600	0.011	1.80	—	6.00	20.0	1.54	
298	15.4	11.7	607	204	5.52	1.79	25.9	2.14	395	3.65	792	1425	98.2	22.5
350	10	15	1000	60	1.5	1.7	19	2	200	2	1200	1200	70	10
85	154	78	61	340	368	105	132	107	198	180	66	118	140	225

Nutrient Analysis Form

Quantity	Name	Kcalories	Protein (grams)	Carbohydrate (grams)	Dietary fiber (grams)	Fat total (grams)	Saturated fat (grams)	Monounsaturated fat (grams)	Polyunsaturated fat (grams)	Cholesterol (milligrams)	Sodium (milligrams)	Potassium (milligrams)
Total:												
RDA or minimum requirement*												
% of RDA												

*Values from inside front cover. The values listed are for a male age 19 to 24 years. Note that number of kcalories is just a rough estimate. It is better to base energy needs on actual energy output.

Nutrient Analysis Form—cont'd

Magnesium (milligrams)	Iron (milligrams)	Zinc (milligrams)	Vitamin A (RE)	Vitamin E (milligrams)	Vitamin C (milligrams)	Thiamin (milligrams)	Riboflavin (milligrams)	Niacin (milligrams)	Vitamin B$_6$ (milligrams)	Folate (micrograms)	Vitamin B$_{12}$ (micrograms)	Calcium (milligrams)	Phosphorus (milligrams)	Selenium (micrograms)	Vitamin E (milligrams)

III. Complete the following table as you summarize your dietary intake.

Percentage of Kcalories from Protein, Fat, Carbohydrate, and Alcohol

Intake
Protein (P):   _____ g/day × 4 kcal/g   =   (P)_____   kcal/day
Fat (F):   _____ g/day × 9 kcal/g   =   (F)_____   kcal/day
Carbohydrate (C):   _____ g/day × 4 kcal/g   =   (C)_____   kcal/day
Alcohol (A):   (A)_____   kcal/day*
                               Total kcal (T)/day   =   (T)_____   kcal/day

Percentage of kcalories from protein:

$$\frac{(P)}{(T)} \times 100 = \underline{\quad} \text{ % of total kcalories}$$

Percentage of kcalories from fat:

$$\frac{(F)}{(T)} \times 100 = \underline{\quad} \text{ % of total kcalories}$$

Percentage of kcalories from carbohydrate:

$$\frac{(C)}{(T)} \times 100 = \underline{\quad} \text{ % of total kcalories}$$

Percentage of kcalories from alcohol:

$$\frac{(A)}{(T)} \times 100 = \underline{\quad} \text{ % of total kcalories}$$

NOTE: The four percentages can total 99, 100, or 101, depending on the way in which figures were rounded off earlier.
*To calculate how many kcalories in a beverage are from alcohol, look up the beverage in Appendix A. Determine how many kcalories are from carbohydrate (multiply carbohydrate grams times 4), fat (fat grams times 9), and protein (protein grams times 4). The remaining kcalories are from alcohol.

IV. Use the following table to again record your food intake for one day, placing each food item in the correct categories of the Food Guide Pyramid. Note that a food like toast with margarine would contribute to two categories—(1) the bread, cereals, rice, and pasta group and (2) the fats, oils, and sweets group. You can expect that many food choices will contribute to more than one group.

Indicate the number of servings from the Food Guide Pyramid that each food yielded.

Food or Beverage	Amount Eaten	Milk, Yogurt, and Cheese	Meat, Poultry, Fish, Beans, Nuts, and Seeds	Fruits	Vegetables	Bread, Cereals, Rice, and Pasta	Fats, Oils, and Sweets
Group totals							
Recommended servings							in moderation
Shortages in number of servings							

V. Evaluation. Are there weaknesses suggested in your nutrient intake that correspond to missing servings in the Food Guide Pyramid? Consider improving the latter to help you improve the former.

VI. For the same day you keep your food record, also keep a 24-hour record of your activities. Include sleeping, sitting, and walking, as well as the obvious forms of exercise. Calculate your kcalorie expenditure for these activities using Mosby Diet Simple II software. Try to substitute a similar activity if your particular activity is not listed. Calculate the total kcalories you used for the day (total for column 3). Here is an example of an activity record. A blank form follows for your use. Ask your instructor whether you are to turn that in, or the activity printout from the software.

Weight (lb or kg):				
	Energy Cost			
Activity	Time (minutes); convert to hours	Column 1 kcal/hr (from table)	Column 2 Time	Column 3 (Column 1 × Column 2)
Example for 150 lb. man: Brisk walking	(30 min) 0.5 hr	299	0.5	150

Weight (lb or kg):				
	Energy Cost			
Activity	Time (minutes); convert to hours	Column 1 kcal/hr (from table)	Column 2 Time	Column 3 (Column 1 × Column 2)

Total kcalories used (from adding all column 3 amounts):

The first section of this appendix deals with analyzing your current diet and exercise program. The second section concentrates on planning a diet/exercise program.

WEEKLY MENU MATRIX

In each of the six nutrient chapters, the Menu Matrix Section of In My Diet explains how to use this Menu Matrix to plan healthful meals. You can make several copies of this form so you'll always have some blank ones on hand.

Food Group	Monday	Tuesday	Wednesday	Thursday	Friday	Saturday	Sunday
BREAD, CEREAL, RICE, AND PASTA 6-11 servings/day or 42-77 servings/week							
FRUIT 2-4 servings/day 14-28 servings/week							
VEGETABLES 3-5 servings/day 21-35 servings/week							
MILK, YOGURT, AND CHEESE 2-3 milk servings/day or 14-21 low-fat or nonfat milk or milk substitutes/week							
MEAT AND MEAT SUBSTITUTES 14 3 oz servings/week of fish 2 poultry 10-11 meat 1-2 or a meat substitute							
FATS, OILS, AND SWEETS Use Sparingly							

Adapted from Wardlow GM, Insel PM, Seyler MF: *Contemporary Nutrition*, ed 2, St Louis, 1994, Mosby.

WEEKLY EXERCISE MATRIX

Directions: After reading Chapter 10, Exercise, develop weekly goals for flexibility, aerobic, and strength building exercises. Enter these goals in the left column of the Exercise Matrix. Enter the activity you chose and the actual amount of exercise you performed in each exercise category under the appropriate day of the week. Make several copies of this form so you'll always have some blank ones on hand.

Exercise Category	Monday	Tuesday	Wednesday	Thursday	Friday	Saturday	Sunday
Flexibility							
Strength							
Aerobic							

APPENDIX E

COMMON CAUSES OF FOOD POISONING: SOURCE, SYMPTOMS, AND PREVENTION

Organism	Source of Illness	Symptoms	Prevention Methods
BACTERIA			
Staphylococcus aureus	Lives in nasal passages and in cuts on skin. Toxin is produced when food contaminated by bacteria is left for extended time at room temperature. Meats, poultry, egg products; tuna, potato, and macaroni salads; and cream-filled pastries are likely targets.	Onset: 2-6 hours after eating Diarrhea, vomiting, nausea, and abdominal cramps Mimics flu Lasts 24-48 hours Rarely fatal	• Handle foods in a sanitary manner. • Refrigerate foods promptly and properly. • Keep cuts on skin covered.
Salmonella	Found in raw meats, poultry, eggs, fish, milk, and products made with these items. Multiplies rapidly at room temperature. The bacteria themselves are toxic.	Onset: 5-72 hours after eating Nausea, fever, headache, abdominal cramps, diarrhea, and vomiting Can be fatal in infants, the elderly, and sick persons	• Handle foods in a sanitary manner. • Thoroughly cook foods. • Refrigerate foods promptly and properly. • Watch cross-contamination.
Clostridium perfringens	Widespread in environment. Generally found in meat and poultry dishes. Multiplies rapidly when foods are left for extended time at room temperature. The bacteria themselves are toxic.	Onset 8-24 hours after eating Abdominal pain and diarrhea Symptoms last a day or less	• Practice sanitary handling of foods. • Thoroughly cook and reheat foods. • Refrigerate promptly and properly.
Clostridium botulinum	Widespread in the environment. However, bacteria produce toxin only in low-acid, anaerobic (oxygen-free) environments, such as in cans of green beans, mushrooms, spinach, olives, and beef. Honey may carry spores.	Onset: 12-36 hours after eating Double vision, inability to swallow, speech difficulty, and progressive paralysis of the respiratory system OBTAIN MEDICAL HELP IMMEDIATELY. BOTULISM CAN BE FATAL.	• Use proper methods for canning low-acid foods. • Avoid commercial cans of low-acid foods that have leaky seals or are bent, bulging, or broken.
Campylobacter jejuni	Found on poultry and beef and can contaminate meat and milk. Chief food sources are raw poultry and meat and unpasteurized milk.	Onset: 3-5 days after eating or longer Diarrhea, abdominal cramping, fever, and sometimes bloody stools. Lasts 2-7 days.	• Thoroughly cook foods. • Handle foods in a sanitary manner. • Avoid unpasteurized milk.
Listeria monocytogenes	Found in soft cheeses and unpasteurized milk. Resists acid, heat, salt, and nitrate well.	Onset: 4-21 days Fever, headache, vomiting, and sometimes even more severe symptoms. May be fatal.	• Thoroughly cook foods. • Handle foods in a sanitary manner. • Avoid unpasteurized milk.
Escherichia coli (some forms)	Found in raw ground beef, raw milk, and some types of soft cheeses.	Onset: 1-2 days after eating Diarrhea, abdominal cramps May cause kidney damage and death	• Thoroughly cook meat. • Handle foods in a sanitary manner. • Avoid unpasteurized milk.

Organism	Source of Illness	Symptoms	Prevention Methods
VIRUSES			
Hepatitis A virus	Chief food sources: shellfish harvested from contaminated areas and foods that are handled a lot during preparation and then eaten raw (such as vegetables).	Onset: 30 days Jaundice and fatigue May cause liver damage and death	• Handle foods in a sanitary manner. • Use treated drinking water. • Adequately cook foods.
PARASITES			
Trichinella spiralis	Found in pork and wild game.	Onset: weeks-months Muscle weakness, fluid retention in face, fever, and flulike symptoms	• Thoroughly cook pork and wild game.
Anisakis	Found in raw fish.	Onset: 12 hours Stomach infection and severe stomach pain	• Thoroughly cook fish.
Tapeworms	Found in raw beef, pork, and fish.	Abdominal discomfort and diarrhea.	• Thoroughly cook all animal products.
MYCOTOXINS			
A group of toxic compounds produced by molds, such as aflatoxin	Produced in foods that are relatively high in moisture. Chief food sources: beans and grains that have been stored in a moist place.	May cause liver and/or kidney disease	• Check foods for visible mold and discard those that are contaminated. • Properly store susceptible foods.

APPENDIX F

KITCHEN AND PANTRY ESSENTIALS

BASIC KITCHEN EQUIPMENT

Pots and Pans with Lids

1½- to 2-quart pot
4-quart pot
7- to 10-inch sauté or fry pan
Wok
Coffeepot
Teapot
Pyrex or Corningware casseroles/baking dishes with two
   lids each (a glass lid for cooking and a plastic lid for
   freezing)

Utensils

Nesting mixing bowls: glass/stainless
Measuring spoons
Microwave-proof measuring cups
Colander
Vegetable brush
Vegetable peeler
Grater
Small citrus juicer
Can/bottle opener
Funnel
Kitchen tongs
Eggbeater or wire whisk
Slotted cooking spoon*
Regular cooking spoon*
Spatula*
Long-handled fork
Knives (paring, bread, cleaver or chef's knife)
2 plastic chopping boards with shallow lips (1 for meat, 1
   for produce)

Nice Extras

Microwave
Toaster/toaster oven
Blender
Additional pots and pans
Baking pans (cake/pie/muffin) and equipment
Kitchen timer

Kitchen Linens

Dishcloths and towels
Potholders and oven mitt
Perma-press fabric napkins (save a tree)

BASIC PANTRY AND REFRIGERATED GOODS

Pantry

Cornstarch (for stir-fry)
Salt and pepper
Other herbs and spices of your choice
Canned beans (kidney/garbanzo)
Dried beans
Assorted dried pasta
Quick-cook brown rice and other grains
Assorted dry cereal
Pancake mix
Low sodium, meal-style soups (clam chowder, lentil,
   pasta, and bean)
Low-fat vegetarian chili
Canned fruit in own juice
Canned mixed vegetables
Spaghetti sauce in jars
Assorted low-fat snack crackers, chips, and cookies
Coffee/tea/low-fat instant cocoa
Microwaveable or air-popped popcorn
Canned, water-packed fish: tuna/clams
Onion and garlic
Baking potato
Assorted dried fruit
Peanut butter
Sugar-free preserves
Syrup
Sugar
All-purpose monounsaturated cooking oil like canola
Bouillon cubes or crystals

Refrigerator

Condiments: mustard/ketchup/soy sauce, etc.
Low-fat mayonnaise, salad dressings, and sandwich
   spreads
Cheeses (low-fat varieties and grated)
Low-fat butter or margarine
Milk
Eggs
Juice
Fresh vegetables (lettuce, carrots, celery, etc.)
Frozen mixed vegetables
Whole wheat bread and bagels (keep in freezer)
Assorted nutritious frozen meals

---

*Teflon for nonstick cookware.

What's for Dinner?

Here are some quick and easy meals you can prepare using items from your pantry and refrigerator.

- A large baked potato topped with mixed frozen vegetables and melted cheese; whole wheat bread
- Pasta with garbanzo beans and spaghetti sauce, bread sticks, salad
- Red beans, rice, and mixed vegetables

NUTRITION INFORMATION RESOURCES

WELLNESS AND NUTRITION LETTERS

Reliable reviews of current trends in nutrition are valuable tools for health-conscious consumers. Several institutions publish monthly or bimonthly wellness letters that distill fact from fantasy and provide sound dietary and fitness guidance.

**Center for Science in the Public Interest
Nutrition Action Newsletter
1875 Connecticut Ave, NW, Suite 300
Washington, DC 20009

Harvard Medical School Health Letter
Department of Continuing Education
25 Shattuck St.
Boston, MA 02115

Healthline
830 Menlo Ave. #100
Menlo Park, CA 94025

Johns Hopkins Medical Letter, Health After 50
Subscription Department, Health After 50
P.O. Box 42017
Palm Coast, FL 32124

Tufts University Diet & Nutrition Letter
203 Harrison Ave.
Boston, MA 02111 $20/year

University of California at Berkeley Wellness Letter
Subscription Department
P.O. Box 420163
Palm Coast, FL 32124 $24/year

Vegetarian Journal
P.O. Box 1463, Dept. P
Baltimore, MD 21203

How on Earth! a vegetarian newsletter for teens
c/o VE-NET
P.O. Box 3347
West Chester, PA 19381

**This newsletter is not of the same caliber as the others listed. The editors take a more radical view of nutrition and food policy, and they advocate a good food/bad food philosophy that runs counter to the official position of the American Dietetic Association. However, the health legislation updates and product reports and comparisons are valuable.

PROFESSIONAL AND SERVICE ORGANIZATIONS WITH A COMMITMENT TO NUTRITION EDUCATION

Many professional and service organizations provide free health and nutrition information. Addresses for some of the more common ones are provided below.

American Academy of Pediatrics
P.O. Box 1034
Evanston, IL 60204

American Cancer Society
90 Park Ave.
New York, NY 10016

American Diabetic Association
2 Park Ave.
New York, NY 10016

American Dietetic Association
216 W. Jackson Blvd.
Chicago IL 60606

American Heart Association
7320 Greenville Ave.
Dallas, TX 75231

American Institute of Nutrition
9650 Rockville Pike
Bethesda, MD 20014

The Canadian Diabetes Association
123 Edward St., Suite 601
Toronto, Ontario M5G 1E2 Canada

The Canadian Dietetic Association
480 University Ave., Suite 601
Toronto, Ontario M5G 1V2 Canada

The Canadian Society for Nutritional Sciences
Department of Foods and Nutrition
  University of Manitoba
Winnipeg, Manitoba R3T 2N2 Canada

Food and Nutrition Board
National Research Council
National Academy of Sciences
2101 Constitution Ave. N.W.
Washington, DC 20418

The National Center for Nutrition and Dietetics, sponsored by the American Dietetic Association, has a toll-free nutrition hot line (1-800-366-1655). You can speak directly with a registered dietitian Monday through Friday from 9 A.M. to 4 P.M. central time or listen to a rotating selection of nutrition messages 24 hours a day.
USDA Meat and Poultry Hotline (1-800-535-4555) provides answers to common consumer questions 24 hours a day.
Vegetarian Resource Group
P.O. Box 1463, Dept. P
Baltimore, MD 21203

SCIENTIFIC REPORTS AND BROCHURES

U.S. Government. In a sense, food and nutrient intake standards like the Dietary Guidelines for Americans and the RDA are reviews of current knowledge. They may be criticized for being too conservative, but they will not steer people wrong—just move them slowly toward change. These and other publications are available from the U.S. government. To receive a brochure that lists currently available government publications, send a stamped, self-addressed envelope to

Consumer Information Center
Dept. 514-X
Pueblo, CO 81009

The RDA, which are published by the National Academy Press in Washington, DC, can be ordered through any local bookstore.

COOKBOOKS

One of the best all-around cookbooks for the novice chef is *The New Basics* by Julee Rosso and Shelia Lukins (Workman Publishing). In addition to providing a wealth of recipes, *The New Basics* provides nutrition facts and teaches proper food handling and cooking techniques. See the sections on microwave recipes for grains, legumes, and fresh preserves.

Many excellent health-wise cookbooks are also available. Three good ones to get you started are: *The Wellness Lowfat Cookbook*, written and edited by the staff of the University of California at Berkeley Wellness Cooking School, and *Wellness Letter* (published by Rebus, distributed by Random House); *The New American Diet* by Sonja Conner, MS, RD, and William Conner, MD (Simon & Schuster); and *Jane Brody's Good Food Book* by Jane Brody (Bantam). All three books combine recipes with nutrition and health information. *Sunset Magazine's Low-Fat Cookbook* published in 1992 is a good health-wise recipe book with an eye toward easy-to-prepare meals.

People interested in vegetarian cuisine will enjoy the updated versions of *Diet for a Small Planet* by Frances Lappé (Ballantine Books); *The Moosewood Cookbook* by Mollie Katzen (Ten Speed Press); and *Laurel's Kitchen* by Laurel Robertson, Carol Flinders, and Bronwen Godfrey (Nilgiri Press).

CHILDREN'S COOKBOOKS

Creative Food Experiences for Children (revised edition) by Goodwin and Pollen (Center for Science in the Public Interest, 1980) suggests food activities to use with preschoolers and elementary students. The book integrates nutrition, health, social development, math, art, and nature. *Kitchen Fun for Kids* by Jacobson and Hill (Henry Holt, 1991) contains healthy recipes and nutrition facts for 7- to 12-year-olds.

BASIC NUTRITION BOOKS

The Columbia Encyclopedia of Nutrition
Institute of Human Nutrition
Columbia University
College of Physicians and Surgeons
M. Winick *et al.*
G.P. Putnam's Sons, 1988

Dr. Jean Mayer's Diet and Nutrition Guide
J. Mayer and J.P. Goldberg
Pharos Books, 1990

The Duke University Medical Center Book of Diet and Fitness
Duke Diet and Fitness Center
M. Hamilton *et al.*
Fawcett Columbine, 1991

Eat for Life: The Food and Nutrition Board's Guide to Reducing Your Risk of Chronic Disease
C.E. Woteki and P.R. Thomas
National Academy Press, 1992

Eating on the Run
E. Tribole
Leisure Press, 1992

The Mount Sinai School of Medicine Complete Book of Nutrition
V. Herbert and G.J. Subak-Sharpe
St. Martin's Press, 1990

The Real Life Nutrition Book: Making The Right Food Choices Without Changing Your Lifestyle
S. Finn and L.S. Kass
Penguin Books, 1992

The Tufts University Guide to Total Nutrition
S.W. Gershoff and C. Whitney
Harper & Row, 1990

The Wellness Encyclopedia of Food and Nutrition: How to Buy, Store, and Prepare Every Variety of Fresh Food
S. Margen and the Editors of the *University of California at Berkeley Wellness Letter*
Health Letter Associates, 1992
Distributed by Random House, Inc.

Your Guide to Good Nutrition
F.J. Stare, V. Aronson, and S. Barrett
Prometheus Books, 1991

EXERCISE BOOKS

Walking Off Weight Workbook, a 14-step walking program, is available for $7 from California Prune Board, 55 Union St., San Francisco, CA 94111

Biomarkers: The 10 Determinants of Aging You Can Control by Evans and Rosenberg (Simon & Schuster, 1991).

The Official YMCA Physical Fitness Handbook is available at your local YMCA.

Eating For Endurance by Ellen Coleman, RD, Bull Publishing.

Brochure: "Athlete's Guide To Healthy Eating," free from American Dietetic Association (1-800-366-1655).

EXERCISE VIDEOS

There are dozens of exercise videos on the market. To help you select one that's safe and appropriate for you, you can use the Complete Guide to Exercise Videos Catalog and Consumer Hotline (1-800-433-6769). The catalog is published five times a year and contains descriptions and ratings of about 250 current videos. Subscriptions are free. Send your name and address to Exercise Video Catalog, Dept. G, 5390 Main St. N.E., Minneapolis, MN 55421.

COMPUTERIZED DIET ANALYSIS PROGRAMS

Mosby Diet Simple
Ohio Distinctive Software
DINE

MAGAZINES

Eating Well and *Cooking Light* provide a good selection of fat-wise recipes on a bimonthly basis. Also look for special issues of *Food and Wine, Gourmet,* and *Bon Appetit* magazines. All three publications usually devote one issue a year to lean cuisine.

Three other magazines routinely carry articles written by registered dietitians: *Health, Self,* and *Shape.*

GLOSSARY

AA amino acid

ADA American Dietetic Association

ADH antidiuretic hormone

ADP adenosine diphosphate

AHA American Heart Association

AMA American Medical Association

AMP adenosine monophosphate

ATP adenosine triphosphate

adenosine diphosphate (ADP) an intermediate in energy metabolism that is able to either accept or donate energy

adenosine monophosphate (AMP) an intermediate in energy metabolism that is able to accept energy

adenosine triphosphate (ATP) a chemical end product of energy metabolism that donates energy

adipose of or related to fat (Latin *adip,* "fat"); tissue in which the body stores surplus fat

adrenaline see epinephrine

aerobic (air-OH-bick) in the presence of oxygen

albumin (AL-bue-min) a type of plasma protein

allergen a substance that can produce an allergic reaction in the body but is not necessarily intrinsically harmful, such as pollen and various foods

Alzheimer's (ALLS-high-mers) disease of progressive senility

amenorrhea (a-men-o-REE-a) absence of menstruation

amino acids (AA) building blocks of protein. Amino acid molecules contain both an amine (nitrogen-containing) group and a carboxyl group.

amniotic fluid liquid produced by the fetal membranes and the fetus that surrounds the fetus throughout pregnancy, protecting and helping maintain oxygen and nutrient homeostasis

anabolism metabolic process of building larger molecules and tissue; requires ATP

anaerobic (AN-air-oh-bick) in the absence of oxygen

analgesic drug designed to provide pain relief

android obesity male fat distribution pattern, characterized by accumulation of body fat in the abdominal area

anemia (a-KNEE-me-a) lower than normal red blood cell number, hemoglobin level, or volume of packed red cells in the blood

anorexia loss of appetite (Greek *an-,* "without" + *orexis-,* "longing")

anorexia athletica depressed appetite caused by overexercise; reversible if exercise is cut back

anthropometry (an-throw-PAH-meh-tree) science of measuring the weight, length, width, and circumference of the human body (Greek)

antibody a specialized protein produced by the body that targets and attacks foreign proteins

antidiuretic hormone (ADH) a hormone that causes the kidneys to conserve water

antigen a foreign protein that causes the formation of an antibody and reacts specifically with that antibody

aorta (ay-OR-ta) major artery carrying blood from the heart

appetite hunger for a specific food or foods; believed to stem from environmental as well as internal drives

aromatic having a pleasing smell

arteriosclerosis hardening of the arteries caused by loss of elasticity and calcification of the artery walls; results in decreased blood flow. This condition often develops with aging, and in people with diabetes and/or hypertension.

aspartame sugar substitute made of the amino acids aspartate and phenylalanine

atherosclerosis (ath-er-o-skler-OH-sis) formation of deposits (plaques), composed of cholesterol and minerals, on the internal lining of the blood vessels (Greek *athera,* "soft, fatty, gruel-like" + *skleroun,* "to harden")

autoimmune any of a number of diseases in which the body's immune system attacks the body's own tissues

BMR basal metabolic rate

BV biological value

balance see homeostasis

baryophobia literally, fear of being fat; refers to parental pressure or example that leads to inappropriate weight loss dieting in children

basal metabolism energy required to maintain the body while it is at rest

beriberi thiamin deficiency disease characterized by muscle weakness, loss of appetite, and nerve degeneration

bile an emulsifying substance made by the liver and stored in the gallbladder; released into the intestine to aid in fat digestion and absorption

bioelectrical impedance measurement of body fat using the flow of electricity through tissues

bioengineered foods plant or animal products that have been genetically altered to improve shelf life, fat content, or, in the case of plants, pest resistance

body mass index (BMI) a technique for estimating a person's percentage of body fat based on his/her weight

body weight set point tendency of a person's metabolism to maintain a given body weight

bomb calorimetry a technique used to determine the number of kcalories contained in a given amount of food

bottle mouth extensive tooth decay caused by bacterial fermentation of the sugars from milk or juices that slowly drip from a bottle into a sleeping child's mouth

bran the outer fiber coating of seeds that protects them from insects and dehydration

bulimia an eating disorder characterized by binge eating and purging. The term literally means to eat like an ox (Greek *bous,* "ox," "cow," + *limos,* "hunger" or "famine").

CCK cholecystokinin

CS Chemical Score

CVD cardiovascular disease

calibrated calipers measuring device used to determine body fat content by measuring skinfold thickness at selected body sites

cancer group of diseases characterized by unchecked cellular growth

carbohydrate loading the process of consuming a very high-carbohydrate diet for several days before an athletic event to increase muscle glycogen stores

carcinogen (car-SIN-o-jin) any substance that promotes development of cancer

cardiovascular pertaining to the heart and blood vessels

caries dental cavities

carnitine a substance used by the body to move fatty acids into the cell's mitochondria where they are burned for energy; often used as an ergogenic aid by athletes

carotene a yellow-orange plant pigment that is a precursor for vitamin A

casein a protein found in milk

catabolism metabolic process within cells that breaks chemical bonds and releases stored energy (a source of ATP)

catalyst a chemical that speeds up a reaction without becoming part of the reaction

chylomicron a lipoprotein containing mostly triglycerides

chyme the semiliquid food mass that leaves the stomach

cis/trans fatty acids cis: configuration of the double bond in a natural oil; trans: configuration of double bonds after partial hydrogenation of oils

chelate to chemically bind an element

chemically engineered foods food items that have been chemically altered to improve shelf life, texture, or nutrient content. Examples are margarine and sugar and fat substitutes.

chlorophyll the light-sensitive pigment in plants that absorbs solar energy (Greek *khloros*, "green" + *phyllon*, "leaf")

chloroplast (KLOR-o-plast) the structure within a plant cell that contains the pigment chlorophyll and the enzyme systems that are responsible for photosynthesis

cholesterol waxy fatlike substance found only in animal tissue, where it is an essential part of cell membranes and the precursor for various hormones and vitamin D

coenzyme a molecule that combines with an inactive protein to create an active enzyme; required for essential metabolic reactions

cofactor a mineral element necessary for the functioning of an enzyme

collagen a water-soluble protein that is integral to connective tissue and the bone matrix; it acts as an intercellular "glue"

colostrum the antibody-rich fluid secreted in the breasts during late pregnancy and the first days after birth before lactation (milk production) begins

complementary protein a protein that contains the essential amino acids that are deficient in another protein so the two can produce a complete protein

complete protein a protein that contains all of the essential amino acids

complex carbohydrate a carbohydrate that contains more than a few saccharide units; examples are starch and fiber

compound (chemistry) a substance composed of two or more different elements, chemically combined in certain proportions, that cannot be separated by physical means

congregate meal a meal served to many people at a central location such as a senior center

connective tissue fibrous body tissue that supports and connects internal organs, lines blood vessels, and connects muscles to bones

control a standard of comparison for verifying the results of an experiment

convenience food a food that is prepared and packaged so it is easy to cook at home

correlation the relation between two findings in an experiment

cortisol stress hormone that promotes gluconeogenesis (production of glucose from protein and glycerol)

cretinism a combination of severe mental and physical retardation resulting from a congenital deficiency of thyroid hormone

cruciferous (crew-SIH-fer-us) plants belonging to the cabbage family, such as turnips, broccoli, and bok choy, whose blossoms form a cross-like pattern

cyanocobalamin scientific name for vitamin B_{12}

DIT dietary-induced thermogenesis

dehydration loss or removal of water from the body or a tissue

Delaney clause the portion of the 1958 Food Additives Amendment to the Pure Food and Drug Act that forbids the intentional addition to foods of any substance that has been shown to cause cancer in animals or humans

dementia loss of intellectual function

deoxyribonucleic acid (DNA) the material in the chromosomes that carries genetic information

dermatitis inflammation of the skin

diabetes mellitus a disorder in which blood glucose is elevated; IDDM (insulin dependent or Type I); NIDDM (noninsulin dependent or Type II)

Dietary Guidelines for Americans a publication of the U.S. government that describes recommended food intake patterns

dietary-induced thermogenesis (DIT) the energy used by the body to digest, absorb, transport, and initially metabolize food

digestible food that contains chemical bonds that can be broken by enzymes in a person's small intestine

diglyceride a glycerol with two fatty acids attached

dipeptide two amino acids joined by a peptide bond

direct calorimetry a direct method for measuring the amount of energy used by the human body at rest

disaccharidases enzymes that digest the disaccharides sucrose, maltose, and lactose

disaccharides sugars that contain two saccharide units (sucrose, lactose, maltose)

diuretics (die-yur-ET-ticks) chemical substances like caffeine or alcohol that increase urine production

diverticulitis (die-ver-tick-u-LIE-tis) painful inflammation of pouches that line the walls of the intestine

diverticulosis (die-ver-tick-u-LOW-sis) formation of pouches in the walls of the large intestine

EAA essential amino acid

EFA essential fatty acid

ectomorph body type associated with long, slender bones

edema (eh-DEE-ma) abnormal accumulation of fluid in the intercellular spaces of the body

electrolyte a substance that dissociates into ions in water and thus becomes electrically charged (capable of conducting electricity)

electron transport system a series of chemical reactions that occur in the mitochondria of cells and generate ATP

elements the more than 100 primary, simple substances that cannot be broken down by chemical means into any other substance; the mineral nutrients are elements

emetic a medication that induces vomiting

emulsifier a substance that can suspend fat in tiny droplets within a watery fluid

endogenous (en-DAH-jin-us) produced or caused by factors within the body

endomorph a body type characterized by short thick bones and a short trunk, neck, and fingers

endorphins natural tranquilizers produced by the body that appear to be involved in the feeding response and are known to reduce perception of pain

endosperm the starchy part of a grain

energy the ability to do work. Chemical energy is released as the result of a chemical reaction, as in the metabolism of food. Energy also occurs in the forms of heat, light, movement, sound, and radiation.

enrichment the process of adding vitamins and minerals back to a food from which they were lost during processing

enzyme a protein that facilitates specific chemical reactions without itself being used up in the reaction

epidemic a prevalent disease that spreads rapidly among many people in a community at the same time

epidemiologists (ep-i-deem-ee-OLL-i-jists) scientists who study trends in disease within populations

epidermal pertaining to the outermost, nonvascular layer of skin

epinephrine an adrenal hormone, sometimes referred to as adrenaline, or the fight/flight hormone, that promotes glucose release from glycogen in the liver during stress (gluconeogenesis)

epithelial   outside tissue such as skin and linings of the reproductive, respiratory, digestive, and urinary tracts

equilibrium   any condition in which all acting influences are canceled by others, resulting in a stable, balanced, or unchanging system (Latin *equi*, "equal" + *libra*, "balance")

ergogenic   an energy-producing substance or reaction

essential (nutrition)   refers to a compound or element that is not synthesized in the body in adequate amounts to support life and therefore must be provided by the diet

estrogen   one of a group of steroid hormones that promotes the development of female secondary sex characteristics

exchange lists   a system of grouping food into six lists such that all the foods on a given list have essentially the same number of kcalories and other nutrients and thus can be exchanged for each other

exogenous   (ex-AH-jin-us) originating outside the body

extracellular   situated or occurring outside of the cells

extrinsic factor   dietary vitamin B_{12}

FA   fatty acid

FAO   Food and Agriculture Organization of the United Nations

FAS   fetal alcohol syndrome

FDA   Food and Drug Administration

fatty acids   acids found in fat; ranging from 4 to more than 20 carbons linked to hydrogens with an acid group at one end

fermentation   the enzymatic decomposition of organic material, especially carbohydrates

Fetal Alcohol Syndrome (FAS)   a set of congenital psychological, behavioral, cognitive, and physical abnormalities that tend to appear in infants whose mothers consumed alcoholic beverages during pregnancy

fiber   material in plants that humans are unable to digest; roughage. Dietary fiber is used to describe the total fiber in a food; crude fiber represents only insoluble fiber.

fortify   to add vitamins and/or minerals to a food at a higher level than was present in the original product

g   gram(s)

GRAS   generally recognized as safe

germ (of wheat)   the part of a grain kernel that will germinate or begin to grow into a new plant

glucagon   a hormone produced in the pancreas that increases blood glucose concentration

glucogenic   glucose generating; requires three-carbon fragments—about half of the amino acids may produce glucose

gluconeogenesis   (glue-co-knee-o-JEN-e-sis) the synthesis of glucose from noncarbohydrate sources such as some of the amino acids (glycogenic amino acids) and glycerol

glycogen   a branched-chain polysaccharide composed of glucose units that is stored in liver and muscle tissue; sometimes referred to as animal starch

gram   a measure of weight in the metric system; $\frac{1}{28}$ ounce

gynoid obesity   female fat distribution pattern characterized by fat deposits in the buttocks and thighs

HDL   high-density lipoprotein

heme iron   iron associated with the proteins hemoglobin and myoglobin. Found exclusively in animal tissue, heme iron accounts for about 50% of the iron in meat.

hemoglobin   the iron-containing protein in red blood cells that carries oxygen to the cells and carbon dioxide away from them

hemorrhagic anemia   (hem-ore-A-jick a-KNEE-me-a) anemia that results from blood loss caused by long-term internal bleeding

herbivore   an animal that eats only plants

high-density lipoprotein   (HDL) a lipoprotein made up of half protein, half lipid, and containing 20% to 30% of total plasma cholesterol; also known as "good cholesterol"

homeostasis   (hoe-mee-o-STAY-sis) state of equilibrium of the internal environment of the body (Latin *homeo*, "same" + *stasis*, "state")

honey botulism   an infection seen in infants who consume honey contaminated with botulism

hormone   a chemical produced by the body and secreted in the bloodstream that controls the function of distant cells

hunger   the term used to describe an internally generated (physiological) need to eat

hydrogenation   (high-drah-gen-A-shun) the addition of hydrogens to the double bonds of unsaturated fatty acids resulting in the production of a saturated fat

hydrolysis   (high-DROLL-i-sis) breaking apart with the help of a water molecule (Latin *hydro*, "water" + *lyse*, "to break apart")

hydroxyapatite   (high-drocks-i-AH-pah-tight) the hydroxyl (OH)-rich calcium and phosphorus crystal part of bone and teeth

hypercholesterolemia   (high-per-ko-lester-roll-EE-mi-a) high blood cholesterol level

hyperglycemia   high blood glucose level

hyperhydration   the practice of drinking extra fluid before an athletic event

hyperplasia   (high-per-PLAY-si-a) increase in number of cells

hypoallergenic   (*hypo* means low) a substance with a minimal potential of causing an allergic reaction

hypoglycemia   low blood glucose level

IF   intrinsic factor

IDDM   insulin-dependent diabetes mellitus

incidental additives   substances such as packing material or insect parts that unintentionally make their way into the food supply

incomplete protein   a protein lacking one or more essential amino acids. In general, plant proteins are incomplete, whereas animal proteins are complete.

indigestible   materials that human enzymes do not break down

inorganic   composed of matter that is not animal or vegetable and contains no carbon

insoluble fiber   fiber that does not dissolve in the intestinal environment and that intestinal bacteria cannot ferment

insulin   a hormone produced by specialized pancreatic cells, the islets of Langerhans; required for cells to absorb glucose and convert it to energy

insulin-dependent diabetes mellitus   IDDM (Type 1) see *diabetes*

intentional additives   substances purposely added to a food to maintain or increase nutritional value, enhance appearance and flavor, aid in processing, or serve as a preservative

intermediates   molecules that are created in the process of forming another chemical (such as glucose and acetyl CoA in energy metabolism within the cells)

International Units   (IU) measurement of activity determined by a biological method; used with fat-soluble vitamins

interstitial fluid   (in-ter-STIH-sholl) fluid contained between cells

intracellular fluid   fluid contained within a cell

intrinsic factor   (IF) protein-like compound produced in the stomach that is required for the absorption of vitamin B_{12}

ion   electrically charged particles in solution. A cation has a positive charge; an anion has a negative charge.

irradiation   the process of sanitizing food and extending its shelf life with the application of radiant energy

kcal   kilocalorie(s)

kg   kilogram(s)

ketones or ketone bodies   intermediate products of fatty acid catabolism containing three to four carbons

ketosis   a condition in which the absence of plasma glucose results in partial oxidation of fatty acids (ketones)

kidneys organs that filter the blood; they excrete wastes and retain useful substances in the blood

kilocalorie the amount of heat energy required to raise 1000 grams of water 1 degree Celsius; the measure of energy for food and in exercise. It is abbreviated kcal, kcalorie, or Calorie with a capital C.

kilogram 1000 grams or 2.2 pounds

koshering ritual of food cleansing practiced by Jews

kwashiorkor protein deficiency that may be accompanied by inadequate kcalorie intake

LDL low-density lipoprotein

labeling terms see Box 2-6 in Chapter 2.

lactase enzyme that digests lactose (milk sugar) into glucose and galactose

lactation the synthesis and secretion of milk from the breasts in the nourishment of an infant or child; breastfeeding; to nurse a baby

lactic acid a by-product of anaerobic metabolism during intense exercise

lacto-ovo-vegetarian a semivegetarian food plan in which milk, eggs, and plant products are consumed

lacto-vegetarian a semivegetarian food plan in which milk and plant products are consumed

lactose milk sugar; disaccharide containing glucose and galactose

lactose intolerance disorder in which the milk sugar lactose cannot be digested

lanugo (la-NEW-go) fine, long, soft body hair that appears during starvation (Latin, *lanugo*, "down," from *lana*, "wool"). The hair strands erect to trap body heat and act as an insulating device in the absence of body fat.

laxative a medication that promotes bowel movements

lecithin a naturally occurring emulsifying chemical refined from egg yolk and soybeans and used extensively in processed food; a phospholipid

legume any of a large group of plants of the pea family, including dried beans and peas such as lentils, kidney beans, and pinto beans

lesion an injury or wound

lignin a noncarbohydrate substance found with fiber in the walls of cells

limiting amino acid the most deficient essential amino acid in a protein

linoleic acid essential fatty acid; contains 2 double bonds and is an omega-6 fatty acid (a fatty acid in which the endmost double bond occurs 6 carbons back along the chain)

lipase a fat-digesting enzyme that breaks apart triglycerides and lecithin

lipid a chemical composed of carbon, hydrogen, and some oxygen that is insoluble in water and soluble in organic solvents; commonly known as fat and oil

lipogenic a chemical that can be used by the body to synthesize fat

lipoprotein a combination of fats (lipids) and protein in the blood

low birth weight (LBW) less than 5.5 pounds

low-density lipoprotein (LDL) a lipoprotein that contains mostly cholesterol; 60% to 70% of total plasma cholesterol. The blood fat that seems to increase the risk of heart attack when present in excess.

lymph transparent, slightly yellow opalescent liquid, about 95% water, that circulates in the lymphatic system

lyse to break apart or cause the disintegration of a compound, substance, or cell

MFP nutrition shorthand for meat, fish, and poultry

MFP factor a substance in meat, fish, and poultry that enhances iron absorption

mg milligram(s)

μg microgram(s)

MSG monosodium glutamate

MUFA monounsaturated fatty acid

maltase enzyme that digests maltose

maltose a disaccharide that contains 2 glucose units; found in corn syrup and malt; also a breakdown product of starch digestion

mannitol a sugar substitute made from naturally occurring plant alcohol

marasmus energy deficiency with or without adequate protein intake

megadose a supplement that supplies 10 times or more of the RDA for a given nutrient

menopause cessation of menstruation

mesomorph a body type characterized by powerful muscle or a predominant skeletal framework

metabolism chemical reactions that occur in the cells, enabling them to release energy from foods, convert one substance to another, and prepare end products for excretion; the sum of anabolism and catabolism

metalloenzyme an enzyme system that includes a mineral

metastasize to form a new site of disease in a distant part of the body, as in cancer

milk anemia a disorder that may occur in children who receive most of their kcalories from milk and thus develop iron deficiency anemia

mill to grind grain into flour

monoglyceride a glycerol with one fatty acid attached

monosaccharide a single sugar; the hexose (6 carbons) is the common dietary monosaccharide. Mono, *1; saccharide,* sugar.

monounsaturated fatty acid (MUFA) a fatty acid that contains one double bond

myelin sheath the lipid-dense wrapping around nerve cells that insulates the electrical charge

myoglobin the form of hemoglobin found in muscle tissues

NAS National Academy of Science

NEAA nonessential amino acid

NIDDM noninsulin-dependent diabetes mellitus

NIH National Institutes of Health

NPU Net Protein Utilization

negative energy balance fewer kcalories are consumed than are required to meet basal metabolic and activity needs

neutraceutical a food or a component of a food that is used to cure or treat a disease

nitrogen a chemical element found in air, compounds in the soil, and protein

nonheme iron iron from plant sources and animal tissues not associated with hemoglobin (e.g., egg yolk)

noninsulin-dependent diabetes mellitus (NIDDM) (Type 2) see *diabetes*

norepinephrine an adrenal hormone that increases blood pressure

nutrient density (ND) a measure that compares the nutrients in a food to the kcalories in the food

nutrients chemical substances in food that provide the body with vital energy, building materials, and substances that regulate metabolism

obesity excess body fat

olfactory (ol-FAC-tor-ee) pertaining to the sense of smell (Latin *olfacere*, "to smell")

oligosaccharide (oll-i-go-SACK-a-ride) an undigestible sugar that contains a known small number of monosaccharide units (Greek *oligos*, "few, little" + *sakkharon*, "sugar")

omega (oh-MAY-ga) the last letter of the Greek alphabet, used to refer to the position of the endmost double bond in a fatty acid

omega-3-linolenic acid an essential fatty acid found abundantly in fish oils and required for the synthesis of hormones

omega-6-linoleic acid an essential fatty acid found abundantly in vegetable oils and required for the synthesis of hormones

omnivore a person or animal that eats both plant- and animal-derived foods

organic a substance that contains carbon, specifically in carbon-to-hydrogen and carbon-to-carbon bonds

organically grown produce produce grown with the use of fertilizers and mulch composed only of animal or vegetable matter, with no use of synthetic fertilizers or pesticides

osteomalacia adult rickets caused by vitamin D or calcium deficiency; demineralization of bone (Greek *osteo,* "bone," + Latin *mal,* "bad")

osteoporosis a bone disease characterized by a decrease in bone density; occurs most commonly in women after menopause

oxalic acid/oxalate substance in spinach, rhubarb, and other vegetables that binds (chelates) calcium and iron and makes them nonabsorbable

oxygen debt the amount of oxygen required to clear the buildup of lactic acid after cessation of exercise

PEM protein energy malnutrition
PER protein efficiency ratio
PKU phenylketonuria
PMS premenstrual syndrome
PUFA polyunsaturated fatty acid
palatable appealing to eat

pancreatic amylases the group of carbohydrate-digesting enzymes that are produced in the pancreas and secreted to the small intestine

pellagra niacin deficiency disease; characterized by inflammation of the skin, diarrhea, dementia, and eventual death

pepsin a protein-digesting enzyme in the stomach

peptide bond the chemical bond that connects one amino acid to another

periodontal (pair-e-o-DON-tal) the tissue that supports teeth, including the jawbone, ligaments, and gums (Greek *peri,* "around" + *odous,* "teeth")

peristalsis wavelike contractions of the walls of the intestine that move food along the gastrointestinal tract

pernicious anemia the anemia that results from a lack of intrinsic factor in the stomach with which to absorb vitamin B$_{12}$

phenylketouria (PKU) the genetic inability to metabolize the amino acid phenylalanine

photosynthesis the formation of carbohydrates in the chloroplasts of plants from carbon dioxide and water under the influence of ultraviolet light

phytates compounds found in wheat bran that chelate (bind) certain minerals, preventing their absorption

phytochemicals nonnutritive substances in plant-based foods that appear to have disease-fighting properties

pica (PIE-ka) the consumption of nonnutritive foods, such as clay, cornstarch, and ice, that seems to correspond to a need for zinc and/or iron

placebo (plah-SEE-boh) a substance that contains no medication and is given merely to humor a patient or used as a control in an experiment (Latin, "I shall please")

placenta a highly vascular fetal organ through which the fetus absorbs oxygen, nutrients, and other substances and excretes carbon dioxide and other wastes

plasma the fluid portion of the blood in which blood cells are suspended

polypeptide many amino acids joined by peptide bonds

positive energy balance more kcalories are taken in than are needed for basal metabolic and activity energy needs

potable (POE-ta-bul) fit to drink
ppm parts per million
prophylactic a preventive measure

protein-calorie malnutrition (PCM) or protein-energy malnutrition (PEM) malnutrition caused by a combination of insufficient protein and energy (kcalories)

pseudovitamins substances in food that are known to be necessary in the diets of some animals but whose benefit to humans is unproven

pulmonary pertaining to lung tissue and function

quick-weight-loss diet any diet that causes a person to lose more than 2 pounds per week

RBC red blood cell
R.D. Registered Dietitian
RDA Recommended Dietary Allowances
REE resting energy expenditure
RQ respiratory quotient

radiation literally, energy emitted in all directions from a central source. Examples include X-rays, radioactive chemicals (such as those used to produce nuclear energy), and the ultraviolet light from the sun

reactant a participant in a chemical reaction

reactive hypoglycemia low blood glucose levels as a result of limited food intake or irregular eating patterns

Recommended Dietary Allowances (RDA) standards of nutrient intake developed by the Food and Nutrition Board of the National Academy of Sciences

refining the process of purifying a food substance (such as flour) by selective removal of some of its constituent parts

rehydration adding water back to a substance from which it has been removed

respiratory quotient (RQ) method of measuring energy use by determining the ratio of oxygen used to carbon dioxide produced

retinol-binding protein transports vitamin A in the blood

ribonucleic acid (RNA) material that is a copy of the DNA message and carries it to the protein-manufacturing center in the cell

rickets severe vitamin D deficiency characterized by soft bones

SFA saturated fatty acid

saccharide (SACK-a-ride) a single sugar unit that contains five or six carbons; the pentose (five carbons) is part of DNA; the hexose (six carbons) is the common dietary monosaccharide

saccharin synthetic sugar substitute

saliva the watery fluid in the mouth

salivary amylase the oral enzyme that digests carbohydrate

salt sodium chloride or any product of a reaction between an acid and a base (Latin *sal, salis*)

satiated, satiety full or satisfied

saturated fatty acid (SFA) a fatty acid that has no double bonds and contains the maximum number of hydrogens

scurvy severe vitamin C deficiency; characterized by degeneration of the connective tissue and sores or wounds that will not heal

serotonin a neurotransmitter that is a naturally occurring derivative of the amino acid tryptophan; found in platelets and in cells of the brain and the intestine

serum blood with cells and clotting factors removed

set point term describing the tendency of an individual's metabolism to maintain itself in terms of body fat accumulation

simple carbohydrate mono- or disaccharides, the sugars

Simplesse® a synthetic fat substitute composed of milk protein

soluble fiber fiber that forms a gel in water; fiber that intestinal bacteria will ferment

solute a substance dissolved in another substance

solvent the liquid in which another substance (the solute) is dissolved to form a solution

sorbitol sugar substitute made of naturally occurring sugar alcohol

sphincter (SVINK-tur) a circular muscle that surrounds and is able to contract or close a bodily opening

spina bifida congenital neural tube defect

spontaneous hypoglycemia very low blood sugar

sports anemia low concentration of red blood cells caused by increased blood volume

starch many glucose units bonded together; a complex carbohydrate

status quo   existing situation

steroid   any of a large number of hormonal substances with a similar basic chemical structure, produced mainly in the adrenal cortex and gonads, such as sterols and bile acids, many hormones, certain natural drugs, such as digitalis compounds, and the precursors of certain vitamins

sterols   a group of fatlike chemicals such as cholesterol and plant sterols that serve as precursors of steroid hormones

stress   any emotional, physical, social, economic, or other factor that requires a response or change

sucrase   enzyme that digests sucrose

sucrose   disaccharide found in fruit, sugarcane, and sugar beets and commonly known as table sugar

sugar alcohols   sugar substitutes made from naturally occurring plant alcohols

Sunette®   (acesulfame-K) a kcalorie-free synthetic sugar substitute

synthesize   to combine so as to form a new, complex product

TCA   tricarboxylic acid cycle

tannin   substance obtained from the bark and fruit of many plants, including tea and red wine grapes

thermogenesis   the process of heat production by the human body (Greek *therme,* "heat" + *genesis,* "birth, beginning")

thirst   conscious desire for water

tricarboxcylic acid cycle   (TCA) or Kreb's cycle   cellular reactions that liberate energy from fragments of carbohydrate, protein, and liquid

tripeptide   three amino acids joined by peptide bonds

turgor   rigidity of form or structure

USDA   United States Department of Agriculture

USDHHS   United States Department of Health and Human Services

U.S. RDA   United States Recommended Dietary Allowances

unsaturated fatty acid   a fatty acid that contains fewer than the maximum number of hydrogens

urea   a substance made in the liver and excreted in the urine; contains one carbon and two amino groups; the major pathway for excretion of toxic nitrogen excesses

urine   a fluid that contains water, urea, and other waste products as well as excesses of some vitamins and minerals. It is produced and secreted by the kidneys, stored in the bladder, and voided by the urethra

very-low-density lipoprotein   (VLDL) a lipoprotein that contains mostly endogenous triglycerides and constitutes 10% to 15% of total plasma cholesterol

voluntary physical activity   purposeful motion; one of three possible normal energy uses by the body; others are basal metabolism and dietary-induced thermogenesis

WHO   World Health Organization

whey   liquid remaining when cheese has been made from milk, as in: "Little Miss Muffet sat on a tuffet, eating her curds and whey"

xylitol   sugar substitute made from natural plant alcohols

PHOTO CREDITS

Cover

Andrew J. Zito, The Image Bank

Chapter 1

p. 1, Barbara Bourne
p. 3, Barbara Bourne
p. 6, Barbara Bourne

Chapter 2

p. 15, PhotoDisc ©1994

Chapter 3

p. 31, PhotoDisc ©1994
p. 33, Lewis & Neale, Inc.
p. 39, Barbara Bourne
p. 40, Barbara Bourne

Chapter 4

p. 43, PhotoDisc ©1994
p. 54, New Zealand Apple and Pear Marketing Board
p. 56, Barbara Bourne
p. 59, Barbara Bourne
p. 62, Barbara Bourne
p. 63, Barbara Bourne

Chapter 5

p. 69, Barbara Bourne
p. 75, Barbara Bourne
p. 86, Barbara Bourne
p. 88, Barbara Bourne
p. 89, Barbara Bourne

Chapter 6

p. 95, Barbara Bourne
p. 107, Barbara Bourne

Chapter 7

p. 115, Barbara Bourne

Chapter 8

p. 141, Barbara Bourne
p. 150, from Thibodeau G, Patton K: *Anatomy and physiology*, ed 2, St Louis, 1993, Mosby
p. 152, National Dairy Council
p. 155, Barbara Bourne
p. 159, Barbara Bourne

Chapter 9

p. 165, Barbara Bourne
p. 179, from Wardlaw G, Insel P, Seyler M: *Contemporary nutrition: issues and insights*, ed 2, St Louis, 1993, Mosby

Chapter 10

p. 185, Barbara Bourne
p. 188, Barbara Bourne
p. 198 *(top)*, Barbara Bourne
p. 198 *(bottom)*, Courtesy of YMCA of Greater St. Louis
p. 201, Courtesy of YMCA of Greater St. Louis

Chapter 11

p. 205, Barbara Bourne
p. 208, Barbara Bourne
p. 215, Barbara Bourne

Chapter 12

p. 219, Barbara Bourne
p. 244, from Williams S: *Basic nutrition and diet therapy*, ed 10, St Louis, 1995, Mosby
p. 227, Barbara Bourne
p. 231, Barbara Bourne

Looking to the Future

p. 239, Barbara Bourne

Index

Page numbers followed by *f* indicate figures; page numbers followed by *t* indicate tables.